MEDICAL RADIOLOGY

Diagnostic Imaging and Radiation Oncology

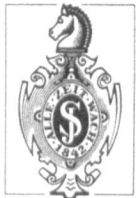

Radiology of the Upper Urinary Tract

Contributors

L. R. Bigongiari · J. Clayton · L. Dalla-Palma · S. Dorph
L. Ekelund · R. M. Friedenberg · S. M. Goldman · R. W. Günther
S.-O. Hietala · J. Kofod Larsen · E. K. Lang · A. J. LeRoy
W. S. McDougal · C. Müller-Leisse · T. Mygind · J. H. Newhouse
N. Papanicolaou · R. C. Pfister · R. Pozzi-Mucelli
H. S. Thomsen · F. Wang · W. Wells · A. C. Winfield · H. Zarnow

Edited by
Erich K. Lang

Foreword by
Martin W. Donner and Friedrich Heuck

With 418 Figures and 14 Tables

Springer-Verlag
Berlin Heidelberg New York
London Paris Tokyo
Hong Kong Barcelona
Budapest

ERICH K. LANG, M. D.
Professor and Chairman

Department of Radiology, School of Medicine
Medical Center, Louisiana State University
1542 Tulane Avenue, New Orleans, LA 70122-2822, USA

MEDICAL RADIOLOGY · Diagnostic Imaging and Radiation Oncology

Continuation of
Handbuch der medizinischen Radiologie
Encyclopedia of Medical Radiology

ISBN-13: 978-3-642-84191-0   e-ISBN-13: 978-3-642-84189-7
DOI: 10.1007/978-3-642-84189-7

Library of Congress Cataloging-in-Publication Data
Radiology of the upper urinary tract/contributors, L. R. Bigongiari . . . [et al.] ; edited by Erich K. Lang: foreword by Martin
W. Donner and Friedrich Heuck. p. cm. - (Medical radiology) Includes bibliographical references and index.

1. Kidneys - Imaging. 2. Kidneys - Radiography. 3. Urinary organs - Radiography. I. Bigongiari, L. R. (Lawrence R.) II. Lang,
Erich K. (Erich Karl), 1929-. III. Series.[DNLM: 1. Kidney - radiography. 2. Urography. WJ 141 R1285] RC904.5.I42R34
1991 616.6'10757-dc20 DNLM/DLC 91-4648

© Springer-Verlag Berlin Heidelberg 1991
Softcover reprint of the hardcover 1st edition 1991

Reproduction of the illustrations: Gustav Dreher, Württembergische Graphische Kunstanstalt GmbH, Stuttgart
Typesetting and printing: Appl, Wemding

10/3130-543210 - Printed on acid-free paper

Foreword

The advent in recent years of several new imaging modalities for the application in diagnosis and patient management has had an unprecedented impact on patient care. By permitting the acquisition of information without intervention, these new modalities have made the diagnostic process more humane. They have also made possible the treatment of many disorders of the upper and lower urinary tract by means of interventional techniques, replacing a number of surgical procedures.

The editor of this volume has engaged international experts in radiology to describe the state of the art of radiolog y of the upper urinary tract. Local and regional abnormalities are covered, but so too is the involvement of urinary structures in systemic disease. The radiologic approach and interpretation are combined with the presentation of pertinent clinical observations and important pathophysiologic concepts. The text is concise and the illustrations are appropriate. Up-to-date international bibliographies are provided. Both the text and the illustrations will serve as sources of information for the radiologists, urologists, nephrologists, gynecologists, and oncologists. Most importantly, the material is presented in such a way that practicing specialists dealing with urologic disorders, as well as physicians in training will benefit. We feel that it is timely to publish a present day treatise on urinary tract radiology in order to convey the contributions made by various newer imaging modalities to the diagnosis of urinary disorders. The contributions cover very well the opportunities for noninvasive evaluation as well as for cost containment in recommending diagnostic pathways and the selection of the most appropriate techniques to alleviate the patient's problem.

Volumes dealing with the lower urinary and genitourinary tracts will follow shortly, using the same approach of presentation as the current volume of the upper urinary tract.

Baltimore/Stuttgart, May 1991   M. W. DONNER · F. HEUCK

Preface

The past two decades have witnessed an unprecedented growth in the subspecialty of uro-radiology. The advent of new imaging modalities, such as magnetic resonance imaging, computed tomography, transrectal ultrasonography, Doppler ultrasound, real-time ultra-sonography, and digital angiography, has, in conjunction with technical advances in nu-clear medicine scanning such as SPEC scanning, reoriented the diagnostic approach to problems of the genitourinary tract. New concepts and algorithms for diagnostic evalu-ation have evolved, in line with the cost-conscious approach dictated by a rapidly chang-ing environment in health insurance coverage. Definitive diagnostic assessment on an out-patient basis is often obligatory and can be achieved by appropriate deployment of the now available diagnostic examinations. In addition to the remarkable advances in diag-nostic techniques, innumerable interventional and therapeutic uroradiology procedures have been introduced. The marriage of diagnostic modalities with techniques developed for angiography has made possible nonsurgical management of complex conditions that in the past mandated major surgical interventions with attendant prolonged hospitaliza-tion. Percutaneous nephrostomy, antegrade placement of ureteral stents, dilatation of strictures of the ureter or ureteropelvic junction, embolotherapy of both benign and malig-nant renal neoplasms, superselective chemotherapy to neoplasms, embolotherapy of anomalous veins in the management of male impotence, sclerotherapy in the management of varicoceles, percutaneous transluminal recanalization of the fallopian tubes, percuta-neous lithotripsy and stone removal, and a plethora of ultrasound- or CT-guided biopsies for diagnostic purposes as well as ultrasound- and CT-guided drainage procedures for ab-scesses, urinomas, lymphoceles, hygromas, and hematomas are but a few pertinent exam-ples indicative of the trend in respect to interventional uroradiologic procedures.

Our goal has been to provide a work that comprehensively covers the field of uroradio-logy in its broadest context. The orientation of this work is from a radiologic point of view; however, pertinent clinical observations, important pathophysiologic concepts, and key urologic surgical considerations have been included. A detailed text complemented by ap-propriate illustrations and an up-to-date bibliography will serve as a source of information for radiologists, urologists, nephrologists, gynecologists, and oncologists in particular. However, physicians of other specialty interest such as pediatricians, surgeons, obstetri-cians, and generalists will also find information needed in their practice. Moreover, this book should be useful to physicians in training and specialists alike as a reference source during preparation for certifying examinations and in-house conferences. The bibliog-raphy should readily satisfy the needs of radiologists, urologists, gynecologists, and onco-logists as regards both daily practice and research.

To ensure that the information provided is completely up-to-date, the publishers, the contributors, and the editor have made a special effort to assemble and print the material as rapidly as possible, while simultaneously ensuring that the end product is of the re-quired high quality. Two subsequent volumes on the lower urinary tract and the female pelvic organs will follow in the near future.

The editor has carefully respected the opinions of each contributor and editorial changes have been made only to enhance readability. The idiosyncrasies of individual contributors, and often differing points of view with regard to the same problem, have been respected and maintained. This is reflected in a variable writing style and some degree of repetition. In the editor's opinion the comprehensiveness that this approach ensures more than justifies the resulting minimal redundancy.

Acknowledgments pose a vexing problem, since a many have played a large role in the creation of the final product. I would like to acknowledge the dedication and understanding of each contributor and I thank all of them sincerely. Ms. Tammy Garner, my secretary, has played a major role in the final assembly and transmission of material to the publishers. Last but not least, I would like to acknowledge the special understanding, tolerance, and support that my wife has provided during the busy and stressful time spent compiling these volumes.

New Orleans, May 1991   ERICH K. LANG

Contents

1 Imaging of Medical and Surgical Adrenal Lesions
  ROLF W. GÜNTHER and CHRISTOPH MÜLLER-LEISSE (With 26 Figures)   1

2 Renal Developmental Anomalies
  FELIX WANG and RICHARD M. FRIEDENBERG (With 67 Figures) 33

3 Parenchymal Diseases of the Kidneys
  HILARY ZARNOW and LAWRENCE R. BIGONGIARI (With 17 Figures) 71

4 Inflammatory Renal Disease
  STANFORD M. GOLDMAN (With 73 Figures) 103

5 Urinary Obstruction
  NICHOLAS PAPANICOLAOU and RICHARD C. PFISTER (With 20 Figures) 151

6 Therapy for Calculus Disease of the Kidney and Ureter
  ANDREW J. LEROY (With 9 Figures) 177

7 Renal Trauma
  ERICH K. LANG (With 46 Figures) 189

8 Benign Renal Tumors
  JEFFREY H. NEWHOUSE (With 9 Figures) 215

9 Renal Cystic Disease
  ERICH K. LANG (With 35 Figures) 227

10 Malignant Renal Neoplasms
  LUDOVICO DALLA-PALMA and ROBERTO POZZI-MUCELLI (With 24 Figures) . . . 251

11 Renal Cell Carcinoma
  ALAN C. WINFIELD and W. SCOTT MCDOUGAL (With 32 Figures) 275

12 Renovascular Hypertension
  LEIF EKELUND and SWEN-OLA HIETALA (With 15 Figures) 295

13 Radiology of the Transplant Kidney
  SVEN DORPH, JAN KOFOD LARSEN, THORKILD MYGIND, and
  HENRIK S. THOMSEN (With 31 Figures) 311

14 Ultrasound Diagnosis of Neonatal Conditions of the Genitourinary Tract
  JANE CLAYTON and WILLIAM WELLS (With 13 Figures) 339

Subject Index 351

List of Contributors 369

1 Imaging of Medical and Surgical Adrenal Lesions

Rolf W. Günther and Christoph Müller-Leisse

CONTENTS

1.1	Introduction	1
1.2	Imaging Techniques	2
1.2.1	Abdominal Plain Film and Urography	2
1.2.2	Computed Tomography	2
1.2.3	Ultrasound	2
1.2.4	Magnetic Resonance Imaging	3
1.2.5	Radioisotope Scanning	3
1.2.6	Arteriography	5
1.2.7	Venography and Selective Venous Sampling	5
1.2.8	Percutaneous Adrenal Biopsy	5
1.3	Normal Adrenals	6
1.4	Pathology	7
1.4.1	Developmental Abnormalities	7
1.4.2	Adrenal Lesions Without Endocrine Activity	7
1.4.2.1	Cysts	8
1.4.2.2	Metastases/Adrenal Lymphoma	9
1.4.2.3	Other Miscellaneous Rare Adrenal Lesions	10
1.4.2.4	Bleeding	14
1.4.2.5	Inflammation	15
1.4.2.6	Adrenal Necrosis	16
1.4.2.7	Calcifications	16
1.4.2.8	Wolman's Disease (Primary Familial Xanthomatosis)	17
1.4.3	Adrenal Lesions Associated with Adrenal Hypofunction	17
1.4.4	Adrenal Lesions Associated with Adrenal Hyperfunction	17
1.4.4.1	Conn's Syndrome	18
1.4.4.2	Cushing's Syndrome	19
1.4.4.3	Adrenogenital Syndrome	21
1.4.4.4	Adrenal Carcinoma	21
1.4.4.5	Pheochromocytoma	22
1.4.4.6	Neuroblastoma	25
1.5	Conclusion	27
	References	27

1.1 Introduction

The function of the adrenals has long been obscure and it was not until the twentieth century that the endocrine activity of the gland was fully understood. Originally, the Roman anatomist Bartholomaeus Eustachius discovered the gland and described it in

Rolf W. Günther, M.D.; Christoph Müller-Leisse, M.D.; Department of Diagnostic Radiology, Medical School, RWTH Aachen, University of Technology, Pauwelsstraße 30, W-5100 Aachen, FRG

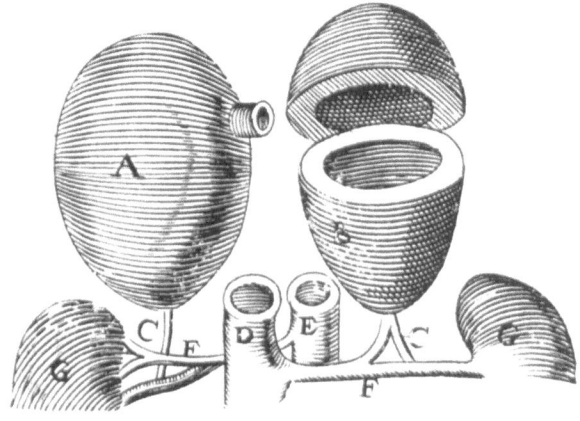

Fig. 1.1. Illustration from *Anatomia Bartholiana* (1641) by Thomas Bartholin (1616–1680): Adrenal glands referred to as "receptacles of the black bile," i.e., "capsulae atrabiliariae" (Nürnberg 1677). *A, B,* right and left adrenal gland; *G,* kidney

his *Libellus de renibus* in 1563. Thomas Bartholin (1616–1680), misunderstanding the function of the gland, described the adrenals as "capsules of the black bile" (Fig. 1.1) in accordance with Vesalius' concept of the human body fluids, and even in the classic textbook by Joseph Hyrtl (1887) the adrenal gland was referred to as "capsulae atrabiliariae" or "capsulae Bartholini." Following the discovery of epinephrine by the end of the nineteenth century, the function of the adrenals was gradually unveiled. Morphologic in vivo diagnostics started with abdominal plain roentgenogram, urography, and nephrotomography, which were later supplemented by retroperitoneal pneumography, adrenal arteriography, and phlebography. Since the advent of the new imaging modalities such as ultrasound, computed tomography (CT), magnetic resonance imaging (MRI), and radioisotope studies, direct visualization of the adrenals has considerably improved. CT, MRI, and ultrasound are currently the most important modalities for adrenal imaging, permitting visualization of the normal adrenal glands and tumors larger than 5 mm in diameter. However, due to the small thickness of the gland, differentiation of adrenal cortex and medulla in the adult is not feasible; also, atrophy and hyperplasia may be difficult to diagnose because of the wide range of normal adrenal size. Density measurement, signal intensity, echogenicity, and contrast behavior permit classification of adrenal tumors to a limited degree. In addition to the various morphologic modalities, functional studies, such as radioisotope scanning and selective venous sampling, are also available, and are supplemented by percutaneous biopsy.

1.2 Imaging Techniques

The following imaging modalities for adrenal diagnostics are currently in use:

1. Abdominal plain film and urography
2. Computed tomography (CT)
3. Ultrasound
4. Magnetic resonance imaging (MRI)
5. Radioisotope scanning
6. Arteriography
7. Venography and selective venous sampling
8. Percutaneous adrenal biopsy

1.2.1 Abdominal Plain Film and Urography

Abdominal plain film and urography used to be the initial radiographic procedures for patients suspected of having adrenal disease. This has changed considerably. Plain film is no longer used as a routine imaging modality to detect adrenal pathology such as calcifications or large adrenal masses. Urography continues to be used in the workup of patients with arterial hypertension, which may also imply renal disease, pheochromocytoma, and Conn's syndrome.

1.2.2 Computed Tomography

Computed tomography is the primary imaging technique of the adrenal gland in the adult and provides the best morphologic information. It permits detection of tumors with a high success rate (BERLAND et al. 1988), allows classification of adrenal lesions to a certain degree, and is most helpful in the assessment of tumor extent.

Contiguous 2-mm slices of the adrenals with small masses and 8-mm slices in tumors larger than 3 cm are used. Small adrenal pheochromocytomas do not differ in density from the surrounding adrenal tissue. Since opacification of these tumors tends to

be transient, dynamic CT following bolus injection of contrast medium has to be performed. In the search for an extraadrenal pheochromocytoma in the abdomen, contiguous 8-mm precontrast and dynamic postcontrast scans are obtained from the diaphragm to the symphysis (glucagon shold not be given in suspected pheochromocytoma because it may provoke hypertensive crisis).

The mean attenuation value of the normal adrenal gland is 25 HU (Hounsfield units). Calcifications are detected on CT with unsurpassed sensitivity. The surrounding retroperitoneal fat makes possible clear delineation of the adrenals and any contour-altering masses larger than 5 mm in diameter. Adrenal cortex and medulla, however, cannot be distinguished. In suspected small tumors such as aldosteronomas, thin section CT (section thickness 2 mm) is mandatory. Owing to their smooth outline and fat content, adrenal myelolipomas and lipomas can be diagnosed, but these are rare. Cysts are more frequent and characterized by low density values (0–15 HU) and by the absence of contrast enhancement on dynamic CT scans. Small, homogeneous tumors with slightly negative attenuation values can be diagnosed reliably as cortical adenomas (MIYAKE et al. 1989). On non-contrast-enhanced scans, cortical adenomas with values of 0–25 HU may resemble cysts, small pheochromocytomas, or metastases. Masses with density values of 20–60 HU are more difficult to classify. Dynamic CT may be useful for differentiating hypervascular tumors such as pheochromocytoma or hemangioma. CT features that suggest benignity are homogeneous low attenuation, possibly with punctate contrast enhancement, an enlarged gland with preserved configuration, a thin or absent rim, and an oval or round shape with sharp margins. In contrast, a thick rim with irregular and poorly defined margins, inhomogeneous attenuation, and invasion of the neighboring structures are indicative of malignancy (BERLAND et al. 1988). It has been reported that dynamic CT features may permit prediction of malignancy in 72% and benignity in 100% (BERLAND et al. 1988). However, even with meticulous analysis quite a number of lesions remain indeterminate on CT (HUSSAIN et al. 1985).

1.2.3 Ultrasound

Ultrasound has been widely used as a screening procedure for abdominal pathology and adrenal lesions in children and adults. In the neonate, infant, and child, ultrasound is also the primary technique in adrenal pathology because in these age groups the adrenals are readily accessible to ultrasound, which, however, is supplemented by CT in large masses to define tumor extent and to enable differentiation of neuroblastomas from. Wilms' tumor. In adults, visualization of the normal adrenal gland and small tumors is more difficult. Using a 3.5-MHz transducer, several approaches may serve to delineate the organ. The most effective access to the normal gland is provided by the intercostal longitudinal approach, which may demonstrate the adrenal area as a hyperechoic structure in up to 82% on the right side and in up to 41% on the left (GÜNTHER et al. 1984a, b). However, in adults visualization of the gland itself is hardly possible. In a series of 60 normal subjects we were able to image the normal glands in only one with real-time ultrasound. In contrast, using the compound scanning technique visualization of the gland was successful in 78%–85% on the right and in 44%–85% on the left (SAMPLE 1978; YEH 1980).

Although small masses may be visualized in up to 97% in experienced hands (YEH 1980), in practice, ultrasound of the adrenals may be time consuming and is less reliable than CT (ABRAMS et al. 1982). Adrenal masses smaller than 1 cm in diameter are easily missed, whereas lesions larger than 3 cm in diameter are usually detected (GÜNTHER et al. 1984 a, b; YEH 1980).

In neonates, the adrenal gland can be identified by ultrasound in 97% on the right side and in 83% on the left. Cortex and medulla can be distinguished (OPPENHEIMER et al. 1983).

1.2.4 Magnetic Resonance Imaging

Using T1- and T2-weighted spin-echo MR images the normal adrenals and adrenal tumors can be visualized with similar resolution as with CT. Imaging in different planes is an additional advantage of MRI (McGAHAN 1988). Based on signal intensity behavior, MRI provides tissue characterization to a certain degree, but is inferior to CT in evaluating calcifications. Anatomic resolution is best on T1-weighted images, but these are nonspecific regarding tissue characterization. Nearly all adrenal masses are hypointense. T2-weighted images are reported to be more specific at 0.5 T: nonfunctioning adenomas and hyperfunctioning adenomas have a low signal intensity, similar to that of the liver; metastases and other tumors are moderately intense or very intense (REINIG et al. 1986; CHEZMAR et al. 1988). However, in about 20% of the cases metastases with low signal intensity cannot be distinguished from functioning adenomas. Pheochromocytomas have a high signal intensity on T2 images, but this may also be seen with adrenal carcinomas and metastases. CHANG et al. (1987) stress the usefulness of the adrenal mass/fat signal intensity ratio in distinguishing adenomas from malignancies. KIER and McCARTHY (1989), however point out that at 1.5 T signal intensity ratios (adrenal/liver; adrenal/fat) are unreliable for differentiating adenomas from nonadenomas; the calculated T2 relaxation time is more useful (BAKER et al. 1989). Fast gradient-echo sequences and Gd-DTPA-enhanced scans may also improve differentiation and reduce total examination time (KRESTIN et al. 1989). After administration of Gd-DTPA, adenomas show a mild enhancement and a quick washout; malignant tumors and pheochromocytomas display strong enhancement and slower washout (Fig. 1.2, see p. 4). Hyperfunctioning and nonhyperfunctioning cortical adenomas display some variability in signal intensity and seem to be indistinguishable on the basis of their signal behavior (REMER et al. 1989). Overall, the precise role of MRI in the diagnosis of adrenal lesions has still to be defined.

MR spectroscopy has been reported to be capable of distinguishing adrenal adenomas larger than 15 mm from carcinomas due to the higher lipid content in adenomas (LEROY-WILLIG et al. 1989; SMITH et al. 1989).

1.2.5 Radioisotope Scanning

Scintigraphy is the only technique basing visualization of lesions on their endocrine activity. SPECT may further improve resolution of small lesions (ISHIMURA et al. 1989). There are two different tracers available for imaging in adrenocortical and adrenomedullary hyperfunction.

Of the agents that have been advocated for adrenocortical imaging, [131]I-19-iodo-norcholesterol (NP-59) is the most widely used (CONN et al. 1976; MILES et al. 1979). The tracer (7–9 MBq) is given intravenously and images are obtained after 4–7 days.

In order to increase the specificity of adrenocortical scintigraphy the dexamethasone suppression scan was introduced (GROSS et al. 1987). Adrenocortical imaging has two disadvantages: NP-59 requires up to 1 mCi (37 MBq) of ^{131}I, which results in considerable radiation exposure, and necessitates 2 days of patient preparation and up to 7 days' delay in the completion of scanning (MILES et al. 1979). Adrenocortical radionuclide scanning is recommended for aldosteronomas not detected on CT. In

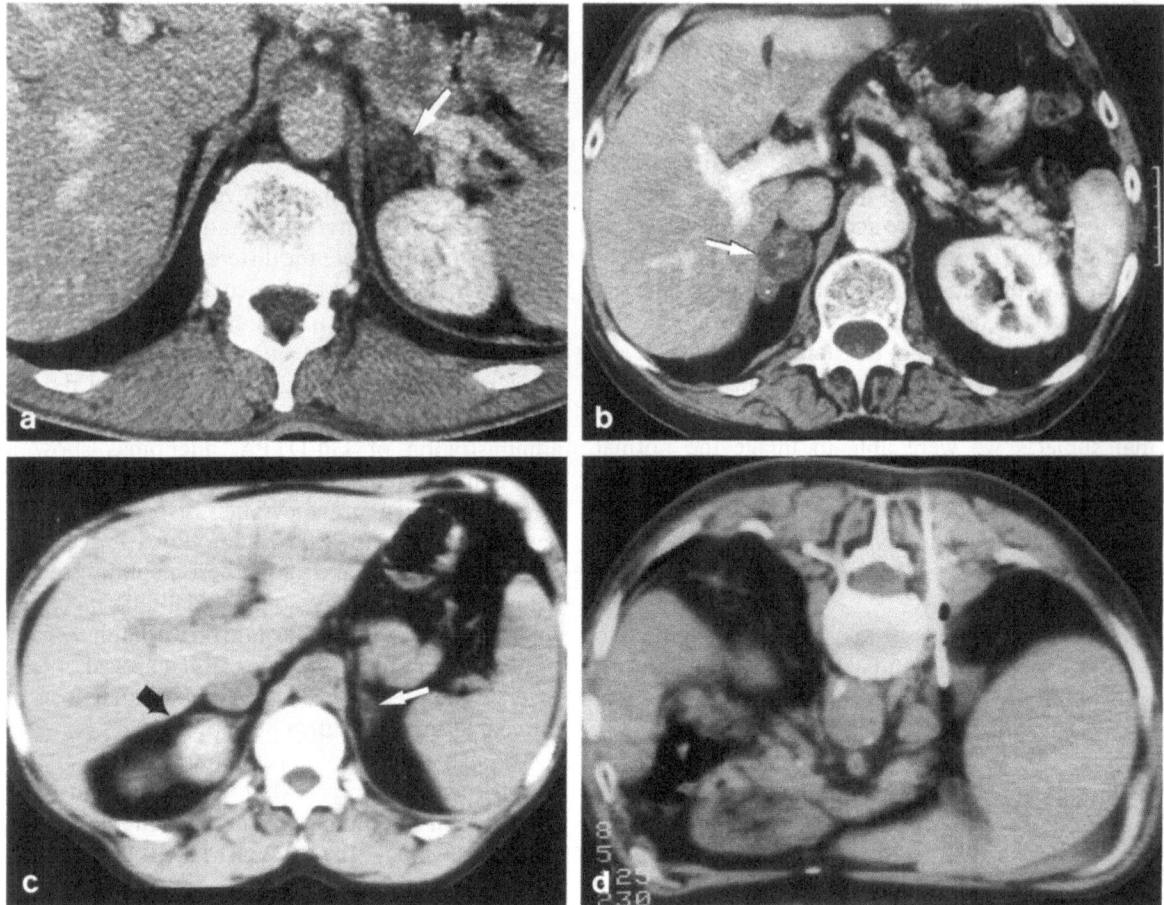

Fig. 1.2 a–d. Varying CT features of nonhyperfunctioning adrenal adenomas. **a** Dynamic CT showing left adrenal adenoma (10 HU) without noticeable contrast enhancement. **b** Precontrast scan demonstrating bilateral adenomas – unusually hyperdense on the right side (80 HU) and hypodense on the left. **c** Dynamic CT displaying heterogeneous hypodense adenoma in a tumor patient. **d** CT-guided Tru-Cut biopsy revealed an adenoma

Cushing's syndrome radioisotope scanning is controversial and limited to selected cases (MILES et al. 1979).

Iodine 131-metaiodobenzylguanidine (^{131}I-MIBG) is an adrenergic tissue localizing agent that has mainly been used in adrenal and extraadrenal pheochromocytomas and neuroblastomas. It is a physiologic analogue of norepinephrine and guanethidine and is taken up predominantly by the neuronal uptake system (TOBES et al. 1985) and stored in the noradrenergic neurosectory granules. MIBG may be labeled with iodine 123 or iodine 131 and is used for imaging of the adrenal medulla and related tumors such as pheochromocytomas, other paraganglomas, and neuroblastomas; carcinoids also may incorporate the substance.

For scanning 18–37 MBq ^{131}I-MIBG is administered intravenously and scintigrams are obtained after 24, 48, and 72 h. ^{123}I-MIBG seems to be superior to ^{131}I-MIBG in effectiveness and dosimetry (LYNN et al. 1984; SHAPIRO et al. 1985). One advantage of scintigraphy is that the entire body is imaged. Thus, it is the primary technique in the search for extraadrenal pheochromocytomas, tumor recurrence, and metastases of malignant pheochromocytomas. Sensitivity in the detection of pheochromocytomas is reported to be 86%–90%, with a specificity of 96%–99% (QUINT et al. 1987; SHAPIRO et al. 1985; SWENSON et al. 1984). ^{131}I-MIBG is also important in the staging of neuroblastomas.

Radiation exposure for adrenal scintigraphy may be considerable: estimates of the absorbed adrenal dose are 0.3 Gy/mCi with NP-59, 1 Gy/mCi with ^{131}I-MIBG, and 0.008 Gy/mCi with ^{123}I-MIBG (GROSS and SHAPIRO 1990). Because of the high degree of radionuclide uptake, malignant adrenergic tumors such as metastatic pheochromocytoma and neuroblastoma may also be treated selectively with high doses of ^{131}I-MIBG (SISSON et al. 1984).

1.2.6 Arteriography

Arteriography of the adrenal glands (KAHN et al. 1971) has lost its previously important role and has been nearly completely replaced by noninvasive techniques. Occasionally, however, it may be used in the search for extraadrenal pheochromocytomas, for preoperative demonstration of blood supply in large adrenal tumors such as adrenal carcinomas, or for therapeutic interventions such as transcatheter embolization of such neoplasms. In suspected abdominal pheochromocytoma, flush aortography and pelvic arteriography are followed by selective arteriography of the adrenals or other suspicious regions. Patients scheduled for angiography for suspected pheochromocytomas, particularly with selective catheterization, should be treated with phenoxybenzamine 1–2 mg/kg daily for 2–3 days before angiography to prevent hypertensive crisis. In marked tachycardia, β-blocking agents may be necessary in addition. It is also advisable to have a stand-by internist in case uncontrolled hypertension develops (phentolamine should be prepared). A venous access prior to the procedure is a prerequisite. The angiographic features of pheochromocytomas vary from hypo- to mostly hypervascular, and detection rate varies from 85% to 100% according to the size of the tumor (CHRISTENSON et al. 1976; ZELCH et al. 1974).

1.2.7 Venography and Selective Venous Sampling

Prior to the advent of the new noninvasive imaging techniques, venography used to be the most important technique for directly visualizing the adrenal gland (REUTER et al. 1967; KAHN et al. 1971). Venography is possible because there is a single draining vein which can be catheterized, more easily on the left than on the right side (GEORGI et al. 1975). On the right side one should be aware of small hepatic veins joining the inferior vena cava and simulating the adrenal gland on injection. Adrenal venography is not without risks: extravasation, also associated with subsequent adrenal infarction, following vigorous injection of contrast medium with the catheter in a wedged position and thrombosis of the adrenal vein have been reported (EAGEN and PAGE 1971). However, according to our personal experience in more than 250 adrenal phlebographies and to that

of others, these complications are avoidable if a careful technique is employed. In pheochromocytoma, hypertensive crisis may be induced by forceful injection into the adrenal vein.

Venography for detection of adrenal pathology has become obsolete and its importance is negligible for that purpose. But using the same catheterization techniques as for venography, venous blood sampling from the adrenal veins still remains a valuable technique for hormonal characterization of adenomas (aldosteronomas) and for localization of questionable adrenal and suspected extraadrenal pheochromocytomas or medullary hyperplasia. It is used only rarely in cortisol-producing tumors and in differentiating the source of the adrenocorticotropic hormone (ACTH)-producing tumors. In this context simultaneous bilateral selective venous sampling of the inferior petrosal sinus should also be mentioned. It is used in suspected pituitary microadenomas in Cushing's disease undetected by CT or MRI and for differentiation of an ectopic ACTH-producing tumor (DOPPMAN et al. 1984; BOHNDORF et al. 1988).

Selective adrenal venous sampling is easy to perform, but sometimes tedious and time consuming. Systemic heparinization (4000 IU heparin) should be given intravenously to prevent thrombosis. This is also helpful if blood samples cannot be withdrawn from the small veins with a syringe. Blood is then collected by gravity drainage from the catheter. It should be taken into account that injection of contrast medium may considerably increase catecholamine value but not so much cortisol values (CORDES et al. 1979). Thus, verification of the catheter position within the adrenal vein should be performed only after blood sampling. Additional cortisol determination helps to establish that the adrenal veins have been, in fact, selected. In suspected extraadrenal pheochromocytomas blood samples are obtained from the adrenal veins and all major veins from the neck to the pelvis. Selective venous sampling is highly accurate in the detection of hormonally active adrenal lesions such as aldosteronomas and pheochromocytomas (sensitivity 91%–100%) (EL SHERIEF et al. 1982; WEINBERGER et al. 1979).

1.2.8 Percutaneous Adrenal Biopsy

Needle biopsy is a well-established technique for tissue diagnosis. Because of the better display of the anatomy, CT guidance is superior to ultrasound in adrenal lesions (KOENKER et al. 1988). Although the combination of CT, MRI, and ultrasound provides a definitive diagnosis in a number of adrenal masses, some lesions (primary tumor, metastasis) remain unclear. If an adrenal mass suspected of being a metastasis is the only evidence of metastatic disease, confirmation may be obtained by fine-needle aspiration biopsy, which usually yields sufficient material for the diagnosis. In suspected primary tumors Tru-Cut biopsy is recommended. The sensitivity of fine-needle aspiration cytology is reported to be 90%–100% (BERNARDINO et al. 1985; WELCH et al. 1989; KLOSE and GÜNTHER 1988). With a complication rate of 5.3% and with bleeding more often encountered than in other biopsies, adrenal biopsy seems to be more problematic than biopsies of other regions (WELCH et al. 1989). Hormonally active adrenal tumors are usually not an indication for percutaneous puncture. In addition, percutaneous puncture of a pheochromocytoma may provoke a potentially fatal hypertensive crisis (MCCORKELL and NILES 1985), whereas similar risks are unknown in adenomas.

1.3 Normal Adrenals

The adrenal glands are thin retroperitoneal structures enclosed within Gerota's fascia. On the right side the gland is triangular and is located directly medial and cranial to the upper pole of the kidney. Sometimes it may be located several centimeters above the upper pole of the kidney in the perirenal fat. The gland lies immediately behind and slightly lateral to the inferior vena cava, between the right crus of the diaphragm medially and the right lobe of the liver laterally. On the left side the adrenal gland is of semilunar shape and is usually more closely related to the upper pole of the kidney. Its cephalad extent is most often seen just anterior and medial to the upper pole of the left kidney; it is noteworthy that the left adrenal gland may extend down to the renal vein. Cross-sections demonstrate the thin wings of the adrenals in a linear, inverted "Y" or "V," or triangular shape within the retroperitoneal fat (MONTAGNE et al. 1978). The adrenals measure 4–6 cm in length and 2–3 cm in width, and are 2–6 mm thick.

The adrenal glands are usually surrounded by a sufficient amount of fat to allow good CT identification. Using optimal scanning technique, both adrenal glands can be clearly identified in nearly 100% of patients. Sometimes, however, the differentiation of the right adrenal gland from the adjacent liver and crus of the diaphragm may be difficult. This is especially true for children, in whom there is a paucity of retroperitoneal fat. Volume measurements on CT in normal adrenals show a wide range: 2.8–6 cm³ for the left and 2.5–5.4 cm³ for the right adrenal gland (HÜBENER et al. 1984). However, the absolute measurements of the adrenals have not proved of great value in evaluating adrenal disease. Rather the shape of the glands, i.e., nodularity or a prominent mass, is a valuable criterion. In children, measurements of the normal adrenals vary with age. Comparison of the adrenal limb thickness with the adjacent diaphragmatic crura is helpful as the thickness of normal adrenal limbs is equal to or less than the thickness of the crura in older children but equal to or greater than that of the crura in normal neonates or older children with adrenal hyperplasia (DANEMAN 1987).

In neonates, the adrenal gland can be identified by ultrasound (6- to 7.5-MHz transducer) in 97% on the right side and in 83% on the left, ranging from 0.2 to 0.5 cm in size; also cortex and medulla can be distinguished (OPPENHEIMER et al. 1983). The gland is characterized by a thin echogenic core surrounded by a thick sonolucent zone with convex borders. With increasing age, the cortex becomes smaller and the medulla relatively larger. The cortex remains hypoechoic and the medulla hyperechoic until age 5–6 months, by which time the whole gland becomes hyperechoic and smaller, with poor or absent sonographic differentiation between cortex and medulla. After 1 year of age, the appearance of the gland is similar to that of the adult gland, with straight or concave borders and a hypoechoic character (KANGARLOO et al. 1986). However, in adults visualization of the gland itself is hardly possible. Sonographic imaging of the adrenal gland in the fetus can readily be accomplished beginning at a gestational age of approximately 25 weeks (LEWIS et al. 1982; ROSENBERG et al. 1982).

As with CT, the retroperitoneal fat provides excellent contrast for MRI of the adrenal gland, which normally has a homogeneous MRI appearance. Sometimes the adrenal cortex can be differentiated from the medulla because the latter has a lower signal intensity (MOON et al. 1983). On all pulse sequences, the adrenals have a signal intensity greater than that of the diaphragmatic crura and less than that of fat (DAVIS et al. 1984). The difference in signal intensity between the adrenal gland and surrounding fat is greater on T1-weighted images than on T2-weighted images. The adrenal glands are easily distinguished from the inferior vena cava and splenic vessels because of the lack of signal from the flowing blood.

1.4 Pathology

Diseases of the adrenal gland may be classified according to their etiology (Table 1.1) and may be divided into lesions with normal function, hypofunction, and hyperfunction. In the following, the characteristics of the various lesions on CT, MRI, and ultrasound and relevant diagnostic steps are described.

1.4.1 Developmental Abnormalities

Agenesis of the adrenal glands, congenital hypoplasia, and heterotopia of adrenal tissue (cortex and medulla) are rare entities (PETERSON 1987; LAMPRECHT and KORTMANN 1984). Bilateral agenesis is incompatible with life, whereas unilateral agenesis is tolerated and leads to contralateral hyperplasia of the adrenal gland. Congenital hypoplasia is regularly encountered in anencephaly secondary to failure or abnormalities of the hypophysis. In addition primary congenital adrenal hypoplasia may occur, resulting in death soon after birth unless adequate therapy (cortisol and sodium substitution) is initiated. True heteropia of the adrenal gland in a location other than the adrenal region is very rare. Accessory adrenal tissue near to the parent gland or somewhere else in the retroperitoneum, the gonads, or the inguinal canal may be found more often, mostly as an incidental finding at surgery or autopsy (LAMPRECHT and KORTMANN 1983). Imaging of these congenital abnormalities has not yet been described in the literature and is assumed to remain a serendipitous event.

1.4.2 Adrenal Lesions Without Endocrine Activity

Adrenal adenomas without endocrine activity, which are very often found on CT incidentally, have been referred to as incidentalomas (SEDDON et al. 1985). Their incidence ranges between 0.6% and 2.9% (ABECASSIS et al. 1985; GLAZER et al. 1982; MITNICK et al. 1983; OLIVER et al. 1984). CT features of these benign tumors, which are homogeneous and usually 1.4 cm in size, do not differ from those of tumors with endocrine activity (hyperaldosteronism, hypercortisolism). Density values vary considerably from −20 to 40 HU (Fig. 1.2) (BERLAND et al. 1988; HAERTEL et al. 1980). On dynamic CT, only slight enhancement is present. With increased density values of 20–40 HU on a precontrast scan, these lesions are indistinguishable from metastases. This

Table 1.1. Survey on adrenal pathology

1. Adrenocortical tumors
2. Adrenomedullary tumors
3. Adrenal hyperplasia
4. Adrenal metastases, lymphoma
5. Adrenal cysts
6. Rare tumors
   Hemangioma, lymphangioma, myelolipoma, teratoma, ganglioneuroma, liposarcoma
7. Inflammation
   Tuberculosis, adrenalitis of other origin, abscess
8. Circulatory disturbances
   Adrenal vein thrombosis, adrenal necrosis
9. Bleeding
10. Others
    (e.g., xanthomatosis, amyloidosis)

often presents a diagnostic dilemma, particularly in patients with malignant disease (OLIVER et al. 1984). Percutaneous biopsy is most useful to clarify these lesions (Fig. 1.2).

Adrenal hyperplasia can rarely be diagnosed definitely on ultrasound. As normal adrenal glands, in our experience, are not visualized in most cases on real-time sonography, a hypoechoic, triangular structure, which is normal in neonates, is suggestive of adrenal hyperplasia in the child and adult. Small hypoechoic and focal adrenal masses (1–4 cm in size) frequently represent benign adenoma, although it cannot be differentiated from a metastatic malignant tumor. There is no way of differentiating functioning from nonfunctioning adenoma, or multiple adenoma from bilateral nodular hyperplasia, or a solitary hyperplastic nodule from a small adenoma. Tumors 1.5 cm or less in diameter may fail to be visualized.

Magnetic resonance imaging seems of be of value in differentiating nonfunctioning adenomas from silent metastases, since most adrenal metastases have a higher signal intensity than nonfunctioning adenomas (DOPPMAN et al. 1987; SMITH et al. 1989) (Fig. 1.3). Percutaneous biopsy may also be applied in these cases (KOENKER et al. 1988). The large majority of nonfunctioning adenomas are more or less isointense to the liver in all spin-echo sequences (FALKE et al. 1986, 1987), but cannot be differentiated from hyperfunctioning adenomas (REMER et al. 1989). Application of Gd-DTPA may improve differentiation of such lesions (Fig. 1.4) (KRESTIN et al. 1989).

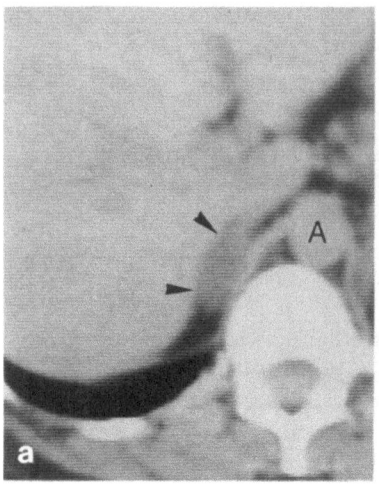 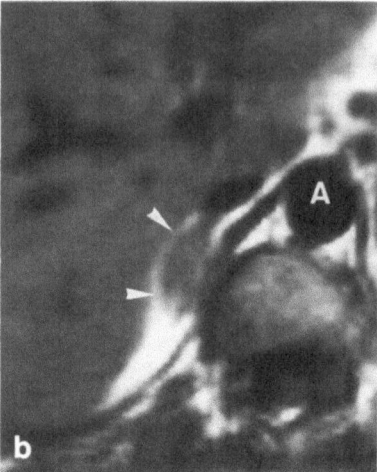 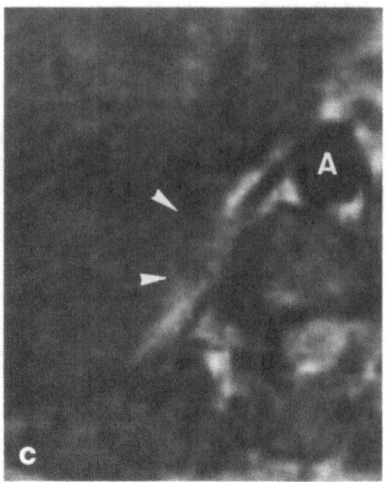

△

Fig. 1.3 a–c. Nonhyperfunctioning right adrenal adenoma *(arrowheads)*. **a** On CT an oval-shaped and hypodense right adrenal mass is seen as an incidental finding in a 50-year-old woman with tracheal carcinoma. On T1- and T2-weighted spin-echo images (TR 600/TE 15, TR 2000/TE 70) **(b, c)** at 1.5 T the lesion is of low signal intensity, indicative of an adenoma *(arrow)*

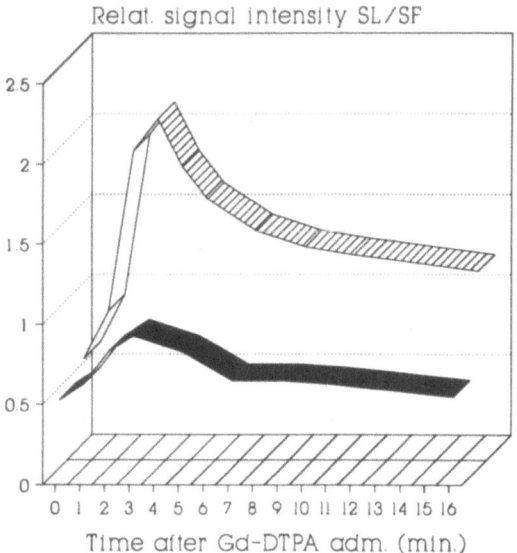

Fig. 1.4. Time-related enhancement of adrenal adenomas *(lower curve)* and malignancies and pheochromocytomas *(upper curve)* following intravenous Gd-DTPA on MRI (mean values and range of standard deviation). *SL/SF,* ratio of signal intensity of lesion to signal intensity of fat. (KRESTIN et al. 1989)

1.4.2.1 Cysts

Cysts of the adrenal gland are rare and are mainly detected incidentally either during abdominal imaging or at autopsy. Various modalities of pathogenesis have been suggested (ABESHOUSE et al. 1959):

1. Endothelial cysts
2. Epithelial cysts
3. Pseudocysts
4. Parasitic cysts

Endothelial cysts represent the most common variety of all adrenal cysts (45%) (FOSTER 1966). They are predominantly of lymphangiomatous and rarely of angiomatous origin and are usually small (KEARNEY et al. 1977). They include those cysts usually described as cystic lymphangiectasia. Epithelial cysts (9%) are of various etiologies, i.e., true glandular or rentention cysts, or cysts of embryonal origin caused by embryonic malformation, or cystic adenomas as a result of cystic degeneration of benign tumors.

Pseudocysts represent the second most common variety of all adrenal cysts (39%) but they are the most common clinically recognized type of adrenal cyst found at operation (FOSTER 1966). They usually occur as a result of hemorrhage, which may occur in a wide variety of pathologic conditions. Parasitic cysts are mostly of echinococcal origin and part of a generalized hydatid disease. In less than 0.5% of all patients with echinococcal disease is the adrenal involved (BARNETT 1942).

Adrenal cysts may be of any size and are usually unilateral with near-water density on CT and do not display contrast enhancement (Fig. 1.5 a). If the cyst contains debris, a higher protein content, or intracystic hemorrhage, the density may increase beyond 20 HU. The wall of an adrenal pseudocyst may contain calcification and may be enhanced after administration of contrast material (YAMAKITA et al. 1976). A pseudocyst may have multiple septations. Differentiation between a cyst and a low density adenoma can be difficult with CT; if ultrasound or MRI are also equivocal guided cyst puncture and biochemical and cytologic examination can be added to affirm the diagnosis (TUNG et al. 1989).

On ultrasound, adrenal cysts are easily detected when they are larger than 3 cm in diameter. They are roundish, well defined, and devoid of internal echoes, and through-transmission is excellent. Differentiation of a cyst from a solid tumor is usually not difficult, though sometimes there may be difficulties in differentiating very low echogenic metastases from cysts. Difficulties arise with complex cysts leading to internal echoes. As large adrenal cysts may compress the adrenal to a high degree, it may be impossible to differentiate them from hepatic cysts (Fig. 1.5 b, c). If ultrasound yields conclusive evidence of a simple adrenal cyst devoid of internal echoes, there is no need for CT.

On MRI, adrenal cysts are of very low signal intensity on T1-weighted and very high, usually homogeneous signal intensity on T2-weighted images, which is not encountered in other pathologic conditions. Hemorrhage results in increase in signal intensity in T1-weighted images.

1.4.2.2 Metastases/Adrenal Lymphoma

The most common primary tumors metastasizing to the adrenal gland are lung and breast malignancies, but thyroid, renal, gastric, colon, pancreatic, and esophageal carcinomas, as well as melanomas, not infrequently metastasize to the adrenals.

Lymphomatous involvement of the adrenals is more common with non-Hodgkin's lymphoma than with Hodgkin's disease and may occur in 1%–4% of patients with non-Hodgkin's lymphoma (GLAZER et al. 1983; JAFRI et al. 1983; PALING and WILLIAMSON 1983). Both adrenals are usually involved. Infiltration of the adrenal gland by Kaposi sarcoma in AIDS has been reported as an autopsy finding (GROLL et al. 1990).

On CT, adrenal metastases are demonstrated as soft tissue masses that vary considerably in size and density (20–45 HU) (Fig. 1.6). They are frequently bilateral and most commonly have a round or ovoid shape. They have well-defined smooth contours or may have irregular, lobulated margins. Larger masses frequently appear inhomogeneous as a result of focal areas of necrosis or hemorrhage. On rare occasions, adrenal metastases may even calcify or their appearance may be modified by hemorrhage (SHAH et al. 1989).

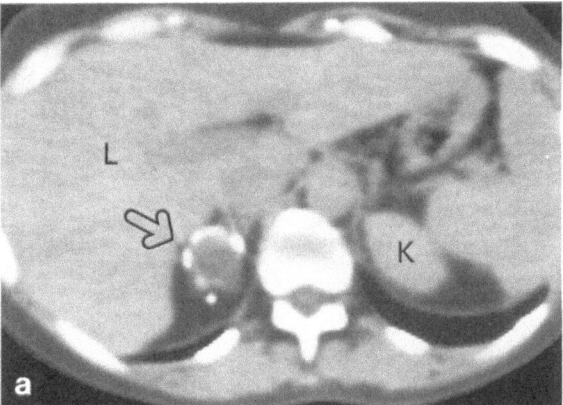

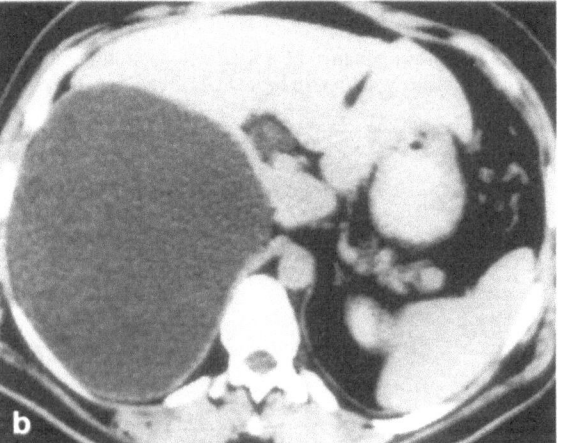

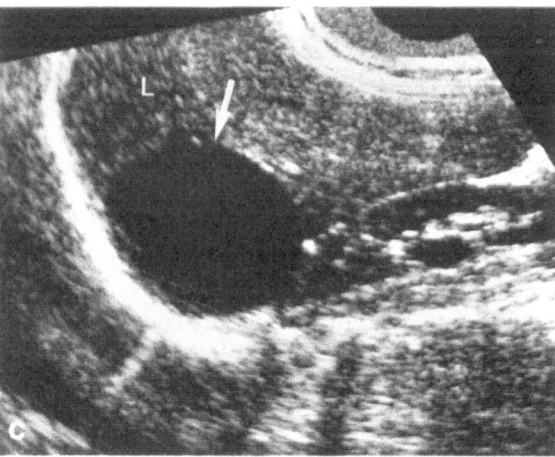

Fig. 1.5 a–c. Adrenal cysts. **a** Small partially calcified cyst *(arrow)* displaying high attenuation values on CT (cyst subsequently proven by percutaneous puncture). **b** Large right adrenal cyst simulating liver cyst on CT. **c** Large adrenal cyst on ultrasound *(arrow)* (different patients). *L,* liver; *K,* kidney

With lymphoma of the adrenals there is enlargement of one or both glands, usually concomitant with retroperitoneal lymphadenopathy, although lymphoma limited to the adrenal glands can occur (FELDBERG et al. 1986; VICKS et al. 1987). The den-

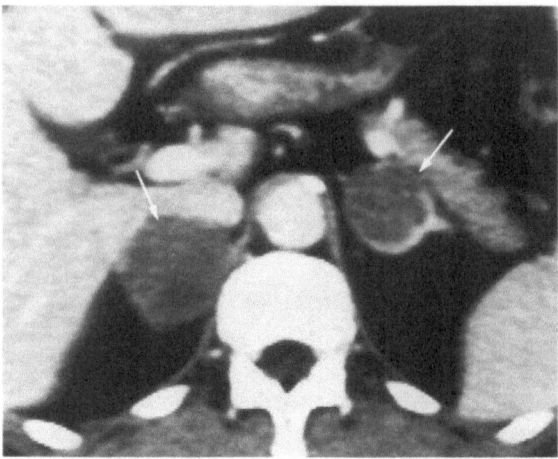

Fig. 1.6. Contrast-enhanced CT scan demonstrating bilateral adrenal metastases *(arrow)* in bronchial carcinoma

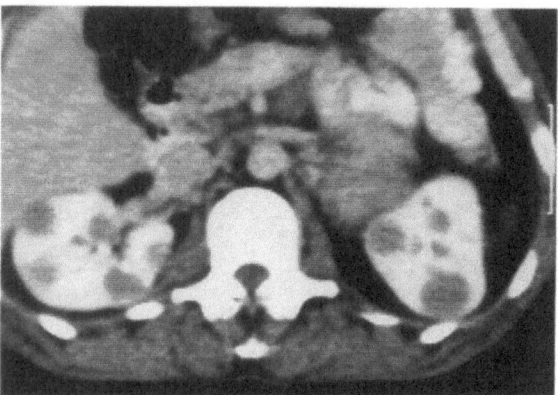

Fig. 1.7. Contrast-enhanced CT scan showing bilateral adrenal and renal involvement in non-Hodgkin's lymphoma

sity of most masses is described as varying between 40 and 60 HU (JAFRI et al. 1983) and the masses are described as solid or low density compared to the kidneys after intravenous contrast. In general, CT findings of adrenal lymphoma are not specific but in large bilateral nonmetastatic lesions without calcifications or necrosis this diagnosis may also be considered, particularly when additional lymphomas are present (Fig. 1.7). GLAZER et al. reviewed the CT scans in 400 patients with newly diagnosed or recurrent non-Hodgkin's lymphoma. Adrenal involvement was seen in four patients. The CT appearances demonstrated soft tissue masses, 3–6 cm in size (GLAZER et al. 1983).

On ultrasound, metastases of the adrenal gland vary from hypoechoic to hyperechoic (Table 1.2). There is no known correlation between the sonographic appearance and the type of the primary

tumor. There is no way to differentiate between a benign and a malignant solid lesion by ultrasound.

Primary involvement of one adrenal gland by lymphoma demonstrated on ultrasonograms is rare and there are but few sonographic descriptions of its appearance. VICKS et al. (1987) reviewed three cases reported in the literature and presented one case of their own. There does not seem to be a special sonographic characteristic of primary lymphomatous involvement of the adrenal on ultrasonograms though cystic components were seen in three of the four cases presented (VICKS et al. 1987). FELDBERG et al. (1986) showed massive bilateral non-Hodgkin's lymphoma limited to the adrenals in two patients, in all four adrenals presenting as a predominantly echolucent mass.

With MRI adrenal metastases appear either hypointense or isointense to the liver on T1-weighted images. On T2-weighted images all adrenal metastases are reported to appear hyperintense as compared with the liver and frequently have a signal intensity equal to or greater than that of fat (CHANG et al. 1987; FALKE et al. 1986; REINIG et al. 1986). If hemorrhage has occurred within the tumor, the metastasis may have areas of high signal intensity on both T1- and T2-weighted images depending on the age of the hemorrhage. Although adrenal metastases may simulate nonhyperfunctioning adrenal adenomas on T1-weighted images, they usually can be differentiated from the latter on T2-weighted sequences by virtue of their long TR/TE images.

However, long TR/TE images have also occasionally been shown with nonhyperfunctioning adenomas (BAKER et al. 1987). Moreover, high signal intensity on T2-weighted images can also be encountered with pheochromocytoma, neuroblastoma and carcinomas (Table 1.2; Fig. 1.23). The MRI appearance of adrenal lymphoma is nonspecific and is indistinguishable from that of metastatic disease to the adrenals.

1.4.2.3 Other Miscellaneous Rare Adrenal Lesions

Myelolipoma. Adrenal myelolipoma is a rare benign lesion, consisting of bone marrow and fatty elements (VON GIERKE 1905), with an autopsy incidence of 0.08%–0.2% (OLSSON et al. 1973; NOBLE et al. 1982). Individuals range in age from 17 to 93. Males and females are equally affected. The tumor arises in the adrenal cortex, and since cortical tissue may be present outside the adrenal capsule in periadrenal fat, myelolipomas may also arise there (PLAUT 1958). Myelolipomas are usually unilateral, asymptomatic,

Table 1.2. Imaging characteristics of adrenal lesions. (BEHAN et al. 1977; BERLAND et al. 1988; FALKE et al. 1987; HAERTEL et al. 1980; HOCHHAUSER et al. 1982; MIYAKE et al. 1989; REMER et al. 1989)

Lesion	CT: density	Ultrasound: echogenicity	MRI: signal intensity[a]	
			T1	T2
Myelolipoma	−20 to −100 HU, also soft tissue densities (50 HU)	Highly hyperechoic	Hyperintense	Hyperintense
Adenoma				
Nonfunctioning	−20 to 40 HU	Hypoechoic	Iso-/hypointense	Isointense
Aldosteronoma	−20 to 15 HU	Hypoechoic	Iso-/hypointense	Slightly hyperintense
Cushing adenoma	0–46 HU	Hypoechoic	Iso-/hypointense	Iso-/hyperintense
Cyst	0–25 HU	Sonolucent	Hypointense	Superintense
Pheochromocytoma	20–60 HU	Hypo-/or moderately hyperechoic, heterogeneous in large tumors	Iso-/hypointense	Hyper-/superintense
Carcinoma	30–60 HU	Hypoechoic/heterogeneous	Iso-/hypointense	Hyperintense
Neuroblastoma	20–60 HU	Hyperechoic/heterogeneous	Hypointense	Hyperintense
Metastases	20–40 HU	Variable: hypoechoic to hyperechoic	Iso-/hypointense	Hyperintense

[a] Signal intensity relative to the liver on spin-echo T1- and T2-weighted images at 0.35–0.5 T (intensity characteristics change when hemorrhage, cystic degeneration, and calcifications occur).

and, when small, commonly are diagnosed incidentally during cross-sectional imaging for other reasons. However, they may enlarge to 10–12 cm in diameter and patients occasionally develop flank or abdominal pain secondary to hemorrhage or necrosis within the mass (FINK and WURTZEBACH 1980).

On CT images, myelolipomas usually are well-defined masses with at least some areas of density equivalent to or slightly higher than normal fat (MUSANTE et al. 1988; VICK et al. 1984). Depending on their amount of fatty tissue, they vary in appearance from a predominantly fatty mass with a surrounding thin rim of soft tissue to a lesion that is predominantly of soft tissue density but contains small regions of fat density (Fig. 1.8a). High density areas may be secondary to prior hemorrhage; occasionally calcification may be present. A myelolipoma containing widespread hemorrhage or myeloid elements may have unrecognizable fat on CT and may be indistinguishable from other adrenal tumors (FINK and WURTZEBACH 1980). The differential diagnosis of a fatty mass in the suprarenal area includes lipoma, lymphangioma, myelolipoma, angiomyolipoma of the kidney, increased intraabdominal fat deposition, retroperitoneal teratoma, and liposarcoma (BEHAN et al. 1977; LIEBMANN and STRIKANTASWAMY 1981; FRIEDMAN et al. 1981).

If, on ultrasound, a lesion contains a uniform pattern of high amplitude echoes in suprarenal position, one may suggest the presence of fatty tissue and thus make the presumptive diagnosis of myelolipoma (Fig. 1.8d). However, other adrenal tumors containing fatty tissue as mentioned above may look similar.

As with CT, the MRI appearance of myelolipomas varies with the amount of fat contained in the tumor. The fatty component of myelolipoma shows signal intensity characteristics similar to those of retroperitoneal fat in all pulse sequences (Fig. 1.8b, c) (Table 2).

Teratoma. Teratomas of extragonadal origin are very rare (MCMILLAN and HORWICH 1987). Even if teratoma histology is found in an extragonadal tumor, a metastasis of an occult testicular teratoma is the most likely cause. CT features of adrenal teratomas have not been described in the literature yet. In our series of 60 primary adrenal tumors studied by CT, we observed one teratoma, which was a well-encapsulated fat density mass containing calcifications and soft tissue elements (Fig. 1.9). DAVIDSON et al. (1989) described a series of 23 retroperitoneal teratomas presenting as complex masses containing a well-circumscribed fluid component, adipose tissue and/or sebum in the form of a fatty fluid level, and calcifications.

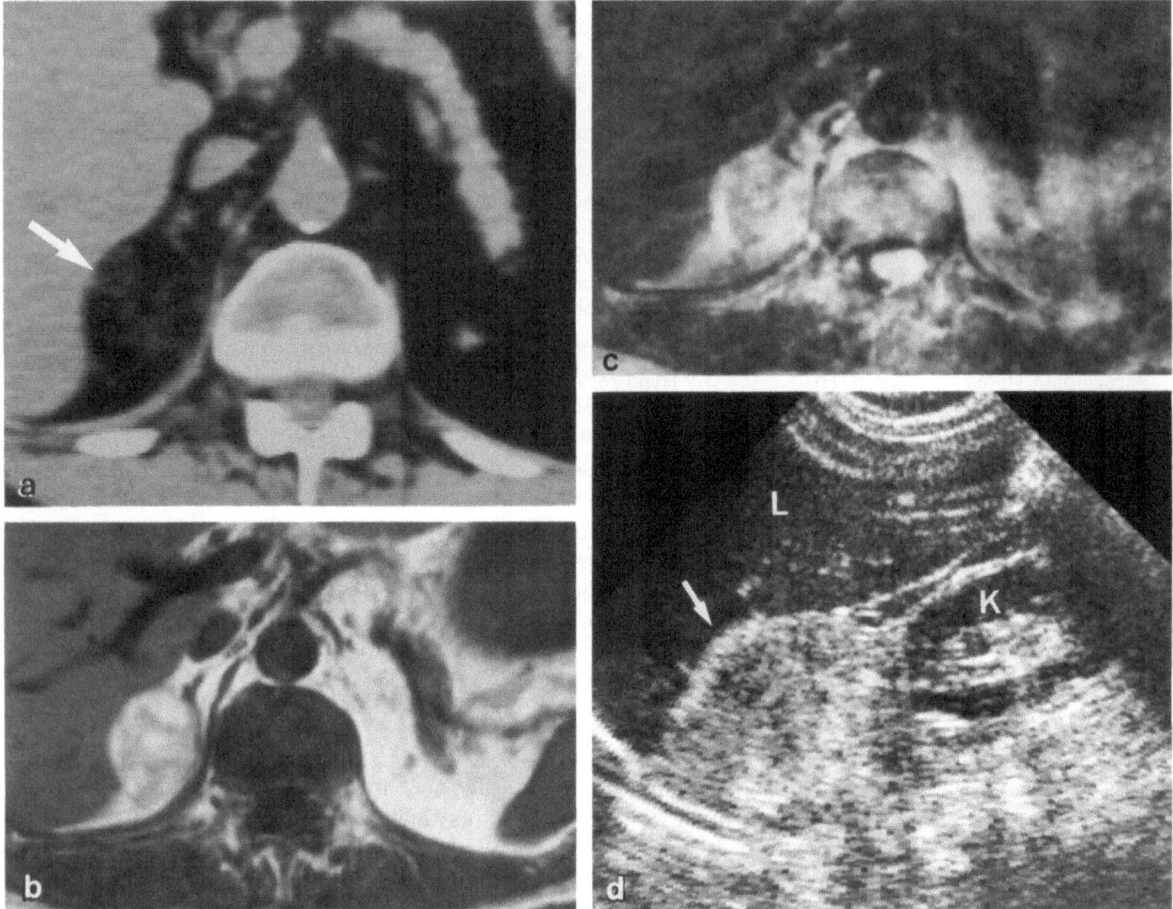

Fig. 1.8 a–d. Adrenal myelolipoma. **a** CT scan showing large right adrenal mass with fat density values *(arrow)*. **b** On MRI a heterogeneous hyperintense tumor is present (T1-weighted image). **c** T2-weighted image. **d** Ultrasonogram (different patient) showing a homogeneous hyperechoic adrenal mass *(arrow)*. *L*, liver; *K*, kidney

Ganglioneuroma. Ganglioneuroma is a rare, relatively mature benign tumor of the sympathetic system. It may arise from the adrenal medulla or from other sites of the sympathetic system (neck, posterior mediastinum, retroperitoneum) and, in the majority of cases, is found incidentally in young patients (BUNN and KING 1961).

There are only a few reports on CT appearances of ganglioneuromas (DANEMAN 1987). In our series of 60 primary adrenal tumors we observed three patients with adrenal ganglioneuromas 5–12 cm in size. CT showed an ovoid tumor and two longish, well-encapsulated tumors with density values of 28 and 40 HU on precontrast scans and only slight contrast enhancement (Fig. 1.10). Ultrasound was available in two cases and the features were inconstant: one tumor was hypoechoic with scattered circumscribed bright echoes (GÜNTHER and MÜLLER-LEISSE 1989), while the second tumor was homogeneously hypoechoic. MRI features have not been reported in the literature. In one of our cases the tumor was hypointense on T1- and hyperintense on T2-weighted spin-echo sequences (Fig. 1.10).

Hemangioma, Lymphangioma. Adrenal hemangiomas are very rare tumors, found mostly incidentally and resembling hemangiomas in other areas of the body (DERCHI et al. 1989; ROTHBERG et al. 1978; VERGAS 1980) (Fig. 1.11 a, b). The presence of phleboliths is characteristic of this tumor. Adrenal cystic lymphangioma is rather an exotic tumor, and as yet there has been no description of its appearance on imaging studies (Fig. 1.11 c, d).

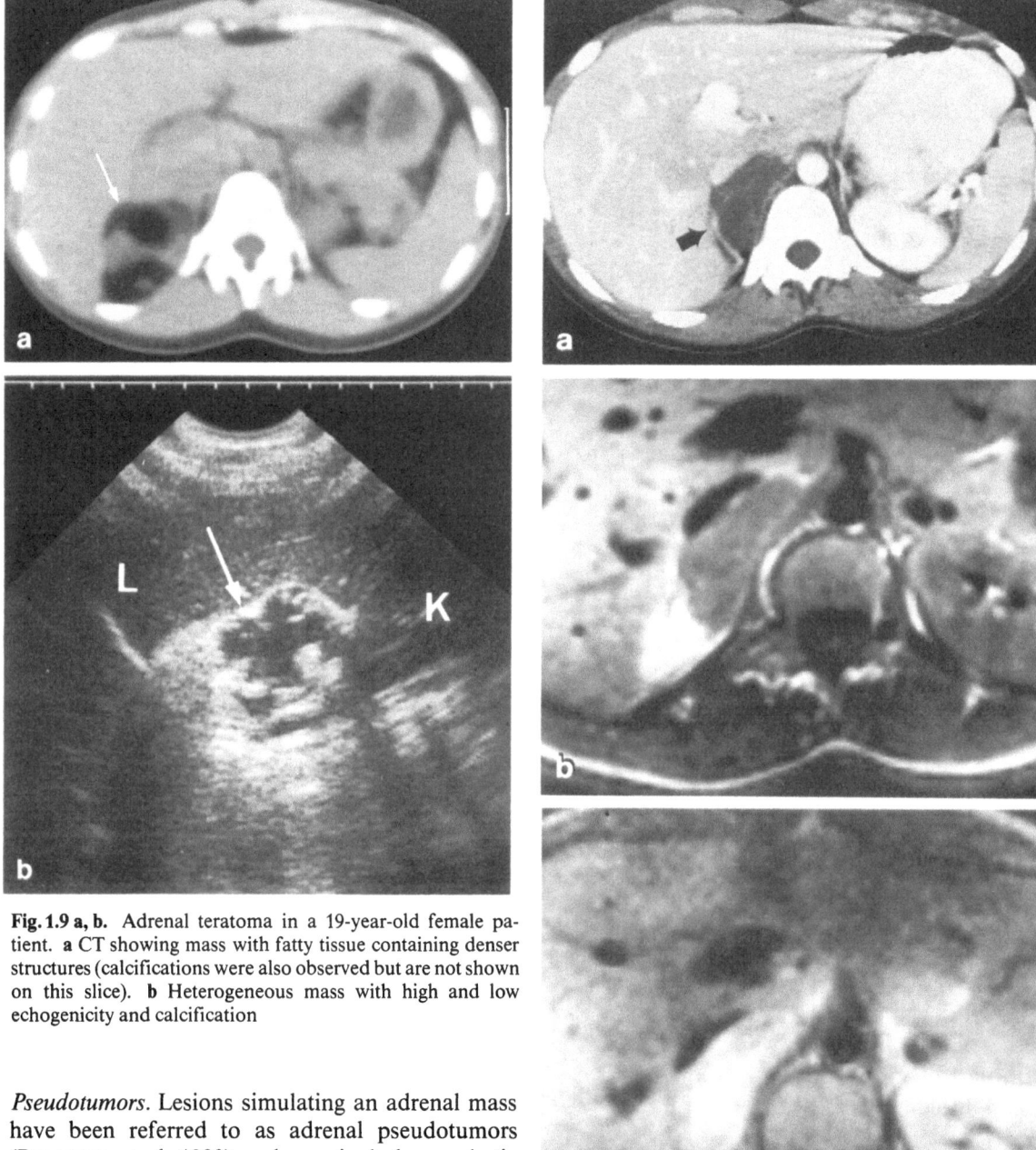

Fig. 1.9 a, b. Adrenal teratoma in a 19-year-old female patient. **a** CT showing mass with fatty tissue containing denser structures (calcifications were also observed but are not shown on this slice). **b** Heterogeneous mass with high and low echogenicity and calcification

Pseudotumors. Lesions simulating an adrenal mass have been referred to as adrenal pseudotumors (BERLINER et al. 1982) and may include exophytic renal mass, splenic lobulations, accessory spleen, tortuous splenic artery and retroperitoneal vessels, fundus of the stomach, or gastric diverticulum. Misdiagnosis can usually be avoided by a meticulous technique and careful analysis of sequential slices.

Fig. 1.10 a–c. Adrenal ganglioneuroma in a 26-year-old female patient. **a** Dynamic CT scan showing hypodense, well-defined, longish right adrenal mass with fine septations *(arrow)*. **b, c** On MRI the tumor is hypointense on T1-weighted images (**b**) and hyperintense on T2-weighted images (at 1.5 T) (**c**)

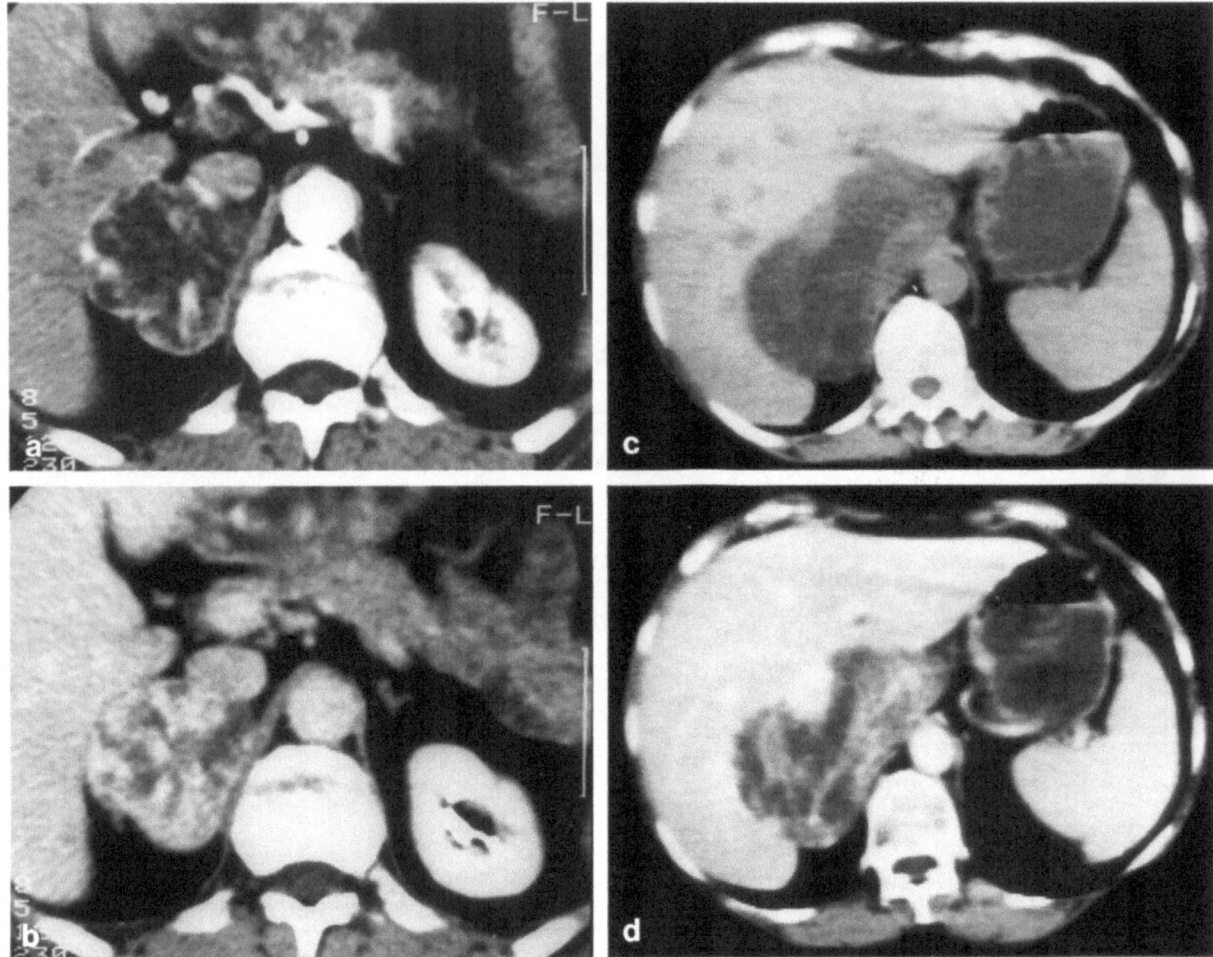

Fig. 1.11 a–d. Large adrenal hemangioma (**a, b**) and cystic lymphangioma (**c, d**) on dynamic CT scans. **a, b** Hemangioma: gradual enhancement of the tumor from the periphery to the center. **c** Cystic lymphangioma on precontrast scan; irregular and spotty and striped contrast enhancement (**d**)

1.4.2.4 Bleeding

Unilateral or bilateral adrenal hemorrhage is not uncommon in the perinatal period as a consequence of perinatal hypoxia. Adrenal hemorrhage is often asymptomatic and may be detected on routine abdominal ultrasound. In adults, adrenal hemorrhage may be secondary to septicemia, anticoagulation therapy, or pregnancy. Furthermore, posttraumatic adrenal hemorrhage (in 85% on the right side) has been reported in up to 25% of severely traumatized patients (SCULLY et al. 1984).

Typically bilateral adrenal bleeding presents as bilateral masses (MURPHY et al. 1988). Unilateral focal involvement with preservation of the normal configuration of the gland was seen in neonates (COHEN et al. 1986). In the acute stage, the attenuation values vary between 50 and 70 HU. During follow-up, the adrenal mass decreases in size (LING et al. 1983) and in density (varying between 10 and 15 HU) and may also calcify (WILMS et al. 1987). The sonographic appearance also depends on the age of the hemorrhage (WILLEMSE et al. 1989). Early in the course of the bleeding, an echogenic mass is demonstrated in the suprarenal region. With increasing liquefaction, the hematoma becomes more sonolucent and cystic (Fig. 1.12). On MRI, subacute and chronic adrenal bleeding is manifested by areas of high and low signal intensity on T1-weighted images and hyperintense areas on T2-weighted images (BAKER et al. 1989; KOCH and CORRY 1986).

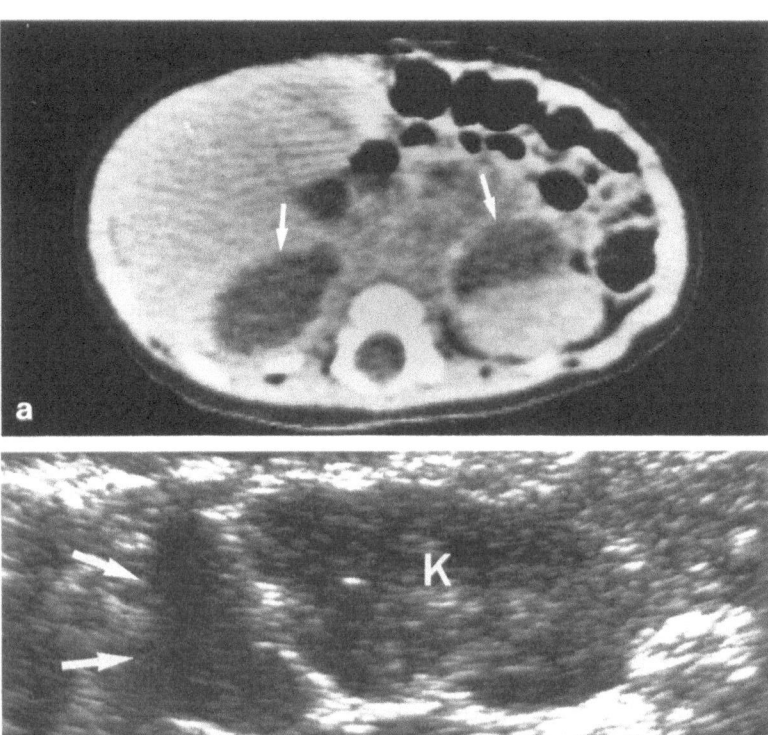

1.4.2.5 Inflammation

Bilateral tuberculous involvement of the adrenal gland is well known as the classic cause for Addison's disease. Unilateral involvement is also possible but remains endocrinologically silent. Connatal syphilis may manifest itself in the adrenals. Disseminated histoplasmosis and North American blastomycosis have also been reported to involve the adrenals (WILSON et al. 1984). Adrenal pathology in AIDS includes adrenalitis due to cytomegalovirus infection in up to 50%–89% (GROLL et al. 1990; REICHERT et al. 1983), which may progress to a necrotizing adrenalitis. Also other opportunistic infections such as toxoplasmosis, cryptococcosis neoformans, or atypical mycobacteriosis may occur in AIDS.

Active granulomatous disease such as tuberculosis of the adrenals may lead to a gross enlargement of the adrenals with cystoid areas of caseous necrosis surrounded by a thick wall (HAUSER and GURRET 1986; SAWCZUK et al. 1986; WILMS et al. 1983) (Fig. 1.13). Later on, atrophy of the gland and calcifications are seen (KTA et al. 1985) (Fig. 1.14). In histoplasmosis the range of CT findings includes slight

Fig. 1.12 a, b. Adrenal bleeding. **a** CT scan in a 4-week-old child showing bilateral peripartal adrenal hematoma. **b** On ultrasound a hypoechoic left adrenal mass *(arrow)* is shown (longitudinal view, posterior approach)

enlargement with faint flecks of calcium, moderate enlargement with focal low attenuation nodules, and massive enlargement with large areas of necrosis or dense calcifications. The changes are bilateral and symmetric (WILSON et al. 1984). Autoimmune adrenalitis leads to atrophy of the organ without calcifications (Fig. 1.15).

Bacterial abscess formation within the adrenals is very uncommon and may be secondary to infection of adrenal hematomas in the neonatal period (ATKINSON et al. 1985; O'BRIEN et al. 1987). Ultrasound may display a mass with low level echoes and good through-transmission or a complex mass. A well-encapsulated mass with rim enhancement may be seen on CT. Atrophy of the gland in autoimmune adrenalitis cannot be diagnosed with ultrasound.

Magnetic resonance imaging reports of adrenal tuberculosis are rare; BAKER et al. (1987) reported

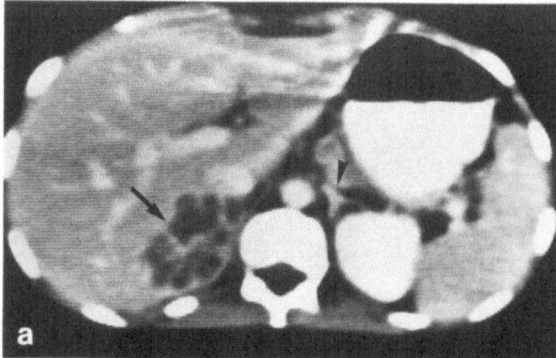

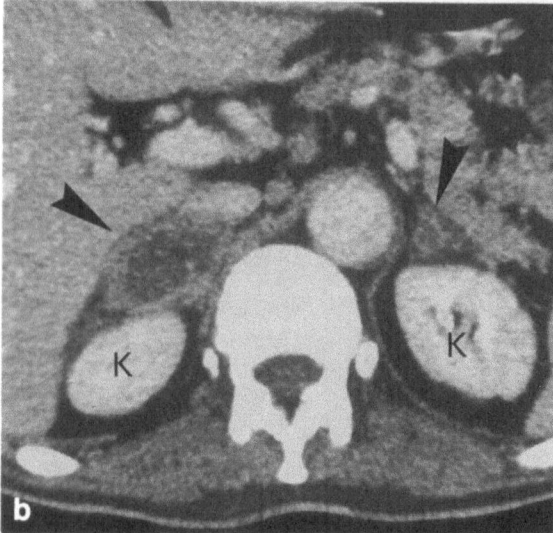

Fig. 1.13 a, b. Unilateral and bilateral adrenal tuberculosis on contrast-enhanced CT. **a** Unilateral multiseptated adrenal mass *(arrow)* with normal contralateral gland *(arrowhead)* (courtesy of Dr. A. HALBSGUTH, Frankfurt). **b** Bilateral adrenal mass *(arrowheads)* with a thick wall on contrast-enhanced CT. CT-guided Tru-Cut biopsy revealed tuberculosis. (The patient presented with signs of adrenal insufficiency.) *A*, aorta; *C*, inferior vena cava; *K*, kidney

one case of adrenal tuberculosis showing a bilateral mass with a signal intensity equal to the liver on T1-weighted images and a high signal intensity similar to fat on T2-weighted images.

1.4.2.6 Adrenal Necrosis

Adrenal necrosis may be due to circulatory disturbances or inflammatory disease. In the Waterhouse-Friderichsen syndrome extensive hemorrhagic necrosis may develop as a complication of septic meningococcal meningitis or pneumoccocal-streptococcal-gonococcal sepsis in children. Adrenal necrosis has also been described in AIDS (TAPPER et al. 1984). Hemorrhagic adrenal infarction may occur following local cytomegalovirus infection of the adrenals (REICHERT et al. 1983). Iatrogenic thrombosis of the adrenal vein with subsequent hemorrhagic necrosis and adrenal insufficiency is a rare iatrogenic complication of adrenal venography following forceful injection of contrast medium (EAGEN and PAGE 1971).

1.4.2.7 Calcifications

Calcifications of the adrenals are common in neuroblastomas, cysts, tuberculosis, and histoplasmosis and following adrenal hemorrhage (Fig. 1.14). They may also be found in carcinomas, pheochromocytomas, adenomas, ganglioneuromas, and teratomas and are rare in myelolipoma, hemangioma, and Wolman's disease (HILL et al. 1983; KENNEY and STANLEY 1987; MITTY and YEH 1982; WOLMAN et al. 1961).

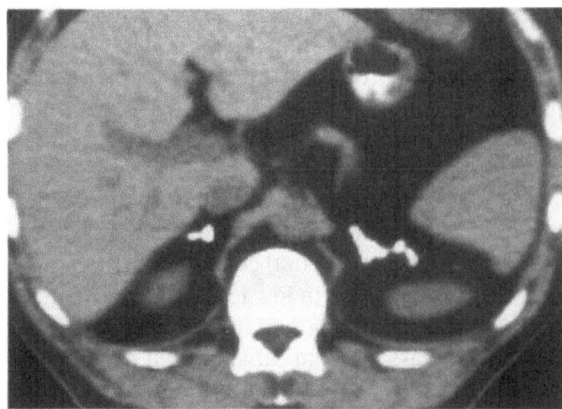

Fig. 1.14. Bilateral adrenal calcifications following adrenal tuberculosis associated with Addison's disease

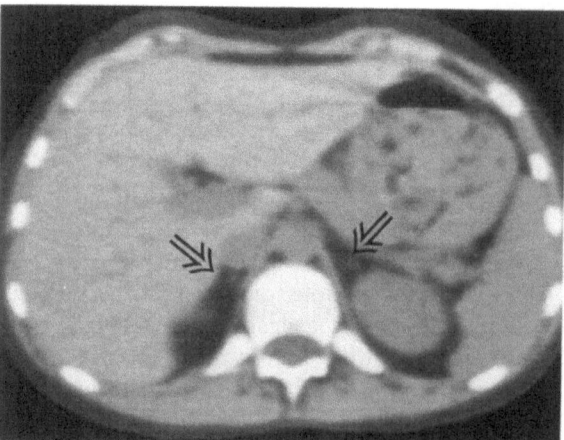

Fig. 1.15. Marked atrophy of both adrenals in autoimmune adrenalitis associated with Addison's disease. Hardly visible adrenals on CT *(arrows)*. There are no calcifications

The presence of calcium within an adrenal mass is nonspecific and it is an indicator of neither malignancy nor benignity. When the pattern of calcification is combined with other morphologic characteristics in the various imaging modalities and with clinical features, the diagnosis may be clearly evident. In reviewing 106 adrenal masses of which 33 contained calcium, KENNEY and STANLEY (1987) came to the conclusion that one pattern of calcification seems characteristic: in all their cases of adrenal cysts, the calcium was only present in the periphery and was often densest at the base as measured with CT.

Gross calcifications are easily detected on abdominal plain film or on ultrasound. CT, however, is the most sensitive technique to detect even faint calcifications and at the same time to evaluate the surrounding tissue. MRI does not visualize calcifications.

1.4.2.8 Wolman's Disease (Primary Familial Xanthomatosis)

Wolman's disease is a rare autosomal recessive metabolic disease in neonates that is usually fatal at the age of 6 months (WOLMAN et al. 1961). It is characterized by a deficiency of liposomal acid lipase, which results in widespread accumulation of triglycerides and cholesterol esters. The clinical symptoms are failure to thrive, vomiting, diarrhea, anemia, and abdominal distention due to hepatosplenomegaly. Imaging is fairly characteristic, showing normally shaped, enlarged adrenals with diffuse mottled or punctate calcifications (BERDON 1990).

1.4.3 Adrenal Lesions Associated with Adrenal Hypofunction

Primary adrenal insufficiency develops following complete or at least 90% destruction of the adrenal cortex as an acute (e.g., Waterhouse-Friderichsen syndrome) or chronic event. Adrenal tuberculosis has been the classical cause of chronic adrenal insufficiency as described by Addison. Today, the most common cause of Addison's disease in Western countries is autoimmune adrenalitis (idiopathic atrophy); histoplasmosis, metastases, Hodgkin's disease, amyloidosis, hemochromatosis, bilateral hemorrhage, and necrosis due to circulatory disturbances are rare. According to SEIDENWURM et al. (1984), however, the incidence of Addison's disease

due to adrenal metastases and lymphoma may be higher than previously suspected (4 of 21 patients = 19%). Cytomegalovirus infection in AIDS may also result in adrenal insufficiency due to adrenal necrosis (GROLL et al. 1990).

Imaging of adrenal metastases, lymphoma, bleeding, and tuberculosis (Fig. 1.13) has already been described (Sect. 1.4.1). In autoimmune adrenalitis, atrophy of the adrenals without calcification is the morphologic feature in the end-stage of the disease and may be disclosed on CT. Sometimes, atrophy of the adrenal cortex is so severe that the gland may be difficult to find (Fig. 1.15). Because there is no consistent correlation between adrenal size and function, the size of the gland cannot be judged independently of laboratory and clinical findings. CT may provide hints to the underlying etiology in Addison's disease which are usually not obtained by ultrasound. MRI does not seem to be capable of distinguishing between acute inflammatory and metastatic disease of the adrenal glands in Addison's disease, but may be as efficacious as CT in suggesting the diagnosis of adrenal hemorrhage (BAKER et al. 1988).

Diagnostic Workup. The diagnosis of adrenal insufficiency is usually based on clinical, hormonal, and laboratory findings. In acute adrenal insufficiency, CT may be important to substantiate the diagnosis of an addisonian crisis morphologically. In subacute and chronic Addison's disease, CT may provide information on the etiology. In unclear enlargement of the adrenal gland, percutaneous CT-guided biopsy is indicated (Fig. 1.13b).

1.4.4 Adrenal Lesions Associated with Adrenal Hyperfunction

Excess secretion of different adrenal hormones (aldosterone, cortisol, androgens, epinephrine, norepinephrine) results in different clinical signs and symptoms. There are four distinct clinical syndromes:

1. Conn's syndrome (primary hyperaldosteronism)
2. Cushing's syndrome
3. Adrenogenital syndrome
4. Adrenomedullary hyperfunction

In contrast to pheochromocytoma, which is usually caused by hyperfunction of the adrenal medulla, Conn's and Cushing's syndromes as well as adrenogenital syndrome are secondary to adrenocortical hyperfunction.

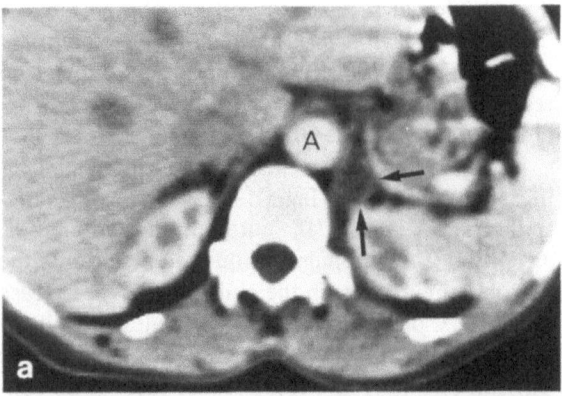

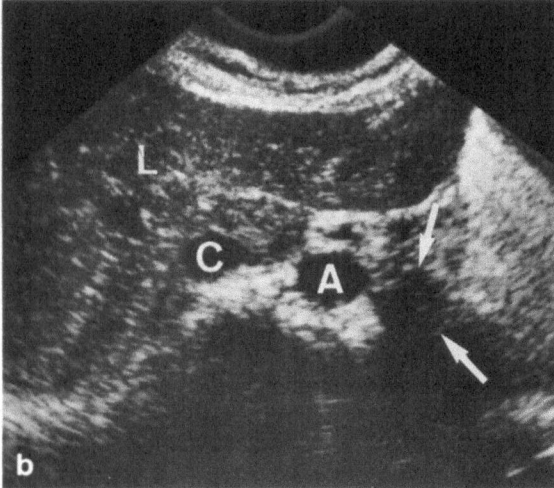

Fig. 1.16 a, b. Left cortical adenoma *(arrows)* in Conn's disease. **a** Low density oval adrenal mass (15 HU) on dynamic ultrasound. *L*, liver; *K*, kidney; *C*, inferior vena cava; *A*, aorta

1.4.4.1 Conn's Syndrome

In Conn's syndrome or primary hyperaldosteronism the underlying morphologic changes vary considerably:

1. Solitary adenoma (aldosteronoma)
2. Bilateral adenoma
3. Bilateral hyperplasia (diffuse and/or micro-, macronodular)
4. Adrenal carcinoma

In 80%–90% of cases, solitary adenomas (usually 1–2 cm in size) are responsible for the syndrome. Bilateral hyperplasia is less often encountered; the presence of several adrenal nodes is indicative of macronodular hyperplasia. Adrenal carcinomas leading to aldosteronism are rare and are usually of considerable size at the time of detection.

On CT, aldosteronomas are indistinguishable from other adenomas. They are usually hypodense

(range −20 to 15 HU) (Table 1.2) or isodense compared to the surrounding adrenal gland and small, measuring 1.5–2 cm in diameter (Fig. 1.16). Moderate enhancement following bolus injection of contrast medium may be seen (BERLAND et al. 1988). Sensitivity of CT in detecting aldosteronomas varies between 61% and 88% (ABRAMS et al. 1982; GEISINGER et al. 1983; DUNNICK et al. 1982b; IKEDA et al. 1989). Since tumors of 10 mm in diameter and less can be easily missed; thin section scans (2 mm) are advocated.

On ultrasound, aldosteronomas are hypoechoic, and tumors as small as 8–10 mm in diameter may be detected (GÜNTHER et al. 1984a, b; YEH 1980). Their appearance is indistinguishable from that of other adenomas (Fig. 1.16b). Visualization of such tumors on the right side is easier than on the left because of the "acoustic window" provided by the liver, but the accuracy of ultrasound is generally inferior to that of CT (ABRAMS et al. 1982).

On MRI, aldosteronomas are reported to be slightly hypointense when compared to the signal intensity of the liver on T1-weighted images and slightly hyperintense or isointense when compared to the liver on T2-weighted images (BAKER et al. 1989; FALKE et al. 1986, 1987; GLAZER et al. 1986; REINIG et al. 1986). In a study of 27 patients, REMER et al. (1989) could not distinguish nonhyperfunctioning cortical adenomas (Fig. 1.3) from benign hyperfunctioning cortical lesions at 0.35 T.

On scintigraphy, aldosteronomas are characterized by radiotracer uptake, which reveals the tumor 4–7 days after administration of the tracer NP-59 (GROSS et al. 1981; ISHIMURA et al. 1989). To enhance radionuclide uptake in the non-ACTH-dependent adrenal tissue the dexamethasone suppression scan was introduced. After 4 mg dexamethasone daily for 7 days prior to iodocholesterol in normal subjects, the adrenals are not visualized at all or are seen faintly at the end of the imaging sequence. Early unilateral adrenal visualization (prior to the 5th day) suggests an adrenal adenoma, whereas bilateral early adrenal visualization (after the 5th day) suggests hyperplasia (GROSS et al. 1981). Using the suppression regimen, the accuracy is said to be 90% and more (FREITAS et al. 1979; MILES et al. 1979). In a series of 17 patients, IKEDA et al. (1989) found CT and NP-59 scintigraphy to be equivalent in the detection of adrenal abnormalities in primary aldosteronism.

In selective venous sampling, the aldosterone concentration in the adrenal vein on the side of the lesion is high and cannot be overlooked, with levels usually more than a fourfold aldosterone step-up

(Fig. 1.17) (HORTON and FINCK 1972). Diagnosis of bilateral hyperplasia may be more difficult, as different catheter placement on each side may lead to admixture of adrenal venous blood with that from other sources. Therefore it is recommended that the aldosterone/ cortisol ratio be used to provide a more reliable basis for quantitative comparison of the two adrenals (DUNNICK et al. 1979). As cortisol secretion is unaffected by aldosterone overproduction this provides a means of compensating for differences in catheter placement. Similar to scintigraphy, seletive venous blood sampling may identify aldosteronomas with a diagnostic accuracy of 91%–100% (WEINBERGER et al. 1979; DUNNICK et al. 1982a). It may therefore be applied as an alternative to scintigraphy.

Diagnostic Workup. In clinically suspected primary hyperaldosteronism CT is the primary technique in localization of the lesion. If CT fails to show the adrenal lesion, selective venous sampling is indicated; alternatively scintigraphy may be applied.

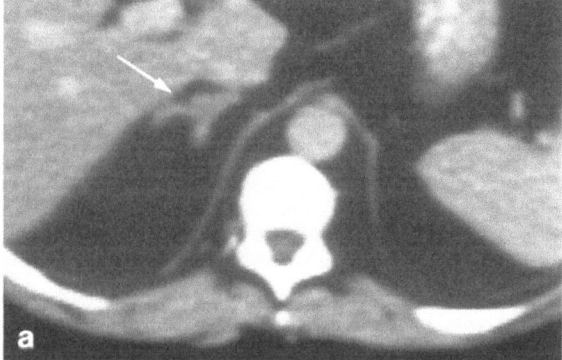

Fig. 1.17. Selective adrenal venography and seletive venous sampling for aldosterone determination. High aldosterone step-up on the left confirming an aldosteronoma. (Also on phlebography a small mass was present in the uppermost part of the left gland) *(arrow)*

1.4.4.2 Cushing's Syndrome

Hypercortisolism (Cushing's syndrome) may be ACTH dependent or may be caused by autonomous adrenal hyperfunction. The following conditions may be encountered (SYMINGTON 1982):

1. Bilateral adrenal hyperplasia (pituitary adenoma; Cushing's disease) (85%)
2. Autonomous adrenal adenoma (10%)
3. Adrenal carcinoma (5%)
4. Ectopic nonpituitary ACTH-producing tumor (rare)

Adrenal hyperplasia may be diffuse; micro- or macronodular hyperplasia is less common (FLATTET and HEDINGER 1980). Primary pigmented nodular adrenocortical disease is a rare cause of Cushing's syndrome in infants, children, and young adults (DOPPMAN et al. 1989), and some of the patients may exhibit stigmas of Carney complex (spotty skin pigmentation, calcified Sertoli cell tumors of the testes, and cardiac and soft tissue myxomas). It should be stressed that, prior to imaging, the diagnosis of Cushing's syndrome first requires a thorough clinical and biochemical workup of the diagnosis.

Computed tomography is the most important modality for imaging of the adrenals in Cushing's syndrome. Increased ACTH production leads to bilateral adrenal hyperplasia and to thickening of the adrenal limbs. Since the thickness of the normal

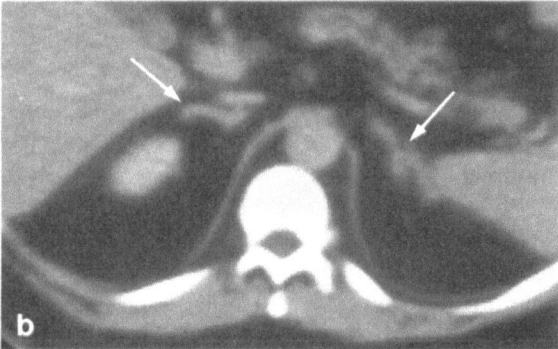

Fig. 1.18 a, b. Bilateral macronodular adrenal hyperplasia *(arrow)* in Cushing's disease (CT scan on two different levels)

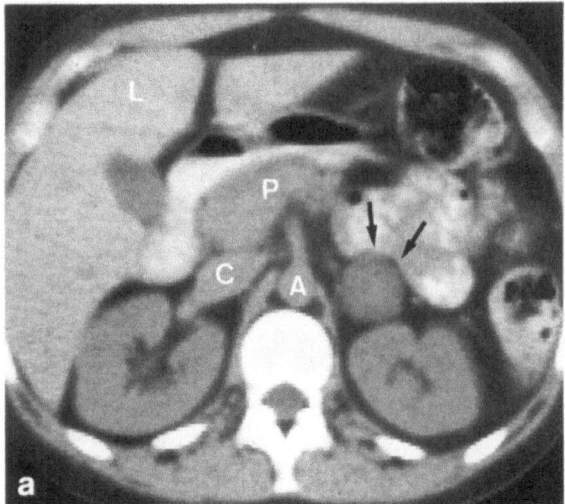

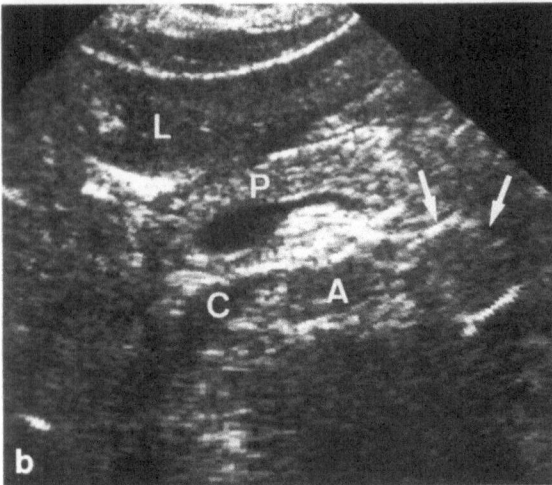

Fig. 1.19 a, b. Left cortical adenoma *(arrow)* in Cushing's disease. **a** On CT a mass is present displaying higher attenuation values (38 HU) than the aldosteronoma in Fig. 1.16. **b** Ultrasound (anterior approach) shows a hypoechoic mass *(arrow)*. *A,* aorta; *C,* inferior vena cava; *L,* liver; *P,* pancreas

mal sized or nodular, hyperplasia is likely to be present. In primary pigmented nodular adrenocortical disease, CT may demonstrate unilateral or bilateral nodularity (DOPPMAN et al. 1989).

Cortisol-producing autonomous adenomas are well-defined roundish masses, usually 2–4 cm in size, and may have higher attenuation values (0.4–46 HU) than aldosteronomas (Fig. 1.19a) (MIYAKE et al. 1989). They are frequently associated with atrophy of the ipsilateral and contralateral gland tissue. Sensitivity of CT for the detection of adrenal adenomas is 70%–75% (GEISINGER et al. 1983).

On ultrasound, Cushing adenomas are all hypoechoic and well defined (Fig. 1.19b); their appearance is indistinguishable from that of other adrenal adenomas. In cortical hyperplasia diffuse hypoechoic enlargement or a mass may be seen, but this is inconstant and very often the adrenals are normal appearing.

On MRI, the signal intensity of adrenal hyperplasia is similar to that of the normal gland. Experience with cortical adenomas in Cushing's syndrome is limited, but signal characteristics are variable (REMER et al. 1989) and similar to those of aldosteronomas (FALKE et al. 1987), i.e., often hyperintense to the liver with T2-weighted sequences or isointense (MCGAHAM 1988) (Table 1.2). The appearance of adrenal carcinomas is described below. On scintiscan with NP-59, adrenal adenomas may be delineated by unilateral increased uptake; bilateral uptake may be indicative of adrenal hyperplasia – provided interpretation is combined with the clinical and biochemical diagnosis. Because of the high radiation dose to the patient and the length of the examination time, scintigraphy has severe limitations.

Venous sampling occasionally may be needed in Cushing's syndrome. Among patients with Cushing's syndrome, CT has been entirely accurate for the detection of functioning adrenal adenoma and carcinoma and the need for adrenal venography and adrenal venous sampling is questionable. However, selective sampling of the inferior petrosal sinus is indicated in suspected ACTH-producing pituitary microadenomas undetected by CT or MRI and for differentiation of an ectopic ACTH-producing tumor (OLDFIELD et al. 1985).

Diagnostic Workup. The diagnostic workup in clinically and biochemically proven Cushing's syndrome includes adrenal CT as the primary modality for the detection of an adrenal adenoma. If a pituitary adenoma is suspected on the basis of laboratory data (dexamethasone suppression test, urine cortisol excretion), evaluation of the pituitary gland by CT

adrenal cortex is only 2 mm, it is conceivable that CT fails to demonstrate diffuse adrenal hyperplasia in about 50% of cases, and perhaps more (KOROBKIN et al. 1979; POJUNAS et al. 1986; DOPPMAN et al. 1988). In nodular hyperplasia (Fig. 1.18), the nodules are usually hypodense because of the high lipid or hormone content. Diffuse hyperplasia and macronodular hyperplasia may also be combined. In a single dominant nodule, the finding may be misinterpreted as a unilateral autonomous adenoma, which may have an important clinical impact on therapy (FALKE et al. 1987). Careful evaluation of the ipsilateral and contralateral adrenal size is necessary to avoid misinterpretation. If the remainder of the gland and the contralateral gland are nor-

(sensitivity 63%, specificity 62.5%) (MARCOVITZ et al. 1987) or MRI (sensitivity 71%, specificity 87%) (PECK et al. 1989) is necessary. Selective venous sampling of the inferior petrosal sinus is indicated in proved Cushing's disease, if no tumor is detected with other imaging modalities.

1.4.4.3 Adrenogenital Syndrome

Adrenal lesions leading to feminization (very rare) or masculinization include congenital adrenal hyperplasia (Fig. 1.20), acquired adrenocortical hyperplasia, or an adrenocortical tumor (adenoma, carcinoma) or can be due to excess secretion of hormones from a virilizing tumor from the ovaries.

In contrast to Conn's syndrome, in the adrenogenital syndrome the CT density values of the hyperplastic gland, adenomas, and carcinomas have been described as varying between 30 and 50 HU (HÜBENER et al. 1984). If the tumors are too small, they may escape detection by palpation or by imaging modalities.

Diagnostic Workup. After clinical examination and a complex biochemical evaluation, CT is the most important morphologic modality and is particularly important for excluding an adrenal tumor. Ultrasonograms have been advocated as an inexpensive screening examination (BRYAN et al. 1988; DAVIES and LAM 1987). In the differential diagnosis, tumors of the testis, in which ultrasonics and MRI are the imaging modalities of choice, and tumors of the ovaries may be considered. If an adrenal tumor is suspected and all noninvasive imaging modalites have been equivocal and the site of the hormone production is unclear, the clinician has to resort to selective venous sampling from the gonadal and adrenal veins in order to identify the source of the increased hormone production (SÖRENSEN and MOLTZ 1981).

1.4.4.4 Adrenal Carcinoma

Adrenal carcinoma is a rare tumor that affects all ages and sexes. It is insidious and of dismal prognosis because the tumor may grow to a large size before it becomes clinically symptomatic (KING and LACK 1979; RICHIE and GITTES 1980). At the time of presentation the tumor usually exceeds 4 cm in diameter and can reach up to 10 cm (BELLDEGRUN et al. 1986; DUNNICK et al. 1982b; HENLEY et al. 1983). Approximately 50% of the tumors are endocrinologically active and may lead to Cushing's syn-

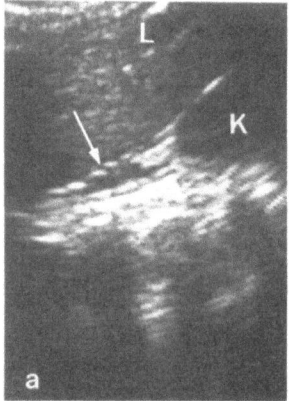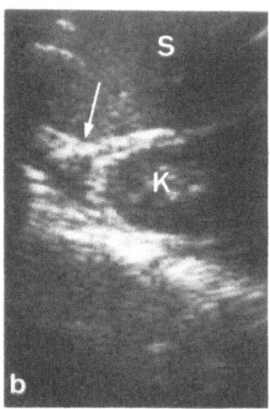

Fig. 1.20 a, b. Ultrasonogram showing bilateral adrenal hyperplasia *(arrow)* in adrenogenital syndrome in a $3^1/_2$-year-old boy (21-hydroxylase deficiency). **a** Right adrenal gland; **b** left adrenal gland. *K,* kidney; *L,* liver; *S,* spleen

drome, feminization, virilization, or, in isolated cases, hyperaldosteronism. Childhood adrenocortical carcinoma, although extremely uncommon, is still the most common tumor occurring in the adrenal cortex in this age group (ZAITOON and MACKIC 1983; DANEMAN et al. 1983) and also may be seen in Beckwith-Wiedemann syndrome. Due to their large size, adrenal carcinomas are easily detected by imaging modalities.

On CT, the tumors are well defined with irregular contours and may exhibit central diminished attenuation, representing central tumor necrosis and calcifications (Fig. 1.21; Table 1.2) (DUNNICK et al. 1982b). Density values vary from 30 to 60 HU and enhancement following bolus injection of contrast medium is inhomogeneous. FISHMAN et al. (1987) found a thin, enhancing, capsule-like rim surrounding the neoplasms, which may add to the specificity of CT diagnosis. Altogether, distinguishing malignant from benign adrenal lesions is difficult because no single criterion is specific. Central necrosis and tumor calcification are seen in a variety of lesions, including small benign adenomas. The only definite criterion for malignancy is the presence of metastases, commonly within the liver.

On ultrasound, the tumors, particularly the large ones, are heterogeneous and exhibit hypoechoic and hyperechoic areas due to tumor necrosis, hemorrhage, and sometimes calcification (19%). However, small carcinomas (3–6 cm) may be rather homogeneous (HAMPER et al. 1987) and indistinguishable from adenomas. The size of the lesion may be an adjunct for differentiation of adrenal carcinoma from adenoma, as larger masses have a greater probability of being malignant than smaller ones. However,

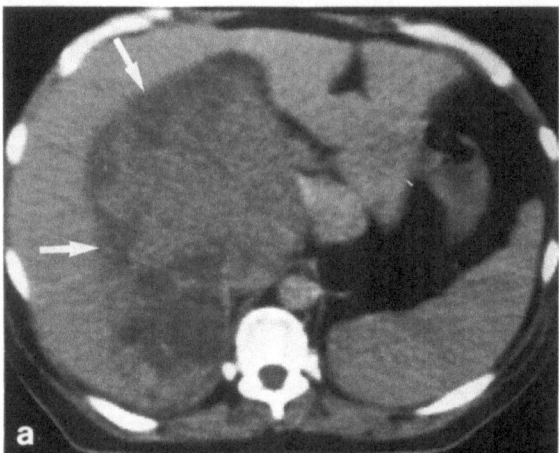

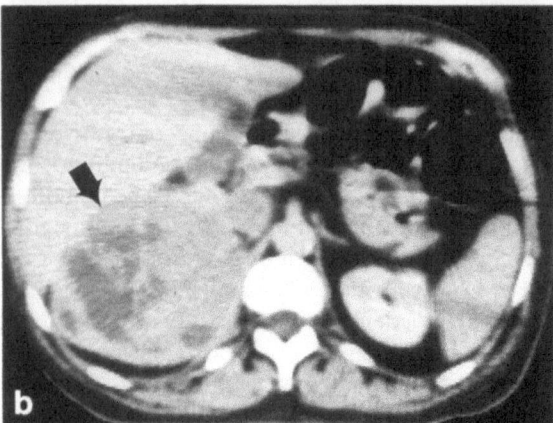

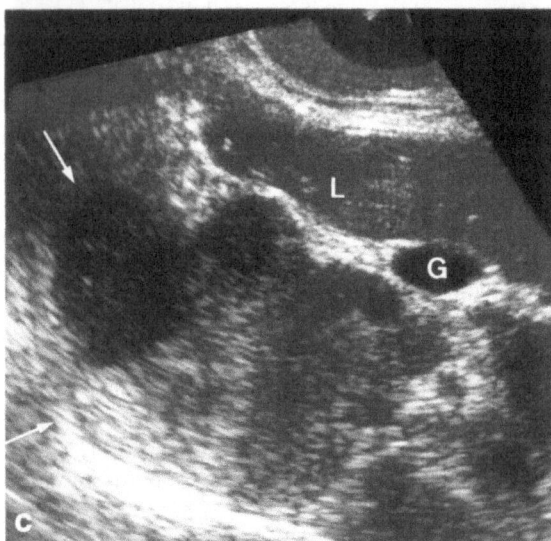

Fig. 1.21 a–c. Large right adrenal carcinoma with inhomogeneous absorption values and irregular margins *(arrow).* **a, b** CT scan; **c** ultrasonogram (subcostal oblique view). *G,* gallbladder; *L,* liver

adenomas can exceed 5 cm in diameter as well. Distinction between an adrenal mass and a tumor originating in the liver or the upper pole of the kidney is usually possible on the basis of the characteristic displacement of the retroperitoneal fat planes. However, if the lesion is large, cleavage planes may not be easily appreciated. In general, adrenal carcinomas do not display characteristic features on ultrasound that permit morphologic differentiation from a large metastasis or a pheochromocytoma, and even adenomas may look similar.

On MRI, adrenal carcinoma usually produces signals of moderately low intensity relative to the hepatic parenchyma in T1-weighted images. Signal intensity increases relative to liver with T2 weighting and is greater than that of fat (CHANG et al. 1987; DOPPMAN et al. 1987; SMITH et al. 1989). As with CT, tumor heterogeneity, best demonstrated by the use of T2-weighted sequences, is seen and represents tumor necrosis and hemorrhage. Due to the low proton density, calcification may go undetected with MRI. CT and MRI are useful in assessing staging parameters such as tumor extent, involvement of regional lymph nodes, hepatic metastases, and renal vein and inferior vena cava extension. If CT shows conclusive evidence of the tumor location and tumor extent, further evaluation by MRI is unnecessary.

1.4.4.5 Pheochromocytoma

Adrenal medullary hyperfunction is usually caused by pheochromocytomas. In isolated cases medullary hyperplasia may be found in conjunction with the multiple endocrine neoplasia type II syndrome (MEN-II) or with a neurocutaneous syndrome (e. G., Hippel-Lindau disease or neurofibromatosis). Pheochromocytomas arise from chromaffin cells of the sympathetic nervous system. Although most pheochromocytomas are found in the adrenal medulla, as many as 10% occur in extraadrenal locations, most frequently in the paracaval or paraaortic regions along the course of the sympathetic ganglia (7%) or near the organ of Zuckerkandl. These tumors also occur in the mediastinum (1%) and the wall of the urinary bladder (1%) (FRIES and CHAMBERLIN 1968). Extraadrenal pheochromocytomas may occur singly or as multicentric lesions (HATTERY et al. 1981). Only approximately 6%–10% of pheochromocytomas are malignant; however, in extraadrenal locations the rate of malignancy is approximately 40% (HUME 1960). Pheochromocytoma has also been referred to as "10% tumor" since approximately 10%

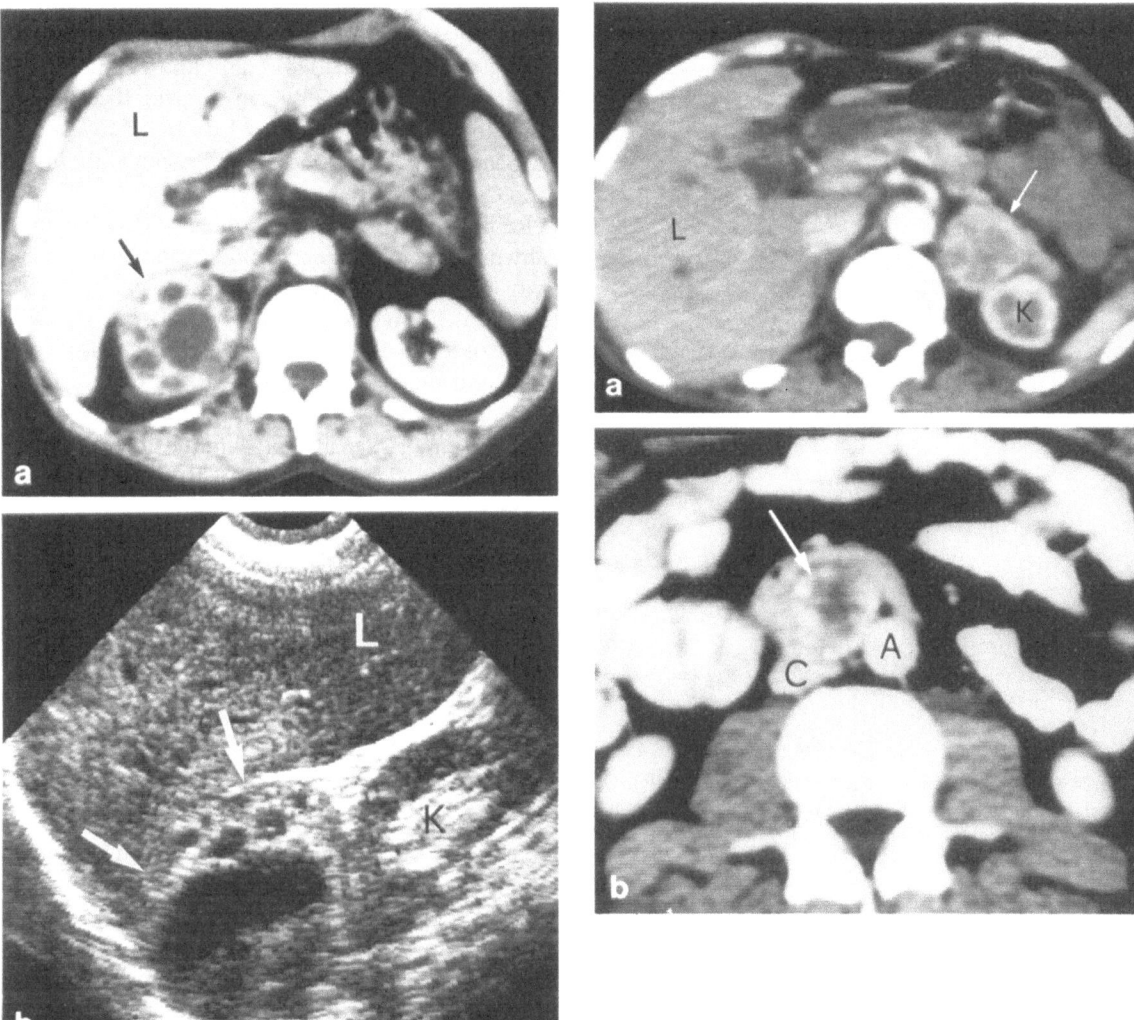

Fig. 1.22 a, b. Right adrenal cystic pheochromocytoma *(arrow).* **a** Contrast-enhanced CT scan showing well-delineated enhancing tumor containing cystic areas ("Swiss-cheese" pattern). **b** Corresponding ultrasonogram. *L*, liver; *K*, kidney

Fig. 1.23. a Solid adrenal pheochromocytoma on left *(arrow).* On dynamic CT there was intense contrast enhancement of the tumor. *L*, liver; *K*, kidney. **b** Extraadrenal pheochromocytoma in the organ of Zuckerkandl. Heterogeneous contrast enhancement

of the tumors are extraadrenal in location, 10% are bilateral, and 10% are malignant. The size of pheochromocytomas varies considerably, from very small (5–10 mm) to 10 cm in diameter. The tumors may be solid or partially necrotic or may have a cystic appearance (Figs. 1.22, 1.23).

On CT, pheochromocytomas present on precontrast scan as round or oval, well-defined tumors that have a solid, homogeneous appearance and are usually greater than 3 cm im diameter; the tumors have density values ranging from 20 to 60 HU (FRANCIS et al. 1983; MIYAKE et al. 1989). Solid tumor parts show intense enhancement in the early phase following bolus injection of contrast medium

(Fig. 1.23). With larger tumors, necrosis is frequently present, producing central regions of low density. Rarely, extensive central necrosis results in a cystic appearance that may resemble an adrenal cyst (BUSH et al. 1985). Sensitivity of CT for detection of adrenal pheochromocytomas is 92%–100% (WELCH et al. 1983; QUINT et al. 1987); false-negative examinations most commonly occur as a result of difficulty in detecting small tumors in patients with little retroperitoneal fat or in those cases in which the tumor is located outside the area surveyed by the CT examination. For suspected mediastinal and other extraadrenal pheochromocytomas, dynamic CT is recommended (Fig. 1.23 b). Extraadrenal pheochro-

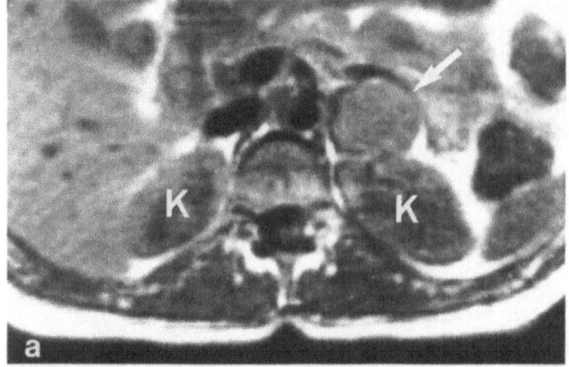

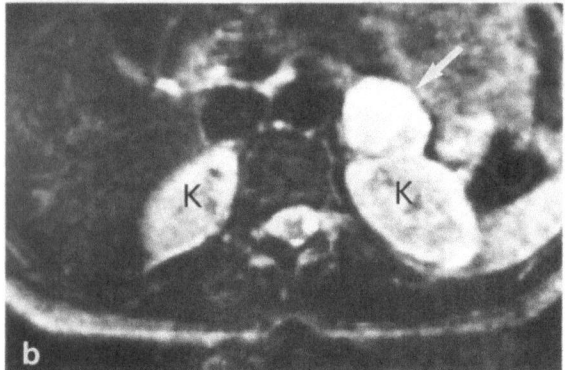

Fig. 1.24 a, b. Left adrenal pheochromocytoma on MRI. On T1-weighted images (SE: TR 600/TE 15) (**a**) the tumor is hypointense T2-weighted images (SE: TR 2200/TE 90) (**b**) it is hyperintense. *K*, kidney

mocytomas, which may be located anywhere from the base of the skull to the pelvis, are much more difficult to detect than a tumor of adrenal origin (Fig. 1.25).

On ultrasound, pheochromocytomas are of moderate to increased echogenicity and often homogeneous. A "Swiss cheese" pattern with cystic areas of necrosis may be seen in large, partially necrotic tumors (Fig. 1.22 b). The tumor cannot be distinguished from other adrenal tumors on the basis of its echogenicity (Table 1.2).

Pheochromocytomas as small as 1.1 cm have been detected by MRI (REINIG et al. 1986). As with CT, small pheochromocytomas often have a homogeneous appearance, whereas the larger tumors appear inhomogeneous. On MRI, pheochromocytomas are hypointense on T1-weighted images, similar to kidney, liver, and muscle and well differentiated from the high signal of fat (FALKE et al. 1986; REINIG et al. 1986). With T2-weighted images they are hyperintense, the signal intensity being markedly greater than that of liver and muscle and sometimes greater than that of fat (Fig. 1.24) (VELCHIK et al. 1989; DOPPMAN et al. 1987; QUINT et al. 1987). Intratumor

bleeding may result in an increase in signal intensity on T1-weighted images. QUINT et al. reported a prospective series of 13 adrenal and extraadrenal pheochromocytomas (3–4 cm in size) 10 of which were detected by CT and 12 by MRI. MRI is also advocated for detection of often small tumors in Sipple's disease (MATHIEU et al. 1987).

Radioisotope scanning with ^{131}I-MIBG has been shown to diagnose pheochromocytoma with a sensitivity of 87%–90% and a specificity of 95%–99% (Fig. 1.25) (SHAPIRO et al. 1985; QUINT et al. 1987; SWENSON et al. 1984, VELCHIK et al. 1989). Both primary and metastatic lesions may be detected successfully. Radioisotope scanning with ^{131}I-MIBG is the single most sensitive technique for evaluating metastatic bone lesions in pheochromocytoma.

On angiography, most pheochromocytomas are hypervascular and demonstrate large feeding vessels and tumor blush. Adrenal pheochromocytomas are detected with a sensitivity of 85%–100% (CHRISTENSON et al. 1976; ZELCH et al. 1974). Large extraadrenal pheochromocytomas are similarly easy to detect, but small ones in the order of 1–2 cm in diameter may be most problematic to detect. KADIR et al. (1981) stress the importance of subtraction angiography in the diagnosis of extraadrenal pheochromocytomas.

Selective venous sampling for determination of epinephrine and norepinephrine selectively in the adrenal veins and in major branches of the inferior and superior vena cava veins has been used in a small number of patients with suspected pheochromocytoma (CORDES et al. 1979; DUNNICK et al. 1982a; GEORGI et al. 1978). Since catecholamine values from the adrenal vein can be considerably adulterated by injection of contrast medium, a very subtle catheterization technique is of the utmost importance; location of the catheter tip should be verified after withdrawal of the blood samples. Definite data regarding the accuracy of this technique are not available due to the small size of the series reported in the literature.

Selective venous sampling is a measure of last resort in suspected pheochromocytoma not detected by other means or in inconclusive small pheochromocytomas on CT or MRI. It is also a technique of second choice in the search for an extraadrenal pheochromocytoma.

Diagnostic Workup. The diagnostic workup in suspected pheochromocytoma will certainly depend on the local facilities. In general, localization of a suspected pheochromocytoma may start with CT and ultrasound. If an adrenal tumor is found, ^{131}I-MIBG

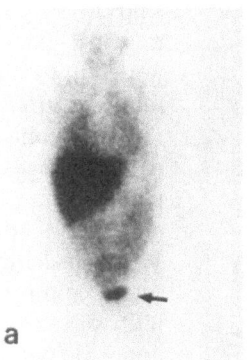
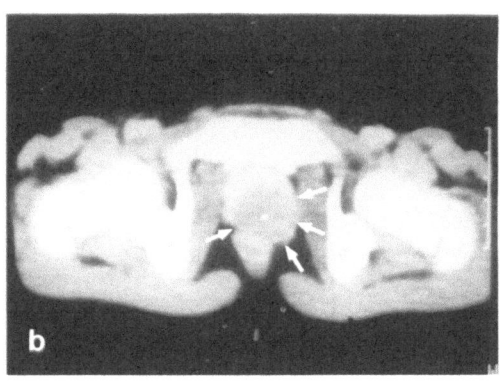

Fig. 1.25 a, b. Extraadrenal pheochromocytoma in the prostate (8-year-old boy). **a** ^{131}I-MIBG scintigraphy disclosing focal radionuclide uptake in the prostate. **b** Dynamic CT scan showing a slightly contrast-enhancing mass in the prostate. (Courtesy of Prof. K. J. KLOSE, Marburg, Germany)

(or ^{123}I-MIBG) scanning may be performed to exclude an additional extraadrenal pheochromocytoma or metastases from a malignant pheochromocytoma. Instead of CT, MRI may be used as the primary procedure since it is at least equally suitable (FRANCIS et al. 1983). Other authors recommend scintigraphy as the primary modality in the search for pheochromocytomas because the entire body is imaged (GLAZER et al. 1988); scintigraphy is then followed by MRI or CT for better anatomic localization (QUINT et al. 1987). In suspected extraadrenal pheochromocytoma or recurrent or metastatic pheochromocytoma, a functional diagnostic test using ^{131}I-MIBG scintigraphy and/or selective venous sampling is recommended as the first step. If there is evidence of an ectopic tumor location, directed CT or MRI is applied to support the diagnosis and to provide precise anatomic localization. Angiography has little place except in the search for extraadrenal pheochromocytomas when noninvasive procedures have failed or are inconclusive. Having found a pheochromocytoma, the clinician must think of the possibility of an associated syndrome.

1.4.4.6 Neuroblastoma

Neuroblastoma arises from primitive sympathetic neuroblasts of the embryonic neural crest. It is the most common extracranial solid malignant tumor in children and the third most common malignancy of childhood, surpassed in incidence only by acute leukemia and primary brain tumors; it accounts for at least 10% of all pediatric neoplasms, with an approximate incidence of 500 new cases diagnosed in the United States each year (EXELBY 1981; HAYES and GREEN 1983). Fifty percent of patients are less than 2 years of age, 75% of patients are less than 4 years of age, and fewer than 10% of neuroblastomas occur in children over age 10 years (EXELBY 1981). More than 50% of neuroblastomas are in the abdomen and two-thirds of them are located in an adrenal gland. Other abdominal or pelvic neuroblastomas almost always originate in the paravertebral sympathetic chain or the presacral area, with an occasional abdominal tumor arising at the celiac axis or organ of Zuckerkandl. Fifteen percent of neuroblastomas are thoracic, usually located in the sympathetic ganglia of the posterior mediastinum. Other anatomic sites include pelvis (5%) and cerebrum (0.2%). Between 10% and 12% of neuroblastomas are disseminated without known site of origin (ANDRESEN et al. 1981; BERGER et al. 1983; HAYES and GREEN 1983; KAJANTI 1983; STY et al. 1984). Patients with neuroblastomas usually present with advanced disease, having a large abdominal mass crossing the midline. At least 70% of patients will have disseminated disease at the time of diagnosis and many present symptoms secondary to metastatic disease. Common sites of metastases are skeleton, bone marrow, liver, lymph nodes, and skin. The pattern of metastases varies greatly with age. Bony metastases are extremely common in children over 1 year of age, usually involving the long bones and orbit, and frequently causing bone pain or exophthalmos. However, bony metastases occur in less than 5% of newborns, while massive hepatomegaly and skin lesions are frequent. Patients of any age may have bone marrow involvement, adenopathy, and liver metastases. Despite the high frequency of increased catecholamines secreted by neuroblastomas, no more than 10% of children have hypertension (HOLLAND et al. 1980). Approximately 80% of patients with neuroblastoma excrete excess catecho-

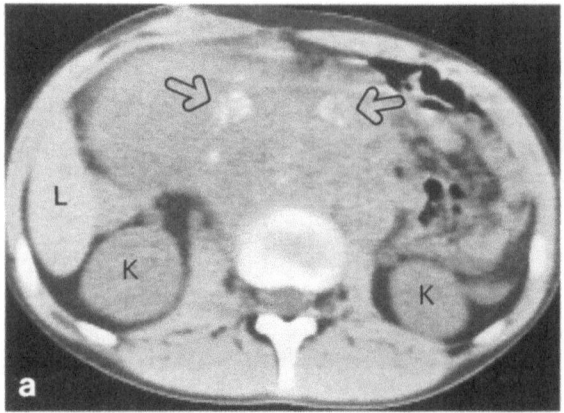

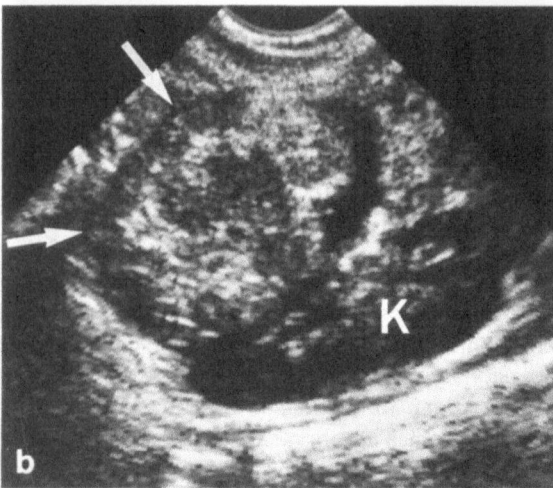

Fig. 1.26 a, b. Neuroblastoma. **a** CT scan demonstrating a large abdominal mass containing typical rim calcifications *(arrow)* in a 12-year-old girl. **b** Ultrasonogram showing a left-sided neuroblastoma with heterogeneous echoes *(arrow)* in a 10-year-old boy. *K*, kidney

lamine metabolites in urine. Increased excretion of these metabolites indicates the presence of a neural crest neoplasm.

With CT, the diagnosis of neuroblastoma can be established even when the lesion is relatively small. The tumor is recognized as an irregular adrenal soft tissue mass. On precontrast scans, the mass usually has a density lower than that of surrounding soft tissues; intravenous contrast medium accentuates this difference. The vast majority of the larger lesions have an inhomogeneous attenuation appearance. Calcifications, usually dense, amorphous, and mottled in appearance, are common (79%) (BOUSVAROS et al. 1986); rim calcifications are most specific and were found by STARK et al. (1983a) in 29% of 38 cases (Fig. 1.26a). Differentiation from Wilms' tumor may sometimes be impossible. CT provides information about tumor extent, including relation-

ships to the great vessels, liver involvement, and intraspinal extension. In addition, CT has been reported to be a most sensitive imaging test (85%) for tumor recurrence (STARK et al. 1983b).

Sonographically, the neuroblastoma is predominately echogenic, being more echogenic than liver parenchyma. Some lesions are relatively homogeneous and others extremely heterogeneous (Fig. 1.26b); calcification may be detected with ultrasound, and cystic zones are rather rare. In the majority of cases of neuroblastoma the margins of the tumor are poorly defined, although in the less malignant forms (i. e., ganglioneuroblastoma) they may be more clearly delineated (BUNN and KING 1961). In the classic case of neuroblastoma arising from the adrenal gland, sonography readily demonstrates the relationship of the tumor to the kidney and its typical downward and outward displacement. Occasionally, neuroblastoma is markedly hypoechoic. The primary tumor or hepatic metastases may even appear cystic with lack of internal echoes, sharp posterior wall margins, and increased through-transmission. In children, the presence of a suprarenal mass with hepatic lesions, regardless of their echogenicity, should strongly suggest the diagnosis of neuroblastoma.

Like CT, MRI may accurately detect and stage neuroblastoma (DIETRICH et al. 1987). On T1-weighted images, neuroblastomas have the same signal intensity as the renal medulla and slightly lower signal intensity than the renal cortex and liver; on T2-weighted images, neuroblastomas show increases in signal intensity, the intensity being higher than that of the liver but similar to that of the kidney (Table 1.2) (DIETRICH et al. 1987; FALKE et al. 1987). The main advantage of MRI as compared to CT is that imaging is possible in several planes, which may facilitate evaluation of tumor resectability. In addition, bone marrow involvement may be detected. However, calcifications, which are important clues to the diagnosis, are not seen on MRI.

Scintigraphy using ^{131}I-MIBG has proved to be highly sensitive for detecting neuroblastoma, its sensitivity being nearly 100% for primary neuroblastoma. For metastases, the specificity of ^{131}I-MIBG is 80% (HIBI et al. 1987).

Diagnostic Workup. Ultrasonography is the screening modality of choice for neonatal or pediatric abdominal masses. If a mass suspicious of a tumor is discovered, a further workup by CT is almost always necessary. CT will show tumor extent and invasion of other organs to better advantage, and this is especially true for extension of extradural or intradural structures and for detection of retroperitoneal and retrocrural lymph nodes. MRI possibly provides some additional information on tumor resectability. Scintigraphy with ^{131}I-MIBG is not the method of choice for detecting the primary tumor but is essential in the initial staging of any patient with neuroblastoma. Skeletal scintigraphy is currently the most sensitive imaging method for detecting skeletal metastases. Bone marrow aspiration and biopsy combined with skeletal scintigraphy will detect over 95% of patients with metastatic disease (BOUSVAROS et al. 1986).

1.5 Conclusion

Adrenal lesions may be clinically silent and found incidentally or may be clinically symptomatic. The history of a previous or existing primary tumor and physical examination are essential in making the diagnosis. Patients should be evaluated for evidence of endocrine activity because this changes the diagnostic strategy and requires additional biochemical evaluation or functional imaging tests. Some adrenal lesions may be classified on the basis of morphologic characteristics alone; others remain indeterminate without additional information. In approaching adrenal lesions there are some important questions: Does the patient have clinical or biochemical evidence of endocrine disease? Is the adrenal lesion an incidental finding? Has the patient clinical symptoms of malignancy or is there a known primary malignant tumor elsewhere? Is there evidence of infectious disease?

Large primary adrenal tumors, where surgery is indicated, usually do not present a diagnostic problem. Small adrenal masses incidentally found in tumor patients (without evidence of metastases elsewhere) and patients without known primary malignancy are more difficult to assess. CT permits morphologic differentiation of these lesions to a certain degree. If the nature of the tumor remains indeterminate. MRI is performed to distinguish between silent adenoma and metastasis. In equivocal cases, percutaneous biopsy may also be performed following CT scan or after MRI evaluation. If a small mass on CT scan is most likely an adenoma in a patient without known malignancy, expectative management and follow-up CT after 3–4 months are acceptable instead of percutaneous biopsy, which may be used alternatively.

References

Abecassis M, McLoughlin MJ, Langer B, Kudlow JE (1985) Serendipitous adrenal masses: prevalence, significance and management. Am J Surg 149: 783–788

Abeshouse GA, Goldstein RB, Abeshouse BS (1959) Adrenal cysts: review of literature and report of three cases. J Urol 81: 711

Abrams HL, Siegelman SS, Adams DF, Sanders R, Finberg HJ, Hessel SJ, McNeill BJ (1982) Computed tomography versus ultrasound of the adrenal gland: a prospective study. Radiology 143: 121–128

Andresen J, Madsen B, Steenskov V (1981) Radiological and clinical evaluation of twenty neuroblastomas. Clin Radiol 32: 191

Atkinson GO, Kodroff MB, Gay BB Jr, Ricketts RR (1985) Adrenal abscess in the neonate. Radiology 155: 101–104

Baker ME, Spritzer C, Blinder R, Herfkens RJ, Leight GS, Dunnick NR (1987) Benign adrenal lesions mimicking malignancy on MR imaging: report of two cases. Radiology 163: 669–671

Baker DE, Glazer GM, Francis IR (1988) Adrenal magnetic resonance imaging in Addison's disease. Urol Radiol 9: 199–203

Baker ME, Blinder R, Spritzer C et al. (1989) MR evaluation of adrenal masses at 1.5 T. AJR 153: 307–312

Barnett I (1942) Hydatid cysts: their location in the various organs and tissues of the body. Aust NZ J Surg 12: 240

Behan M, Martin EC, Muecke EC, Kazam E (1977) Myelolipoma of the adrenal: two cases with ultrasound and CT findings. AJR 129: 993–996

Belldegrun A, Hussain S, Seltzer SE, Loughlin KR, Gittes RF, Richie JP (1986) Incidentally discovered mass of the adrenal gland. Surg Gynecol Obstet 163: 203–208

Berdon WE (1990) Diseases of the adrenal in infancy and childhood. In: Pollack HM (ed) Clinical urography, vol III. Saunders, Philadelphia, pp 2362–2375

Berger MS, Edwards MS, Wara WM, Levin VA, Wilson CB (1983) Primary cerebral neuroblastoma. J Neurosurg 59: 418

Berland LL, Koslin DB, Kenney PJ, Stanley RJ, Lee JY (1988) Differentiation between small benign and malignant adrenal masses with dynamic incremented CT. AJR 95–101

Berliner L, Bosniak MA, Megibow A (1982) Adrenal pseudotumors on computed tomography. J Comp Assist Tomogr 6: 281–285

Bernardino ME, Walther MM, Phillips VM et al. (1985) CT-guided adrenal biopsy: accuracy, safety, and indications. AJR 144: 67–69

Bohndorf K, Günther RW, Vorwerk D et al. (1988) Lokalisation hypophysärer, ACTH-produzierender Mikroadenome mittels bilateraler und simultaner Katheterisierung des Sinus petrosus inferior. Fortschr Röntgenstr 148: 275–278

Bousvaros A, Kirks DR, Grossman (1986) Imaging of neuroblastoma: an overview. Pediatr Radiol 16: 89–106

Bryan PJ, Calbamone AA, Morrison SC et al. (1988) Ultrasound findings in the adreno-genital syndrome (congenital adrenal hyperplasia). J Ultrasound Med 7: 675–680

Bunn ND Jr, King AB (1961) Cervical ganglioneuroma. A case report and review of the literature. Guthrie Clin Bull 30: 5–14

Bush WH, Elder JS, Crane RE, Wales LR (1985) Cystic pheochromocytoma. Urology 25: 332–334

Chang A, Glazer HS, Lee JKT, Ling D, Heiken JP (1987) Adrenal gland: MR imaging. Radiology 163: 123–128

Chezmar JL, Robbins SM, Nelson RC, Steinberg HV, Torres WE, Bernardino ME (1988) Adrenal masses: characterization with T1-weighted MR imaging. Radiology 166: 357–359

Christenson R, Smith CW, Burko H (1976) Arteriographic manifestations of pheochromocytoma. AJR 126: 567–575

Cohen EK, Daneman A, Stringer DA, Soto G, Throner P (1986) Focal adrenal hemorrhage: a new US appearance. Radiology 161: 631–633

Conn JW, Cohen EL, Herwing KR (1976) The dexamethasone-modified adrenal scintiscan in hyporeninemic aldosteronism (tumor vs. hyperplasia). A comparison with adrenal venography and adrenal venous aldosterone. J Lab Clin Med 88: 841

Cordes K, Georgi M, Günther R, Beyer J (1979) Adrenale und extraadrenale Phäochromocytome. Dtsch Med Wochenschr 104: 317–323

Daneman A (1987) Pediatric body CT. Springer, London Berlin Heidelberg New York, p 134

Daneman A, Chan HSL, Martin J (1983) Adrenal carcinoma and adenoma in children: a review of 17 patients. Pediatr Radiol 13: 11–18

Davidson AJ, Hartmann DS, Goldman SM (1989) Mature teratoma of the retroperitoneum: radiologic, pathologic and clinical correlation. Radiology 172: 421

Davies RP, Lam AH (1987) Adrenocortical neoplasm in children: ultrasound appearance. J Ultrasound Med 6: 325–331

Davis PL, Hricak H, Bradley WG Jr (1984) Magnetic resonance imaging of the adrenal glands. Radiol Clin North Am 22: 891–895

Derchi LE, Rapaccini GL, Banderali A et al. (1989) Ultrasound and CT findings in 2 cases of hemangioma of the adrenal gland. J Comput Assist Tomogr 13: 659–662

Dietrich RB, Kangarloo H, Lenarsky C, Feig SA (1987) Neuroblastoma: the role of MR imaging. AJR 148: 937–942

Doppman JL, Oldfield E, Krudy AG et al. (1984) Petrosal sinus sampling for Cushing syndrome: anatomical and technical considerations. Radiology 150: 99–103

Doppman JL, Reinig JW, Dwyer AJ et al. (1987) Differentiation of adrenal masses by magnetic resonance imaging. Surgery 102: 1018–1025

Doppman JL, Miller DL, Dwyer AJ et al. (1988) Macronodular adrenal hyperplasia in Cushing disease. Radiology 347–352

Doppman JL, Travis WD, Nieman L et al. (1989) Cushing syndrome due to primary pigmented nodular adrenocortical disease: findings at CT and MR imaging. Radiology 172: 415–420

Dunnick NR, Castellino RA (1975) Arteriographic manifestations of ganglioneuromas. Radiology 15: 323–328

Dunnick NR, Doppman JL, Mills SR, Gill JR Jr (1979) Preoperative diagnosis and localization of aldosteronomas by measurement of corticosteroids in adrenal venous blood. Radiology 133: 331–333

Dunnick NR, Doppman JL, Gill JR et al. (1982a) Localization of functional adrenal tumors by computed tomography and venous sampling. Radiology 142: 429–433

Dunnick NR, Heaston D, Halvorsen R, Moore AV, Korobkin M (1982b) CT appearance of adrenal cortical carcinoma. J Comput Assist Tomogr 6: 987–982

Eagen RT, Page MI (1971) Adrenal insufficiency following bilateral adrenal venography. JAMA 215: 115–116

Eklöf O, Grotte G, Jorulf H et al. (1975) Perinatal hemorrhagic necrosis of the adrenal gland. A clinical and radiologic evaluation of 24 consecutive cases. Pediatr Radiol 4: 31

El Sherief MA, Hemmingsson A, Loerelius L-E (1983) Computed tomography and angiography in the evaluation of adrenal diseases. Acta Radiol [Diagn] (Stockh) 23: 625–637

Exelby PR (1981) Retroperitoneal malignant tumors. Wilms' tumor and neuroblastoma. Surg Clin North Am 61: 1219

Falke THM, teStrake L, Shaff MI et al. (1986) MR imaging of the adrenals: correlation with computed tomography. J Comput Assist Tomogr 10: 242–253

Falke THM, teStrake L, Sandler MP et al. (1987) Magnetic resonance imaging of the adrenal glands. Radiographics 7: 343–370

Feldberg MAM, Hendriks MJ, Klinkhamer AC (1986) Massive bilateral non-Hodgkin's lymphomas of the adrenals. Urol Radiol 8: 85–88

Fink DW, Wurtzebach LR (1980) Symptomatic myelolipoma of the adrenal. Radiology 134: 451–452

Fishman EK, Deutch BM, Hartman DS, Goldman SM, Zerhouni EA, Siegelman SS (1987) Primary adrenocortical carcinoma: CT evaluation with clinical correlation. AJR 148: 531–535

Flattet A, Hedinger C (1980) La morphologie de la corticosurrénale dans le syndrome de Cushing. Schweiz Med Wochenschr 110: 1300–1306

Foster DG (1966) Adrenal cysts. Arch Surg 92: 131–143

Francis IR, Glazer GM, Shapiro B, Sisson JC, Gross BH (1983) Complementary roles of CT and ^{131}I-MIBG scintigraphy in diagnosing pheochromocytoma. AJR 141: 719–725

Freitas JE, Grekin RJ, Thrall JH, Gross MD, Swanson DP, Beierwaltes WH (1979) Adrenal imaging with iodomethylnorcholesterol (I-131) in primary aldosteronism. J Nucl Med 20: 7–10

Friedman AC, Hartman DS, Sherman J, Lautin EM, Goldman N (1981) Computed tomography of abdominal fatty masses. Radiology 139: 415–429

Fries JG, Chamberlin JA (1968) Extra-adrenal pheochromocytoma: literature review and report of a cervical pheochromocytoma. Surgery 63: 268–279

Geisinger MA, Zelch MG, Bravo EL, O'Donovan PB, Borkowski GP (1983) Primary hyperaldosteronism: comparison of CT, adrenal venography, and venous sampling. AJR 141: 299–302

Georgi M, Günther R, Weigand H (1975) Technique and results of adrenal phlebography. Radiologe 15: 279

Georgi M, Cordes U, Günther R et al. (1978) Phlebographische Diagnostik des Phäochromozytoms. Fortschr Röntgenstr 128: 727–735

Glazer HS, Weyman PJ, Sagel SS, Levitt RG, McClennan BL (1982) Nonfunctioning adrenal masses: incidental discovery on computed tomography. AJR 139: 81–85

Glazer HS, Lee JKT, Balfe DM, Mauro MA, Griffith R, Sagel SS (1983) Non-Hodgkin lymphoma: computed tomographic demonstration of unusual extranodal involvement. Radiology 149: 211–217

Glazer GM, Woodsey EJ, Borello J et al. (1986) Adrenal tissue characterization using MR imaging. Radiology 158: 73–79

Glazer GM, Francis IR, Quint LE (1988) Imaging of the adrenal glands. Invest Radiol 23: 3–11

Groll A, Schneider M, Althoff PH et al. (1990) Morphologische und klinische Bedeutung pathologischer Veränderungen an Nebenniere und Hypophyse bei AIDS. Dtsch Med Wochenschr 115: 483–488

Gross MD, Shapiro B (1990) Scintigraphic localization of adrenal disease. In: Pollack HM (ed) Clinical urography, vol III. Saunders, Philadelphia, pp 2376–2387

Gross MD, Valk TW, Freitas JE, Swanson DP, Schteingart DE, Beierwaltes WH (1981) The relationship of adrenal iodomethylnorcholesterol uptake to indices of adrenal cortical function in Cushing's syndrome. J Clin Endocrinol Metab 52: 1062

Gross MD, Wilton GP, Shapiro B et al. (1987) Functional and scintigraphic evaluation of the silent adrenal mass. J Nucl Med 28: 1401-1407

Günther R, Kelbel C, Beyer J (1984a) Technik der real-time-Ultraschalluntersuchung von Nebenniere und Nebennierentumoren. Fortschr Röntgenstr 141: 292-296

Günther R, Kelbel C, Lenner V (1984b) Real-time ultrasound of normal adrenal gland and small tumors. J Clin Ultrasound 12: 211-217

Günther RW, Müller-Leisse C (1989) Assessment of adrenal lesions by imaging studies. In: Lang EK (ed) Problems in urology. Lippincott, Philadelphia, pp 582-606

Haertel M, Probst P, Bollmann J, Zingg E, Fuchs WA (1980) Computertomographische Nebennierendiagnostik. Fortschr Röntgenstr 132: 31-36

Hamper UM, Fishman EK, Hartman DS, Roberts JL, Sanders RC (1987) Primary adrenocortical carcinoma: sonographic evaluation with clinical and pathologic correlation in 26 patients. AJR 148: 915-919

Hattery RR, Sheedy PF II, van Heerden JA (1981) Computed tomography of the adrenal gland. Semin Roentgenol 16: 290-300

Hauser H, Gurret JP (1986) Miliary tuberculosis associated with adrenal enlargement: CT appearance. J Comput Assist Tomogr 10: 254-256

Hayes FA, Green AA (1983) Neuroblastoma. Pediatr Ann 12: 366

Henley DJ, Van Heerden JA, Grant CS, Carney JA, Carpenter PC (1983) Adrenal cortical carcinoma - a continuing challenge. Surgery 94: 926-931

Hibi S, Todo S, Imashuku S, Miyazaki T (1987) ^{131}I-Meta-iodobenzylguanidine scintigraphy in patients with neuroblastoma. Pediatr Radiol 17: 308-313

Hill SC, Hoeg JM, Dwyer AJ, Vucich JJ, Doppman JL (1983) CT findings in acid lipase deficiency; Wolman disease and cholesteryl ester storage disease. J Comput Assist Tomogr 5: 815-818

Hochhauser L, Louis E St, Gray R et al. (1982) Myelolipom der Nebenniere in der Ganzkörper-Computer-Tomographie. Radiologe 22: 423-428

Hogan MJ, McRae J, Schambelan M et al. (1976) Location of aldosterone-producing adenomas with [131]I-19-iodocholesterol. N Engl J Med 294: 410

Holland T, Donohue JP, Baehner RL, Grosfeld JL (1980) The current management of neuroblastoma. J Urol 124: 579

Horton R, Finck E (1972) Diagnosis and localization in primary aldosteronism. Ann Intern Med 76: 885-890

Hübener K-H, Treugut H (1984) Adrenal dysfunction: CT findings. Radiology 150: 195-199

Hume DM (1960) Pheochromocytoma in the adult and in the child. Am J Surg 99: 458-496

Hussain S, Belldegrun A, Seltzer SE, Richie JP, Gittes RF, Abrams HL (1985) Differentiating of malignant from benign adrenal masses: predictive indices on computed tomography. AJR 144: 61-65

Hyrtl J (1887) Lehrbuch der Anatomie des Menschen, 19th edn. Vienna, p 774

Ikeda D, Francis IR, Glazer GM (1989) The detection of adrenal tumors and hyperplasia in patients with primary aldosteronism: comparison of scintigraphy, CT and MR imaging. AJR 153: 301-306

Ishimura J, Kawanaka M, Fukuchi M (1989) Clinical application of SPECT in adrenal imaging with iodine 131, 6 beta, iodomethyl-19, norcholesterol. Clin Nucl Med 14: 278-282

Jafri SZH, Francis IR, Glazer GM, Bree RL, Amendola MA (1983) CT detection of adrenal lymphoma. J Comput Assist Tomogr 7: 254-256

Kadir S, Robertson D, Coulam CM (1981) Pitfalls in the diagnosis of extraadrenal pheochromocytoma. Cardiovasc Intervent Radiol 4: 99-104

Kahn PC, Kelleter D, Egdahl RH, Melby JC (1971) Adrenal arteriography and venography in primary aldosteronism. Radiology 101: 71-78

Kajanti M (1983) Neuroblastoma in 88 children. Ann Clin Res 15 [Suppl 39]: 1

Kangarloo H, Diament MJ, Gold RH et al. (1986) Sonography of adrenal glands in neonates and children: changes in appearance with age. J Clin Ultrasound 14: 43-47

Kearney GP, Mahoney EM, Maher E, Harrison JH (1977) Functioning and nonfunctioning cysts of the adrenal cortex and medulla. Am J Surg 134: 363-368

Kenney PJ, Stanley RJ (1987) Calcified adrenal masses. Urol Radiol 9: 9-15

Kier R, McCarthy S (1989) MR characterization of adrenal masses: field strength and pulse sequence considerations. Radiology 171: 671-674

King KR, Lack EE (1979) Adrenal cortical carcinoma. A clinical and pathologic study of 49 cases. Cancer 44: 239-244

Klose KC, Günther RW (1988) CT-gesteuerte Punktionen. In: Günther R, Thelen M (ed) Interventionelle Radiologie. Thieme, Stuttgart, pp 474-475

Koch KJ, Corry DA (1986) Simultaneous renal vein thrombosis and adrenal hemorrhage: MR demonstration. J Comp Assist Tomogr 10: 681

Koenker RM, Mueller PR, van Sonnenberg E (1988) Interventional radiology of the adrenal gland. Semin Roentgenol 23: 314-322

Korobkin M, White EA, Kressel HY, Moss AA, Montagne JP (1979) Computed tomography in the diagnosis of adrenal disease. AJR 132: 231-235

Krestin GP, Steinbrich W, Friedmann G (1989) Adrenal masses: evaluation with fast gradient-echo MR imaging and GD-DTPA-enhanced dynamic studies. Radiology 171: 675-680

Lamprecht W, Kortmann K-B (1983) Incidence and significance of accessory adrenal tissue in the inguinal region of children (in German). Chirurg 54: 39-41

Leroy-Willig A, Bittoun J, Luton JP, Louvel A, Lefevre JE, Bonnin A, Roucayrol JC (1989) In vivo MR spectroscopy imaging of the adrenal glands: distinction between adenomas and carcinomas larger than 15 mm based on lipid content. AJR 153: 771-773

Lewis E, Kurtz AB, Dubbins PA, Wapner RJ, Goldberg BB (1982) Real-time ultrasonographic evaluation of normal fetal adrenal glands. J Ultrasound Med 1: 265-270

Liebmann R, Strikantaswamy S (1981) Adrenal myelolipoma demonstrated by computed tomography. J Comput Assist Tomogr 5: 262-263

Ling D, Korobkin M, Silverman PM, Dunnick NR (1983) CT demonstration of bilateral adrenal hemorrhage. AJR 141: 307-308

Lynn MD, Shapiro B, Sisson JC et al. (1984) Portrayal of pheochromocytoma and normal human adrenal medulla by m-[123]Iodobenzylguanidine: concise communication. J Nucl Med 25: 436-440

Marcovitz S, Wee C, Chan J, Haroy J (1987) The diagnostic accuracy of preoperative CT scanning in the evaluation of pituitary ACTH-secreting adenomas. AJNR 8: 641–644

Mathieu E, Despres E, Delepine N et al. (1987) MR imaging of the adrenal gland in Sipple disease. J Comput Assist Tomogr 11: 790–793

McCorkell SJ, Niles NL (1985) Fine-needle aspiration of catecholamne-producing adrenal masses: a possible fatal mistake. AJR 145: 113–114

McGahan JP (1988) Adrenal gland: MR imaging. Radiology 166: 284–289

McMillan A, Horwich A (1987) Case report: malignant teratoma presenting with an adrenal mass. Clin Radiol 38: 327–328

Miles JM, Wahner HW, Carpenter PC, Salassa RM, Northcutt RC (1979) Adrenal scintiscanning with NP-59: a new radioiodinated cholesterol agent. Mayo Clin Proc 54: 321

Mitnick JS, Bosniak MA, Megibow AJ, Naidich DP (1983) Non-functioning adrenal adenomas discovered incidentally on computed tomography. Radiology 148: 495–499

Mitty HA, Yeh H-C (1982) Radiology of the adrenals with sonography and CT. Saunders, Philadelphia

Miyake H, Maeda H, Tashiro M et al. (1989) CT of adrenal tumors: frequency and clinical significance of low-attenuation lesions. AJR 152: 1005–1007

Montagne J-P, Kressel HY, Korobkin M, Moss AA (1978) Computed tomography of the normal adrenal glands. AJR 130: 963–966

Moon KL, Hricak H, Crooks LE et al. (1983) Nuclear magnetic resonance imaging of the adrenal gland: a preliminary report. Radiology 147: 155–160

Murphy BJ, Casillas J, Yrizarry JM (1988) Traumatic adrenal hemorrhage: radiologic findings. Radiology 169: 701–703

Musante F, Derchi LE, Zappasodi F et al. (1988) Myelolipoma of the adrenal gland: sonographic and CT features. AJR 151: 961–967

Noble MJ, Montague DK, Levin HS (1982) Myelolipoma: an unusual surgical lesion of the adrenal gland. Cancer 49: 952–958

O'Brien WM, Choyke PL, Copeland J, Klappenbach RS, Lynch JH (1987) Computed tomograhy of adrenal abscess. J Comput Assist Tomogr 11: 779–783

Oldfield EH, Chrousos GP, Schulte HM, Loriaux DL, Schaaf M, Doppman J (1985) Preoperative localization of ACTH-secreting microadenomas by bilateral and simultaneous inferior petrosal sinus sampling. N Engl J Med 312: 100–107

Oliver TW JR, Bernardino ME, Miller JL, Mansour K, Greene D, Davis WA (1984) Isolated adrenal masses in nonsmall-cell bronchogenic carcinoma. Radiology 153: 217–218

Olsson CA, Krane RJ, Klugo RG, Selikowitz SM (1973) Adrenal myelolipoma. Surgery 73: 665–670

Oppenheimer DA, Carroll BA, Yousem S (1983) Sonography of the normal neonatal adrenal gland. Radiology 146: 157–160

Paling MR, Williamson BRJ (1983) Adrenal involvement in non-Hodgkin lymphoma. AJR 141: 303–305

Peck WW, Dillon WP, Dorman D, Newton TH, Wilson CB (1989) High resolution MR imaging of pituitary microadenomas at 1.5 T: experience with Cushing disease. AJR 152: 145–151

Peterson RO (1987) Urologic pathology. Lippincott, Philadelphia

Plaut A (1958) Myelolipoma in the adrenal cortex. Am J Pathol 34: 487–507

Pojunas KW, Daniels DL, Williams AL, Throsen MK, Haughton VM (1986) Pituitary and adrenal CT of Cushing syndrome. AJR 146: 1235–1238

Powell S, Henry WR, Peckham MJ (1983) Occult germ cell testicular tumours. Br J Urology 55: 440–444

Quint LE, Glazer GM, Francis IR, Spapiro B, Chenevert TL (1987) Pheochromocytoma and paraganglioma: comparison of MR imaging with CT and I-131 MIBG scintigraphy. Radiology 165: 89–93

Reichert CM, O'Leary TJ, Levens DL, Simrell CR, Macher AM (1983) Autopsy pathology in the acquired immunodeficiency syndrome. Am J Pathol 112: 357

Reinig JW, Doppman JL, Dwyer AJ, Frank J (1986) MRI of indeterminate adrenal masses. AJR 147: 493–496

Remer EM, Weinfeld RM, Glazer GM, Quint LE, Francis IR, Gross MD, Bookstein FL (1989) Hyperfunctioning and nonhyperfunctioning benign adrenal cortical lesions: characterization and comparison with MR imaging. Radiology 171: 681–685

Reuter SR, Blair AJ, Schteingart DE, Brokstein JJ (1967) Adrenal venography. Radiology 89: 805

Richie JP, Gittes RF (1980) Carcinoma of the adrenal cortex. Cancer 45: 1957–1964

Rosenberg ER, Bowie JD, Andreotti RF, Fields SI (1982) Sonographic evaluation of fetal adrenal glands. AJR 139: 1145–1147

Rothberg M, Bastidas J, Mathey WE, Bernas E (1978) Adrenal hemangiomas. Angiographic appearance of a rare tumor. Radiology 126: 341–344

Sample WF (1978) Adrenal ultrasonography. Radiology 127: 461–466

Sawczuk IS, Reitelman C, Libby C et al. (1986) CT findings in Addison's disease caused by tuberculosis. Urol Radiol 8: 44–45

Scully RE, Mark EJ, McNeely BU (1984) Hypertension and an adrenal mass after a vehicular accident. Case 38, case records of the Massachusetts General Hospital: weekly clinicopathological exercises. N Engl J Med 311: 783–790

Seddon JM, Baranetzsky N, VanBoxel PJ (1985) Adrenal "incidentalomas". Urology 25: 1–3

Seidenwurm DJ, Elmer EB, Kaplan LM et al. (1984) Metastases to the adrenal glands and the development of Addison's disease. Cancer 54: 552–557

Shah HR, Love L, Williamson MR et al. (1989) Hemorrhagic adrenal metastases: CT findings. J Comput Assist Tomogr 13: 77–82

Shapiro B, Britton KE, Hawkins LA, Edwards CRW (1981) Clinical experience with 75-Se-selenomethylnorchesterol adrenal imaging. Clin Endocrinol 15: 19

Shapiro B, Sisson JC, Lloyd R, Satterlee W, Beierwaltes WH (1984) Malignant pheochromocytoma. Clinical, biochemical and scintigraphic characterization. Clin Endocrinol 20: 189

Shapiro B, Copp JE, Sisson JC, Eyre PL, Wallis J, Beierwaltes WH (1985) Iodine-131 metaiodobenzylguanidine for the locating of suspected pheochromocytoma: experience in 400 cases. J Nucl Med 26: 76–585

Sisson JC, Shapiro B, Beierwaltes WH et al. (1984) Radiopharmaceutical treatment of malignant pheochromocytoma. J Nucl Med 25: 197

Smith SM, Patel SK, Turner DA et al. (1989) Magnetic resonance imaging of adreno-cortical carcinoma. Urol Radiol 11: 1–6

Sörensen R, Moltz L (1981) Diagnostik bei progredientem Hirsutismus. Kathetertechnik und Ergebnisse. Fortschr Röntgenstr 135: 257–266

Stark DD, Moss AA, Brasch RC, deLorimier AA, Albin AR, London DA, Gooding CA (1983a) Neuroblastoma: diagnostic imaging and staging. Radiology 148: 101-105

Stark DD, Brasch RC, Moss AA et al. (1983b) Recurrent neuroblastoma: the role of CT and alternative imaging tests. Radiology 148: 107-112

Sty JR (1984) Neuroblastoma. In: Sty JR, Hernandez R, Starshak RJ (ed) Body imaging in pediatrics. Grune and Stratton, New York, pp 175-184

Swenson SJ, Brown ML, Sheps SG et al. (1984) Use of ^{131}I-MIBG scintigraphy in the evaluation of suspected pheochromocytoma. Mayo Clin Proc 60: 299

Symington T (1982) The adrenal cortex. In: Bloodworth JMB Jr (ed) Endocrine pathology: general and surgical. Williams & Wilkins, Baltimore

Tapper ML, Rotterdam H, Lerner CW, Al'Khafaji K, Seitzman PA (1984) Adrenal necrosis in the acquired immunodeficiency syndrome. Ann Intern Med 100: 239

Tobes MC, Jacques S, Wieland DM et al. (1985) Effect of uptake-one inhibitors on the uptake of norepinephrine and metaiodobenzylguanidine. J Nucl Med 26: 897-907

Tung GA, Pfister RC, Papanicolaou M, Yoder IC (1989) Adrenal cyst: imaging and percutaneous aspiration. Radiology 173: 107-111

Velchik MG, Alavi A, Kressel HY et al. (1989) Localization of pheochromocytoma: MICG, CT and MRI correlation. J Nucl Med 20: 328-333

Vergas AD (1980) Adrenal hemangioma. Urology 16: 389-390

Vick CW, Zeman RK, Mannes E, Cronan JJ, Walsh JW (1984) Adrenal myelolipoma: CT and ultrasound findings. Urol Radiol 6: 7-13

Vicks BS, Perusek M, Johnson J, Tio F (1987) Primary adrenal lymphoma: CT and sonographic appearances. J Clin Ultrasound 15: 135-139

Vita JA, Silverberg SJ, Goland RS et al. (1985) Clinical clues to the cause of Addison's disease. Am J Med 78: 461-466

von Gierke E (1905) Über Knochenmarksgewebe in der Nebenniere. Zieglers Beitr Pathol Anat [Suppl] 7: 311

Weinberger MH, Grim CE, Hollifield JW et al. (1979) Primary aldosteronism. Ann Int Med 90: 386-395

Welch FJ, Sheedy PF, van Heerden JA et al. (1983) Pheochromocytoma: value of computed tomography. Radiology 148: 501-503

Welch TJ, Sheedy PF, Johnson CD et al. (1989) CT-guided biopsy: prospective analysis of 1000 procedures. Radiology 171: 493-496

Willemse APP, Coppes MJ, Feltberg AMM et al. (1989) Magnetic resonance appearance of adrenal hemorrhage in a neonate. Pediatr Radiol 19: 210-214

Wilms GE, Baert AL, Kint EJ, Pringot JH, Goddeeris PG (1983) Computed tomographic findings in bilateral adrenal tuberculosis. Radiology 146: 729-730

Wilms GE, Marchal TJF, Baert AL et al. (1987) CT and ultrasound features of post-traumatic adrenal hemorrhage. J Comput Assist Tomogr 11: 112-119

Wilson DA, Muchmore HG, Tisdal RG, Fahmy A, Pitha JV (1984) Histoplasmosis of the adrenal glands studied by CT. Radiology 150: 779-783

Wolman M, Sterk VV, Gatt S, Frenkel M (1961) Primary fatal xantomatosis with involvement and calcification of the adrenal. Pediatrics 28: 742

Yamakita N, Yasuda K, Goshima E et al. (1976) Comparative assessment of ultrasonography and computed tomography in adrenal disorders. Ultrasound Med Biol 12: 23-29

Yeh H (1980) Sonography of the adrenal glands and small masses AJR 135: 1167-1177

Zaitoon MM, Mackie GG (1983) Adrenal cortical tumors in children: a review of 17 patients. Pediatr Radiol 13: 11-18

Zelch JV, Meaney TF, Belhobek GH (1974) Radiologic approach to the patient with suspected pheochromocytoma. Radiology 111: 279-284

2 Renal Developmental Anomalies

FELIX WANG and RICHARD M. FRIEDENBERG

CONTENTS

2.1   Renal Embryology and Development 33
2.2   Quantitative Anomalies 34
2.2.1   Renal Agenesis 34
2.2.2   Renal Hypoplasia 36
2.2.3   Supernumerary Kidney 37
2.3   Structural Anomalies
        of the Upper Collecting System 37
2.3.1   Duplex Kidneys 37
2.3.2   Extrarenal Pelvis 40
2.3.3   Calyceal Anomalies 40
2.4   Structural Anomalies of the Renal Parenchyma
        (Cystic or Solid Lesions) 43
2.4.1   Congenital Solitary Cysts 43
2.4.2   Multicystic Dysplastic Kidney 43
2.4.3   Multilocular Cystic Nephroma 45
2.4.4   Infantile Polycystic Kidney Disease ... 46
2.4.5   Adult Polycystic Kidney Disease 48
2.4.6   Medullary Sponge Kidney 50
2.4.7   Medullary Cystic Disease 50
2.4.8   Congenital Mesoblastic Nephroma 50
2.4.9   Ask-Upmark Kidney 52
2.5   Fusion Anomalies 53
2.5.1   Horseshoe Kidney 53
2.5.2   Lump Kidney 54
2.5.3   Crossed Ectopy 54
2.5.4   Renal Pseudotumors 58
2.6   Positional Anomalies 60
2.6.1   Ectopy and Ptosis 60
2.6.2   Malrotation 62
2.7   Extrarenal Anomalies 64
2.8   Congenital Hydronephrosis 66
        References 67

2.1 Renal Embryology and Development

The kidney has a complex origin and some familiarity with its development assists in understanding the numerous congenital disorders of the kidney. Two structures, the ureteric bud and the metanephric blastema, must develop and interact in a normal fashion to produce a normal kidney. The earliest precursor to the adult kidney appears at the end of the third gestational week, when a transient cellular condensation forms the *pronephros*. This tissue is nonfunctional and soon involutes.

The second stage of renal development is the *mesonephros*, which develops caudal to the degenerating pronephros. The mesonephric (wolffian) duct develops on the medial side of the nephrogenic cord and develops in a caudal direction towards the cloaca. The nephrogenic cord differentiates into nephrons adjacent to the formed mesonephric duct. However, as the more caudad nephrons form, the craniad nephrons and craniad portion of the duct involute. Eventually all the mesonephric glomeruli, most of the tubules, and most of the mesonephric duct itself degenerate. Remnants form portions of the male genital system and are inconstantly present in the female.

The final phase of renal development is the *metanephros*. This appears prior to the involution of the mesonephros. Two typical types are involved, the ureteric bud, which arises from the caudalmost mesonephric duct, and the metanephric blastema at the caudal end of the nephrogenic cord. The ureteric bud appears at 5 weeks' gestational age and grows and divides dichotomously to eventually form the ureter, renal pelvis, calyces, cribriform plate, and collecting tubules. Although the dividing is dichotomous, the branches may develop to very different degrees. The ureteric bud is necessary to induce nephron formation in the metanephric blastema and eventually communicates with the formed nephrons. If the ureteric bud fails to contact the metanephric blastema, no normal nephron differentiation occurs.

The variations in the number of generations branching in different areas are important in forming the shape of the adult kidney. More extensive ureteral branching occurs in the renal poles than in the mid-third of the kidney, and consequently there is more nephron induction and a thicker renal cortex in the polar regions than in the midportion. The individual calyces are formed when the ureteric bud that will form an infundibulum rapidly divides to form a fan-shaped group of branches. The base of this

FELIX WANG, M.D., Assistant Clinical Professor; RICHARD M. FRIEDENBERG, M.D., Professor and Chairman; Department of Radiological Sciences, University of California, Irvine Medical Center, 101 City Drive, Orange, CA 92668, USA

group gradually expands with urine to obliterate the divisions between branches. Simultaneously, the developing nephrons proliferate and the mass of collecting tubules and loops of Henle are forced into the calyceal space, resulting in a papilla within a cup-shaped calyx. Thus there is some overlap of tissue from the ureteric bud (collecting tubule and cortical rays) and tissue from the metanephric blastema (loops of Henle, connective tissue, and centrally placed nephrons) within the renal parenchyma.

The fetal renal lobes average 14 in number, and each is related to a single calyx. In the later stages of fetal development these lobes fuse, most completely in the renal poles to form compound calyces and compound papillae. The septal cortex that forms the sides of fetal lobes frequently disappears between fused lobes. Surface lobulation generally disappears completely. If the septal cortex remains prominent between lobes, it forms a "column of Bertin." Similarly, fetal lobulation may persist after birth as a normal variant.

The metanephros originates in the caudal portion of the embryo, with the lower poles closer than the upper poles and the renal pelves opening anteriorly. Growth of the caudal region leaves the kidneys behind, carrying them to their normal position. Abnormally, the lower poles move together, and they may fuse; if both renal masses move together they may fuse completely, with both pelves or a single fused pelvis opening generally anteriorly. These fused masses may lie in a renal fossa but are often in the pelvis or midline.

The urogenital system has more congenital anomalies than any other system in the body. Over one-third of all congenital anomalies affect the urinary tract. Many of these anomalies are associated with anomalies of other systems. There frequently is difficulty in differentiating between normal variations and congenital abnormalities. In this chapter, we will follow the outline listed below, divided into the major divisions of: numerical anomalies, structural anomalies of the collecting system, structural anomalies of the renal parenchyma, fusion anomalies, positional anomalies, and extrarenal anomalies.

    I. Quantitative anomalies
      A. Renal agenesis
      B. Renal hypoplasia
      C. Supernumerary kidney
   II. Structural anomalies of the upper collecting system
      A. Extracapsular
        1. Duplex kidney
          a) Complete ureteral duplication
          b) Partial ureteral duplication/bifid pelvis

        2. Extrarenal pelvis
      B. Intracapsular/calyceal
        1. Unicalyceal/bicalyceal kidney
        2. Abortive calyx
        3. Calyceal diverticulum
        4. Ectopic papilla
        5. Congenital megacalyces
 III. Structural anomalies of the renal parenchyma
      A. Cystic lesions
        1. Congenital solitary cyst
        2. Multicystic dysplastic kidney
        3. Multilocular cystic nephroma
        4. Infantile polycystic kidney disease
        5. Adult polycystic kidney disease
        6. Medullary sponge kidney
        7. Medullary cystic disease
      B. Solid lesions
        1. Mesoblastic nephroma
        2. Ask-Upmark kidney
 IV. Fusion anomalies
      A. Major fusion anomalies involving whole kidneys
        1. Horseshoe kidney
        2. Disk/lump kidney
        3. Crossed ectopy
      B. Minor fusion anomalies within one kidney
        1. Fetal lobation
        2. Infra/suprahilar calyces and dromedary hump
        3. Septum of Bertin
        4. Lobar dysmorphism
  V. Positional anomalies
      A. Ectopy and ptosis
      B. Malrotation
 VI. Vascular anomalies
      A. Accessory vessels
      B. Congenital aneurysms
      C. Congenital arteriovenous fistulas
VII. Congenital hydronephrosis

2.2 Quantitative Anomalies

2.2.1 Renal Agenesis

Renal agenesis can be defined as the complete failure of renal development as opposed to abnormal development (dysplasia) or incomplete development (hypoplasia). Bilateral renal agenesis is rare, being reported in 0.04% of autopsy series (male to female ratio, 3:1), and is incompatible with life. Multisystemic abnormalities are usually found in such cases. Since renal development depends on the existence of a ureteric bud and its normal interaction with the metanephric blastema, the failure of either

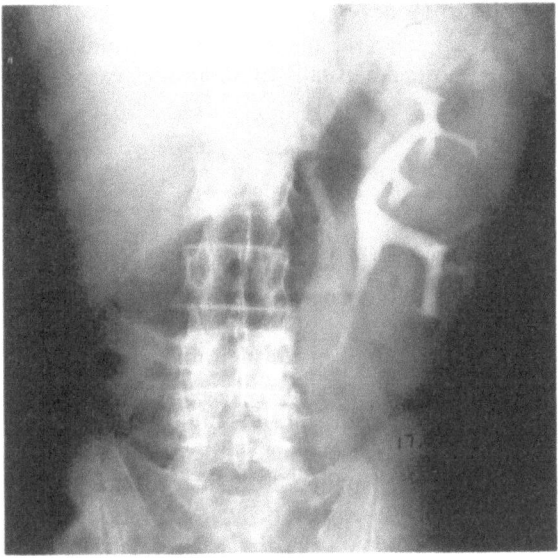

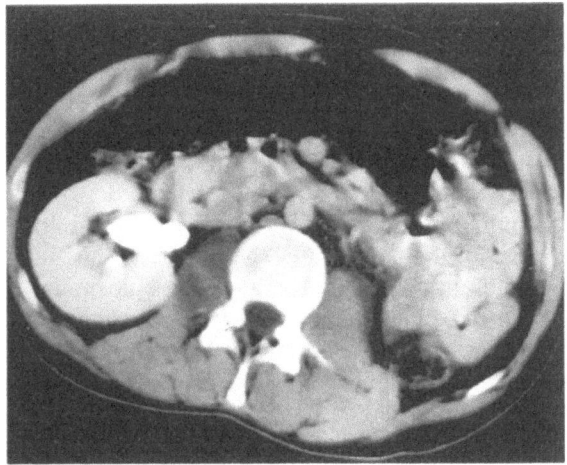

Fig. 2.2. Left renal agenesis and right renal compensatory hypertrophy. CT image at the level of the right renal pelvis with colon and small bowel in the left renal fossa

△

Fig. 2.1. Renal agenesis. There is absence of the right kidney and compensatory hypertrophy of the left kidney

Fig. 2.3 a, b. Renal agenesis and small bowel malrotation. **a** IVP showing absence of the right kidney and small bowel gas in the right renal fossa. **b** Small bowel follow-through confirming duodenal and jejunal malrotation into the right flank. (From NEY and FRIEDENBERG 1981)

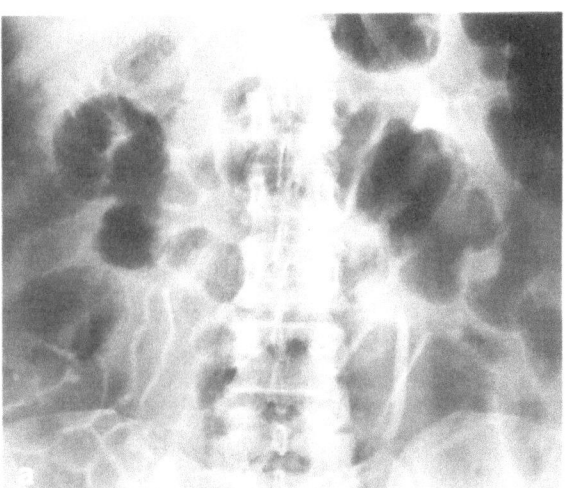

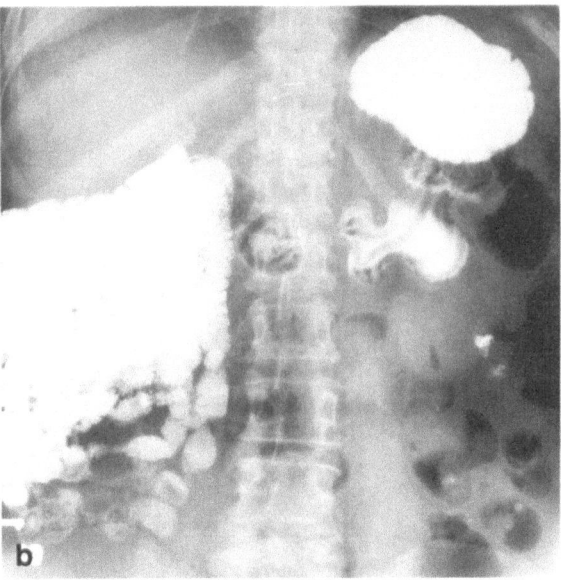

process may lead to renal agenesis. If the ureteric bud fails to develop, the kidney and ipsilateral ureter will be absent, and in over 50% of these cases the ipsilateral hemitrigone will be absent. The presence of an ectopic ureterovesical junction must be excluded before diagnosing renal agenesis. If the ureteric bud does not interact with the metanephric blastema, then a blind-ending ureteral stump may be found (approximately 10% of cases). Although the kidney is absent under these circumstances, the hemitrigone would be present, and therefore the absence of a visible ureteral orifice in the bladder is not conclusive evidence of renal agenesis (Figs. 2.1, 2.2).

Among associated anomalies, special mention should be made of vascular anomalies. In renal agenesis the ipsilateral renal artery is almost always absent. A detectable renal artery usually means some hypoplastic or dysplastic renal tissue exists. The same is not true of the renal veins. Since the left renal vein normally drains the left adrenal gland and the left gonad in addition to the left kidney, a small renal vein may be found in cases of renal agenesis due to these tributaries. However, selective phlebography of such a renal vein should show no traces of intrarenal branches. The right renal vein usually does not receive adrenal or gonadal branches and therefore is more often absent. The inability to catheterize the renal vein is not proof positive of its absence.

Other anomalies may exist related to the absence of a renal mass. In left renal agenesis, the splenic flexure may displace into the left renal fossa. If the right kidney is absent, the duodenum and proximal jejunum may relocate into the right renal fossa (Fig. 2.3). In 10% of cases the ipsilateral adrenal is also absent despite its separate embryonic origin.

The remaining solitary kidney usually shows compensatory hypertrophy and may approximate the mass of two kidneys by the end of the 2nd year. Genital anomalies occur in 50% of females with unilateral agenesis, principally in the vagina and uterus. In males, 20% show genital anomalies, usually in the seminal vesicles, penis, or testes.

In autopsy series, unilateral agenesis was found at a frequency between 1/1000 and 1/500 cases. Clinically, approximately 1/500 cases shows unilateral agenesis (most of these cases are aplastic or small dysplastic kidneys with no function). As already mentioned, bilateral agenesis is rare; multisystemic abnormalities are usually found in such cases.

2.2.2 Renal Hypoplasia

The hypoplastic kidney is a miniaturized normal kidney, usually with a reduced number of renal lobes and calyces. The etiology is unclear. It may be developmental or possibly secondary to vascular insufficiency in utero or during infancy. Diminished blood supply after birth will cause a miniaturized kidney, usually with a normal number of lobes and calyces (Fig. 2.4). Ischemia in the adult can usually be recognized on angiography since the origin of the renal artery from the aorta will be normal in size while the vessel itself will decrease in size, comparable with the size of the kidney (Fig. 2.5). Hypoplasia is generally unilateral and Campbell's series reports it occurring in 1 to 500 autopsies. The opposite kidney will frequently show compensatory hypertrophy, particularly if the lesion producing the small kidney occurred in utero or in infancy.

Aside from its small size, the kidney is essentially normal. It is more medially located, and concentrates contrast normally in the absence of complications. The renal outlines in hypoplasia are smooth,

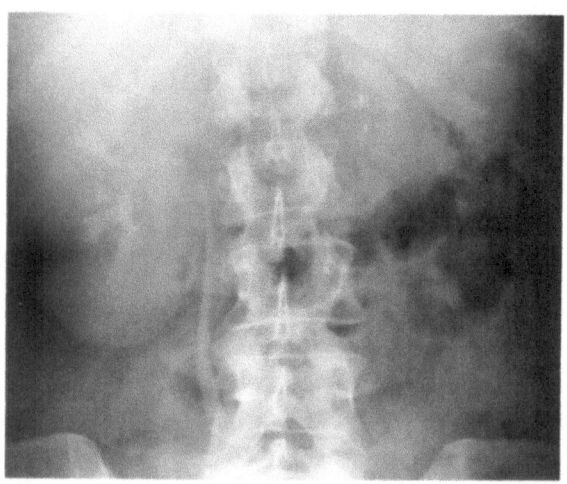

Fig. 2.4. Left renal hypoplasia. The right kidney shows compensatory hypertrophy

Fig. 2.5 a, b. Renal hypoplasia. **a** Urogram with small well-visualized collecting systems. **b** Angiography showing a small renal artery. The adjacent adrenal gland and superior capsular artery suggest the kidney has always been this size. When a kidney shrinks from acquired disease, the superior capsullar artery and adrenal gland maintain their original positions and are not in direct apposition with the capsule
▽

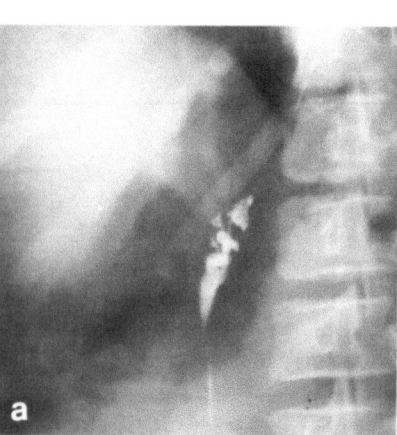
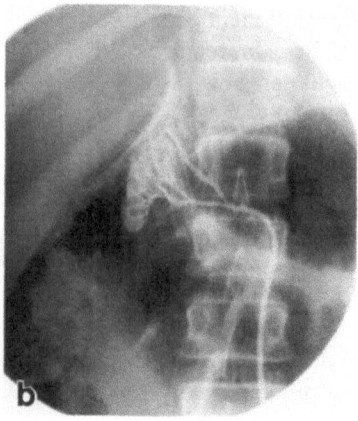

which allows the differentiation of the noncompli-
cated hypoplastic kidney from a pyelonephritic or
infarcted kidney. Occasionally, the histology shows
areas of dysplastic tissue in the hypoplastic kidney.

The hypoplastic kidney is prone to infection and
calculi formation, and once secondary changes have
occurred, differentiation from small kidneys that
have been affected by infection is difficult. Hypertension is a common complication.

2.2.3 Supernumerary Kidney

The supernumerary kidney is a rare anomaly. It may
occur from either division of the ureteric bud from
the wolffian duct, and/or division of the renal an-
lage. The classic supernumerary kidney has a separate blood supply, is completely encapsulated, and is
not connected to the main renal parenchyma. The
ureter may be entirely separate and have an ectopic
orifice, or may join the main ureter at varying levels.
Ectopic ureteroceles may exist in the case of separate ureters. The supernumerary kidneys are generally smaller, often with only a few calyces. More
than one supernumerary kidney may exist, with up
to six reported in a single patient. While they may
function normally, they are liable to infection and
stone disease. They are more common in males and
tend to occur on the left side (Fig. 2.6).

2.3 Structural Anomalies
of the Upper Collecting System

2.3.1 Duplex Kidneys

Duplication of the collecting system ranges from
kidneys with completely separate ureters to a bifid
renal pelvis, the latter being considered a normal
variant.

The most important entity in this spectrum of
anomalies is the duplicated (duplex) collecting system with a single renal mass and completely duplicated ureters. The duplex kidney is usually larger
than normal by 1–2 cm and is the commonest cause
of a unilateral large kidney. There are two renal hila
and pelves (Fig. 2.7). The upper collecting system is
generally smaller and incomplete, while the lower
usually appears to be a total collecting system
(Fig. 2.8). If the ureters are completely separate, they
cross twice below the kidney and the upper pole
ureter enters the bladder caudal to the ureter draining the lower pole, once near the renal pelves and

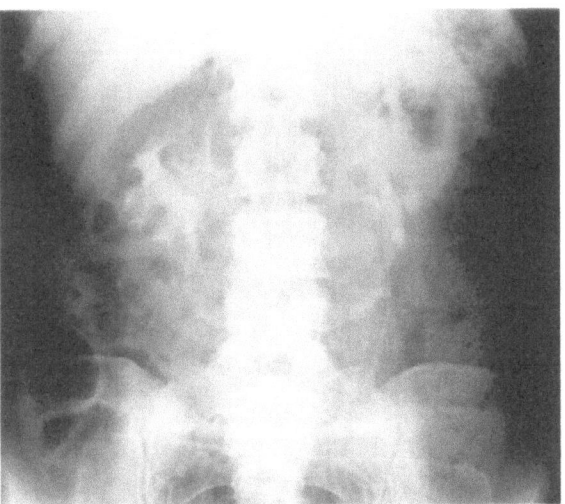

Fig. 2.6. Supernumerary kidney present on the left anteriorly
with malrotation. (From NEY and FRIEDENBERG 1981)

again near the bladder (the "Weigert Mayer" rule).
Bilateral duplication is not uncommon.

Duplex collecting systems are extremely common, being seen in 1 out of 200 intravenous pyelograms (IVPs), more frequently in females. With duplication, there is a one in eight chance that a similar
anomaly exists in siblings/parents.

Three major problems are seen with completely
duplicated ureters: upper pole hydronephrosis,
lower pole reflux, and ectopic ureterocele. The
upper pole system tends to insert ectopically into the
bladder or bladder neck caudal and medial to the
normal ureter and may produce upper pole hydronephrosis secondary to a stenotic orifice. The
mass effect of the dilated upper pole on the lower
pole calyces may produce a "drooping lily" appearance. The dilated nonvisualized upper pole hydroureter may displace the visualized lower pole ureter
laterally. If some parenchyma persists about the
upper pole, a rim sign of hydronephrosis will be
visible.

Vesicoureteral reflux is not uncommon in the
lower system, which is much more likely to reflux
than the upper system. Reflux occurs when the
ureter from the upper system interferes with the normal valve-like structure of the extramural portion of
the lower ureter.

Ectopic ureteroceles may occur whenever there is
a duplicated system with an ectopic ureter. In these
cases the ectopic ureter courses submucosally after
its entrance into the bladder before opening into the
lumen. The compression of the ureter where it enters
the bladder musculature together with the stenotic
ectopic orifice tends to allow dilatation of the sub-

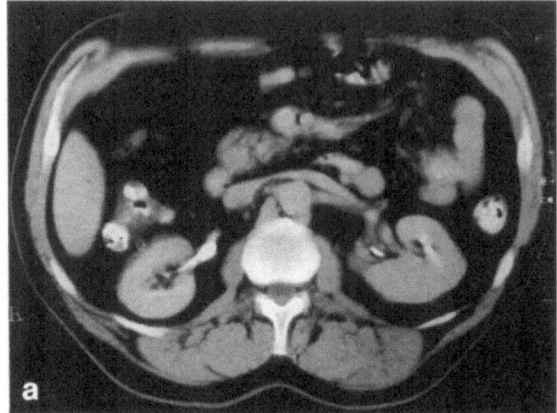

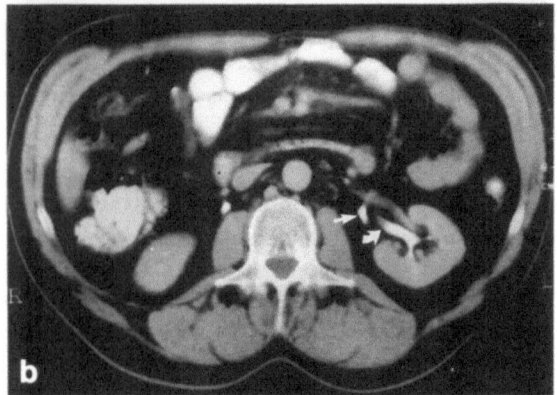

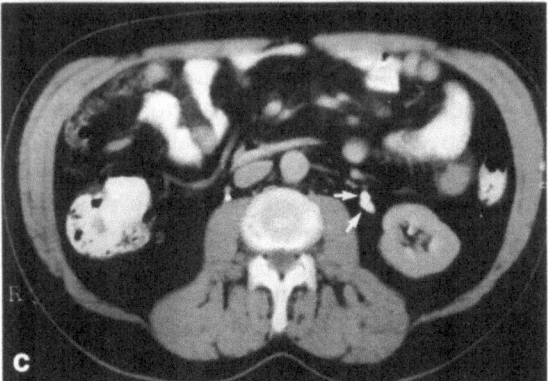

Fig. 2.7 a–c. Left duplex kidney. **a** CT image through the upper pole moiety. **b** CT image through the midleft kidney, showing the upper pole ureter *(arrow)* and the lower pole renal pelvis *(curved arrow)*. **c** CT scan through the lower pole showing two adjacent ureters *(arrows)*

mucosal ureter between these areas, producing the bladder mass.

Renal pseudotumors are common at the junction of the upper and lower systems. In partial duplication, the ureteral fusion may be at varying levels (Figs. 2.9, 2.10). If it is relatively low, a Y-shaped ureter exists; if the fusion is high, there is a bifid renal pelvis.

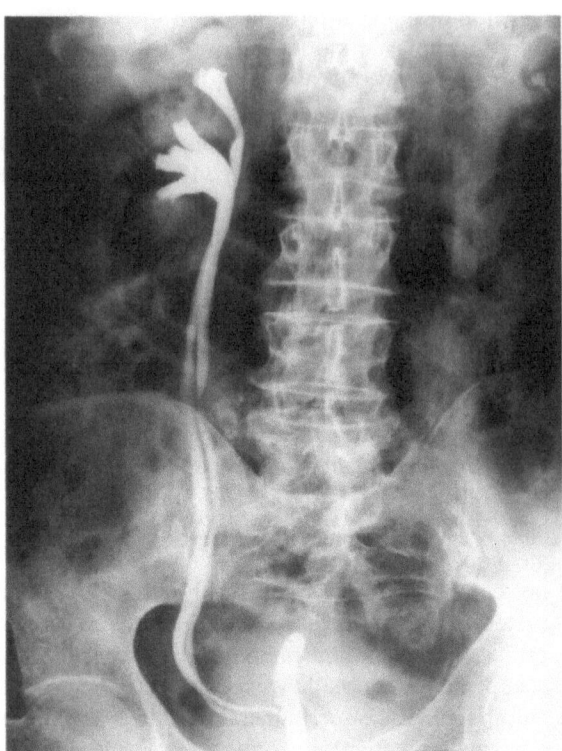

Fig. 2.8. Complete duplex kidney. Complete ureteral duplication can be seen with the ureters crossing twice, once near the ureteropelvic junction and once in the pelvis

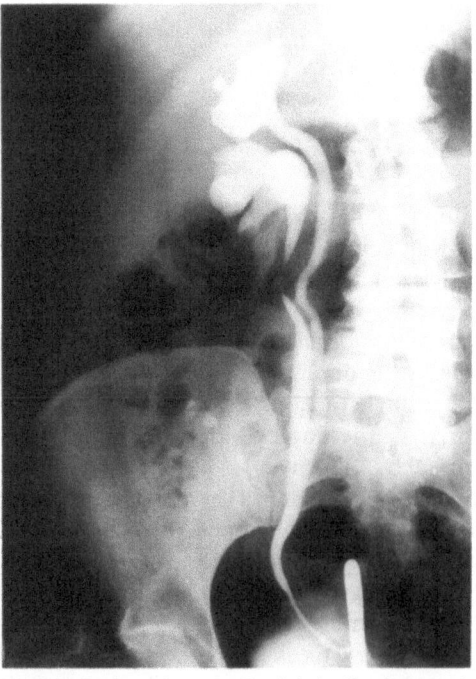

Fig. 2.9. Y-shaped ureter. Partial duplication can be seen of the ureters, which join at the S1 level

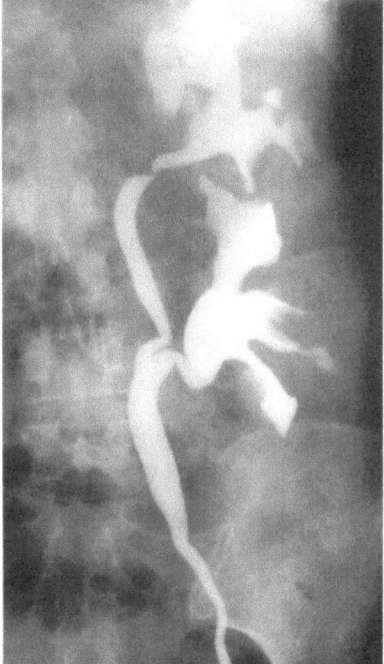
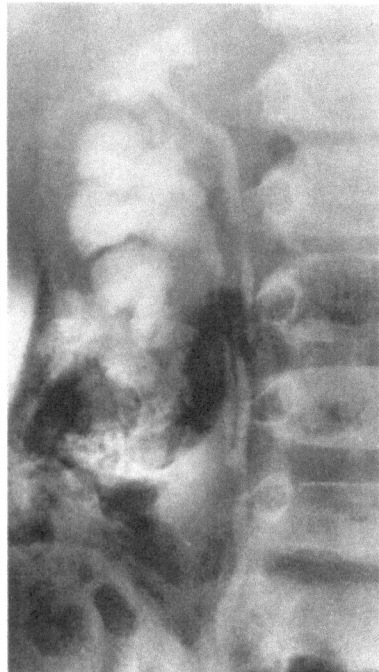

△

Fig. 2.10 (*left*). Partial duplication of the ureter. The ureters join at the L4 level. The patient has autosomal dominant polycystic kidney disease, which distorts the infrarenal collecting system and causes gross renal enlargement

Fig. 2.11 (*right*). Retrograde peristalsis. A duplex kidney with lower pole hydronephrosis and cortical thinning in the lower pole is seen. On fluoroscopy, dysperistalsis could be seen interfering with drainage of the lower pole moiety

One unique feature of partial duplication is abnormal peristalsis. Peristalsis normally originates in the upper infundibulum of the renal pelvis and is propagated myogenically antegrade to the bladder. It is irregular in rate, averaging one to three waves per minute. When partial duplication exists, the peristaltic wave may spread to the junction of the two ureters, and then may propagate not only down the distal common ureter but also retrograde up one of the proximal duplicated ureters. On fluoroscopy, a to-and-fro motion of contrast can be seen. Patients with partial duplication with retrograde peristalsis are more prone to infection and hydronephrosis in the refluxing system (typically the lower pole moiety). This is due to the dysperistalsis causing functional reflux and obstruction in that system (Fig. 2.11).

Segmentation of the renal pelvis is the mildest form of ureteral partial duplication. Bifid pelvis occurs in 10% of the population, and trifid pelvis exists

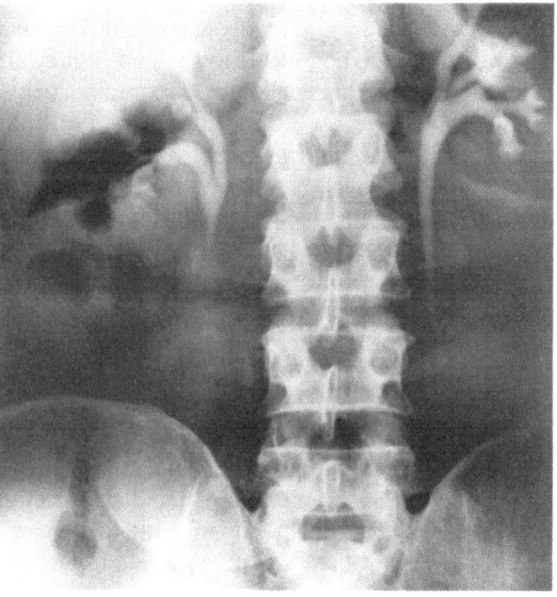

Fig. 2.12. Bifid/ trifid renal pelvis. The right kidney has a bifid renal pelvis, the left kidney a trifid renal pelvis. Note the lowest system on either side has the most calyces. (From NEY and FRIEDENBERG 1981)

but is rare (Fig. 2.12). Other forms of segmentation may occur due to vascular impressions and extrinsic anomalies (see below).

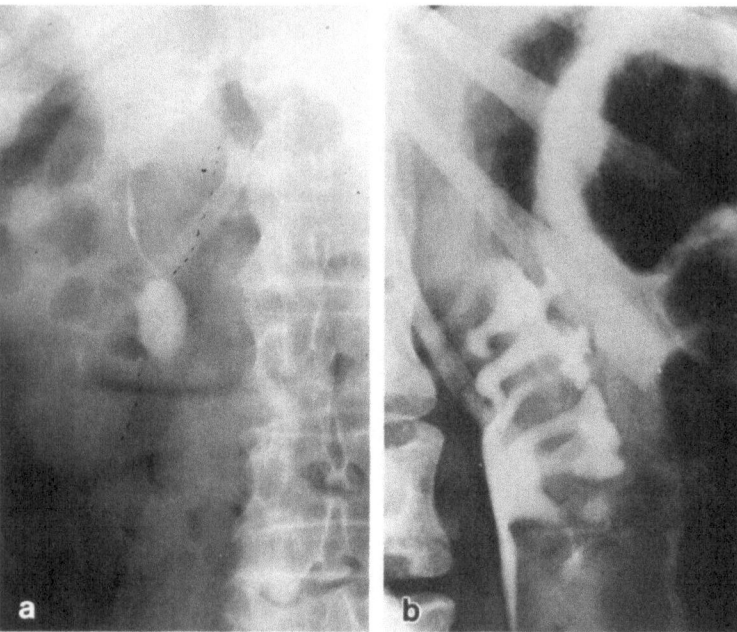

2.3.2 Extrarenal Pelvis

The normal pelvis frequently extends anterior and medial to the kidney, partially extrarenal. This may not be appreciated on the urogram since it may not extend medial to the renal outline. Extrarenal pelves are more common in ectopic, malrotated, or fused kidneys. Rarely, a pelvis may be totally extrarenal, with the infundibula extending outside of the renal shadow to enter the renal pelvis. In such cases there may be an increased problem with drainage, increasing the possibility of hydronephrosis and calculi (Fig. 2.13).

Extrarenal pelves are of no clinical significance. They tend to be larger than average since they can distend easily without being restricted by surrounding tissue. The observer must avoid assuming that this is from obstruction. When extrarenal pelves are involved with obstruction, they dilate significantly before the calyces become significantly dilated and, therefore, protect the renal parenchyma from damage.

2.3.3 Calyceal Anomalies

Unicalyceal kidney is a rare anomaly which is probably due to aborted branching of the ureteric bud in the generations when the renal pelvis and infundibula are formed. The whole kidney is in essence a single renal lobe draining into one calyx which is the pelvis. Contralateral agenesis or bilateral unicaly-

Fig. 2.13 a, b. Extrarenal pelvis. **a** Extrarenal pelvis extending partly beyond renal outline. **b** The rake/claw appearance is seen in total extrarenal pelvis. (From NEY and FRIEDENBERG 1981)

ceal kidneys may be seen, suggesting that the opposite ureter was similarly disturbed during development. The nephrons of such a kidney are reduced in number and hypertrophied. Renal function is often impaired, with proteinuria, azotemia, and hypertension being present (Fig. 2.14).

The *abortive calyx* (blind-ending calyx) is a normal variant whose significance lies in not being mistaken for a calyx amputated by a pathologic process. The abortive calyx is a solitary phenomenon, usually arising in the midportion of the kidney, from the pelvis or from the junction of the upper pole and middle infundibula. It generally points laterally but can be oriented in any direction. The shape of such an abortive calyx varies from a broad-based, blunt protrusion to an elongated, narrow channel with a narrow tip. It has been referred to as a pelvic or infundibular diverticulum. It always lacks a papilla and cupped calyx (Fig. 2.15).

The etiology for the aborted calyx is the cessation of calyceal growth prior to the development of papillary ducts and collecting tubules. Therefore, no papilla or nephron development will occur and a blind-ending protrusion will remain.

The clinical significance of this entity lies in its differentiation from amputated calyces seen in clinical lesions such as tuberculosis, carcinoma, calculi, or other infection.

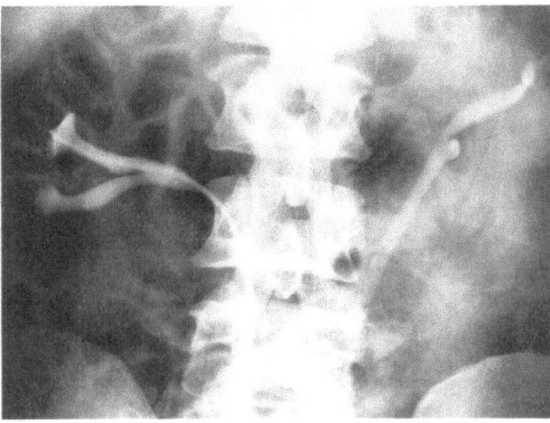

Fig. 2.14. Diminished numbers of calyces. The right kidney shows a bifid renal pelvis with a diminished number of papillae. The left ureter is blind-ending with two stumps. The left kidney was dysplastic. (From NEY and FRIEDENBERG 1981)

▷

Fig. 2.15. Abortive calyx and infundibulum are seen between the upper infundibulum and the middle infundibulum *(arrow)*

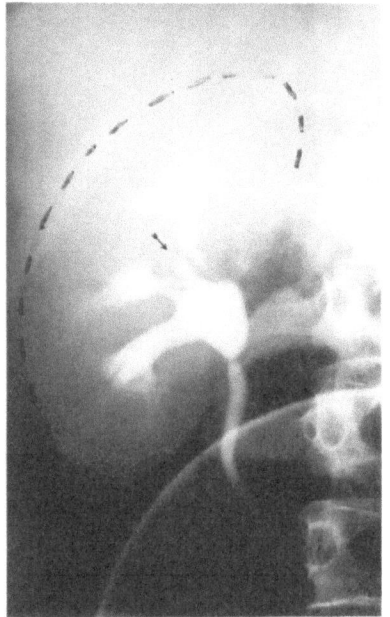

The *calyceal diverticulum* is a solitary cyst-like structure which varies from millimeters up to 3 cm in size and communicates by a narrow channel to the fornix of the calyx (Fig. 2.16). The diverticulum occurs in the cortical column of Bertin rather than the renal pyramid. The calyx which receives the diverticulum is usually normal. Other communicating parenchymal cavities such as in abscess or medullary necrosis occur in the renal pyramid rather than the cortical column and usually deform or destroy the calyx. Complications are uncommon and usually consist of calculi and/or infection secondary to stasis within the diverticulum (Fig. 2.17).

The probable etiology is dilatation of a blind-ending wolffian duct which did not form a calyx during calyceal development. The diverticulum may be confused with a parenchymal cyst which has ruptured into a calyx without distorting it.

An *ectopic papilla* is an intrinsically normal papilla protruding directly into an infundibulum or renal pelvis without a calyx (Fig. 2.18). In the urogram the papilla is seen as a smooth, round or oval mound, mimicking a "calyx en face." The latter has a fine, dense rim of contrast around the lucent defect from contrast in the fornices of the calyx. This is usually not seen in ectopic papilla. This anomaly may be related to failure of differentiation of the wolffian duct forming a calyx in that area. If a minor calyx were too centrally located, the walls of the calyx might similarly be flattened and incorporated into the renal pelvis, creating an ectopic papilla. The defect produced by the ectopic papilla can mimic an intra-luminal filling defect but the ectopic papillae can be shown not to be intraluminal by oblique films.

Congenital megacalyces is a nonobstructive enlargement of the calyces, presumably secondary to malformation of the renal papilla. The renal papilla are undeveloped and shallow, not filling the calyceal cup, with the calyces appearing floppy and oversized and, when seen en face, often polygonal (Fig. 2.19). Although there may be some slightly delay in early calyceal filling, when filled normal concentrations are present. Classically, the infundibula, pelvis, and ureter are usually normal and the renal cortex is of normal thickness.

In the differential diagnosis one must consider nonobstructive hydronephrosis, back pressure atrophy, and hydrocalycosis. In nonobstructive hydronephrosis one would expect a history of infection and evidence of infection deforming cortex and calyces. In back pressure atrophy there is more diffuse dilatation also affecting the pelvis and infundibula, and the cortex appears thin. In hydrocalycosis, the infundibula should be narrow.

Congenital megacalyces does not appear to be familial and is most often unilateral. Males are more commonly affected. In the absence of calculi, the megacalyces are not clinically significant. There have been a few cases described of megaureter accompanying megacalyces. It is not known if this is of any significance.

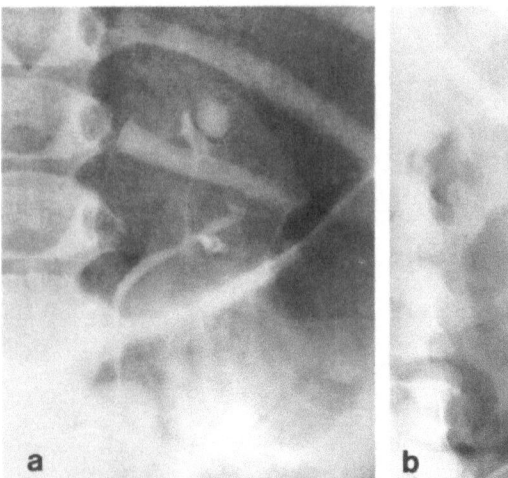
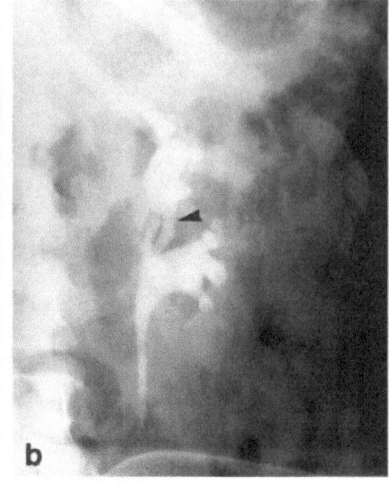

△

Fig. 2.16 a, b. Calyceal diverticulum. **a** An upper pole caly-ceal diverticulum can be seen which fills later than the remain-der of the collecting system. **b** A blind-ending infundibular diverticulum *(arrowhead)* lacks calyces

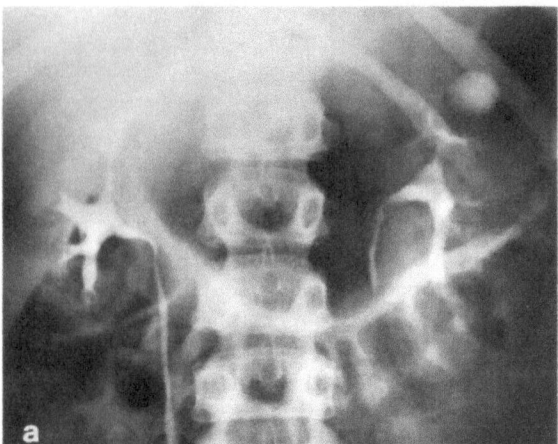

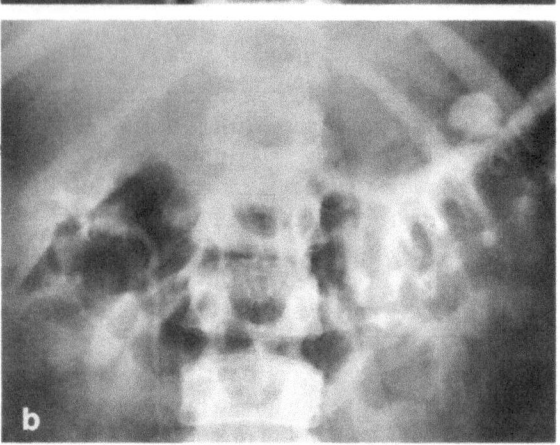

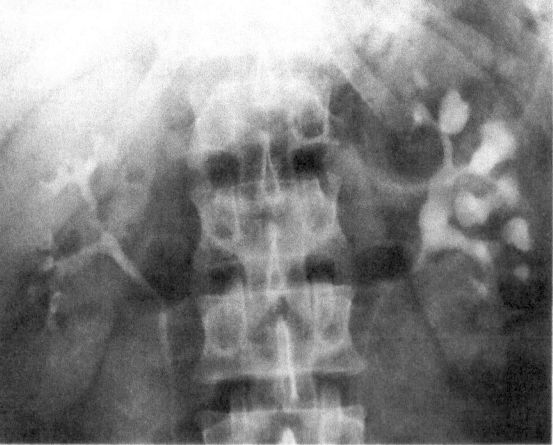

Fig. 2.17 a, b. Calyceal diverticulum. Delayed urogram shows retained contrast agent in the diverticulum. (From NEY and FRIEDENBERG 1981)

Fig. 2.18 see p. 43

Fig. 2.19. Congenital megacalyces. Urogram showing con-genital megacalyces on the left side. The left renal cortex is of normal thickness despite the calyceal dilatation. The right kid-ney has normal calyces

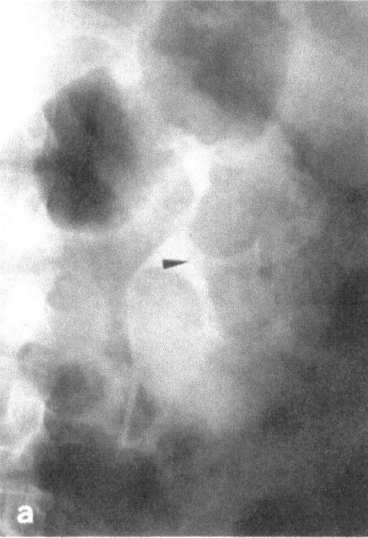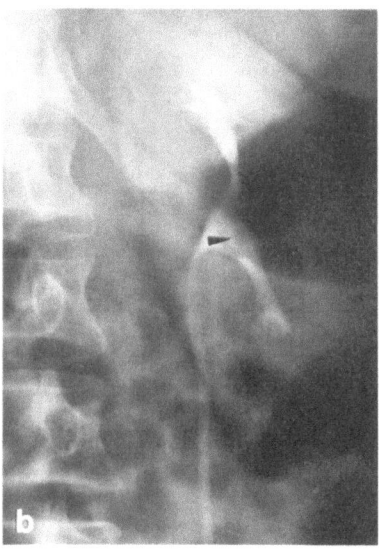

Fig. 2.18 a, b. Ectopic papilla. **a** Anteroposterior image of a urogram showing a filling defect on the renal pelvis *(arrowhead).* **b** Oblique image confirms the papilla extending into the renal pelvis. (From NEY and FRIEDENBERG 1981)

2.4 Structural Anomalies of the Renal Parenchyma (Cystic or Solid Lesions)

2.4.1 Congenital Solitary Cysts

Congenital renal solitary cysts are an occasional finding in autopsies in children (2%–4%). The vast majority of congenital renal cysts are small and it is unclear whether they are developmental, obstructive, or traumatic in nature (Fig. 2.20).

2.4.2 Multicystic Dysplastic Kidney

The subject of cystic disease of the kidney has generated many attempts at classification, with some attendant confusion. The most clinically useful method is to consider congenital multiple cystic disease as consisting of four major entities: the multicystic dysplastic kidney, the multilocular cystic nephroma, infantile polycystic disease, and adult polycystic disease. All of these lesions have more than one name.

The multicystic dysplastic kidney (MCDK) is also referred to as the multicystic kidney or the multicystic degenerative kidney, and is categorized by POTTER (1972) as type II A. The kidney is completely replaced by thin-walled cysts of varying size, lacking any orderly arrangement. The cysts range from mil-

limeters to several centimeters in size and are connected by primitive and dysplastic mesenchymal tissue frequently resembling a bunch of grapes (Fig. 2.21). This is the most frequent form of multicystic kidney and is usually associated with an absent or atretic pelvis and ureter.

A second type of multicystic kidney, classified as the hydronephrotic form of MCDK, has been described in which the renal pelvis is not obliterated and communication occurs between the cystic spaces. In this latter type of multicystic kidney contrast injections may show faint visualization of the parenchyma, but no contrast is seen in the calyces. The nonhydronephrotic form of multicystic kidney may be quite small or very large, while the hydronephrotic form is usually large. Recent sonographic studies by PEDICELLI et al. and KLEINER et al. (1986) have helped to elucidate the natural history of MCDK both prenatally and by serial studies in neonates and infants.

Multicystic dysplastic kidneys are detectable in utero and may both increase and decrease in size (Fig. 2.22). They may disappear entirely, both roentgenographically and even to surgical exploration, suggesting that some cases of presumed renal agenesis are in fact atrophy of MCDK. The second interesting point of prenatal diagnosis of MCDK is the frequency of contralateral renal anomaly. Statistics of prior studies may have been skewed by the mix of pediatric and adult populations. The number of lethal contralateral anomalies would be diminished and nonlethal anomalies increased in adult studies.

Multicystic dysplastic kidney is the most common renal mass in the 1st week of life and second only to hydronephrosis after the 1st week. Approximately

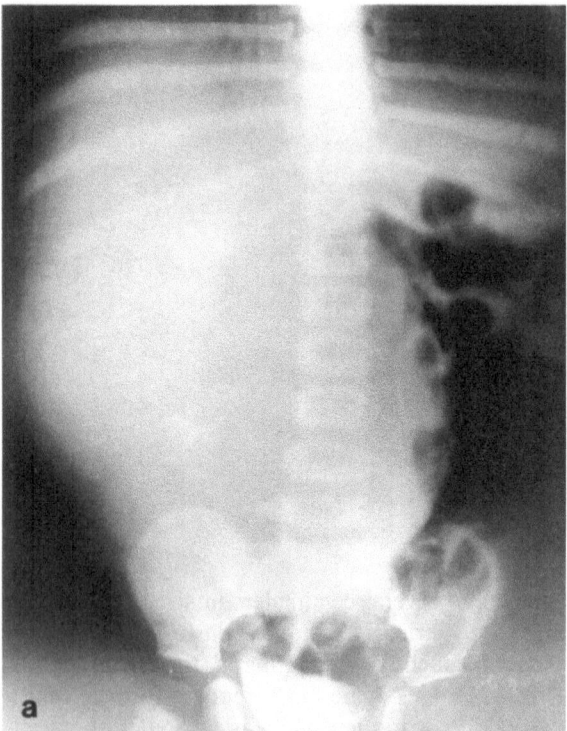

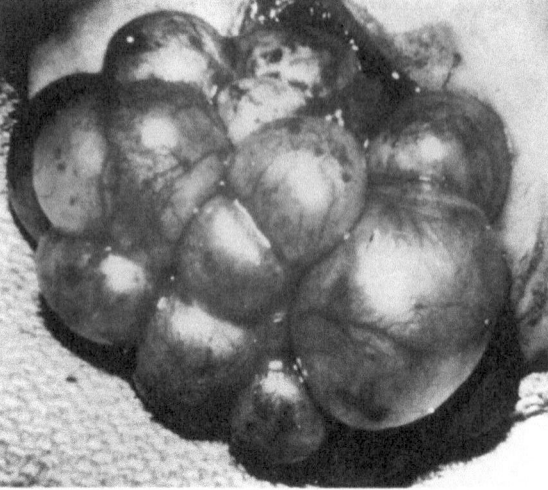

Fig. 2.21. MCDK. Specimen photograph showing the resemblance of the MCDK to a bunch of grapes

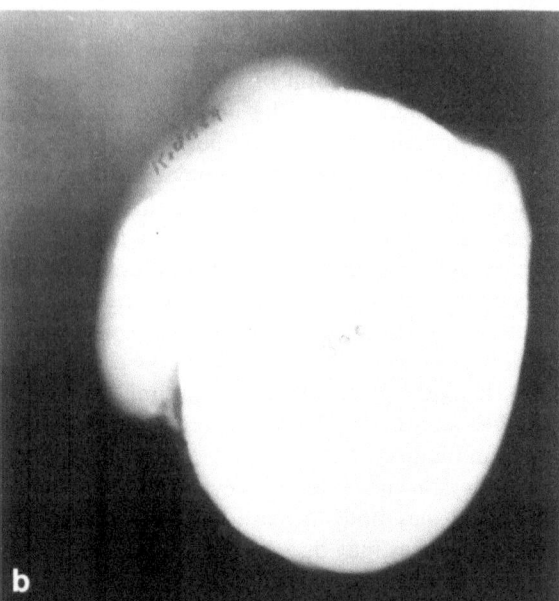

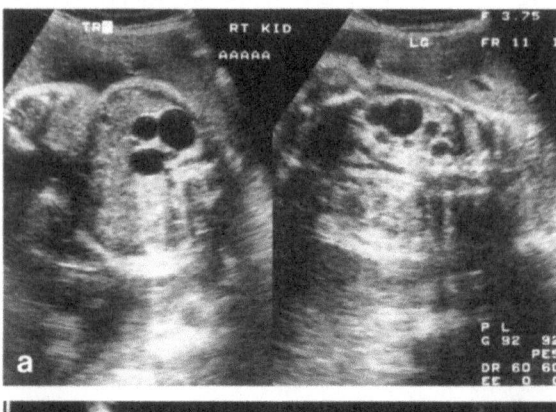

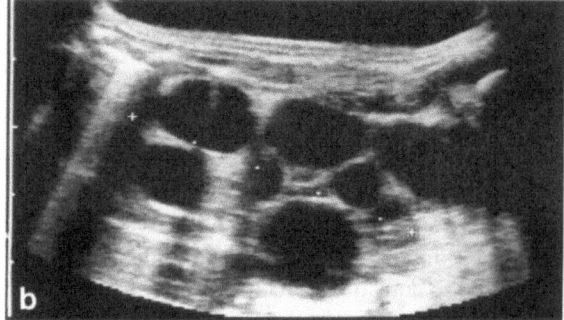

Fig. 2.20 a, b. Congenital renal solitary cyst. a Urogram showing a large mass displacing the bowel gas to the left flank. The left renal collecting system is normal. b Surgical specimen after cyst puncture and injection with contrast showing the large cyst which compresses and flattens the right kidney. (From NEY and FRIEDENBERG 1981)

Fig. 2.22 a, b. Development of the hydronephrotic form of MCDK. a In utero sonogram showing irregularly sized cysts within the kidney. b Postnatal sonogram of the same kidney showing increasing size of the cysts and loss of the parenchyma

40% of patients have a contralateral renal anomaly – either bilateral MCDK (20%), which is incompatible with life, abnormality of the ureteropelvic junction (7%), or occasionally agenesis, hypoplasia, fused or rotated kidneys, etc.

Multicystic dysplastic kidney presents as a non-functional mass in the renal fossa on IVP. There is usually an atretic or absent ureter (Fig. 2.23) and an absent or barely identifiable renal artery. On ultrasound, criteria have been established to distinguish MCDK from gross hydronephrosis (Fig. 2.24). These include: cysts with interfaces among them, location of the largest cyst being noncentral, cysts being multiple in number and noncommunicating, and the absence of identifiable renal parenchyma. Renal scintigraphy shows no function.

As stated above, the hydronephrotic form of MCDK has a dilated renal pelvis and occasionally proximal ureter and may show communication between cystic spaces. It is more likely to have a visible renal artery and some functioning renal parenchyma.

The spectrum of renal dysplasia has been recently introduced to the radiologic literature (SANDERS et al. 1988). The correlation of MCDK with other more distally obstructed renal dysplasias lends credence to the role of obstruction in the genesis of renal dysplasia. Probably the lower the level of obstruction, the lesser the degree of cyst formation that results.

With MCDK, a conservative approach is generally recommended. Complications have been reported, including the development of carcinoma, hypertension, and infection. However, these complications are felt to be uncommon and surgical resection is usually performed in cases with complications.

2.4.3 Multilocular Cystic Nephroma

Multilocular cystic nephroma (MLCN) is an uncommon renal neoplasm that has generated considerable confusion in the literature. MADEWELL et al. (1983) in reviewing this entity, cited over a dozen alternative names. The tumor is an encapsulated mass, well circumscribed, composed of multiple cysts of varying size filled with fluid that ranges from serous to gelatinous. These cysts do not communicate with each other.

Radiographically, MLCN presents as a well-defined mass typically in either pole of the kidney (lower pole more common), with normal function in the remainder of the kidney (Fig. 2.25). The mass does not function on IVP, computed tomography

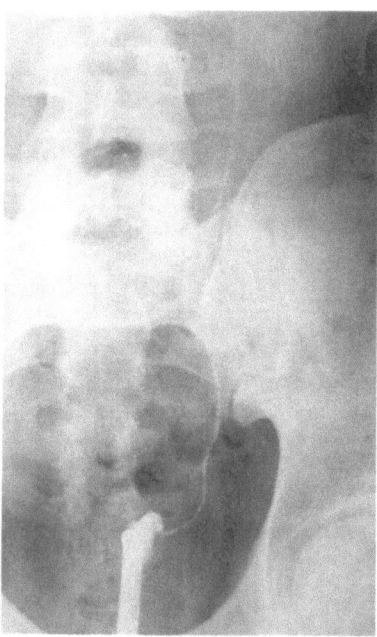

Fig. 2.23. MCDK. Retrograde pyelogram shows an atretic beaded ureter; the beading is felt to be an expression of immaturity

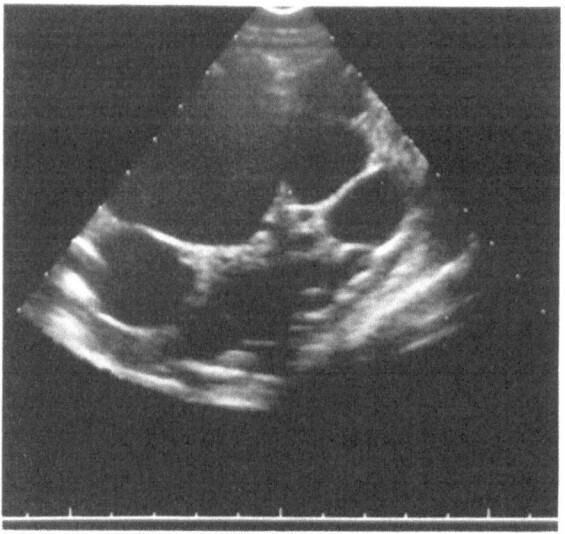

Fig. 2.24. MCDK. Sonogram shows irregular sized cysts without a renal pelvis or orderly arrangement

(CT), or scintigraphy. It occasionally herniates into the renal pelvis and obstructs the collecting systems and, more rarely, has an exophytic growth pattern into the perinephric space. Ultrasound, CT, and nephrotomography generally show multiple cysts. If the cysts are very small, the mass will appear more echogenic (on ultrasound) or more uniformly dense

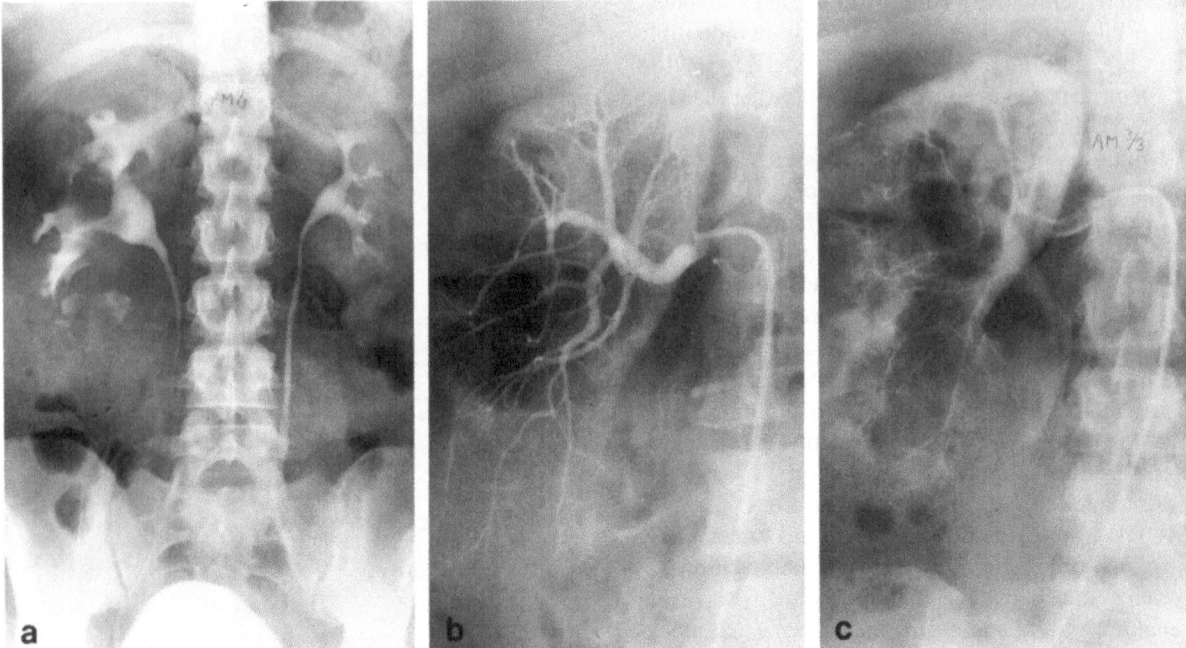

Fig. 2.25 a–c. MLCN. **a** An MLCN is located in the lateral portion of the kidney. A lower pole cyst has ruptured into the collecting system and contrast is seen filling that cyst. **b, c** Angiography better defines the cystic mass, showing spreading of the renal vessels but no neovascularity

(on CT and tomography). Occasional cyst wall calcification is seen (Fig. 2.26). If a cyst puncture is performed, injections of the cyst will fail to show communication with other cysts. On angiography, the mass is usually hypovascular but may show a vague tumor blush.

Multilocular cystic nephroma is a benign neoplasm of the metanephric blastema. It has a bimodal distribution, occurring in males generally less than 24 months of age and in females predominantly in the fifth and sixth decades of life. It is clear that the lesion may grow significantly over weeks to months, and appear in a previously radiographically normal kidney. It is usually unifocal, but rarely multiple and even bilateral. Rarely, malignant elements are seen within it, including microscopic foci of Wilms' tumor, or sarcomatous elements which may metastasize.

2.4.4 Infantile Polycystic Kidney Disease

Infantile polycystic kidney disease (autosomal recessive polycystic kidney disease: ARPKD) is inherited as an autosomal recessive and presents in approximately 1/10000 births. Pathologically, cystic dilatation of the collecting tubules, and to a lesser extent nephrons and glomeruli, extends from the pyramids to the cortical surface of the kidney. ARPKD can be divided into subclassifications which can be displayed as a spectrum of the disease. Some authors utilize three categories, others as many as five. The place on the spectrum relates to the age of the patient at the presentation of the lesion and the extent of kidney and liver involvement.

```
K-++++|__  Neonatal__  Infantile__  Juvenile__  |K-+
L-+|                                             | L-+++
```

If we consider ARPKD as having three subcategories they could be classified as neonatal, infantile, and juvenile. These can be represented on a spectrum with those to the left of the spectrum having primarily renal involvement (over 90% of the nephrons involved with minimal liver disease), while the juvenile form to the right of the spectrum has minimal nephron involvement with primary liver disease. The large majority of the clinically presenting cases are either neonatal or infantile.

The neonatal form (clinically present at birth) has most of the nephrons involved with cystic dilatation of the renal tubules and microcystic formation within the kidney to an extent that renal function does not occur. Most of these children die within the first few weeks of life. Their kidneys may be normal to large in size.

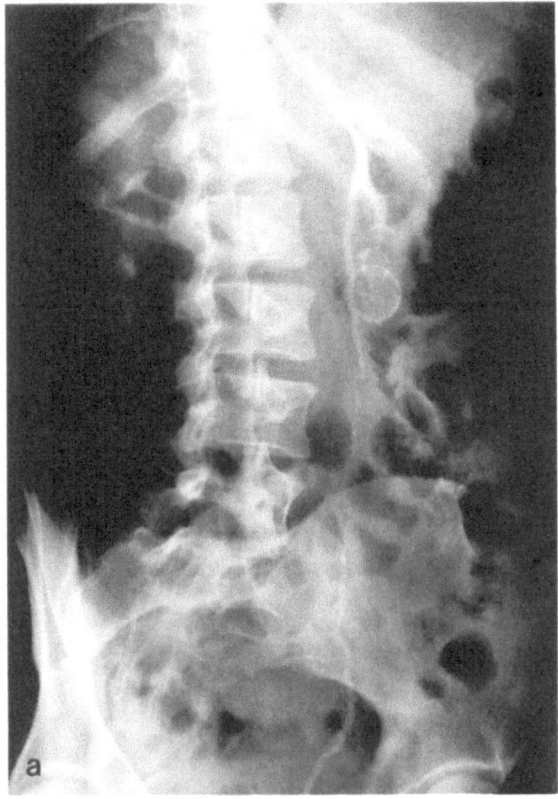

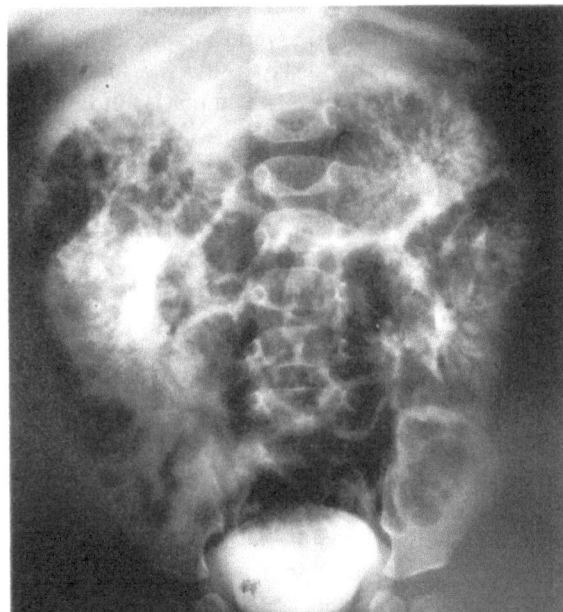

Fig. 2.27. ARPKD. A 3-h film of a urogram shows contrast in the dilated tubules which radiates from the papilla to the cortical surface, a pattern typical of this disease. (From NEY and FRIEDENBERG 1981)

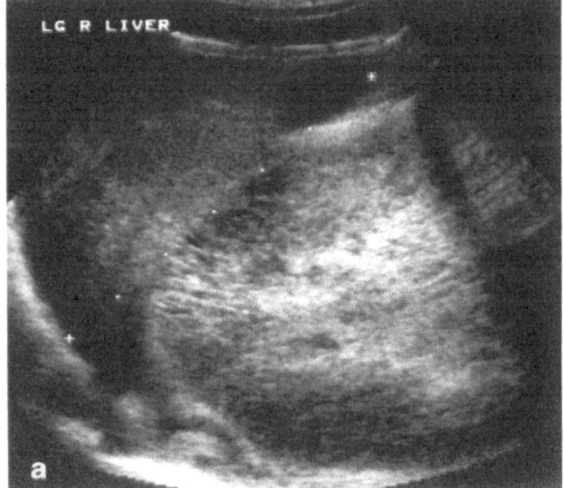

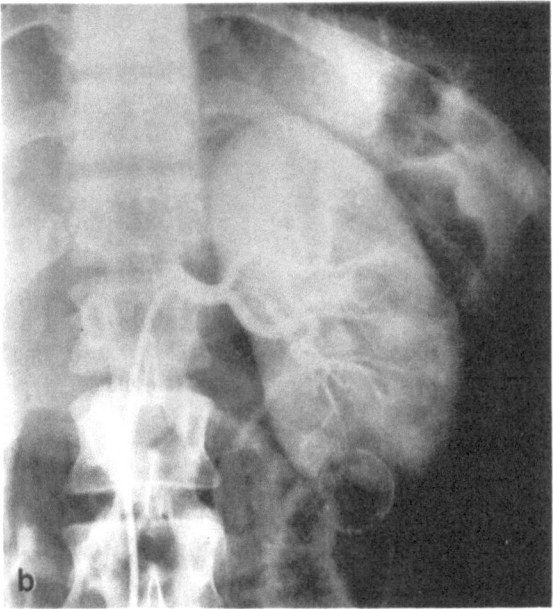

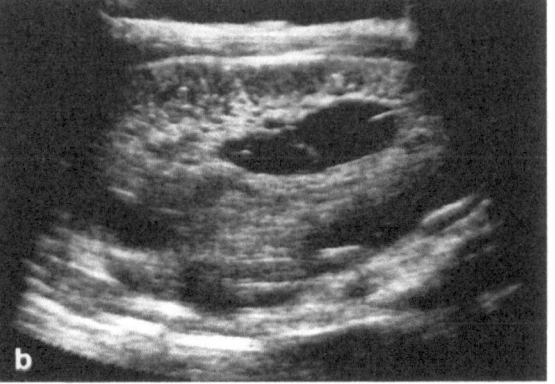

Fig. 2.26 a, b. MLCN. a Cyst wall calcification is seen in an inferior pole MLCN. b Angiogram defines the functional renal mass. Some noncalcified cysts were also present in this lesion

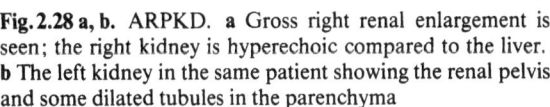

Fig. 2.28 a, b. ARPKD. a Gross right renal enlargement is seen; the right kidney is hyperechoic compared to the liver. b The left kidney in the same patient showing the renal pelvis and some dilated tubules in the parenchyma

In the infantile form, the lesions may present at any time from birth to several months after birth. Function is present and classically cystically dilated tubules are displayed which can be visualized from the collecting tubules to the cortex of the kidney. A peculiar radiating tubular pattern is produced which is distinctive for this disease. In these patients the kidneys are very large and function is poor. Calyceal filling may not occur until 2 or 3 h after injection (Fig. 2.27). There is little periportal fibrosis. Sonographically the kidneys are large and hyperechoic (Fig. 2.28; see also Chap. 19). Usually few or no cysts can be resolved sonographically.

In the juvenile form, the kidney may appear normal or mimic what one expects in a medullary sponge. A bilateral medullary sponge presenting in the first few years of life should arouse suspicion of a juvenile polycystic kidney. Many of these patients do not present with significant hepatic problems, but occasional patients are seen with Riley-Newhouse syndrome, which involves severe periportal fibrosis with secondary varices and bleeding. PREMKUMAR et al. (1988) have reported cases demonstrating that children with ARPKD may show progression and develop hepatic fibrosis and portal hypertension over time. Splenomegaly and variceal bleeding commonly occur.

2.4.5 Adult Polycystic Kidney Disease

Adult polycystic kidney disease (autosomal dominant polycystic kidney disease: ADPKD) is a genetic disease which is transmitted in an autosomal dominant fashion. POTTER (1972) classified this as type III, with cysts of tubular origin in the cortex and medulla. Innumerable cysts of varying size develop in the kidneys, with progressive renal insufficiency resulting. In contrast to infantile polycystic kidney, where the cysts are microcysts and do not significantly alter the renal shape, adult polycystic kidneys have large cysts which markedly deform the cortical outline. The disease affects both kidneys but may present asymmetrically. At times, one kidney may have marked involvement while the other kidney appears roentgenographically normal. Eventually the second kidney will show the changes of the disease. It is rarely present at birth but almost always develops by age 80. The common time of presentation is in the fifth decade, with symptoms of chronic renal failure, hypertension, abdominal mass, or abdominal pain.

At autopsy, the incidence is approximately 1/500 births. The clinical incidence may be lower (as

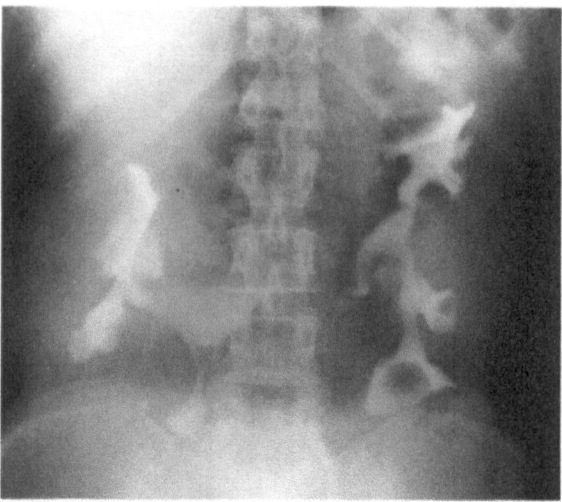

Fig. 2.29. ADPKD. Bilateral renal enlargement and gross distortion of the collecting systems are present

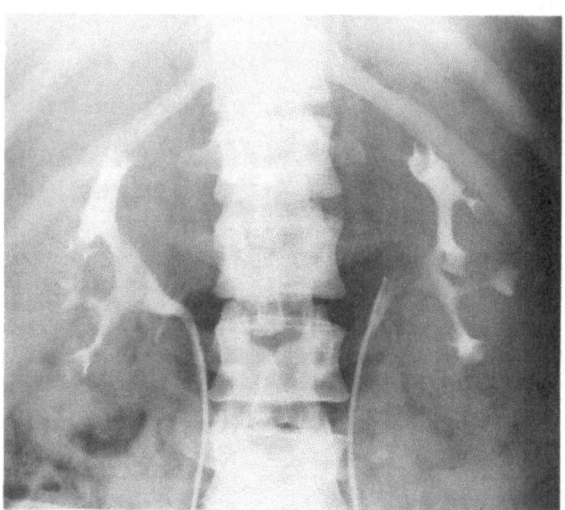

Fig. 2.30. ADPKD. This case shows mild changes of adult polycystic kidney disease; there is some elongation of the infundibula and slight renal enlargement is present

low as 1/1000) due to delayed clinical presentation of the condition. Associated findings include cysts in other organs and aneurysms of the circle of Willis. Hepatic cysts have been reported in one-third to one-half of all patients but CT now suggests that they are present in over 50% of patients. Pancreatic cysts are reported in 9% of the patients, with splenic, pulmonary, and gonadal cysts being less common. Fifteen percent of patients with adult polycystic kidney disease have associated berry aneurysms of the cerebral vascular system and 4% of patients with intracranial aneurysms have polycystic kidney dis-

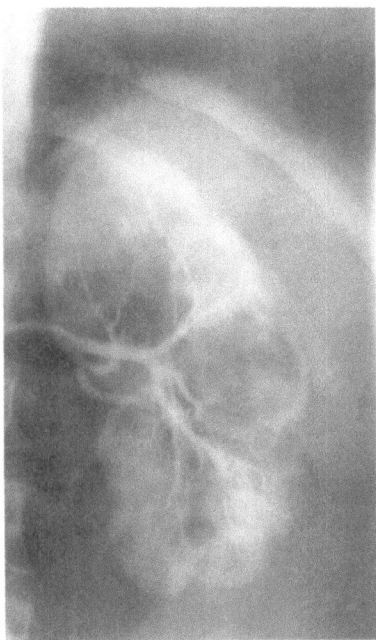

Fig. 2.31. ADPKD. Angiography shows cysts splaying the vessels and there is decreased peripheral branching of the vessels

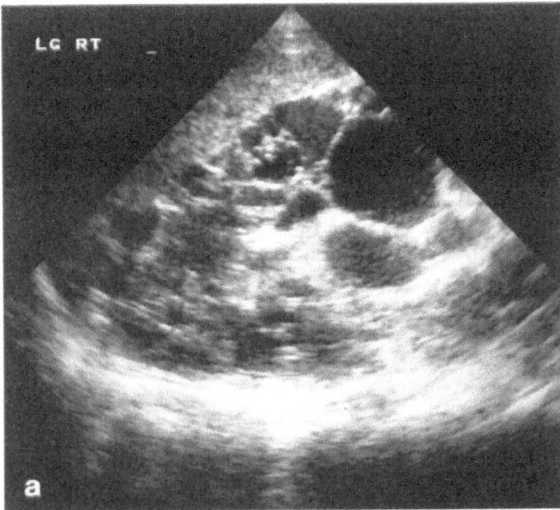

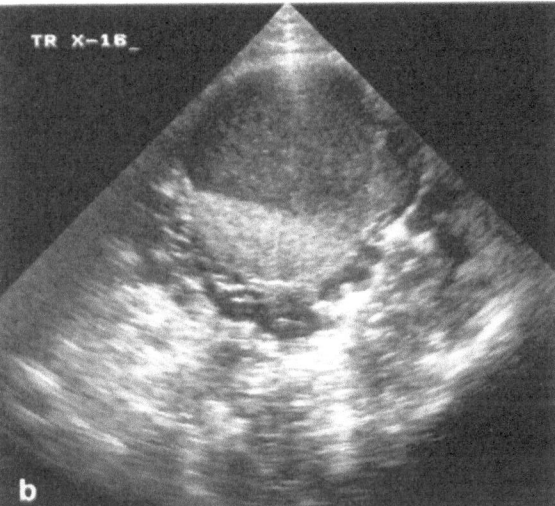

Fig. 2.33 a, b. ADPKD. **a** Numerous cysts of varying size are seen in the kidney. **b** Sonogram of a large cyst with a fluid-fluid level due to hemorrhage complicating adult polycystic kidney disease

◁

Fig. 2.32. ADPKD. CT image shows innumerable macroscopic cysts on either side in no orderly arrangement

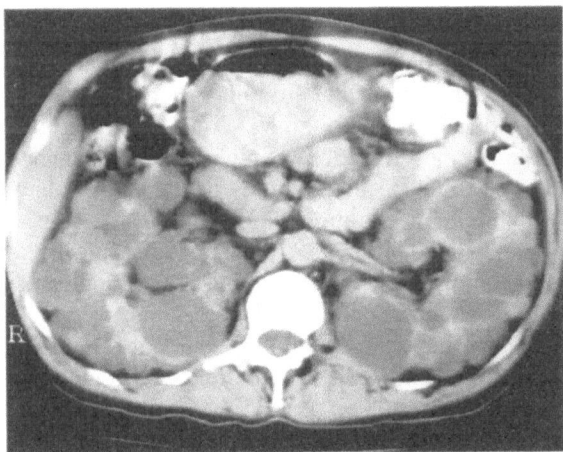

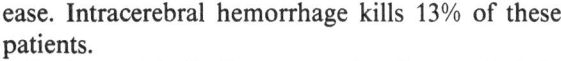

ease. Intracerebral hemorrhage kills 13% of these patients.

Radiographic findings are quite characteristic in advanced cases. The kidneys are enlarged (not necessarily symmetrically) and usually have a lobulated contour. The collecting system is distorted and elongated, with flattening and obliteration of calyces and infundibula from pressure from multiple cysts (Figs. 2.29, 2.30). On angiography the intrarenal vessels will show similar distortion and loss of terminal branching due to cyst pressure (Fig. 2.31). CT and ultrasound generally show enlarged kidneys with irregular outlines due to the multiple cysts (Figs. 2.32, 2.33). Both these modalities may effectively show cysts in other abdominal viscera as well. In ADPKD the cysts are usually larger and the presence of discrete, resolvable cysts on ultrasound can be helpful in excluding ARPKD when ADPKD presents in infants.

Magnetic resonance imaging (MRI) is occasionally useful when patients with ADPKD present with acute abdominal plain. Using T1 and T2 sequences new and old bleeding into cysts can be identified, which frequently correlates with the acute pain.

In the long term, the major complication of adult polycystic kidney disease is renal failure, leading to death. Other complications include hematuria, proteinuria which rarely leads to nephrotic syndrome, infections, and malignancy. Detection of infected cysts can be difficult by CT or ultrasound, and radionuclide scanning (gallium 67 or indium 111 WBCs) or MRI may be helpful. Malignancy is also difficult to locate, although a solid enhancing mass amidst all the cysts is suggestive of tumor. Renal angiography is helpful in locating carcinoma.

2.4.6 Medullary Sponge Kidney

Medullary sponge kidney is a dilatation of the collecting tubules in the distal third of the medullary pyramid. It has been reported to occur in between 0.1% and more than 0.5% of the population. The variation is partially due to the subjective nature of the diagnosis. With the current contrast media, pyramidal blushes are quite common and the observer must differentiate the normal pyramidal blush from the presence of medullary sponge. In the authors' opinion, the best method of reading medullary sponge is to observe the area in question without a magnifying glass and convince yourself that you are able to see individual radiating tubular structures before the condition is diagnosed (Fig. 2.34). There is a spectrum of lesions from minor involvement of a few pyramids in one kidney to severe involvement with cystic changes adjacent to the collecting tubules, which may contain calculi (Fig. 2.35). Various authors have graded medullary sponge from 1 to 3 or 4, depending upon the severity of the lesion. The majority of cases are bilateral, but 30%–40% are unilateral and may involve a few scattered pyramids. The condition is congenital but noninheritable and has been reported in association with hemihypertrophy, Ehlers-Danlos syndrome, hypertrophic pyloric stenosis, and Caroli's disease (Fig. 2.36). The condition manifests itself in young to middle-aged adults. The lesion is usually asymptomatic unless complicated by calculi formation and infection.

Roentgenographically the kidney is usually of normal size. The plain film may show numerous small calculi in the papillae. Urographic appearance is generally diagnostic. Ectatic tubules may be demonstrated in the papilla as discrete structures with or without small cystic rounded collections of contrast. The papilla may be enlarged. On ultrasound, occasional hyperechoic pyramids can be seen secondary to innumerable small stones. Angiography in this condition is not helpful.

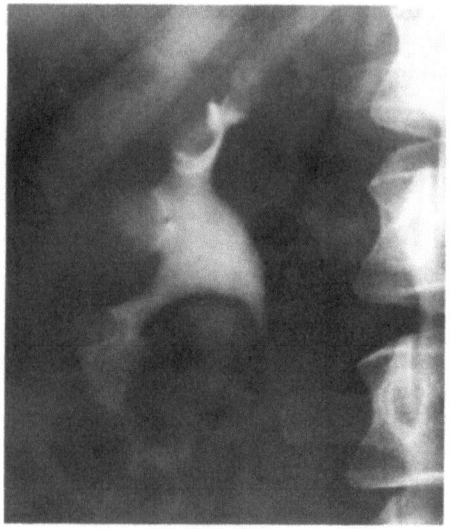

Fig. 2.34. Bilateral medullary sponge kidney with fine dilatation of the collecting tubules in the papillae

2.4.7 Medullary Cystic Disease

Medullary cystic disease is a congenital and familial condition, also referred to as familial juvenile nephronophthisis. It presents in children and young adults with azotemia, salt-wasting, anemia, and eventual hypertension and renal failure. Pathologically cysts occur in and around the corticomedullary junction, with the kidneys eventually becoming shrunken and fibrotic. Roentgenographic signs are few and nonspecific: symmetrically small kidneys with poor concentration in IVP, and frequently nonvisualization (Fig. 2.37). Cysts may be visible on nephrotomography. Angiography shows diminished renal size, a thin cortex, and distortion of vessels by cysts at the corticomedullary junction (Fig. 2.38). Ultrasound shows shrunken kidneys with increased echogenicity and occasional cysts, and decreased differentiation between the cortical and medullary tissues. Occasional cysts may be seen again on ultrasound.

2.4.8 Congenital Mesoblastic Nephroma

Congenital mesoblastic nephroma (CMN) is a benign tumor which presents during the first weeks of life, and is also known as a leiomyomatous or fetal renal hamartoma. It is far more common than a Wilms' tumor at birth. There are no epithelial elements as are usually seen in Wilms' tumor. The tumor is not encapsulated and extends into the normal parenchyuma. BECKWITH (1974) placed this

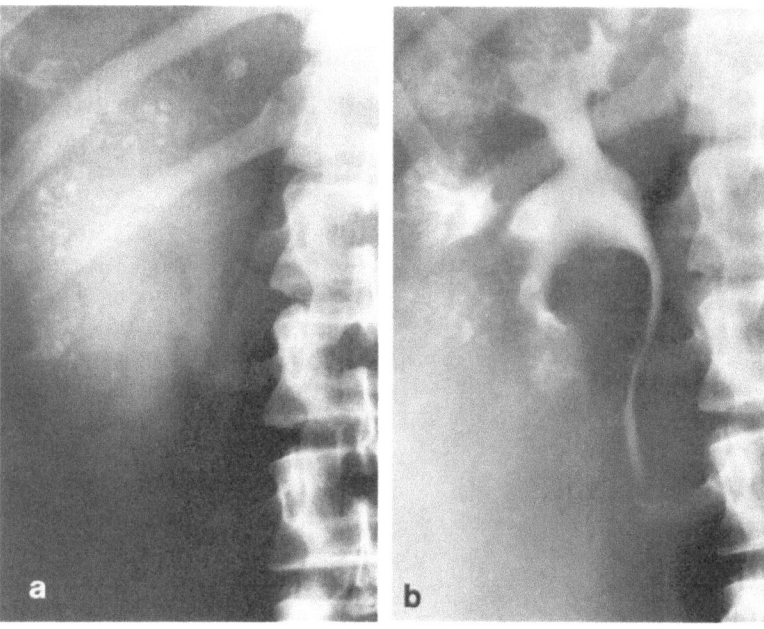

△

Fig. 2.35 a, b. Medullary sponge kidney. **a** Innumerable calculi in the dilated tubules of medullary sponge kidney. **b** Urogram confirming the dilated tubules and cystic spaces which contain the stones seen on plain film. (From NEY and FRIEDENBERG 1981)

Fig. 2.36 a, b. Medullary sponge kidney. **a** Urogram showing medullary sponge changes, particularly in the left kidney. **b** Percutaneous transhepatic cholangiogram shows irregular dilatation of numerous biliary radicles characteristic of Caroli's disease

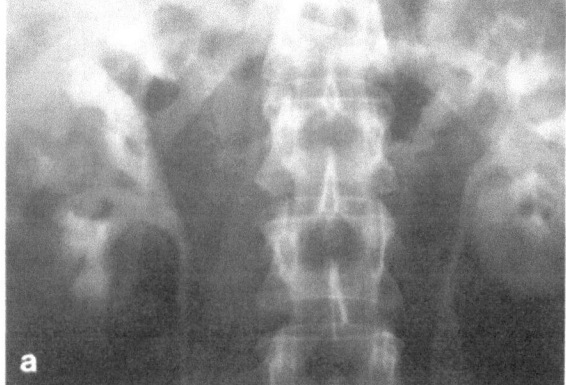

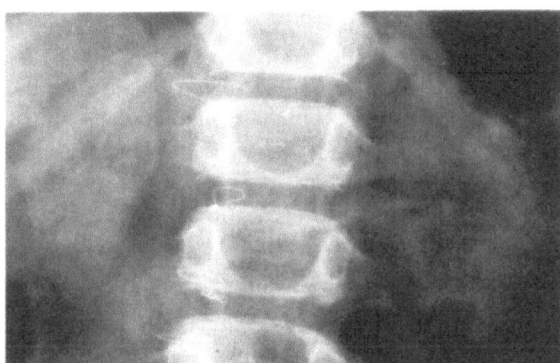

Fig. 2.37. Medullary cystic disease. Urogram with nonfunction of bilaterally small, smoothly contoured kidneys

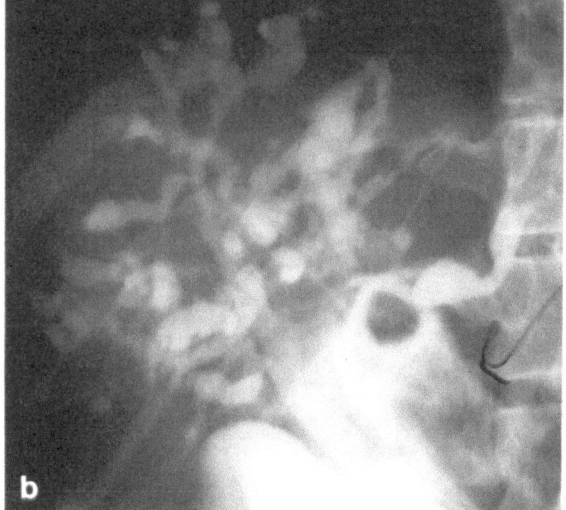

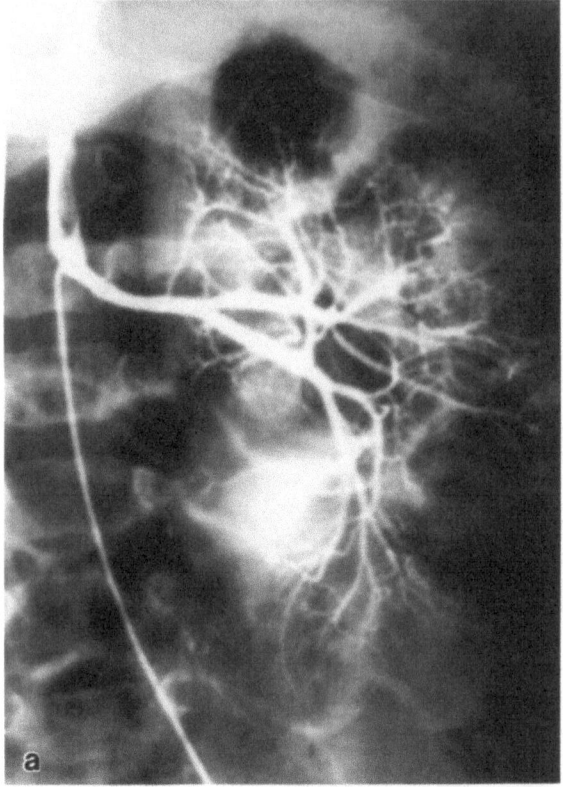

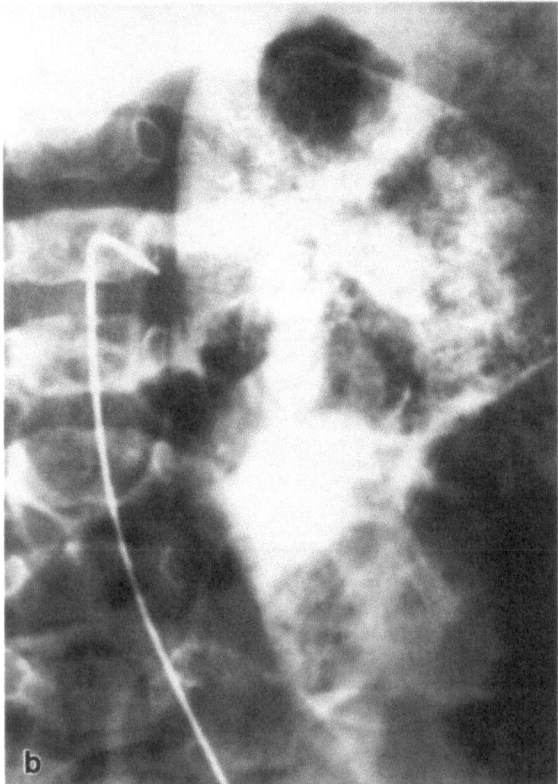

Fig. 2.38 a, b. Angiograms of medullary cystic disease showing cysts of varying size in a smoothly outlined kidney

tumor into a clinical spectrum of benign CMN, cellular/atypical CMN, and clear cell sarcoma. Benign CMN tends to present very early (within the first 3 months of life) as an abdominal mass, often with hypertension, and less often with urinary abnormalities, hematuria, or polyhydramnios. The IVP and CT appearances do not distinguish benign CMN from other solid masses; a sonographic "ring sign," a hyperechoic rim with a hypoechoic outer rim, has been reported as being typical (CHAN et al. 1987). However, since there is some difficulty in making an exact diagnosis on the basis of roentgenographic examinations, surgery is usually performed. Benign CMN may contain small areas of high mytotic rate and even hemorrhage, and may show microscopic extension through the renal capsule into the perirenal fascia. The more aggressive cellular/atypical CMN contains similar tissue elements as a benign lesion but with greater nuclear atypia, larger areas of high mytotic rate, larger areas of necrosis and hemorrhage, possibly local invasion of adjacent organs, and local or distant recurrence. Atypical CMNs tend to be larger tumors and to manifest in older infants than benign CMNs but with similar presenting signs and symptoms. Atypical CMNs may be inhomogeneous on both ultrasound and CT. Benign CMN can be managed by nephrectomy without chemotherapy or radiation, while atypical CMN may warrant adjuvant chemotherapy, particularly if the surgical margins are not clear.

2.4.9 Ask-Upmark Kidney

The Ask-Upmark kidney has previously been classified as a form of renal hypoplasia of developmental origin, but is probably not hypoplastic at all. The lesion as described in 1929 showed focal atrophic glomerular nephritis which formed a deep transverse scar or scars in an otherwise small kidney, with accompanying hypertension (Fig. 2.39). The scar is situated over a dilated calyx, which is typical of reflex nephropathy, and the lesion was originally considered to be developmental in nature due to its histologic appearance, with a near total absence of glomerular elements and a paucity of inflammatory infiltrates being seen on the original specimens. The lesion is more common in females and hypertension is always associated with it. In some cases the renin-angiotension axis is clearly implicated in the hypertension, while in other cases this is not clear-cut. More recent investigators (JOHNSTON und MIX 1976; HODSON 1974) have shown that the lesion can clearly be acquired during the course of childhood, with both hypertension and scars appearing in previously asymptomatic normal patients. Similar lesions can be experimentally induced in pigs. In unilateral Ask-Upmark kidney, nephrectomy is curative of hypertension.

2.5 Fusion Anomalies

2.5.1 Horseshoe Kidney

Horseshoe kidney is the most common of the renal fusion anomalies, occurring in 1/400 to 1/700 of the population. Males appear to be more often affected (2:1) in some series. This anomaly develops at approximately the 7th gestational week, after the ureteric buds have contacted the metanephric blastema, but before the ascent and rotation of the kidneys. At this time the kidneys are relatively close together, and for unknown reasons, the metanephric blastema may fuse. In almost all cases, the fusion is in the lower poles. The isthmus that joins the kidneys is usually parenchymatous but may be a fibrous band. Fusion interferes with renal ascent and rotation of the kidneys. Many other congenital abnormalities have been associated with horseshoe kidney, but there are no specific associations. The increased incidence of this condition has been noted in both trisomy 18 and Turner's syndrome.

Radiologically, plain films will show the kidneys more medially and inferior to the normal position, with the long axis of each of the kidneys more vertical or directed caudomedially (i.e., with the inferior poles closer together). On urography the isthmus can usually be seen during the nephrographic phase unless it is purely fibrous in nature. As in all cases of ectopia or fusion, malrotation is present (Fig. 2.40). The calyces are directed laterally or posteriorly, with the renal pelvis opening anteriorly. The inferior calyces are frequently more medial than the superior calyces. Varying degrees of hydronephrosis may be seen secondary to poor drainage of the renal pelvis or secondary to narrowing of the ureters which course anteriorly over the isthmus (which is anteriorly placed) and frequently dig into the parenchyma, which may restrict flow. High insertion of the ureters in the renal pelvis may contribute to the hydronephrosis. In addition, the vascular supply is from the lower aorta, with numerous anomalous vessels which may cross the ureters and compress them. Aberrant arteries may come from the inferior aorta, inferior mesenteric artery, common iliac arteries, and rarely, external and internal iliac arteries.

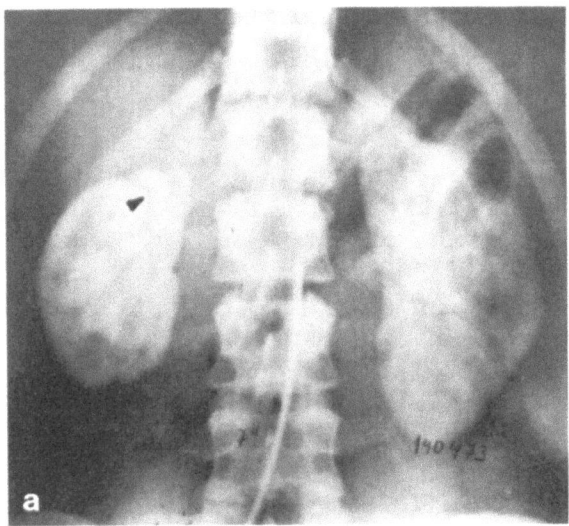

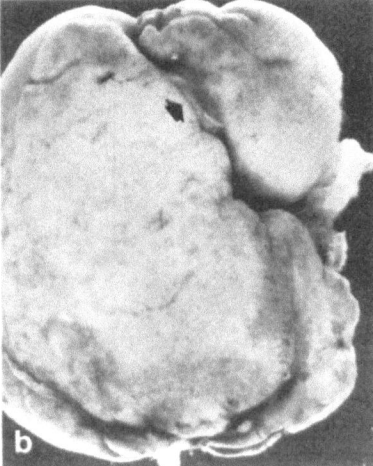

Fig. 2.39 a, b. Ask-Upmark kidney. **a** Nephrogram showing scarring *(arrowhead)* in the upper pole of the right kidney. **b** Specimen photograph showing transverse scar *(arrow)*. (From NEY and FRIEDENBERG 1981)

Additional ureters may exist, as horseshoe kidney can occur with duplication of the collecting systems (Figs. 2.41, 2.42).

The complications of horseshoe kidney are principally related to urinary stasis, infection, and stone formation. In addition, renal cell and squamous cell carcinoma of the pelvis appear to be slightly increased in frequency in these patients, probably related to the greater likelihood of chronic irritation. Virtually all renal lesions have been reported in horseshoe kidney, but they do not appear to occur with increased frequency.

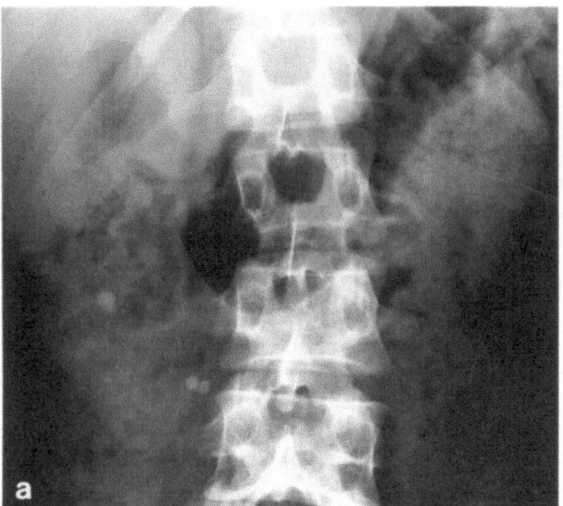

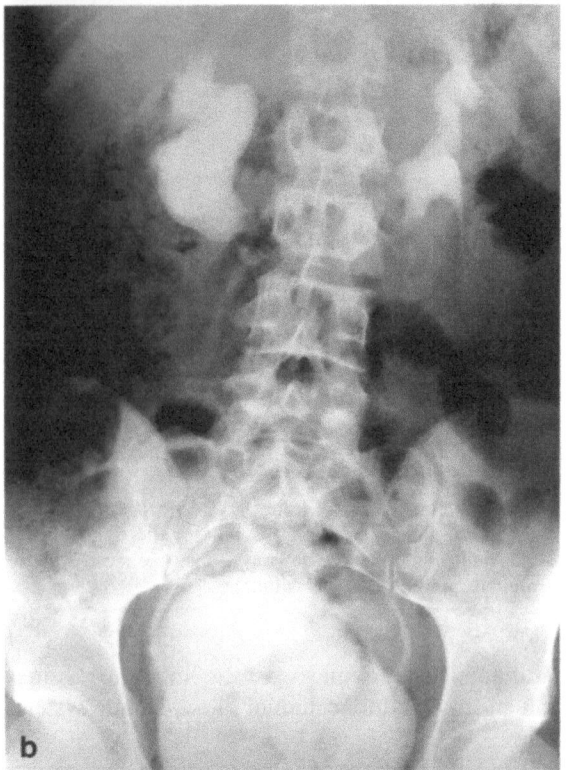

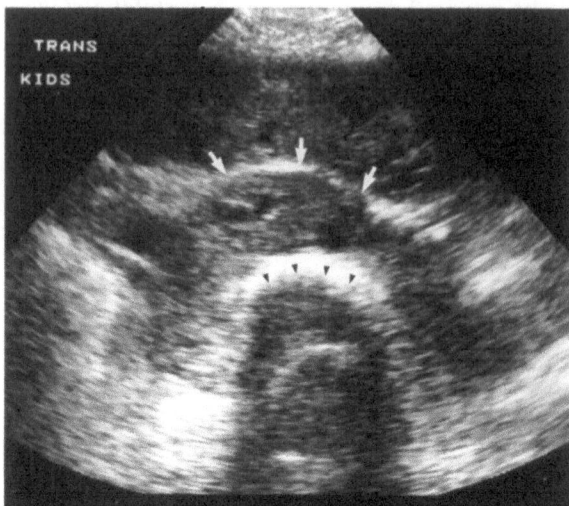

Fig. 2.41. Horseshoe kidney. Sonogram in the midline shows the isthmus of a horseshoe kidney *(arrows)* anterior to the spine *(arrowheads)*

Fig. 2.42 a–c. Horseshoe kidney. **a** CT image at the level of ▷ the upper poles of a horseshoe kidney. **b** CT image through the midthird of a horseshoe kidney showing slight hydronephrosis bilaterally. **c** CT scan through the lower pole of a horseshoe kidney showing the collecting system in the isthmus of functional tissue

This mass usually does not ascend out of the pelvis and generally retains two ureters, although occasionally only one ureter is present (Fig. 2.43). There is no rotation of the kidneys so the ureters emerge anteriorly. Poor drainage due to distortion of the collecting systems may lead to hydronephrosis with stone formation and infection as complications. The parenchyma may show cyst formation and immature elements may be found. Often, this anomaly is seen in association with serious anomalies in other systems of the body, including the cardiovascular, skeletal, and gastrointestinal systems and the CNS.

2.5.3 Crossed Ectopy

A variation of the theme of fusion is seen in crossed ectopy. The frequency of various types of crossed ectopy in autopsy is approximately 1/4000 cases. In all cases, the ureters arise from the bladder in normal fashion (Fig. 2.44). The renal masses are ectopic, usually with both fused and on one side (Fig. 2.45). The lower kidney is the crossed kidney. Rarely, crossed renal ectopy occurs without fusion of the masses. Bilaterally crossed kidneys, with each ureter crossing midline to reach its ureter vesicular junction, is less common. Occasionally there is a solitary

Fig. 2.40 a, b. Horseshoe kidney. **a** Scout film showing calculi in the inferior pole of the right moiety and in the isthmus of a horseshoe kidney. The vertical orientation of the kidneys can be seen. **b** Right hydronephrosis and malrotation of the left half of a horseshoe kidney can be seen

2.5.2 Lump Kidney

Cake/disk/lump kidney is the most extreme form of renal fusion, with the two metanephric blastemas entirely merged into a single more or less midline mass of varying shape (hence the various names).

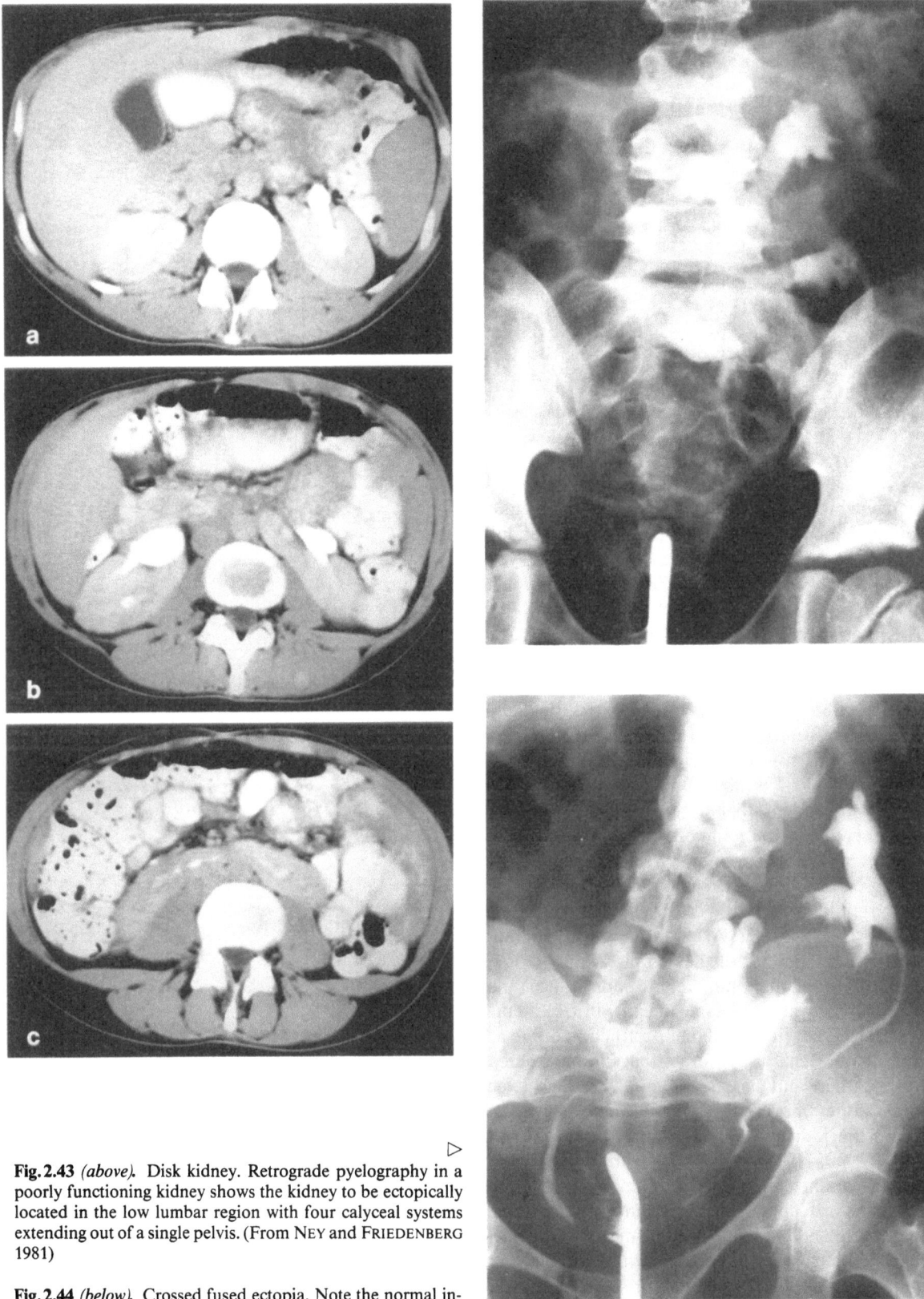

Fig. 2.43 *(above)*. Disk kidney. Retrograde pyelography in a poorly functioning kidney shows the kidney to be ectopically located in the low lumbar region with four calyceal systems extending out of a single pelvis. (From NEY and FRIEDENBERG 1981)

Fig. 2.44 *(below)*. Crossed fused ectopia. Note the normal insertion of the ureters into the bladder. (From NEY and FRIEDENBERG 1981)

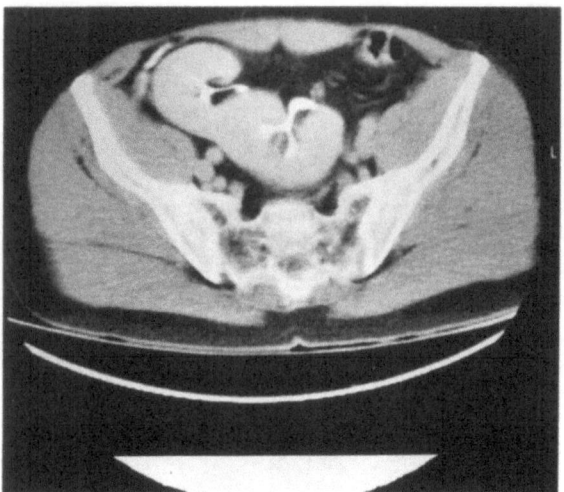

Fig. 2.45. Ectopic fused kidneys. CT image of fused kidneys in the pelvis shows malrotation of the kidneys

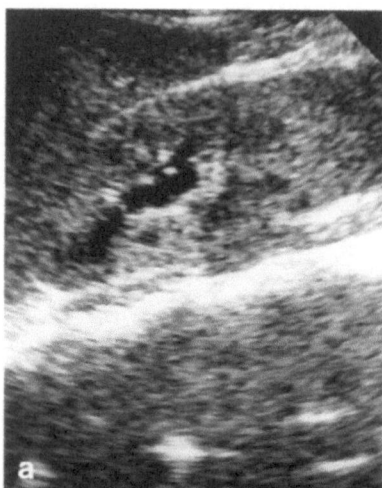

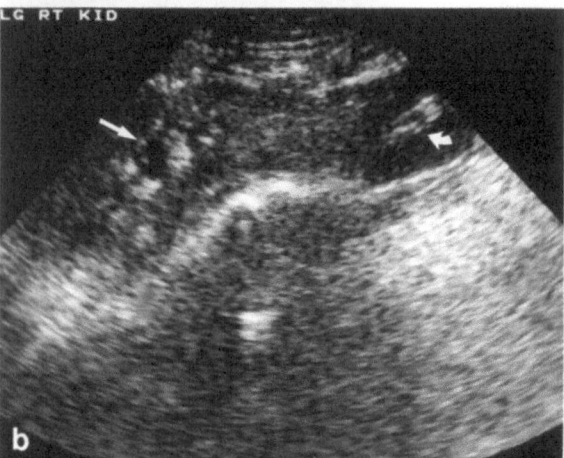

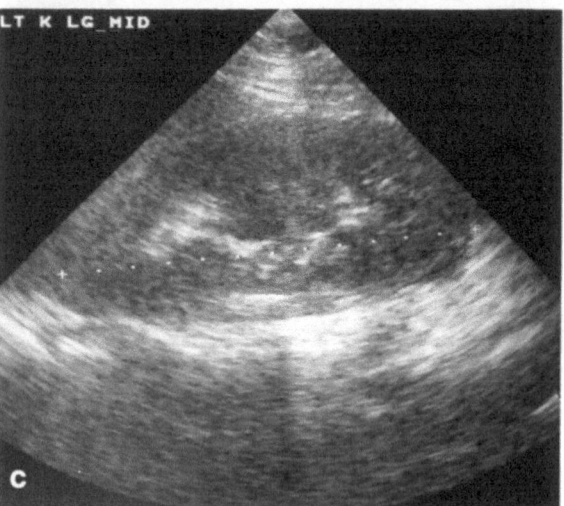

kidney which is crossed (contralateral to its uretero-vesicular junction). The vascular supply is variably abnormal to the ectopic kidneys. Generally the superior kidney is ipsilateral to its ureter and is near normal in location and may be normally rotated. The inferior renal mass has crossed to the opposite side from its ureter; it is usually fused, with its superior pole connected to the inferior pole of the uncrossed kidney, and is always malrotated (Fig. 2.46). The ureter from the superior kidney may be displaced by the crossed ectopic renal mass. The ureter from the crossed kidney crosses over to the contralateral side and inserts normally. Varying degress of hydronephrosis are common. Crossed unfused ectopy is much less common. In such cases the two kidneys are discrete, each within its own capsule.

The etiology of crossed ectopy is an enigma. Some authors (POTTER 1952; ALEXANDER et al. 1950) hold that the ureteric bud of the ectopic kidney crosses the midline and that both ureteric buds induce renal parenchyma within the same metanephric blastema. WILMER (1938) suggested that obstruction of the ascent of one renal mass forces that kidney to cross over. ASHLEY and MOSTOFI (1960) held that the ectopic kidney moves due to an attractive force that draws the kidney to its abnormal location. COOK and STEVENS (1977) suggested that abnormal flexion of the caudal end of the developing fetus might cause the usual buds (which are anterior structures) to develop and grow into a single metanephric blastema (which is a posterior structure). FRIEDLAND and DE VRIES (1975) suggested on the basis of anatomic studies that inhibition of growth of the blastema at the appropriate embryonic stage causes the

Fig. 2.46 a–c. Supernumerary fused kidneys. **a** Sonogram showing the right renal parenchyma extending too far inferiorly. **b** Sonogram at the inferior pole of the right kidney showing parenchyma extending from the inferior right renal collecting system *(arrow)* to the superior end of the supernumerary fused renal collecting system *(curved arrow)*. **c** Sonogram of the normal left renal mass

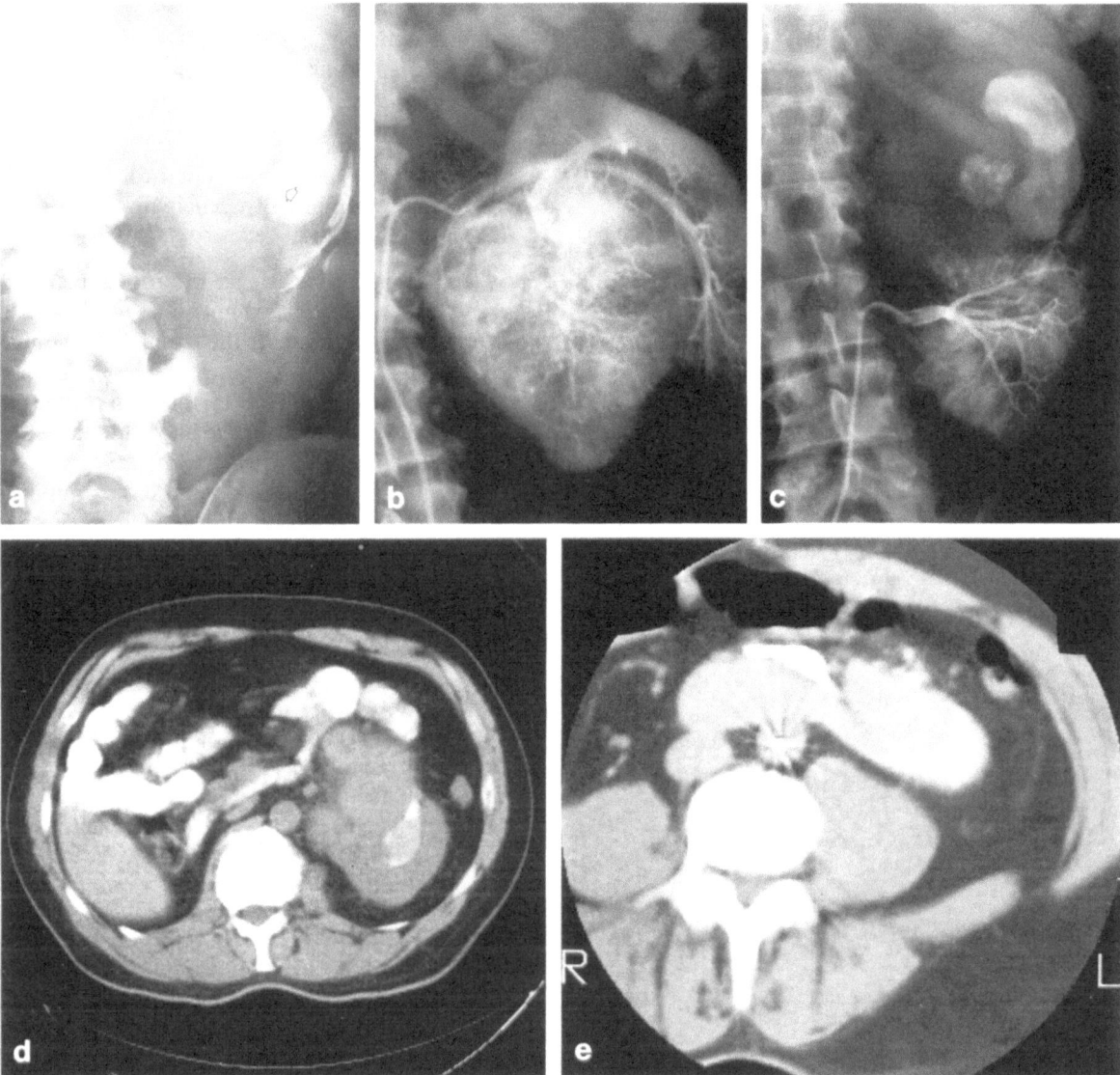

Fig. 2.47. a Intravenous urogram showing a crossed ectopic kidney, hydronephrosis of the superior calyceal group of the left kidney, and effacement of calyces by what appears to be a mass. **b** Selective arteriogram of the left kidney demonstrating a huge renal cell carcinoma central in the left kidney. **c** Selective arteriogram of the upper moiety of the crossed ectopic kidney showing normal renal parenchyma. There are, however, a few abnormal vessels filling from this injection. The anatomy made possible management by heminephrectomy of the crossed ectopic moiety and radical nephrectomy of the left kidney harboring the bulk of the tumor. **d** Computed tomogram demonstrating the centrally located renal cell carcinoma in the left kidney. A small soft calculus is also shown. Note absence of the right kidney. **e** The lower moiety of the crossed ectopic kidney extends across the midline

various ectopies and fusion abnormalities. The adrenal glands, being of unrelated origin, are usually normally placed in cases of renal crossed ectopy. Crossed fused ectopy has been reported to have a higher association with vertebral anorectal anomalies. Renal neoplasms may occur, though not with increased frequency (Fig. 2.47).

Occasionally during the development of the kidney the anterior and posterior renal lobes are malpositioned in relation to each other, leading to various deformities of renal outline. The wolffian duct usually seeks out the various lobes in whatever position they may be, providing a calyx and collecting tubules for the pyramid present within the lobe. One variation of this is the "L-shaped" kidney, where the upper or lower pole may extend perpendicular to

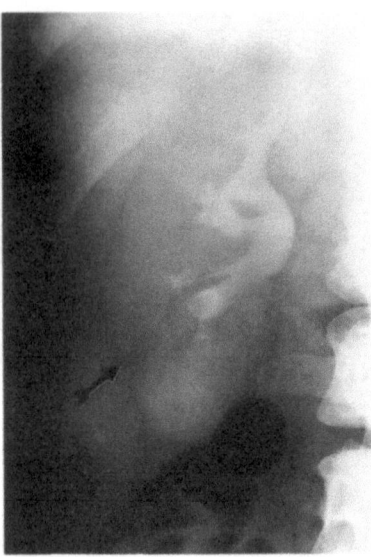

Fig. 2.48. Fetal lobation *(arrow)*. Note the normal thickness of the renal cortex and the absence of calyceal abnormalties

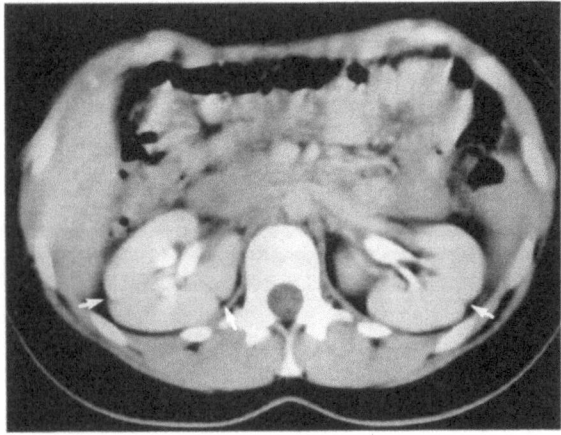

Fig. 2.49. Fetal lobation. CT image shows fetal lobation bilaterally *(arrows)* with preservation of the renal cortex and undilated calyces

the kidney (posteriorly) and will only be visualized in oblique or lateral views.

2.5.4 Renal Pseudotumors

Pseudotumor is defined as a deformation or tumefaction of normal renal tissue which mimics an abnormal mass. They may be classified as congenital and acquired:

Congenital pseudotumor
- Fetal Lobation
- Infrahilar and suprahilar bulges

- Dromedary hump
- Column of Bertin
- Cortical dysmorphism
- Ectopic papilla

Acquired pseudotumor
- Residual normal parenchyma in focal disease
- Hypertrophy of normal parenchyma in areas of focal destruction

Fetal lobation is the persistence of grooves between the renal lobes due to incomplete fusion of these lobes in utero. In such cases the parenchymal bulge is directly over the calyx, and the grooves are directly over the septa of Bertin. Fetal lobation can occur in either kidney and may persist into adult life (4%) (Figs. 2.48, 2.49). *Infrahilar and suprahilar bulges* are unusually prominent areas of renal cortex impinging on the renal pelvis. Since the parenchyma is normally thicker at the poles, any additional tissue on the medial edge of either renal pole will appear comparatively conspicuous. The *dromedary hump* is a normal variant seen in the left kidney, where there is flattening of the curvature of the renal contour from pressure from the adjacent spleen and a bulge just below that level. Upon closer inspection, the cortical thickness between the calyces and the renal outline will be seen to be normal. It is generally felt that the presence of the spleen contributes to the deformity of the renal outline.

A more important minor fusion variant which may mimic a tumor is a prominent *column of Bertin*. This was described by KING et al. (1968) as an unusual prominence of normal cortical tissue usually situated between the upper and middle infundibula of the kidney simulating a mass. HODSON (1972) analyzed the anatomic basis of this finding in detail and concluded that septum ("column") is a mistranslation of the original French and is an unusually prominent remnant of the cortex that lines the sides of renal lobes in the fetus. On urography, the cortical tissue in the column of Bertin near the center of the kidney may displace or compress the collecting system, but appears as normal cortical tissue on the nephrographic phase and has no abnormal vessels on angiography (Figs. 2.50, 2.51). Differentiation from a tumor can be made on scintigraphy with a cortical agent (technetium 99 m glucoheptonate or technetium 99 m DMSA). A mass will be cold while normal renal tissue such as a large cortical column takes up the tracer.

Lobar dysmorphism is a related phenomenon. This represents a malpositioned renal lobe containing cortex and medulla (pyramid and papilla) (Fig. 2.52). The malpositioned lobe may be buried near

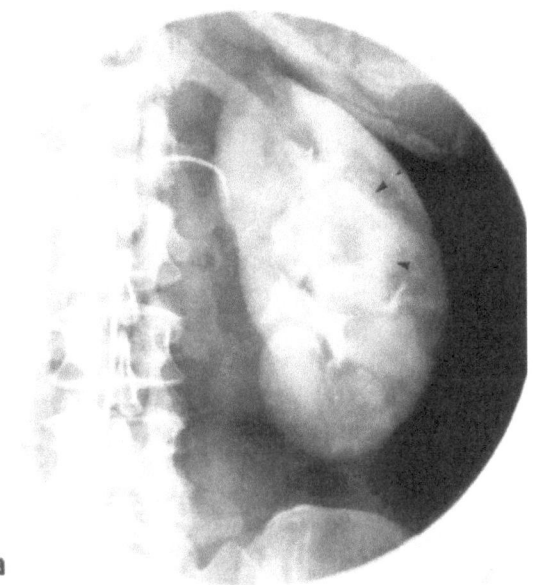

Fig. 2.50. a Nephrographic phase of a selective renal arteriogram demonstrating a tongue of tissue *(arrowheads)* extending between the superior and midcalyceal infundibulum with a staining quality characteristic of cortex, a typical column of Bertin (courtesy of E. K. LANG). b Enhancement phase of a computed tomogram demonstrating the ring-shaped extension of cortical tissues *(arrowheads)* and identical staining quality of these tissue elements with renal cortex (courtesy of E. K. LANG). c Technetium 99 m glucoheptonate scan demonstrating the normal, if not slightly increased, accumulation of radionuclide in the region of the column of Bertin *(arrow)*

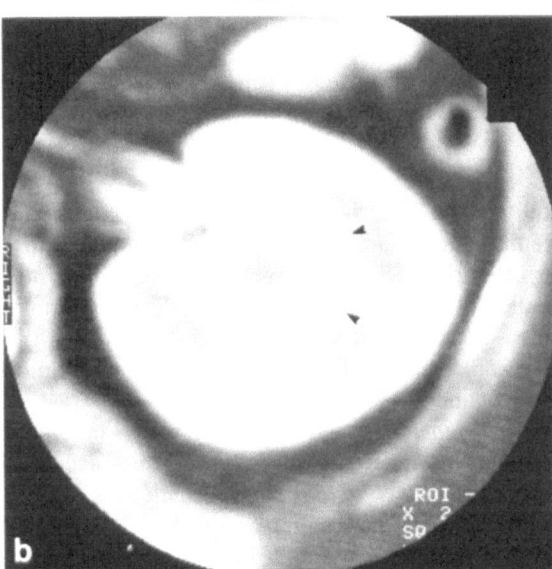

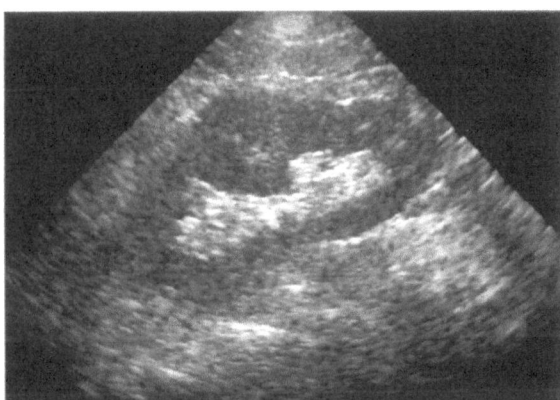

Fig. 2.51. Septum of Bertin. Sonogram shows parenchyma indenting the central echo complex

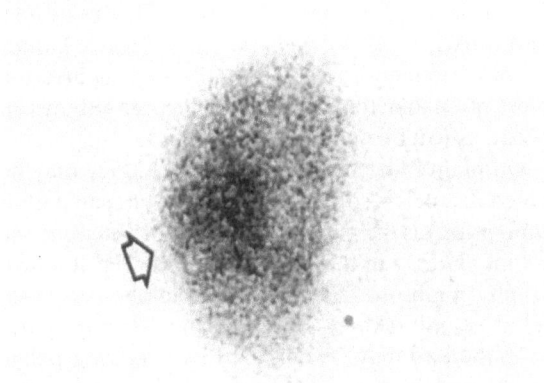

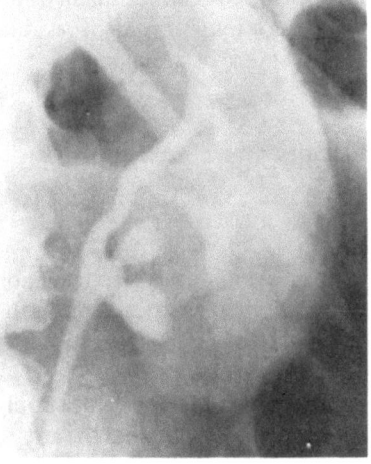

Fig. 2.52. Lobar dysmorphism. Two lobes of the inferior pole drain separately into the renal pelvis. (From NEY and FRIEDENBERG 1981)

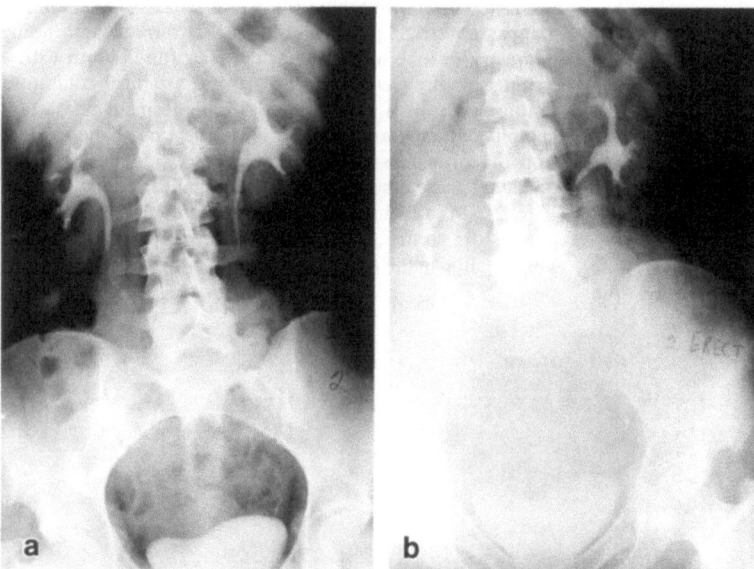

Fig. 2.53a, b. Nephroptosis. **a** Urogram with the patient supine shows the kidneys in normal position. **b** Erect image shows descent of the right kidney, which now overlies the iliac crest

the renal pelvis, in which case it is seen as a mass distorting the collecting system, or it may protrude on the renal surface, where it presents as a cortical mass. In either case, examination of the nephrogram should show both a dense cortical component to the "mass" and a "central lucency" due to the medulla as described by DACIE in 1976. On angiography, no tumor vessels will be present. Scintigraphy will confirm the presence of normal renal parenchyma.

An ectopic papilla is another form of renal pseudotumor. Protrusion of the papilla into an infundibulum or pelvis can mimic an intraluminal mass.

Acquired pseudotumors are most commonly seen in chronic focal pyelonephritis (reflux nephropathy). They are, as stated above, either residual normal parenchyma which appears overly prominent as the kidney around it shrinks or hypertrophy of residual parenchyma in areas of severe destruction.

2.6 Positional Anomalies

2.6.1 Ectopy and Ptosis

An ectopic kidney is one which has a fixed position outside of the renal fossa, whereas in renal ptosis the kidney resides in the renal fossa but fails to stay in its normal position during positional changes.

In *ptotic kidneys* the ureters and vascular supply are normal. When the kidney descends, the ureter becomes redundant. The kidney usually moves positionally by gravity (Fig. 2.53). The ability to move is secondary to loss of anatomic renal supports and a

rather long renal vasculature. It is more common in females and more common on the right side. Ptosis is often defined as movement of at least one and a half to two vertebral bodies. Lesser degrees of movement are common with respiration and normal gravitational change. Ptosis is generally of no clinical significance.

The *ectopic kidney* is a kidney which has never been in the renal fossa. It has either not ascended from the pelvis or partially ascended or overascended, sometimes as high as the chest. The arterial blood supply for ectopic kidneys is variable, arising from the neighboring great vessels in the area of the kidney. Ectopic kidneys in general are malrotated. On autopsy series (DRETLER et al. 1971, ABESHOUSE and BHISITKUL 1959), the frequency of pelvic kidney is approximately 1/1000, with males being affected more often than females. Solitary ectopic kidney can occur, as can bilateral ectopic kidney.

On plain film, the absence of one kidney may be noted or a pelvic soft tissue mass may be seen. Ultrasonography is the method of choice for detecting the ectopic kidney in the pelvis (Fig. 2.54). During urography, nephrotomography may be particularly useful as ectopic kidneys are often small and irregular in shape and may be obscured by overlying pelvic bones and bowel gas. Careful evaluation is suggested prior to implicating the pelvic kidney as the site of disease (Fig. 2.55). Reports have suggested an increased incidence of genital abnormalities in these cases, with up to 45% of females (DOWNS et al. 1973) and 20% of males (THOMPSON and PACE 1937) being thus affected (Fig. 2.56).

Special mention must be made of thoracic kidneys. Renal ascent may continue past the renal fossa and into the chest on rare occasions. The diaphragm at 7–8 weeks is in the form of a pleural peritoneal membrane and only later acquires mesenchymal elements. In this relatively thin form, pressure of an ascending kidney may create an eventration or perhaps even perforation of the membrane. A distinction should be made between thoracic kidneys and diaphragmatic hernia (either congenital or acquired) when several viscera may be present in the chest and not the kidney alone.

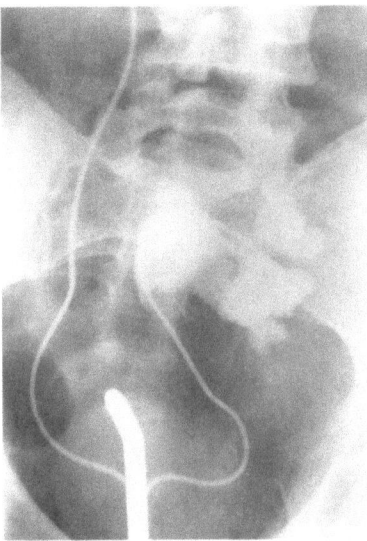

Fig. 2.55. Ectopic kidney. The left kidney is ectopic anterior to the sacrum with changes of chronic pyelonephritis and pyonephrosis present. Calculi can be seen inferior to the lower calyces

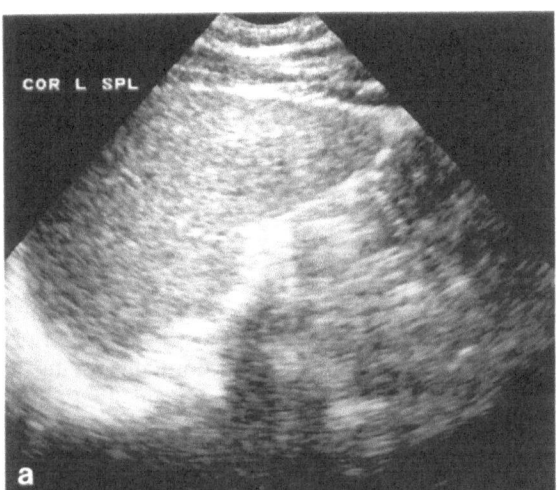

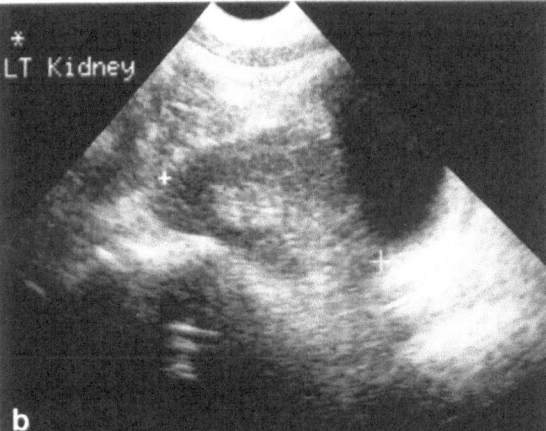

Fig. 2.54 a, b. Ectopic kidney. **a** The left renal fossa adjacent to the spleen is empty. **b** Pelvic image in the same patient showing the left kidney to lie adjacent to the bladder

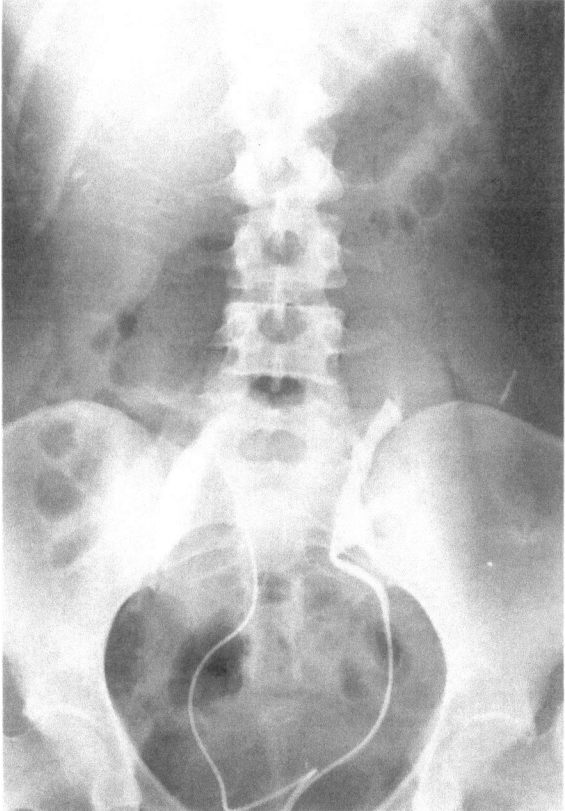

Fig. 2.56. Bilateral ectopic kidneys. Bilateral uncrossed nonfused kidneys are seen. The right kidney is nonrotated and the ureteropelvic junction on the right is abnormally high. Note the appropriate length of the ureters to their position, indicating that they have not decended to this position

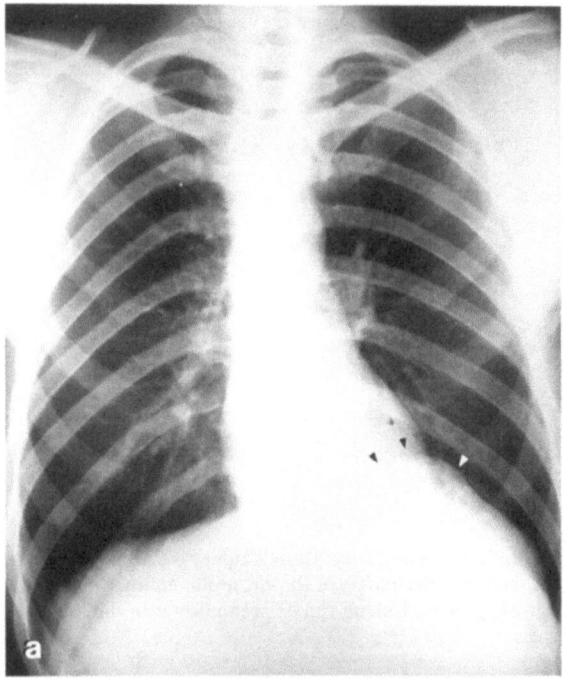

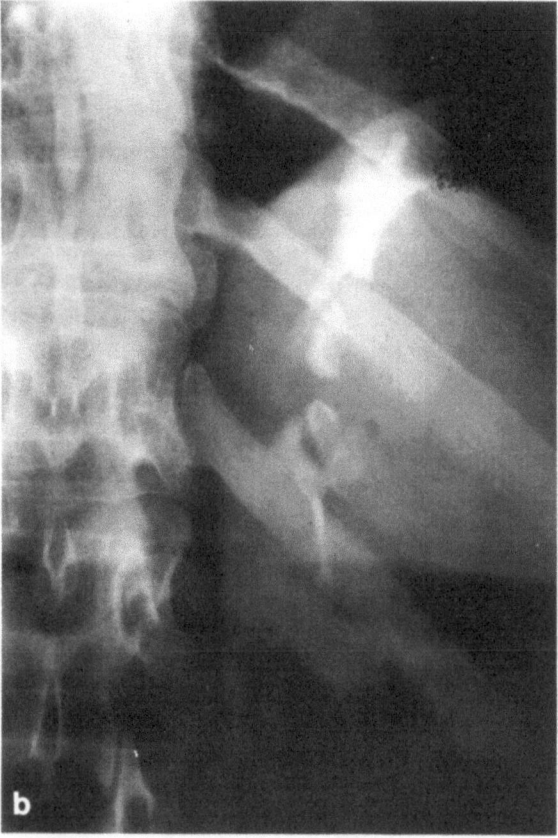

Fig. 2.57. **a** Thoracic kidney. Posteroanterior chest radiograph shows the superior pole of a thoracic kidney as a posterobasal mass in the left chest *(arrowheads)*. **b** Urography confirms the presence of the collecting system in this mass. (From NEY and FRIEDENBERG 1981)

Thoracic kidney occurs primarily on the left side of the chest, posteromedially in the area of the foramen of Bochdalek. Right-sided thoracic kidneys are less likely for similar reasons that right-sided diaphragmatic hernias are less common, i.e., early fusion of the pleural peritoneal membrane on that side and/or the presence of the liver serves as an obstacle to ascent. There is a male preponderance in thoracic kidneys of 3:1 or 4:1 (LOZANO and RODRIGUEZ 1975; MALTER and STANLEY 1972). Thoracic kidneys have been described at all ages, being usually discovered as an incidental finding.

The thoracic kidney on chest x-ray is a smoothly contoured, rounded, homogeneously dense mass in the posteromedial aspect of the left hemithorax (Fig. 2.57). IVP will confirm the diagnosis and show a long but otherwise unremarkable ureter. The kidney is usually malrotated. A thin membrane may cover the top of the kidney and separate it from the pleural space, excluding the diagnosis of true herniation. Such a membrane is best demonstrable by pneumoperitoneum, but this is rarely necessary for the diagnosis. The adrenal gland may or may not accompany the kidney in its ascent.

2.6.2 Malrotation

In the normal course of development, the kidneys prior to ascent have the renal pelvis facing anteriorly. During ascent, the kidneys normally rotate on their long axes so the pelves open medially. Failure of normal rotation is common and probably underdiagnosed, being of little clinical significance. CAMPBELL in 1963 found malrotation in 1/900 autopsies, with a male preponderance of 2:1. Several varieties of malrotation can occur, i.e., around the long axis of the kidney, along the anteroposterior axis of the kidney, or along the transverse axis of the kidney. The latter two types of malrotation are less common and of less importance as the relationship of the ureter and renal vessels vis-à-vis the parenchyma is relatively unchanged by these types of malrotation.

Long axis rotation abnormalities are those of nonrotation, underrotation, overrotation, and reverse rotation. In the first instance the renal pelvis continues to open anteriorly and calyces point medially and laterally (Figs. 2.58–2.60), while in underrotation the pelvis is partially medial but some calyces point laterally. Overrotation results in the renal pelvis turning past its medial position to end up dorsally. In these cases the renal vessels also pass dorsal to the parenchyma to enter the hilus. Reverse rotation results in the pelvis turning laterally to end up

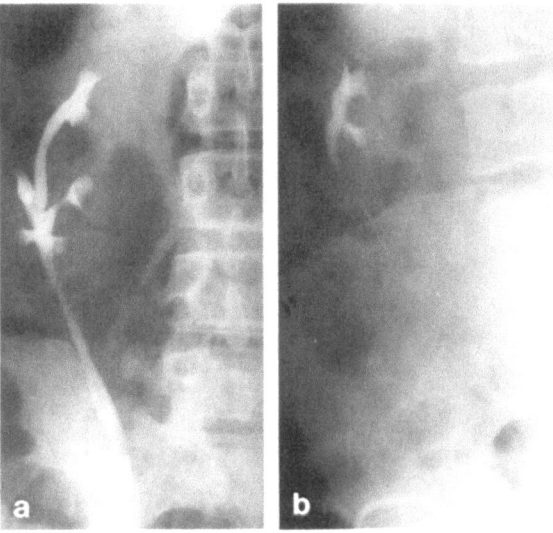

Fig. 2.58. Malrotation of the kidneys. A nonrotated right kidney with a narrow renal outline can be seen. The collecting system is directed anteriorly and the ureter exits anteriorly. (From NEY and FRIEDENBERG 1981)

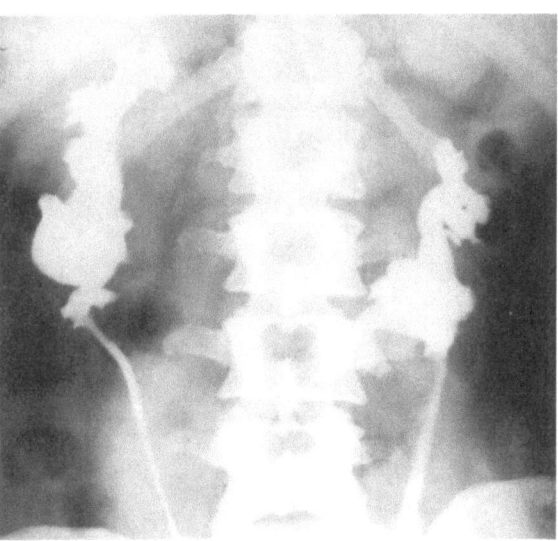

Fig. 2.60. Bilateral nonrotation. Both kidneys show shortened infundibula with the calyces directed both medial and lateral to the pelvis due to nonrotation. (From NEY and FRIEDENBERG 1981)

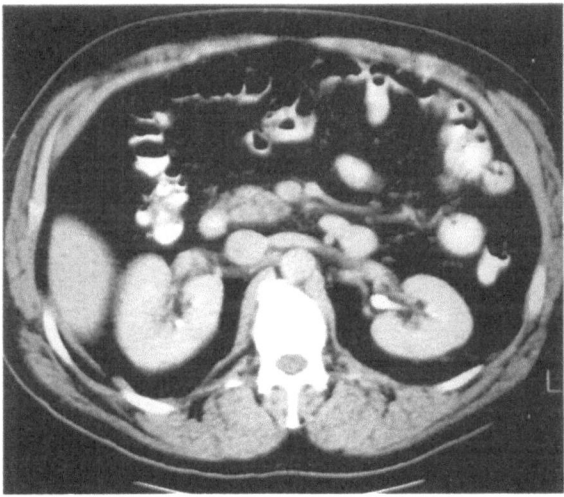

Fig. 2.59. Nonrotated right kidney. CT image shows the renal pelvis opening anteriorly

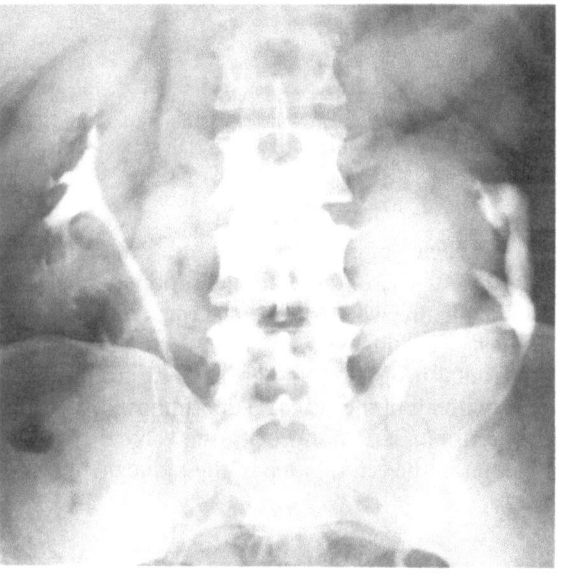

Fig. 2.61. Reverse rotation. The left kidney shows reverse rotation with the collecting system directed laterally. Slight pyelectasis is seen

facing lateral, with the renal vessels passing anterior to the renal mass to reach the hilus (Fig. 2.61). In addition to change in orientation, some distortion of the normal anatomy frequently occurs. The renal mass will be of variable shape with flattening of the anterior and posterior surfaces (Fig. 2.62). Fetal lobation may well be visible. Distortion of the renal pelvis and ureteropelvic junction may occur due to an excess of fibrous tissue in the hilus. The renal vas-

cular supply not only varies with the type of rotation but may include accessory renal vessels. No specific symptoms result from malrotation, but poor drainage of the collecting system along with possible vascular compression by accessory vessels may produce hydronephrosis. In addition to hydronephrosis, infection and stone formation may occur.

Rotation along the anteroposterior *axis* of the kidney is unimportant and usually results in the supe-

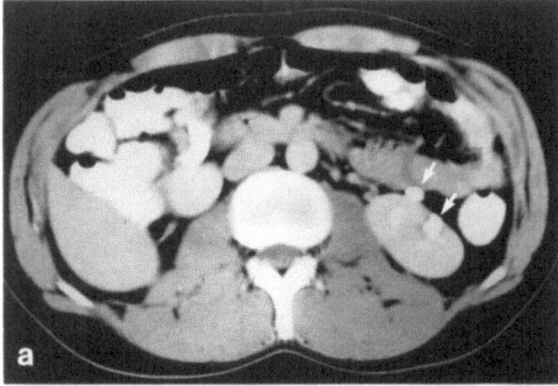

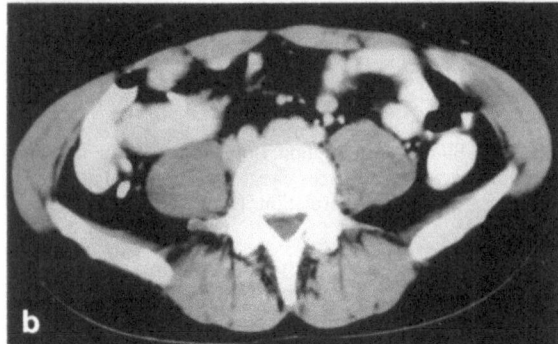

Fig. 2.62 a, b. Malrotation and ectopy. **a** The left kidney is seen to be malrotated with the collecting system and ureter lying anterolaterally *(arrows)*. **b** The right kidney is ectopic with its lower pole overlying the iliac wing

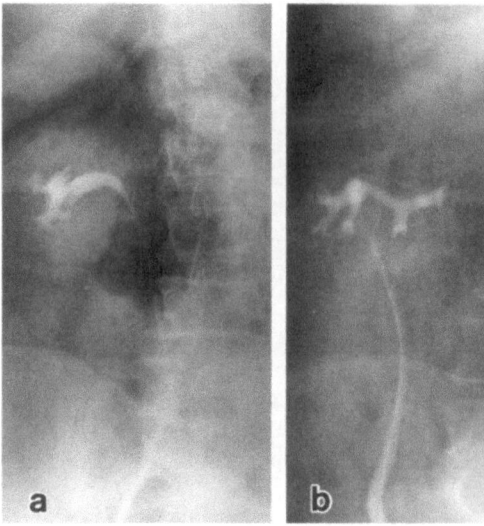

Fig. 2.63. Transverse axis malrotation. The collecting system is viewed "on-end" on the anteroposterior image. The lateral view shows the lower pole to be more anterior than usual. (From NEY and FRIEDENBERG 1981)

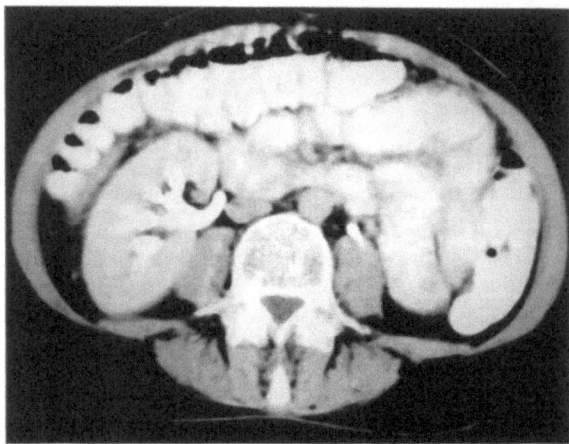

Fig. 2.64. Transverse axis malrotation. The right kidney is malrotated on its transverse axis with the lower pole directed anteriorly on the CT image

rior pole being more laterally placed. Rotation along the *transverse axis* of the kidney produces a characteristic picture, which has been termed a "tennis ball kidney". The kidney rotates in such a manner that in the frontal projection you are looking from pole to pole, with all of the calyces superimposed. The kidney then appears round, with the calyces bunched together in the central area of the kidney (Figs. 2.63, 2.64).

2.7 Extrarenal Anomalies

Vascular anomalies of the kidney are extremely common, particularly in association with fusion and positional anomalies. As the kidneys ascend in the embryo, they connect with successive pairs of arteries along their course, the connection disappearing as the kidneys ascend past that level. Thus the numerous unusual vascular paths described for unusually placed fused kidneys reflect the embryonic circulation at the stage when renal ascent is halted. Even in the normal position, 15%–29% of all kidneys have more than one renal artery (GEYER and POUTASSE 1962; MERKLIN and MICHAELS 1958). The most common additional vessels are polar arteries, particularly to the lower pole of the kidney.

Vascular anomalies are principally of interest to the surgeon. However, on occasion the accessory lower pole artery may cross the ureter or the ureteropelvic junction. This probably is not in itself a primary cause of obstruction but may contribute to hydronephrosis if other factors are present. The IVP will show a bandlike oblique defect at the level of the obstruction (Figs. 2.65, 2.66).

Aneurysms of the renal arteries are not uncommon, being reported in 1/8000 autopsies. Most of these

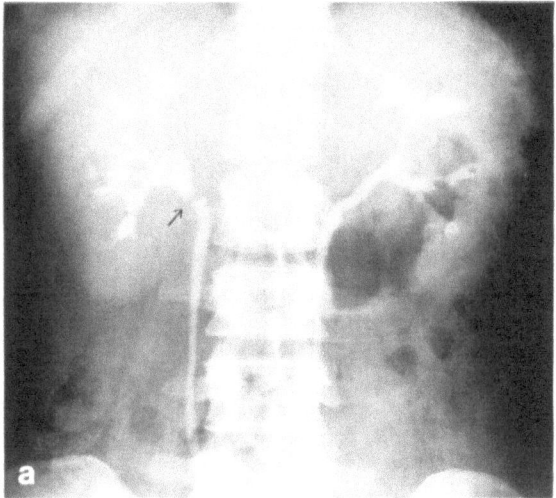

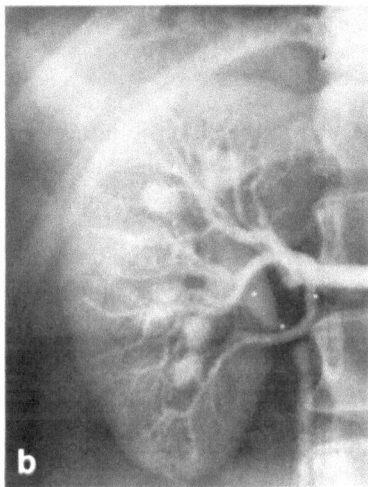

Fig. 2.65 a, b. Vascular impressions on the renal pelvis. **a** Urogram shows a band-like defect in the renal pelvis *(arrow)*. **b** Angiography shows a lower pole artery which crosses the renal pelvis at the same level. (From NEY and FRIEDENBERG 1981)

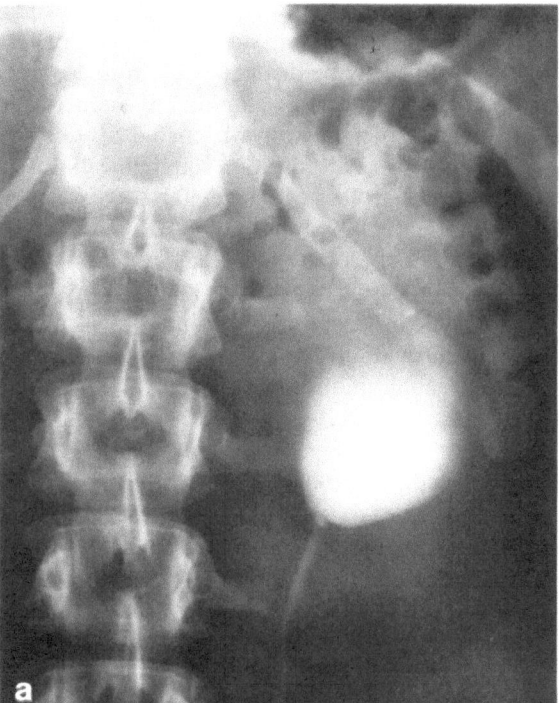

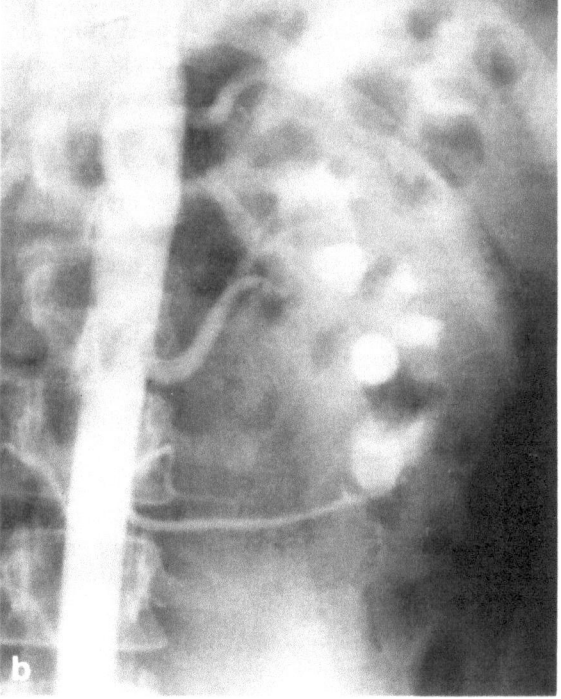

Fig. 2.66 a, b. Vascular impression at the ureteropelvic junction. **a** Hydronephrosis is seen with abrupt tapering of the renal pelvis at the level of the ureteropelvic junction. **b** Aortography shows an aberrant lower pole artery that crosses at the level

are acquired due to vascular disease, trauma, or inflammation, but perhaps one-third are felt to be congenital in origin, particularly those located at branch points of the renal arteries.

Congenital arteriovenous (AV) fistulas are uncommon, most renal fistulas being posttraumatic or idiopathic (tumor, aneurysm, etc.). The distribution of AV fistulas is equal in both sexes (MESSING et al. 1976; THOMPSON 1972), with a slight predilection for the right kidney and the upper polar region. The symptoms of congenital AV fistulas are identical to those of acquired lesions: abdominal bruit (75%), renin-induced hypertension due to ischemia caused by shunting of blood (50%), cardiac failure (50%), and macroscopic or microhematuria (75%). These lesions are not generally symptomatic until adulthood, although the presumed origin is a congenital aneurysm that erodes into an adjacent vein. These lesions can usually be distinguished from acquired AV fistulas by their angiographic appearance. The congenital AV fistulas have a cirsoid appearance with numerous small tortuous communicating vessels, which is typical of congenital AV fistulas in other locations. Urography may show a mass defect, clots in the collecting system, and/or diminished function in the ischemic areas of the kidney. Unlike acquired AV fistulas, true congenital lesions do not spontaneously resolve and require resection and/or possibly embolization and occlusion.

2.8 Congenital Hydronephrosis

Congenital hydronephrosis is a rapidly evolving field. Ultrasonography supplemented by scintigraphy has become the primary means of discovering and evaluating antenatal and postnatal dilatation of the collecting systems. Progress in the development of intrauterine intervention as well as postnatal surgery has made understanding this problem more important. The lesions causing congenital collecting system dilatation can be classified as follows:

1. *Mechanical obstruction*
   a) Upper collecting system
      - Intimal thickening of the ureteropelvic junction
      - Congenital stricture at the ureteropelvic junction
      - Aberrand vessel or band
   b) Lower collecting system
      - Ureteral valves
      - Ureterovesical junction stricture
      - Ureterocele
      - Urethral valve
2. *Functional obstruction*
   a) Aperistaltic ureteropelvic junction abnormality
   b) Aperistaltic ureterovesical junction abnormality (congenital megaloureter)
   c) Loss of abdominal muculature (prune-belly syndrome)
3. *Vesicoureteral reflux*

On IVP the signs of congenital obstruction are similar to those of obstruction in other cases, ranging from an obstructive nephrogram with moderate caliectasis, to a rim sign of parenchyma, to complete nonvisualization of the obstructed system. Voiding cystourethrography is the standard method of evaluation for vesicoureteral reflux.

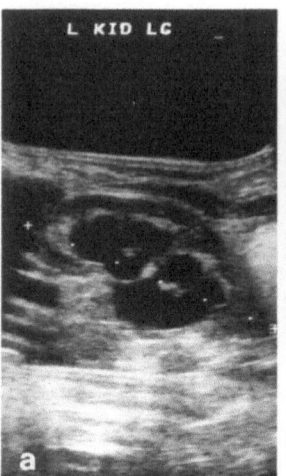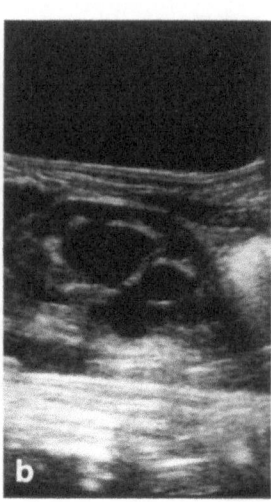

Fig. 2.67. Congenital hydronephrosis. Neonatal hydronephrosis is seen with a dilated renal pelvis and calyces and thinning of the parenchyma

With the advent of routine obstetric ultrasound and widespread neonatal ultrasound, many more cases of congenital hydronephrosis are being recognized than were seen in earlier years (Fig. 2.67). BROWN et al. (1987) reported 142 cases in the period 1979-85 ("sonography era") as compared to 146 cases in the period 1947-77 ("presonography era"). Most of the cases now being discovered are asymptomatic, when previously they presented as an abdominal mass or with signs of urosepsis. Surgical data have accumulated favoring early (within the first year of life) rather than later repair of obstructive lesions so as to maximize the recoverability of the parenchyma. However, it has also been shown that many cases of dilatation will spontaneously resolve, which creates a dilemma between maximizing recoverability of the parenchyma and avoiding unnecessary surgery. One problem is that the radiologic evaluation for this condition is imperfect. Ultrasound criteria for hydronephrosis are not uniform, although severe or increasing dilatation seems to be a clear indication for surgery. Renal scintigraphy is useful in detecting residual function in severely dilated systems and in quantifying the relative amount of renal function between the two kidneys. Studies which are designed to distinguish dilatation from obstruction are unsatisfactory – the Whittaker test is invasive and was designed to evaluate adult urinary systems, while the furosemide radionuclide washout study suffers from a lack of standardization in technique for neonates. Serial sonograms to monitor congenital hydronephrosis are necessary. The indications for and timing of surgical repair are still being evaluated.

References[1]

Abeshouse BS, Bhisitkul I (1959) Crossed renal ectopia with and without fusion. Urol Int 9: 63–91

Afonso DN, Oliveira AG (1988) Medullary sponge kidney, and congenital hemihypertrophy. Br J Urol 62: 187–188

Alexander JC, King KB, From CS (1950) Congenital solitary kidney with crossed ureter. J Urol 64: 230–234

Ambrose SS (1977) Unilateral multicystic renal disease in adults. Birth Defects 13: 349–353

Ashley DBJ, Mostofi FK (1960) Renal agenesis and dysgenesis. J Urol 83: 211–230

Athanasoulis CA, Brown B, Baum S (1973) Selective renal venography in differentiation between congenitally absent and small contracted kidney. Radiology 108: 301–305

Avni EF, Thoua Y, Van Gansbeke D, Matos C, Didier F, Droulez P, Schulman CC (1987) Development of the hypodysplastic kidney: contribution of antenatal US diagnosis. Radiology 164: 123–125

Beckwith JB (1974) Mesenchymal renal neoplasms of infancy revisited. J Pediatr Surg 9: 803–805

Bernstein J (1987) Hepatic involvement in hereditary renal syndromes. Birth Defects 23: 115–130

Boatman DL, Cornell SH, Kolln CP (1971) The arterial supply of horseshoe kidneys. AJR 113: 447–451

Boatman DL, Kolln CP, Flocks RH (1972) Congenital anomalies associated with horseshoe kidney. J Urol 107: 205–207

Bosniak MA, Ambos MA (1975) Polycystic kidney disease. Semin Roentgenol 10: 133–143

Braedel HU, Schindler E, Moeller JF, Polsky MS (1976) Renal phlebography: an aid in the diagnosis of the absent or nonfunctioning kidney. J Urol 116: 703–707

Brown T, Mandell J, Lebowitz RL (1987) Neonatal hydronephrosis in the era of sonography. AJR 148: 959–963

Buntley D (1976) Malignancy associated with horseshoe kidney. Urology 8: 146–148

Campbell MF (1928) Congenital absence of one kidney unilateral renal agenesis. Ann Surg 88: 1039–1044

Campbell MF (1963) Anomalies of the kidney. In: Campbell MF (ed.) Urology, 2nd ed., vol.2, p.1584, WB Saunders, Philadelphia

Castro JE, Green NA (1975) Complications of horseshoe kidney. Urology 6: 344–347

Chan HS, Cheng MY, Mancer K, Payton D, Weitzman SS, Kotecha P, Daneman A (1987) Congenital mesoblastic nephroma: a clinicoradiologic study of 17 cases representing the pathologic spectrum of the disease. J Pediatr 111: 64–70

Chevalier RL (1989) Obstructive nephropathy in early development. Semin Nephrol 9: 5–9

Charghi A, Dessureault P, Droiun G, Gauthier GE, Perras P, Roy P, Charbonneau J (1971) Malposition of a renal lobe (lobar dysmorphism): a condition simulating renal tumor. J Urol 105: 326–329

Cook WA, Stephens FD (1977) Fused kidneys: morphologic study and theory of embryogenesis. Birth Defects 13: 327–340

Cope JR, Trickey SE (1982) Congenital absence of the kidney: problems in diagnosis and management. J Urol 127: 10–12

Craver R, Dimmick J, Johnson H, Nigro M (1986) Congenital obstructive uropathy and nodular renal blastema. J Urol 136: 305–307

Dacie JE (1976) The "central lucency" sign of lobar dysmorphism (pseudotumor of the kidney). Br J Radiol 49: 39–42

Dajani AM (1966) Horseshoe kidney: a review of 29 cases. Br J Urol 38: 388–402

Diard F, Le Dosseur P, Cadier L, Calabet A, Bondonny JM (1984) Multicystic dysplasia in the upper component of the complete duplex kidney. Pediatr Radiol 14: 310–313

D'Alton M, Romero R, Grannum P, DePalma L, Jeanty P, Hobbins JC (1986) Antenatal diagnosis of renal anomalies with ultrasound. IV. Bilateral multicystic kidney disease. Am J Obstet Gynecol 154: 532–537

Davidson AJ (1985) Radiology of the kidney. W.B. Saunders, Philadelphia

Davies CH, Stringer DA, Whyte H, Daneman A, Mancer K (1986) Congenital hepatic fibrosis with saccular dilatation of intraphepatic bile ducts and infantile polycystic kidneys. Pediatr Radiol 16: 302–305

Diard F, Le Dosseur P, Cadier L, Calabet A, Bondonny JM (1984) Multicystic dysplasia in the upper component of the complete duplex kidney. Pediatr Radiol 14: 310–313

Dimmick JE, Johnson HW, Coleman GU, Carter M (1989) Wilms tumorlet, nodular renal blastema and multicystic renal dysplasia. J Urol 142: 484–485; discussion 489

Donaldson JS, Shkolnik A (1988) Pediatric renal masses. Semin Roentgenol 23: 194–204. Erratum: Semin Roentgenol (1989) 24: 142

Downs RA, Lane JW, Burns E (1973) Solitary pelvic kidney. Its clinical application. Urol 1: 51–56

Dreter SP, Olsson C, Pfister RC (1971) The anatomic, radiologic and clinical characteristics of the pelvic kidney: an analysis of 86 cases. J Urol 105: 623–627

Elkin M (1975) Renal cystic disease – an overview. Semin Roentgenol 10: 99–102

Elkin M (1980) Radiology of the urinary system. Little Brown & Co, Boston

Evans JA, Stranc LC (1989) Cystic renal disease and cardiovascular anomalies. Am J Med Genet 33: 398–401

Feldman AE, Pollack HM, Perri AJ jr, Karafin L, Kendall AR (1978) Renal pseudotumors: an anatomic-radiologic classification. J Urol 120: 133–139

Felson B, Cussen LJ (1975) The hydronephrotic type of unilateral congenital multicystic disease of the kidney. Semin Roentgenol 10: 113–123

Fernbach SK, Feinstein KA, Donaldson JS, Baum ES (1988) Nephroblastomatosis: comparison of CT with US and urography 166: 153–156

Fikri E, Hanrahan JB, Stept LA (1973) Renovascular hypertension in a child: Ask-Upmark kidney. J Urol 110: 728–731

Fridland GW, De Vries P (1975) Renal ectopia and fusion – embryologic basis. Urology 5: 698–706

Garcia CJ, Taylor KJ, Weiss RM (1987) Congenital megacalyces. Ultrasound appearance. J Ultrasound Med 6: 163–165

Gary R, Cass AS, Johnson CF (1988) Computed tomography diagnosis of traumatic rupture of congenital hydrohephrotic renal pelvis. Urology 32: 65–66

Geyer JR, Poutasse EF (1962) Incidence of multiple renal arteries in aortography. JAMA 182: 118

Gillerot Y, Koulischer L (1988) Major malformations of the urinary tract. Anatomic and genetic aspects. Biol Neonate 53: 186–196

Gormely TS, Skoog SJ, Jones RV, Maybee D (1989) Cellular congenital mesoblastic nephroma: what are the options? J Urol 142: 479–485; discussion 489

---

[1] This reference list contains not only those works cited in the text but also others likely to be of interest to the reader.

Graham JM Jr, Boyle W, Troxell J, Cullity GJ, Sprague PL, Beckwith JB (1987) Cystic hamartomata of the lung and kidney: a spectrum of developmental abnormalities. Am J Med Genet 27: 45–59

Greene LF, Feinzaig W, Dahlin DC (1971) Multicystic dysplasia of the kidney: with special reference to the contralateral kidney. J Urol 105: 482–487

Griscom NT, Vawter GF, Fellers FX (1975) Pelvoinfundibular atresia: the usual form of multicystic kidney: 44 unilateral and two bilateral cases. Semin Roentgenol 10: 125–131

Gunn TR, Mora JD, Pease P (1988) Outcome after antenatal diagnosis of upper urinary tract dilatation by ultrasonography. Arch Dis Child 63: 1240–1243

Guys JM, Borella F, Monfort G (1988) Ureteropelvic junction obstructions: prenatal diagnosis and surgery in 47 cases. J Pediatr Surg 23: 156–158

Hanna MK, Gluck R (1988) Ureteropelvic junction obstruction during the first year of life. Urology 31: 41–45

Harrison JH, Gittes RF, Perlmutter AD, Stamey TA, Walsh PC (1979) Campbell's urology, 4th edn, vol.2. W. B. Saunders, Philadelphia

Hartman GE, Smolik LM, Shochat SJ (1986) The dilemma of the multicystic dysplastic kidney. Am J Dis Child 140: 925–928

Hashimoto BE, Filly RA, Callen PW (1988) Multicystic dysplastic kidney in utero: changing appearance on US. Radiology 159: 107–109

Hayden CK Jr, Swischuk LE, Smith TH, Armstrong EA (1986) Renal cystic disease in childhood. Radiographics 6: 97–116

Hendren WH, Donahoe PK, Pfister RC (1976) Crossed renal ectopia in children. Urology 7: 135–144

Himmelfarb E, Rabinowitz JG, Parvey L, Gammill S, Arant B (1975) The Ask-Upmark kidney - roentgenographic and pathologic features. Am J Dis Child 129: 1440–1444

Hodson J (1972) The lobar structure of the kidney. Br J Urol 44: 246–261

Hodson CG (1974) Vesico-ureteric reflux and renal scarring with and without infection. In: Villareal H (ed.) Proceedings of the Fifth International Congress of Nephrology, Mexico. Karger, New York, Abstract p. 598

Hodson CJ, Mariani S (1982) Large cloisons. AJR 139: 327–332

Hsueh C, Hsueh W, Gonzalez-Crussi F (1987) Bilateral renal dysplasia with features of nephroblastomatosis. Pediatr Pathol 7: 437–446

Javadpour N, Chelouhy E, Moncada L, Rosenthal IM, Bush IM (1970) Hypertension in a child caused by a multicystic kidney. J Urol 104: 918–921

Javadpour N, Dellon AL, Kumpe DA (1973) Multilocular cystic disease in adults - imitator of renal cell carcinoma. Urology 1: 596–599

Johnson DE, Ayala AG, Medellin H, Wilbur J (1973) Multilocular renal cystic disease in children. J Urol 109: 101–103

Johnson HW, Gleave M, Coleman GU, Nadel HR, Raffel J, Weckworth PF (1987) Neonatal renomegaly. J Urol 138: 1023–1027

Johnston JH, Mix LW (1976) The Ask-Upmark kidney: a form of ascending pyelonephritis? Br J Urol 48: 393–398

Jordon D, Harpaz N, Thung SN (1989) Caroli's disease and adult polycystic kidney disease: a rarely recognized association. Liver 9: 30–35

Kaariainen H, Jaaskelainen J, Kivisaari L, Koskimies O, Norio R (1988) Dominant and recessive polycystic kidney disease in children: classification by intravenous pyelography, ultrasound, and computed tomography. Pediatr Radiol 18: 45–50

Kaplan BS, Kaplan P, deChavarevian JP, Jequier S, O'Regan S, Russo P (1988) Variable expression of autosomal recessive polycystic kidney disease and congenital hepatic fibrosis within a family. Am J Med Genet 29: 639–647

Kaplan N, Elkin M (1968) Bifid renal pelves and ureters. Radiographic and cinefluorographic observations. Br J Urol 40: 235–244

Kelalis PP, Malek RS, Segura JW (1973) Observations on renal ectopia and fusion in children. J Urol 110: 588–592

King MC, Friedenberg RM (1968) Normal renal parenchyma simulating tumor. Radiol 191: 217–222

Kleiner B, Filly RA, Mack L, Callen PW (1986) Multicystic dysplastic kidney: observations of contralateral disease in the fetal population. Radiology 161: 27–29

Koyle MA, Ehrlich RM (1988) Management of ureteropelvic junction obstruction in neonate. Urology 31: 496–498

Kunin M (1982) The abortive calyx: variations in appearance and differential diagnosis. AJR 139: 931–934

Lafortune M, Constantin A, Breton G, Vallee C (1986) Sonography of the hypertrophied column of Bertin. AJR 146: 53–56

Lam AH (1988) Familial megacalyces with autosomal recessive inheritance. Report of 3 affected siblings. Pediatr Radiol 19: 28–30

Lozano RH, Rodriguez C (1975) Intrathoracic ectopic kidney. Report of case. J Urol 114: 601–602

Mackie GG, Stephens FD (1977) Duplex kidneys: a correlation of renal dysplasia with position of the ureteric orifice. Birth Defects 13: 313–321

Madewell JE, Goldman SM, Davis CJ, Hartman DS, Feigin DS, Lichtenstein JE (1983) Multilocular cystic nephroma: a radiographic-pathologic correlation of 58 patients. Radiology 146: 309–321

Malek RS, Panayotis PK, Stickler GB, Burke EC (1972) Observations on ureteral ectopy in children. J Urol 107: 308–313

Malone PS, Duffy PG, Ransley PG, Risdon RA, Cook T, Taylor M (1989) Congenital mesoblastic nephroma, renin production, and hypertension. J Pediatr Surg 24: 599–600

Malter IJ, Stanley RJ (1972) The intrathoric kidney. With a review of the literature. J Urol 107: 538–541

McAlister WH, Siegel MJ (1989) Pediatric radiology case of the day. Congenital hepatic fibrosis with saccular dilatation of the intrahepatic bile ducts and infantile polycystic kidneys. AJR 152: 1329–1330

McFarland WL, Wallace S, Johnson DE (1972) Renal carcinoma and polycystic disease. J Urol 107: 530–532

Merklin RJ, Michels NA (1958) The variant renal and suprarenal blood supply with data on the inferior phrenic, ureteral and gonadal arteries. A statistical analysis based on 185 dissections and review of the literature. J Int Coll Surg 29: 41

Messing E, Kessler R, Kavaney PB (1976) Renal arteriovenous fistulas. Urology 7: 101–107

Muren C, Wikstad I (1988) Unilateral hydronephrosis with congenital absence of contralateral kidney in children. Report of six cases and review of literature. Acta Radiol 29: 679–683

Ney C, Friedenberg RM (1981) Radiographic atlas of the genitourinary system, 2nd edn. Lippincott, Philadelphia

N'Guessan G, Stephens FD (1983) Supernumerary kidney. J Urol 130: 649–653

Nussbaum AR, Hartman DS, Whitley N, McCauley RGK, Sanders RC (1987) Muticystic dysplasia and crossed renal ectopia. AJR 149: 407–410

O'Reilley PH (1989) Relationship between intermittent hydronephrosis and megacalicosis. Br J Urol 64: 125-129

Pedicelli G, Jequier S, Bowen A'D, Boisvert J (1986) Multicystic dysplastic kidneys: spontaneous regression demonstrated with US. Radiology 160: 23-26

Peterson JE, Pinckney LE, Rutledge JC, Currarino G (1982) The solitary renal calyx and papilla in human kidneys. Radiology 144: 525-527

Pettinato G, Manivel JC, Wick MR, Dehner LP (1989) Classical and cellular (atypical) congenital mesoblastic nephroma: a clinicopathologic, ultrastructural, immunohistochemical, and flow cytometric study. Hum Pathol 20: 682-690

Potter EL (1972) Normal and abnormal development of the kidney. Year Book Medical Publishers, Chicago

Premkumar A, Berdon WE, Levy J, Amodio J, Abramson SJ, Newhouse JH (1988) The emergence of hepatic fibrosis and portal hypertension in infants and children with autosomal recessive polycystic kidney disease - initial and follow-up sonographic and radiographic findings. Pediatr Radiol 18: 123-129

Rothermel FJ, Miller FJ Jr, Sanford E, Drago J, Rohner TJ (1977) Clinical and radiographic findings of focally infected polycystic kidneys. Urology 10: 580-585

Sander HM 3rd, Heoyman S, Keller M, Kaplan JM, Norman ME (1987) Association of congenital megacalycosis and ipsilateral segmental megaureter. Pediatr Radiol 17: 28-33

Sander RC, Blakemore K (1989) Lethal fetal anomalies: sonographic demonstration. Radiology 172: 1-6

Sanders RC, Nussbaum AR, Solez K (1988) Renal dysplasia: sonographic findings. Radiology 167: 623-626

Shaffer SE, Norman ME (1989) Renal function and renal failure in the newborn. Clin Perinatol 16: 199-218

Shanbhogue LK, Gray E, Miller SS (1986) Congenital mesoblastic nephroma of infancy. Study of four cases and review of the literature. J R Coll Surg Edinb 31: 171-174

Stuck KJ, Koff SA, Silver TM (1982) Ultrasonic features of multicystic dysplastic kidney: expanded diagnostic criteria. Radiology 143: 217-221

Takehara Y, Takahashi M, Naito M, Kato T, Nishimura T, Isoda H, Kaneko M (1989) Caroli's disease associated with polycystic kidney: its noninvasive diagnosis. Radiat Med 7: 13-15

Terada T, Nakanuma Y (1988) Congenital biliary dilatation in autosomal dominant adult polycystic disease of the liver and kidneys. Arch Pathol Lab Med 112: 1113-1116

Thompson GJ, Pace JM (1937) Ectopic kidney: A review of 97 cases. Surg Gynecol Obstet 64: 935-943

Thompson IM, Rodriguez FR, Spence CR (1987) Medullary sponge kidney and congenital hemihypertrophy. South Med J 80: 1455-1456

Tomooka Y, Onitsuka H, Goya T et al. (1988) Congenital hemihypertrophy with adrenal adenoma and medullary sponge kidney. Br J Radiol 61: 851-853

Tridenti G, Armanetti M, Flisi M, Benassi L (1988) Uterus didelphys with an obstructed hemivagina and ipsilateral renal agenesis in teenagers: report of three cases. Am J Obstet Gynecol 159: 882-883

Vargas B, Leibowitz RL (1986) The coexistence of congenital megacalyces and primary megaureter. AJR 147: 313-316

Vinocur L, Slovis TL, Perlmutter AD, Watts FB Jr, Chang CH (1988) Follow-up studies of multicystic dysplastic kidneys. Radiology 167: 311-315

Webb JAW, Fry IK, Charlton CAC (1975) An anomalous calyx in the midkidney: an anatomical variant. Br J Radiol 48: 674-677

Whitaker J, Danks DM (1966) A study of the inheritance of duplication of the kidneys and ureters. J Urol 95: 176-178

Whitehouse GH (1975) Some urographic aspects of the horseshoe kidney anomaly - a review of 59 cases. Clin Radiol 25: 107-114

Wilmer HA (1938) Unilateral fused kidney. A report of five cases and a review of the literature. J Urol 40: 551-571

Worthington JL, Shackelford GD, Cole BR, Tack ED, Kissane JM (1988) Sonographically detectable cysts in polycystic kidney disease in newborn and young infants. Pediatr Radiol 18: 287-293

Zeier M, Geberth S, Ritz E, Jaeger T, Waldherr R (1988) Adult dominant polycystic kidney disease - clinical problems. Nephron 49: 177-183

3 Parenchymal Diseases of the Kidneys

HILARY ZARNOW and LAWRENCE R. BIGONGIARI

CONTENTS

3.1   Introduction 71
3.2   Basic Anatomy 72
3.3   Imaging Modalities: Value and Limitations ... 74
3.3.1   Excretory Urography 74
3.3.2   Retrograde Pyelography 74
3.3.3   Ultrasound 74
3.3.4   Computed Tomography 74
3.3.5   Angiography and Venography 75
3.3.6   Nuclear Medicine 75
3.3.7   Magnetic Resonance Imaging 75
3.4   Glomerular Diseases 76
3.4.1   Acute Glomerulonephritis 76
3.4.1.1   Clinical Background 76
3.4.1.2   Pathologic Findings 76
3.4.1.3   Radiologic Evaluation 76
3.4.2   Chronic Glomerulonephritis 77
3.4.3   Polyarteritis Nodosa 77
3.4.3.1   Pathology 77
3.4.3.2   Radiologic Evaluation 77
3.4.4   Systemic Lupus Erythematosus 78
3.4.4.1   Pathological Findings 78
3.4.4.2   Radiologic Evaluation 79
3.4.5   Goodpasture's Syndrome 79
3.4.5.1   Clinical Background 79
3.4.5.2   Pathologic Findings 80
3.4.5.3   Radiologic Evaluation 80
3.4.6   Henoch-Schönlein Syndrome 80
3.4.7   Wegener's Granulomatosis 80
3.4.8   Scleroderma 81
3.4.8.1   Clinical Background 81
3.4.8.2   Pathologic Findings 81
3.4.8.3   Radiologic Evaluation 82
3.4.9   Nephrosclerosis 82
3.4.9.1   Clinical Background 82
3.4.9.2   Pathologic Findings 82
3.4.9.3   Radiologic Findings 82
3.5   Bilateral Renal Cortical Necrosis 83
3.5.1   Pathologic Findings 83
3.5.2   Radiologic Findings 83
3.6   Tubulointerstitial Diseases 84
3.6.1   General Considerations 84
3.6.2   Acute Interstitial Nephritis 85
3.6.2.1   Acute Tubular Necrosis 85
3.6.3   Chronic Interstitial Nephritis 87
3.6.3.1   Radiologic Evaluation 87
3.6.3.2   Papillary Necrosis 88

3.6.3.3   Analgesic Abuse 88
3.6.4   Nephropathy of Hematopoietic Disorders ... 89
3.6.4.1   Sickle Cell Hemoglobinopathies 89
3.6.4.2   Multiple Myeloma 90
3.6.4.3   Lymphoma and Leukemia 90
3.6.5   Fanconi's Syndrome 91
3.6.6   Uric Acid Nephropathy 92
3.6.7   Radiation Nephritis 93
3.6.8   Hepatorenal Syndrome 94
3.7   AIDS and Drug Abuse Nephropathy 94
      References 97

3.1 Introduction

Radiologic evaluation does not currently play a primary role in the definitive diagnosis of diseases of the kidney. Specific diagnosis is based upon clinical pattern, laboratory findings, and renal biopsy. Imaging techniques are ancillary procedures used to detect anatomy, assess function, and evaluate for complications or associated abnormalities. The combination of excellent anatomic delineation and information regarding functional status provided by urography, retrograde pyelography, nuclear medical examinations, ultrasound, computed tomography, magnetic resonance imaging, and angiography does not provide results distinctive enough to allow definitive diagnosis. There is significant overlap of findings on any given examination so that even the most specific pattern, i. e., the microaneurysms seen on renal angiograms in polyarteritis nodosa, is also seen in several other entities, such as systemic lupus erythematosus (SLE) and intravenous drug abuse (LONGSTRETCH et al. 1974; HALPERN 1971; LIGNELLI and BUCHHETI 1971).

The use of multiple procedures does not significantly increase the specificity of diagnosis. The key information the clinician requires from the radiologist is anatomic. The overall size and countour of the kidney are basic information used to establish major categories relevant to differential diagnosis (Table 3.1). Establishing the presence or absence of obstructive uropathy as the cause of renal functional impairment is mandatory in all classes of significant renal disease. Ultrasound is now the standard

---

HILARY ZARNOW, M. D., Chairman; LAWRENCE R. BIGONGIARI, M. D., Clinical Professor; Department of Radiology, St. Francis Regional Medical Center, University of Kansas, 929 North St. Francis, Wichita, KS 67214, USA

Table 3.1. Differential diagnosis of renal parenchymal diseases

Differential diagnosis of bilateral large kidneys	*Differential diagnosis of bilateral small kidneys*
1. Acute glomerulonephritis	*With smooth renal contour:*
2. Acute pyelonephritis (when bilateral)	1. Chronic glomerulonephritis
3. Polycystic kidneys	2. Bilateral renal artery stenosis
4. Leukemia and lymphoma	3. Chronic stages of bilateral tubular and cortical necrosis
5. Multiple myeloma	4. Congenital hypoplastic kidneys
6. Kidneys of chronic alcoholics and cirrhotics	5. Medullary cystic disease of the kidneys
7. Bilateral renal vein thrombosis (acute)	6. Radiation nephritis
8. Bilateral renal masses (benign or malignant)	7. Alport's syndrome (hereditary chronic nephritis)
9. Bilateral hydronephrosis	
10. Acute tubular necrosis	*With irregular renal contour:*
11. Acute bilateral renal cortical necrosis (early)	1. Chronic pyelonephritis (when bilateral)
12. Infectious mononucleosis	2. Nephrosclerosis
13. Acromegaly	3. End-stage kidneys from any chronic parenchymal disease
14. Hemophilia	4. Infarcted kidneys (when bilateral)
15. Diabetes (glomerulosclerosis)	
16. Hyperalimentation	
17. Sickle cell disease (homozygous)	
18. Amyloidosis (early)	
19. Von Gierke's disease	
Differential diagnosis of unilateral large kidneys	*Differential diagnosis of unilateral small kidneys*
1. Acute pyelonephritis (when unilateral)	1. Chronic pyelonephritis (when unilateral)
2. Unilateral renal vein thrombosis	2. Unilateral renal artery stenosis
3. Hydronephrosis (when unilateral)	3. Congenital hypoplastic kidney
4. Compensatory hypertrophy due to acquired and congenital causes	4. Partial nephrectomy
5. Kidney with double collecting system (duplex)	5. Radiation nephritis (when unilateral)
6. Unilateral renal mass (benign or malignant)	6. Postobstructive renal atrophy
7. Multicystic kidney	7. Focal renal infarction

screening examination used to provide this information. Other studies are performed as clinically required to answer specific questions, such as whether the renal veins are patent. The selection of the best procedure to evaluate a given problem is most effectively accomplished by a direct dialogue between radiologist and clinician concerning that specific case. The general principle is that the least invasive and safest procedures should be considered first, especially for severely ill patients, except where specific circumstances dictate otherwise.

The next two sections will discuss basic anatomy and the status and role of current radiologic imaging modalities. This will be followed by sections describing specific diseases of the kidneys. These diseases have been divided into two major categories based on their clinical and pathologic findings, which in turn determine their basic radiologic patterns. The first grouping is characterized by the centering of the major pathologic findings around the glomerulus and the renal vasculature. The second grouping is characterized by the centering of the pathologic findings around the tubulus and the renal interstitium. Many entities exhibit combined glomerular and tubular pathology, but with one component predominating in the early stages of the disease. Most conditions exhibit combined pathologic changes in their later stages. Our characterization is based on the predominant changes in the early stages.

3.2 Basic Anatomy

A basic understanding or renal anatomy is necessary to utilize all radiologic modalities effectively. The kidney is grossly divided into a cortex, a medulla, and the renal sinus containing the main renal vasculature. The cortex contains the basic functional units, nephrons, whose function is to provide filtration. The medulla is composed of the collecting tubules, which drain the nephrons into the pelvocalyceal collecting system.

The renal lobe is the major anatomic unit of the kidney (HODSON 1972). A lobe consists of medulla, cortex, and a vascular system (Fig. 3.1). The medulla is conical in its configuration. It is composed of collecting tubules, which arise from the ureteric bud embryologically, and proximal and distal convoluted tubules, loops of Henle, and connective tissue, which arise from the metanephros embryologically. The arterial blood supply of the medulla comes from the vasa recta, a system of postglomerular vessels whose origin is the efferent arterioles of the juxtamedullary cortex (Fig.3.1). These vessels parallel the descending limbs of Henle's loops as they go through the medulla into the papilla. They return with the ascending limbs of Henle's loops to the medulla, where they drain into the interlobar and arcuate veins. This system perfusing the medulla receives 20% of total renal blood flow.

The difference in perfusion between medulla and cortex (cf. THORBURN et al. 1963) is the physiologic basis which allows radiologic demonstration of cortex and medulla on dynamic contrast examinations such as CT or angiography. Corticomedullary definition is also readily achieved by ultrasound and MRI without the use of contrast agents. The status of corticomedullary definition is of great importance clinically in the correlation of anatomic and functional findings (MAROTTI et al. 1987); it contributes to rational management decisions and assists in differential diagnosis in some situations, such as helping to distinguish acute tubular necrosis from rejection in patients with renal transplants (HRICAK et al. 1986).

The renal cortex is primarily made up of nephrons, which are of metanephric origin. The cortex is a dense mantle of tissue which surrounds the medulla, except at the tip of the papilla. The lateral surface of the cortex is divided at regular intervals by linear bands called medullary rays, which are actually terminal branches of collecting tubules, which extend into the cortex from the medulla. HODSON (1972) called the portion which forms the base of the lobe the centrilobar cortex. The portion which surrounds the sides of the medulla he called the septal cortex. The septal cortex is identical with what is commonly called the "column of Bertin." Each lobe ends in a papilla which is invaginated into a renal calyx. These structures mark the central deepest extent of the renal lobe.

In contrast to the medulla, the renal cortex receives 80% of the renal blood flow. The blood supply for a lobe arise from the interlobar arteries. Each interlobar artery supplies two adjacent lobes. The interlobar arteries branch into the arcuate arteries as they pass through the renal sinus fat. Several arcuate vessels provide perfusion to the entire lobe. The arcuate artery enters the renal parenchyma adjacent to the papilla and courses along the corticomedullary junction, giving off interlobar branches at regular intervals. The interlobular arteries branch and form the afferent arterioles which supply the glomeruli. These vessels also supply the juxtamedullary cortex and give rise to the vasa recta, which supply the cortex (Fig.3.2).

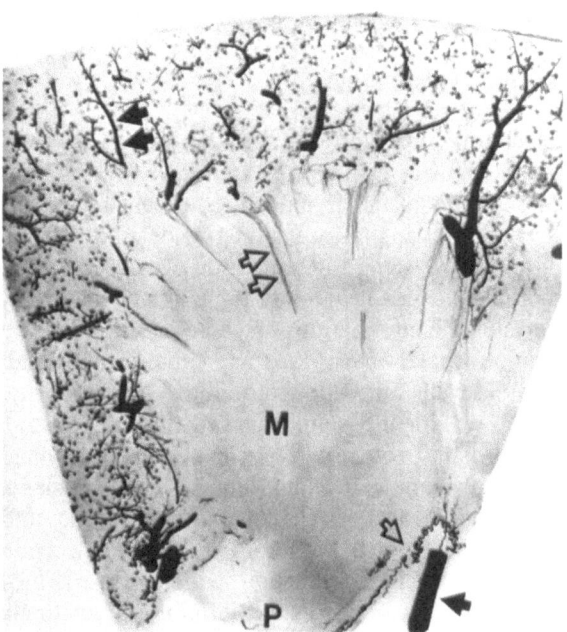

Fig.3.1. Specimen microradiograph of an injected kidney. Cortical vasculature is well defined and predominates. Vasa recta are only poorly opacified. *Single solid arrow,* arcuate artery; *double solid arrow,* interlobular artery; *single open arrow,* spiral artery to papilla; *double open arrow,* vasa recta; *M,* medulla; *P,* papilla. (DAVIDSON 1977)

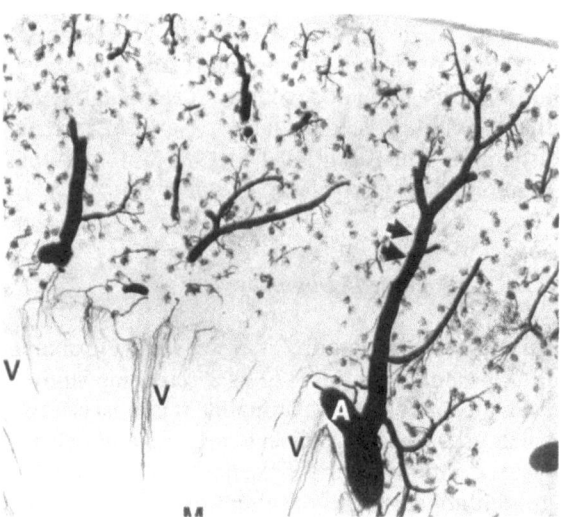

Fig.3.2. Enlarged view of the specimens in Fig.3.1 to better demonstrate renal cortical vascular anatomy. Multiple afferent arterioles branch off each interlobular artery to supply the glomeruli. *Double solid arrow,* interlobular artery; *V,* vasa recta; *M,* medulla; *A,* arcuate artery. (DAVIDSON 1977)

3.3 Imaging Modalities: Value and Limitations

3.3.1 Excretory Urography

Excretory urography is still the basic radiologic method for assessing renal anatomy. Urography is superior to all other modalities except retrograde pyelography in illustrating the fine detail of the pelvocalyceal system, and retrograde pyelography does not provide visualization of the parenchyma or any physiologic information. An excretory urogram will demonstrate the overall size and contours of the kidneys, as well as the amount of functioning parenchyma. It will identify significant obstructive uropathy. Abnormalities of the calyces will allow specific diagnoses of some conditions such as nephrolithiasis, polycystic kidney disease, papillary necrosis, and medullary sponge kidney. Use of body section radiography in conjunction with excretory urography greatly improves the definition of anatomic detail (BECKER 1966, 1967; POLLACK and BANNER 1985).

Today, excretory urography is no longer used as the primary examination for the diagnosis of obstruction or for assessing kidney size as an index of the chronicity of a patient's impaired renal function. This role has been taken over by ultrasound, which provides similar information in a totally noninvasive fashion. The new nonionic contrast agents have significantly decreased the morbidity and mortality of intravenous iodinated contrast examinations and there should be no reluctance to perform excretory urography when additional anatomic information is required (TALIERCIO and BURNETT 1988).

3.3.2 Retrograde Pyelography

Retrograde pyelography is a secondary examination. It should not be used as a screening study to evaluate for obstructive uropathy. It is most effective when used to better delineate ureteral and pelvocalyceal anatomy in the presence of excretory urographic abnormalities or suboptimal visualization. It is important in the evaluation of patients with transitional cell tumors and stone disease to obtain maximum distension of the upper urinary tract.

3.3.3 Ultrasound

Ultrasound has clearly replaced both excretory urography and retrograde pyelography as the primary radiologic examination in the patient with impaired

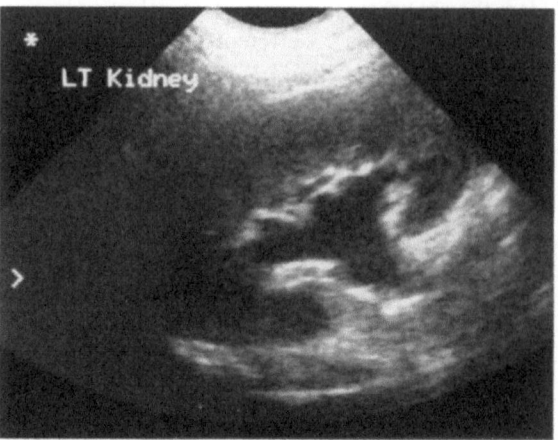

Fig. 3.3. Ultrasonogram showing hydronephrosis with normal cortical size and echo pattern

renal function. It is accurate and sensitive in measuring renal size, in defining corticomedullary relationships, and in assessing the presence or absence of obstructive uropathy. It will also demonstrate incidental findings, such as stones, cysts, or tumors (Fig. 3.3).

There has been great interest in using high resolution ultrasound to define abnormalities in the renal parenchyma in many diseases of the kidney. A number of studies have demonstrated sensitivity with abnormal cortical echo patterns, but specificity has been relatively low (ROSENFIELD and SIEGEL 1981). Studies have shown no correlation between specific sonographic appearance and type of renal disease (HRICAK et al. 1982). There is still some controversy in the literature about sonographic ability to detect parenchymal disease (PLATT et al. 1988).

3.3.4 Computed Tomography

Computed tomography (CT) has some major advantages in the evaluation of the kidneys; its superior sensitivity for density discrimination with a high spatial resolution and presentation in the axial plane allow excellent visualization of the renal anatomy. Because the kidney axis is actually in the coronal plane, the perpendicular axial plane allows definition of structures in the renal hilus and along the anterior and posterior surfaces of the kidney. The psoas muscles and the retroperitoneum are especially well imaged by CT. CT not only provides specific tissue characterization for calcifications in and around the kidney, but also clearly defines fat, fluid, and hemorrhage. The addition of bolus intravenous contrast injection with rapid scanning techniques allows CT-angiographic studies of the renal vasculature and fine definition of the renal parenchyma with good corticomedullary definition and some assessment of perfusion and function. In spite of these many technical advantages, CT seldom makes possible specific diagnosis of parenchymal disease (HEIBERG et al. 1988; LOVE et al. 1989). It is most effective in the evaluation of renal tumors and trauma (SANDLER et al. 1985; LANG 1983).

3.3.5 Angiography and Venography

Renal angiography was once thought to provide specific diagnosis of parenchymal disease (HERSCHMAN et al. 1970; ESSINGER and BONARD 1971). However, even with high resolution magnification and pharmacoangiographic techniques, specific diagnosis of renal parenchymal disease is not possible (MENA et al. 1973; DAVIDSON and TALNER 1973). The angiographic pattern of most medical diseases is strikingly similar. Renal angiography is most useful in the evaluation of renal tumors. Renal venography is used to confirm the diagnosis of renal vein thrombosis and to determine tumor extension into the renal vein and the vena cava in patients with hypernephroma. Digital vascular images can be used in renal angiography of patients with impaired renal function to minimize the contrast load to the kidneys (Fig. 3.4).

3.3.6 Nuclear Medicine

Radionuclide studies provide some information about renal anatomy, but mainly provide physiologic data that reflect renal blood flow, nephron function, and urine drainage (Fig. 3.5). The techniques are simple, safe, and rapid. They are clinically most important for evaluating renal function and to screen for renovascular hypertension. Gallium 67 scintigraphy was reported by BAKIR et al. (1985) to be useful in evaluating and following patients with lupus nephritis. Further studies have shown that gallium scanning is not useful in patients with glomerulonephritis (MOULIN et al. 1988) or in patients with various other glomerular diseases (BAKIR et al. 1988).

3.3.7 Magnetic Resonance Imaging

Magnetic resonance imaging (MRI) provides anatomic, angiographic, and functional metabolic data for the evaluation of the kidneys. To date, true MR-

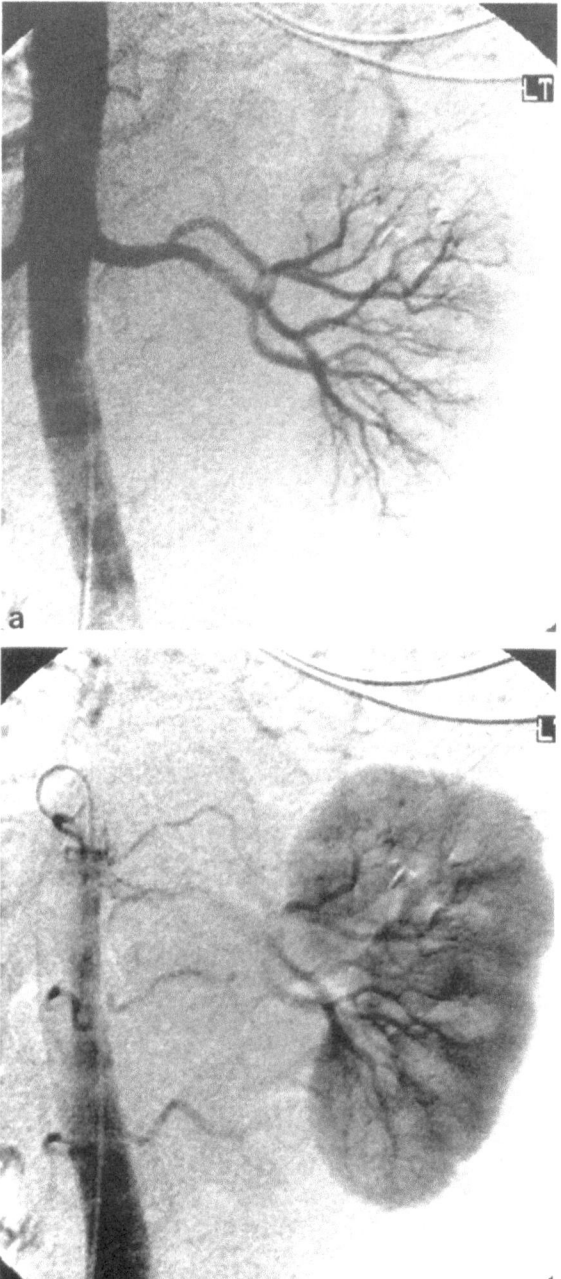

Fig. 3.4 a, b. Normal renal digital subtraction angiogram. **a** Arterial and **b** nephrographic phase

angiography and MR spectroscopy are still only research tools. MR is most useful as an alternative means for assessing renal tumors, especially in children. It has also been shown to be useful as a means of evaluating renal transplants (HHRICAK et al. 1986; WINSETT et al. 1988). MR techniques currently in use do not allow specific diagnosis of renal

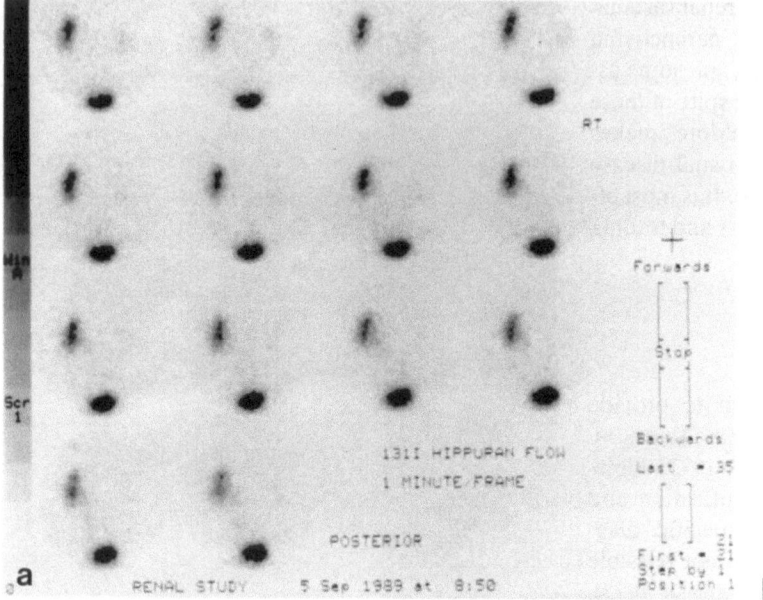

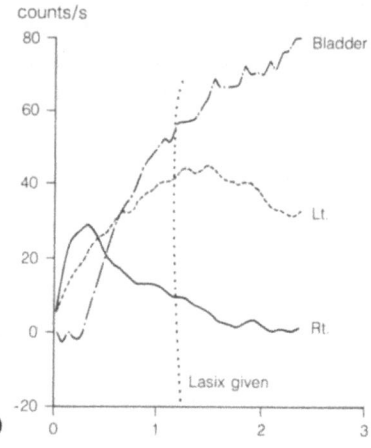

Fig. 3.5. a Renal 131 I-hippuran scan with diuretic (Lasic 40 mg i.v.) injection demonstrating obstruction on the left. This is accentuated by the normal washout with diuresis on the right side. **b** Corresponding renogramm curve showing left obstruction

parenchymal diseases. Some of the current areas under research, most notably MR spectroscopy, do offer some promise of specificity (CHOYKE and POLLACK 1988; ROSS et al. 1986; HONDA et al. 1988; CHOYKE et al. 1989).

3.4 Glomerular Diseases

3.4.1 Acute Glomerulonephritis

3.4.1.1 Clinical Background

Typical acute glomerulonephritis (Bright's disease) has its onset 1 to several weeks following an infection of the skin or respiratory tract with certain strains of group A β-hemolytic streptococcus. The clinical course is characterized by fever, abdominal pain, and hypertension, and many patients exhibit the nephrotic syndrome. Urinalysis shows hematuria, proteinuria, and hemoglobin casts. Most patients, especially children and young adults, go on to complete healing, but some develop chronic disease.

3.4.1.2 Pathologic Findings

In the acute phase, the kidneys are grossly enlarged due to interstitial edema and multiple petechial hemorrhages are seen on the surface. Microscopically, the findings are those of proliferation and necrosis of cellular elements about the glomeruli with increased lobulation. There is also a fibrinous and proteinaceous deposition in the capsular space. The afferent arterioles and interlobular arteries show focal medial necrosis with perivascular cellular infiltrates and collagenous thickening of the intima.

These pathologic findings reflect the immune complex origin of this disease and there are similar patterns in all the immune related diseases: polyarteritis, SLE, Wegener's granulomatosis, Goodpasture's syndrome, and Henoch-Schönlein syndrome.

3.4.1.3 Radiologic Evaluation

Ultrasound is used to assess renal size and contour and to exclude significant obstruction. Renal blood flow and function are best evaluated by radionuclide studies. Gallium 67 scintigraphy may be positive, but is not clinically accurate enough to be useful (LINTON et al. 1985). Urographic contrast studies only show enlarged poorly functioning kidneys and should not be performed because of the danger of inducing acute tubular necrosis (Fig. 3.6). CT is only useful in evaluating for complications such as retroperitoneal hemorrhage. Angiography shows no

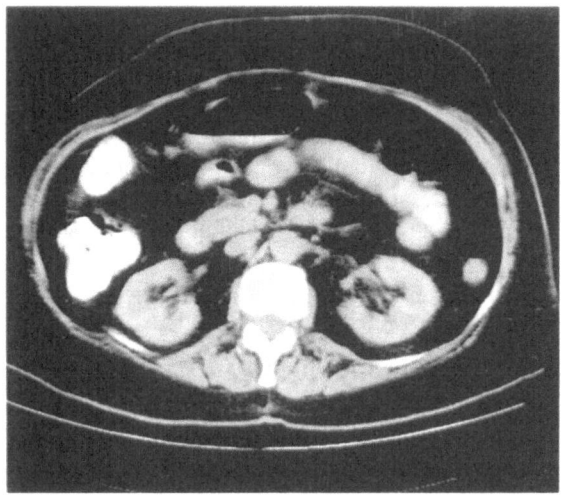

Fig.3.6. Contrast-induced renal failure: CT scan of abdomen the next day shows persistent nephrogram. Patient went into clinical renal failure following this emergency examination

specific changes. No experience is available with MRI.

3.4.2 Chronic Glomerulonephritis

End-stage glomerulonephritis is dominated clinically by chronic renal insufficiency and chronic hypertension. Only a small percentage of patients have a documentable history of prior acute glomerulonephritis. Pathologically, the kidneys are small and symmetrical with a smooth, granular surface. The cortex is thinned. The pelvocalyceal structures are normal.

Ultrasound is again the procedure of choice for evaluating size, contour, and cortical thickness and for excluding obstruction. Because of the renal failure, urographic and radionuclide studies are not useful. Angiography shows cortical thinning with smooth regular outlines and pruning of the interlobular vessels at their origins from poorly perfused arcuate vessels. Intrarenal circulation time is prolonged. These findings, however, primarily reflect the severe hypertension that these patients develop, rather than specific changes attributable to the glomerulonephritis (CUTTINO and CLARK 1988).

3.4.3 Polyarteritis Nodosa

Classic polyarteritis nodosa (PAN) is a multisystem necrotizing vasculitis of small and medium size muscular arteries in which involvement of the renal and visceral arteries is characteristic. Nonspecific signs and symptoms are the hallmarks of PAN. Fever, weight loss, and malaise are present in over half of all cases. Patients usually present with vague symptoms, such as weakness, headache, abdominal pain, and myalgia. Hypertension may dominate the clinical picture. PAN can involve any organ system and clinical findings will vary accordingly.

3.4.3.1 Pathology

Renal involvement most commonly manifests as ischemic change in the glomeruli. Proliferative glomerulonephritis is seen in about 30% of patients. The vascular lesion in classic PAN is a necrotizing inflammation of small and medium sized muscular arteries. The lesions are segmental and tend to involve bifurcations and branchings of arteries. They may spread circumferentially to involve adjacent veins. Involvement of venules is usually not seen and its presence suggests the polyangiitis overlap syndrome. In the acute phase of PAN, polymorphonuclear neutrophils infiltrate all layers of the vessel and perivascular areas, which results in intimal proliferation and degeneration of the vessel wall. In the subacute and chronic stages, mononuclear cells infiltrate the area. As lesions progress, fibrinoid necrosis of the vessels compromises the lumen. Thrombosis then occurs, which causes infarction of the tissue supplied by the involved vessel, or in some cases, hemorrhage. As lesions heal, there is collagen deposition which can also lead to vascular occlusions. Aneurysmal dilatations up to 1 cm in size along the involved artery are characteristic of classic PAN. The pathology of the kidney is mainly arterial, but glomerulitis occurs in up to 30% of patients (HEPTINSTALL 1983). In patients with significant hypertension, typical pathologic features of glomerulosclerosis may be seen alone or superimposed on lesions of arteries and glomerulonephritis.

3.4.3.2 Radiologic Evaluation

The diagnosis of classic PAN is based on biopsy findings of vasculitis. In the absence of easily accessible tissue for biopsy, the angiographic demonstration of involved vessels (Fig.3.7), specifically aneurysms of small and medium sized arteries in the renal, hepatic, or visceral vasculature, is sufficient to make the diagnosis (PADOVANI et al. 1974). Aneurysms are not pathognomonic of PAN and may be seen in systemic lupus erythematosus and in drug

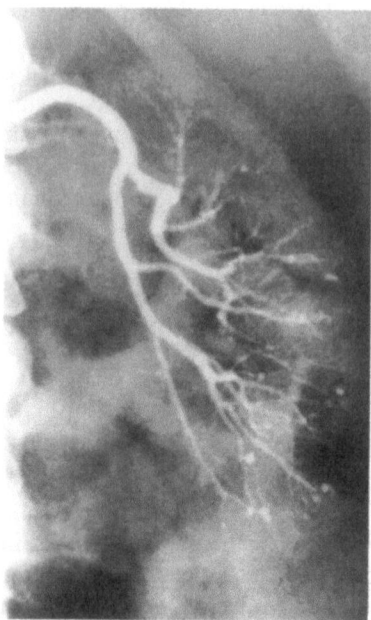

Fig. 3.7. Angiogram showing multiple arcuate artery micro-aneurysms throughout the kidney in a patient with polyarteritis. (DAVIDSON 1985)

addicts who inject amphetamines (LONGSTRETCH et al. 1974; HALPERN and CITRON 1971).

Aneurysms may rupture, causing intrarenal or perinephric hematomas (HORNER et al. 1966; TA-SEDEMIR et al. 1988). Massive hemorrhage of involved kidneys has also been reported (CORNFIELD et al. 1988). CT and MRI are the best means of evaluating renal hemorrhagic complications of PAN (WILMS et al. 1986; CHOYKE and POLLACK 1988). Ultrasound and radionuclide studies play no direct role in managing these cases. Urography may show enlarged smooth kidneys or focal areas of scarring secondary to infarctions. Pelvocalyceal structures are normal. Notching of the proximal ureters, presumably by collateral vessels, has been described, but is both nonspecific and uncommon.

3.4.4 Systemic Lupus Erythematosus

Systemic lupus erythematosus is an immunologically mediated multisystem disease in which renal involvement is common: clinical evidence of renal involvement has been reported in 35%–90% of patients in different series. SLE may present clinically as acute glomerulonephritis, latent nephritis, nephrotic syndrome, or chronic glomerulonephritis. It is predominantly a disease of women of all ages. Its time course is also quite variable, ranging from a

rapidly progressive glomerulonephritis to an indolent chronic glomerulonephritis (MUEHRCKE et al. 1957). Long-term prognosis has considerably improved for patients with SLE with renal involvement. Patients with SLE are currently satisfactory candidates for dialysis and transplantation. The major cause of morbidity and mortality is cerebral involvement secondary to immune suppression therapy.

3.4.4.1 Pathological Findings

Systemic lupus erythematosus is currently classified pathologically into five categories by the World Health Organization (SCHRIER and GOTTSCHALK 1988):

Class I (normal kidneys)
1. Only rarely do patients with SLE have entirely normal kidneys by light microscopy, immune fluorescence, and electron microscopy.
2. The patients have no clinical evidence of glomerular disease.

Class II (minimal or mesangial lupus nephritis)
1. This is the earliest and mildest form of renal envolvement.
2. It is characterized by mesangial deposits of immunoglobulin and C3 with (class II B) and without (class II A) focal proliferative changes on light microscopy.
3. Most patients have hematuria and proteinuria, but nephrotic syndrome and renal insufficiency are uncommon unless progression to a more severe lesion occurs, which happens in about 20% of patients.
4. Five-year survival is over 90%.

Class III (focal proliferative lupus nephritis)
1. This is a continuum between focal *mesangial* involvement and diffuse proliferative lupus nephritis.
2. Focal proliferative changes are present in less than 50% of the glomeruli.
3. Deposits are primarily mesangial, but may also be subendothelial.
4. All patients have proteinuria, but only 20% have nephrotic syndrome and renal insufficiency.
5. Response to treatment is good, and the 5-year survival rate is 90%.
6. Unfortunately, progression to class IV is common.
7. The best predictor for this is the presence of subendothelial deposits.

Class IV (diffuse proliferative lupus nephritis)
1. This is the severest form of lupus nephritis, with over 50% of glomeruli involved, including crescent formation and necrosis.
2. Extensive mesangial, subendothelial, and subepithelial deposits are all seen by electron microscopy. All specimens contain immunoglobulin, C3, and fibrin.
3. Proteinuria is present in all patients, and is in the nephrotic range in 90% of the cases.
4. Renal function is decreased in 75% of the cases.
5. Long-term prognosis has improved with aggressive therapy and is now about 75% at 5 years.
6. Patients who respond to treatment with remission in the 1st year have the best prognosis.

Class V (membranous lupus nephritis)
1. About 15% of patients with SLE will develop a glomerular lesion that is indistinguishable from idiopathic membranous nephropathy, with extensive subepithelial deposits of all immunoglobulins and C3.
2. Nephrotic syndrome and slowly progressive renal disease are common.
3. The incidence of systemic manifestations of SLE and serologic abnormalities in general is lower in these patients.
4. The long-term prognosis is similar to class II disease.
5. There appears to be an increased incidence of renal vein thrombosis, similar to idiopathic membranous nephropathy.

3.4.4.2 Radiologic Evaluation

Radiologic findings are largely related to the state of renal function. Patients with acute nephritis have enlarged smooth kidneys, but function is markedly diminished. Pelvocalyceal structures are normal on retrograde examination. Ultrasound is the technique of choice for evaluating renal size and contour and possible hydronephrosis. Angiographic findings are variable and usually reflect hypertensive changes. SLE can create an angiographic appearance identical to PAN with microaneurysms present, making this a nonspecific pattern (LONGSTRETCH et al. 1974). CT and MRI are useful mainly in assessing nonrenal involvement by SLE, primarily in the CNS. They can also be used to detect a complicating renal vein thrombosis (GLAZER et al. 1984; HONDA et al. 1988). They can also demonstrate spontaneous renal or retroperitoneal hemorrhages (Fig. 3.8).

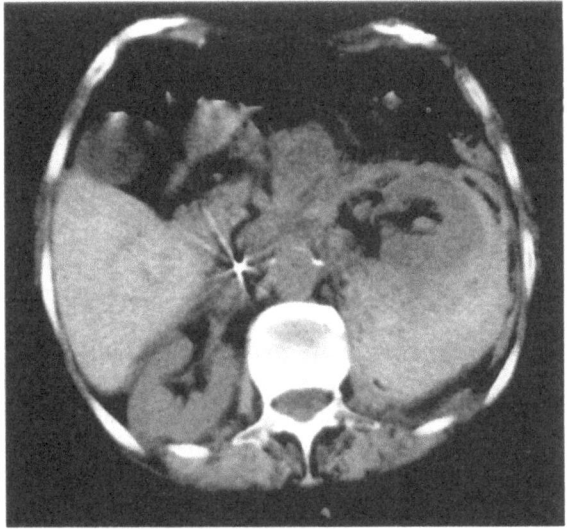

Fig. 3.8. Spontaneous hemorrhage into the subcapsular and perirenal spaces in a patient with SLE

3.4.5 Goodpasture's Syndrome

3.4.5.1 Clinical Background

Goodpasture's syndrome is characterized by pulmonary hemorrhage, glomerulonephritis, and antibody to basement membrane antigens. The etiology is unknown. Goodpasture's syndrome typically affects young males, but it may appear at any age and an increasing number of affected women are being recognized. Pulmonary hemorrhage may be mild and easily overlooked or severe and life threatening. The initial manifestations of pulmonary involvement are cough, mild shortness of breath, and hemoptysis. Hypoxia is a frequent finding. Chest x-ray findings are variable. The changes of pulmonary hemorrhage or pulmonary hemosiderosis are seen in almost all patients. At a certain stage of the disease there are frequent poorly marginated alveolar infiltrates due to acute pulmonary hemorrhage, or there may be a diffuse reticulonodular miliary interstitial pattern from hemosiderin deposition. The pulmonary infiltrates frequently spare the apices and the costophrenic angles. They are characterized by rapidly changing patterns, often going from severe pulmonary edema to a dramatic clearing, with a frequent short-term shifting of infiltrates being typical. The heart is usually normal and these infiltrates are not associated with pulmonary vascular congestion (BENOIT et al. 1964).

Pulmonary hemorrhage may also be seen in association with (a) renal failure in SLE, PAN, Wegener's granulomatosis, Henoch-Schönlein syndrome, pulmonary embolism secondary to renal vein thrombosis, and legionnaires' disease and (b) congestive heart failure in patients with chronic renal failure (DUNCAN et al. 1965). These disorders can usually be differentiated by their clinical features and laboratory findings, most specifically by circulating anti-basement membrane antibodies.

3.4.5.2 Pathologic Findings

The kidneys are usually enlarged with smooth surfaces at autopsy, but if the clinical course is prolonged the kidneys may become small. Initially on biopsy there is a mild focal nephritis, which will progress to a diffuse proliferative and necrotizing glomerulonephritis, with extensive extracapillary proliferation ("crescents"). There is no associated arteritis. Immunofluorescence studies show typical linear deposits of anti-basement membrane antibody and also frequently C3 deposition; these findings are diagnostic of Goodpasture's syndrome. Electron microscopic studies do not demonstrate electron-dense deposits.

3.4.5.3 Radiologic Evaluation

The greatest usefulness of radiologic imaging in patients with Goodpasture's syndrome is in evaluating and following the status of the lungs with chest x-rays. Not infrequently, the pattern of rapidly changing infiltrates in a patient with hemoptysis will suggest the diagnosis before renal involvement is apparent. The radiologic findings in the kidneys are the nonspecific findings of glomerulonephritis. Early in the disease, urography is normal. Later in the course, the findings reflect renal insufficiency and ultrasound remains the best means of anatomically visualizing the kidneys as required clinically. Renal venography is useful to exclude renal vein thrombosis as a differential consideration, although this can also be accomplished by MRI (HONDA et al. 1988). Angiography, CT, and MRI are only useful to evaluate associated complications and further delineate regional anatomy, as required clinically.

3.4.6 Henoch-Schönlein Syndrome

Henoch-Schönlein syndrome or anaphylactoid purpura is a systemic necrotizing vasculitis of small vessels, usually seen in childhood. It is characterized by palpable purpura, most commonly distributed over the buttocks and lower extremities. Symptoms are primarily gastrointestinal complaints, commonly colic, abdominal pain associated with nausea, vomiting, and diarrhea with blood, and arthralgias of the large joints, usually the knees and ankles. About 30% of the patients exhibit renal involvement with hematuria and acute nephritis. Renal involvement tends to be much less severe in children. Up to 25% of adults will develop rapidly progressive glomerulonephritis and progressive renal failure. The nephrotic syndrome is reported to develop in over 50% of cases (BALLARD et al. 1970). Hypertension is seen but is usually mild and self-limited. Most patients have a benign course with full recovery; however, recurrences are common. Laboratory features are not distinctive and are very similar to IgA nephropathy.

Renal biopsy shows a spectrum of lesions, ranging from a focal mesangial proliferation to diffuse crescentic glomerulonephritis. The most typical lesion is a multifocal necrotizing glomerulonephritis with fibrin deposition. Electron microscopy shows diffuse mesangial deposits of IgA with lesser amounts of IgG2 complement. IgA deposits are also seen in dermal capillaries in involved and uninvolved regions. This disease is felt to be an IgA immune mediated progress, but the etiology is unknown.

Radiographic studies are most useful in evaluating the gastrointestinal complaints of these patients. Submucosal hemorrhages may be demonstrated on barium examination of stomach, small bowel, or colon as "thumbprinting" etc. Barium studies are also useful to find intussusceptions which occur as a complication of this disease. Radiologic evaluation of the kidneys shows findings similar to acute glomerulonephritis. Intramural hematomas have been described in the wall of the bladder (McPHERSON 1974). Testicular involvement may occur, and painful scrotal hematomas may mimic testicular torsion (SAHN and SCHWARTZ 1972).

3.4.7 Wegener's Granulomatosis

Wegener's granulomatosis is a distinct clinicopathologic entity. It is a granulomatous and necrotizing vasculitis, which also involves large vessels. Its primary involvement is in the upper respiratory tract, the tracheobronchial tree, the lungs, and the kidneys. However, widely disseminated vasculitis does occur. The disease presents most frequently in the fourth and fifth decades and affects males more than females. Presenting symptoms are usually respiratory. Sinusitis, otitis, keratoconjunctivitis, and purulent rhinorrhea are most common. Skin lesions, such as papules, purpura, or subcutaneous nodules, are fairly frequent. Cardiac involvement also occurs, usually with pericarditis and coronary vasculitis and only rarely cardiomyopathy. Central nervous system manifestations are cranial neuritis or cerebral vasculitis usually associated with hematuria, proteinuria, and glomerulonephritis. Renal involvement occurs in 85% of patients and generally dominates the clinical picture. Once impairment of renal function is present, progressive renal failure will follow without proper therapy.

Renal biopsy shows a focal necrotizing proliferative glomerulonephritis, usually without immune deposits. A severe diffuse necrotizing and crescentic glomerulonephritis may develop rapidly. Necrotizing vasculitis is seen in biopsies of the respiratory tract but is not usually seen in kidney biopsies. The presence of granulomas is the feature which distinguishes Wegener's granulomatosis from PAN pathologically (GOODMAN and CHURG 1954).

Radiologic evaluation of the lungs by chest radiography and CT typically demonstrates multiple parenchymal nodules, some or all of which are cavitating. The major differential diagnoses are metastatic disease and a disseminated inflammatory process, such as pulmonary fungal infection. Occasionally, a solitary lesion will mimic a lung carcinoma. The extensive paranasal sinus and nasal involvement seen with this disease can be well delineated by either CT or MRI, as required clinically (SIMMONS et al. 1987). There are no specific radiologic findings in renal involvement by Wegener's granulomatosis. The kidneys are normal in size or are moderately small. The urographic and angiographic appearance is similar to glomerulonephritis, either acute or chronic. Hypertensive changes tend to dominate the angiographic findings (BAMBERY et al. 1988).

3.4.8 Scleroderma

3.4.8.1 Clinical Background

Scleroderma, or progressive systemic sclerosis (PSS), is a multisystem disorder characterized by inflammatory, vascular, and fibrotic changes of the skin (scleroderma) and multiple viscera, most commonly the gastrointestinal tract, lungs, heart, and kidneys. The course, pattern of involvement, and severity of the disease are highly variable. Scleroderma has a female preponderance (4 to 1) with a peak incidence in the third to fifth decades. Skin changes are the primary clinical manifestation in most patients. This might be the only involvement for many years in some patients, while others may develop progressive visceral involvement over several years with survival being determined by the extent of disease within the heart, lungs, and kidneys. Rarely the disease will present with visceral involvement without skin changes (TUFFANELLI and WINKELMANN 1961).

Raynaud's phenomenon is the first symptom of PSS in over 90% of patients with skin changes. Symptoms of "esophageal" involvement, epigastric fullness with or without pain with regurgitation of gastric contents, occur most noticeably when the patient is lying flat or bending over. Abdominal pain, bloating and malabsorption, and constipation are seen with intestinal and or colonic involvement. Extensive gastrointestinal PSS may occur without other skin or visceral involvement. Pulmonary fibrosis, with or without hypertension, is seen clinically and radiographically. Cardiomyopathy is seen secondary to myocardial fibrosis and may be complicated by pericardial effusion.

Renal failure is the leading cause of death in PSS, accounting for half the mortality. Proteinuria, an abnormal urine sediment, hypertension (often progressive and malignant), and microangiopathic hemolytic anemia are all features of progressive renal disease. The onset of renal involvement is usually within 3–5 years after initial diagnosis. Acute renal failure can occur abruptly at any time, even in an apparently stable patient. The onset of microangiopathic anemia may serve as an indicator of a pending renal failure, which usually follows several weeks later.

3.4.8.2 Pathologic Findings

The primary event in PSS is postulated to be an endothelial cell injury in vessels ranging in size from small arteries to capillaries. The cause of this damage is not known, but a serum cytotoxic factor, a serine protease, has been found in some patients with PSS. Humoral and cell mediated immune phenomena are frequent findings, with laboratory evidence of autoantibodies to fibroblast cell membranes and to type I and IV collagen.

Hypergammaglobulinemia and antinuclear antibodies are frequent findings in PSS. Grossly, kidneys are typically normal or slightly enlarged, although they may be slightly decreased in size depending on the clinical course. Frequently, there are multiple petechial hemorrhages with small in-farctions microscopically. The most striking feature is marked intimal hyperplasia of the interlobular ar-teries, which are severely narrowed or occluded by fibrin clots. There is fibrinoid necrosis of the affer-ent arterioles, including the glomerular tuft, with thickening of the glomerular basement membrane. These lesions result in cortical infarctions and glomerular sclerosis. These renal pathologic changes are indistinguishable from those of malig-nant hypertension but in PSS the lesions may be present in the absence of hypertension.

3.4.8.3 Radiologic Evaluation

Radiologic evaluation is not necessary for estab-lishing the diagnosis of PSS, which is already known clinically in the vast majority of cases. Chest radio-graphic findings of pulmonary fibrosis and/or pul-monary hypertension or the classic gastrointestinal findings in the esophagus and small and large intes-tines may first suggest the diagnosis in patients with-out skin manifestations. Radiologic evaluation is largely a clinical adjunct to assist management. Vas-cular contrast studies should generally be avoided, as they may further impair compromised function. Ultrasound and non-contrast-enhanced CT are the basic anatomic diagnostic procedures. Radionu-clide studies may be used to assess renal blood flow or to demonstrate infarcts. Angiography shows vas-cular constrictions and pruning of intrarenal (figure) vessels similar to advanced nephrosclerosis (LESTER and KOEHLER 1971). Constriction of the interlobular arteries is a finding which parallels the vasospasm of the digital arteries seen in Raynaud's phenomenon.

3.4.9 Nephrosclerosis

3.4.9.1 Clinical Background

Small vessel changes occur in the kidneys as part of the normal aging process. At least some degree of small vessel lesion is found at autopsy in about 70% of normotensive individuals who die after the age of 60 years. These vascular changes presumably ac-count for most of the loss of renal glomerular func-tion which accompanies aging (BONOMINI and VAN-GELISTA 1988) and for the loss of functional reserve seen in older individuals, making them more prone to develop renal failure due to volume depletion, stress such as trauma or surgery, or metabolic in-sults. This loss of function also impairs the ability of

the elderly to clear and detoxify drugs, causing an increased incidence of drug complications. Further-more there is a definite reduction in concentration capacity, indicating some tubular dysfunction sec-ondary to arterial involvement. These patients also have a mild proteinuria.

Hypertension and diabetes mellitus intensify and accelerate this physiologic degenerative process. The longer the duration and the more severe the hypertension, the more severe is the nephrosclerosis which eventually results in small shrunken kidneys and chronic renal failure (BLYTHE 1985). Malignant hypertension can produce an accelerated nephro-sclerosis with acute renal failure. These patients frequently exhibit hypertensive encephalopathy, including papilledema and seizures. Severe retino-pathy is almost always present and congestive heart failure is common. Patients frequently have gross and microscopic hematuria and a fairly marked pro-teinuria.

3.4.9.2 Pathologic Findings

The kidneys are small and somewhat irregular. Large and medium sized arteries at the interlobar and arcuate levels show intimal thickening of vari-able degree. The involvement seen in the small ar-teries and arterioles is more widespread and more severe. These vessels exhibit an eosinophilic hyaline thickening which causes significant vascular ob-struction. The end result is renal ischemia and atrophy. In malignant hypertension, there is a hyperplastic endarteritis of the interlobular and ac-tuate arteries. Fibrinoid necrosis of the afferent ar-terioles subsequently occurs with infarction or atrophy distal to these vessels, depending upon their degree of involvement. The amorphous material in the vessel walls has been demonstrated to be fibrin. It is postulated that severe hypertension causes en-dothelial injury with leakage of fibrin and other plasma components into the vessel wall which then leads to vascular necrosis, a mechanism somewhat similar to that postulated in PSS.

3.4.9.3 Radiologic Findings

Radiological evaluation in patients with nephroscle-rosis is most useful for diagnosing the presence of renal artery stenosis as a cause of hypertension. Screening is done by nuclear radionuclide Hippuran renogram. Timed pyelography is still used, but it is not as sensitive or as accurate a technique. Renal angiography, including digital imaging techniques, is the definitive means for defining renal artery stenosis. For appropriate lesions, therapeutic angioplasty may be carried out immediately following the diagnostic procedure.

Ultrasound is the procedure of choice for assessing renal size and contour and for excluding occult hydronephrosis. Urography, CT, and MRI are used primarily as clinical adjuncts in evaluating for hypertensive complications, such as renal or retroperitoneal hemorrhage. Angiography again is clinically useful to assess for renal artery stenosis in hypertensive patients. In patients with mild nephrosclerosis, angiography is normal. In more severe cases, the main renal arteries are normal whereas the intrarenal vessels are narrowed and show tortuosity of the interlobar arteries, the so-called corkscrew appearance (FRIEDENBERG et al. 1965; GILL and PUDVAN 1970; MENA et al. 1973). The arcuate vessels appear prominent. In late stages, the main renal arteries decrease in caliber proportionate to the loss of renal parenchyma. There is marked reduction in the size and tortuosity of the interlobar vessels with pruning of their branches (fig.). There is poor cortical opacification with loss of corticomedullary definition. The pattern is strikingly similar to that seen in chronic glomerulonephritis or in severe scleroderma and PSS.

3.5 Bilateral Renal Cortical Necrosis

Bilateral renal cortical necrosis (BRCN) is a rare condition which is characterized by death of cells of all types in the renal cortex with progressive acute renal failure. Classically, this occurs in young females as a complication of pregnancy in association with abruptio placentae, but it can also be seen with preeclampsia, eclampsia, septic abortion, placenta previa with hemorrhage, or postpartum hemorrhage. It has also been associated with severe trauma such as burns, multiple fracture, hemorrhagic shock, severe dehydration, systemic toxins such as bacteremia or snakebite, transfusion reactions, PAN, and peptic ulcer (WHELAN et al. 1967). Patient symptomatology is predominantly related to acute anuria and renal failure. Patients may have severe flank pain and gross hematuria with marked proteinuria. The renal damage is irreversible.

3.5.1 Pathologic Findings

The pathogenesis is tissue death due to deficiency of cortical blood flow. The outer 2 mm of the peripheral cortex, which is supplied by capsular vessels, is spared. Gross examination shows the infarcted cortex and columns of Bertin to be pale yellow, in contrast to the pink viable subcapsular rim and the dusky red congested medulla. Early in the course, the kidneys are mildly enlarged, but with time they show a progressive reduction in volume. No gross thrombi are seen in the large vessels and they are only sporadically seen in the arcuate and more peripheral branches. Within 1 week, calcium is seen microscopically within the necrotic tissue concentrated near the interface of the adjacent viable medulla and the capsular supplied cortical rim. Within 3 weeks, calcification can be identified radiographically. At 6–8 weeks, this pattern evolves into the classic radiographic cortical tram track sign of cortical necrosis.

The etiology of the renal cortical ischemia is not established. Thrombosis is not a significant pathologic finding. The current theory most favored is that ischemia is secondary to prolonged vasospasm of the interlobar and interlobular arteries. The resulting diversion of blood flow from the cortex for as little as 2–4 h will produce cortical infarction. The more sustained the vasospasm, the more extensive the infarction. It is postulated that these renal vasomotor changes are mediated by endogenous catecholamine secretion (THAL 1955).

3.5.2 Radiologic Findings

Urographic studies in the early stage of the disease in the past have shown mildly enlarged kidneys with markedly decreased function. A characteristic nephrogram with a hypodense zone of cortex between a dense subcortical rim is sometimes seen with a dense perimedullary rim. This finding can also be seen on ultrasound, CT, and angiographic examinations (LAUPACIS et al. 1983; PAPO et al. 1985). Angiography shows poor peripheral perfusion and slow emptying of the major vessels. Urography and angiography or other contrast examinations should not be performed when BRCN is suspected. Ultrasound, CT without contrast, radionuclide studies, or MRI should provide the clinically needed anatomic information without additional risk to the impaired kidneys. Plain nephrotomography later in the course should nicely demonstrate the pathognomonic cortical tram tracks (CRAMER and FUGLESTAD 1965;

Table 3.2. Principal causes of tubulointerstitial disease of the kidney

I. Toxins
   A. Exogenous toxins
      1. Analgesic nephropathy
      2. Lead nephropathy
      3. Miscellaneous nephrotoxins (e. g., antibiotics, radiographic contrast media, heavy metals)
   B. Metabolic toxins
      1. Acute uric acid nephropathy
      2. Gouty nephropathy
      3. Hypercalcemic nephropathy
      4. Hypokalemic nephropathy
      5. Miscellaneous metabolic toxins (e. g., hyperoxaluria, cystinosis, Fabry's disease)

II. Neoplasia
   A. Lymphoma
   B. Leukemia
   C. Multiple myeloma

III. Immune disorders
   A. Hypersensitivity nephropathy
   B. Sjögren's syndrome
   C. Sarcoidosis
   D. Amyloidosis
   E. Transplant rejection
   F. Tubulointerstitial abnormalities associated with glomerulonephritis

IV. Vascular disorders
   A. Arteriolar nephrosclerosis
   B. Atheroembolic disease
   C. Sickle cell nephropathy
   D. Acute tubular necrosis

V. Hereditary renal diseases
   A. Hereditary nephritis
   B. Medullary cystic disease
   C. Medullary sponge kidney
   D. Polycystic kidney

VI. Infectious injury
   A. Acute pyelonephritis
   B. Chronic pyelonephritis

VII. Miscellaneous disorders
   A. Chronic urinary tract obstruction
   B. Vesicoureteral reflux
   C. Radiation nephritis
   D. Balkan nephropathy

Table 3.3. Manifestations of renal tubulointerstitial diseases

I. Tubular dysfunction disproportionate to reduction in glomerular filtration rate

II. Tubular abnormalities
   A. Reduced maximal urinary concentrating ability (polyuria, nocturia)
   B. Renal tubular acidosis (hyperchloremic metabolic acidosis)
   C. Partial or complete Fanconi's syndrome
      1. Phosphaturia
      2. Bicarbonaturia
      3. Aminoaciduria
      4. Uricosuria
      5. Glycosuria
   D. Sodium wasting
   E. Hyperkalemia

III. Renal endocrine deficiencies
   A. Hyperreninemic hypoaldosteronism (hyperkalemia, metabolic acidosis)
   B. Calcitriol deficiency (renal osteodystrophy)
   C. Erythropoietin deficiency (anemia)

IV. Urinalysis
   A. May be normal but urine usually contains cellular elements
   B. Proteinuria is usually modest (< 3.5 g per day) and consists largely of low molecular weight "tubular" proteins such as lysozyme and β-microglobulin

3.6 Tubulointerstitial Diseases

3.6.1 General Considerations

There is a large and diverse group of condition which can be characterized clinically by tubular functional abnormalities, which are associated with histologic changes, primarily in the interstitium, as against the glomerulus and renal vasculature. These diseases may be acute or chronic and are quite common. Approximately 30% of all cases of chronic renal insufficiency in the United States are caused by tubulointerstitial disease (COTRAN et al. 1986). In most cases, the specific cause can be determined. There are many possible causes, the most common of which are exogenous toxins and metabolic and immunologic derangements (Table 3.2).

In tubulointerstitial disease, functional tubular abnormalities are disproportionately prominent relative to reduction in overall function, as measured by the glomerular filtration rate. Reduction in renal concentration ability is manifested by polyuria and nocturia. Tubular acidosis, sodium depletion, or hyperkalemia may be present on laboratory examinations (Table 3.3).

A specific diagnosis of a renal tubular disease is made by a thorough patient history, physical exam-

WHELAN et al. 1967). BRCN is most often clinically differentiated from acute tubular necrosis, but in difficult cases, serial isotope renograms will usually demonstrate relatively rapid recovery in ATN, whereas BRCN damage is typically irreversible with very slow or no recovery.

ination, and laboratory evaluation. Renal biopsy confirms the diagnosis of interstitial disease but is often nonspecific. The specific type may be revealed by the clinical findings. Radiologic studies are of importance in evaluating for obstructive uropathy or for diagnosing polycystic disease. Contrast examinations should be used only where clinically necessary, and not as a primary investigation. Ultrasound and radionuclide scans are the basic techniques employed. CT and MRI may be useful for additional noninvasive anatomic delineation. Angiography and renal venography are used only as specifically indicated by clinical findings.

3.6.2 Acute Interstitial Nephritis

Acute interstitial nephritis (AISN) is characterized by infiltration of mononuclear cells into the interstitium, particularly in the renal cortex. Eosinophils (especially in drug related cases) and polymorphonuclear leukocytes may also be present. Inflammatory cells may invade tubular walls and may be seen around frank tubular necrosis in more severe cases. This infiltration may be diffuse or patchy. The amount of functional impairment is proportionate to the extent of this infiltration. The interstitial edema is diffuse. Interstitial fibrosis is not seen unless there is progression into chronic interstitial nephritis. The predominant mononuclear cell present is the T cell. Both helper/inducer and suppressor/cytotoxic T cells are present in variable numbers. These findings suggest that both T cell mediated delayed hypersensitivity reactions and cytotoxic T cell injury play a role in pathogenesis. Immunoglobulins and complement, as well as immune complex and anti-basement membrane antibody, have also been identified on biopsy specimens. These findings indicate that humoral immune mechanisms also play a role in the pathogenesis of AISN. The relative importance and actual mechanism of initiation of injury are not yet understood. The many causes of AISN are listed in Tables 3.4 and 3.5. Acute tubular necrosis is a good example of AISN.

3.6.2.1 Acute Tubular Necrosis

Clinical Background. Acute tubular necrosis produces acute reversible renal failure and oliguria. It is caused by exposure to toxic agents – most commonly bichloride of mercury, carbon tetrachloride, ethylene glycol, bismuth, arsenic, or uranium. Exposure to urographic contrast material, especially in pa-

Table 3.4. Causes of acute interstitial nephritis

1. Drug related (see Table 3.5)

2. Systemic infections

Brucellosis	Mycoplasmal pneumonia
Cytomegalovirus	Polyomavirus
Diphtheria	Rocky Mountain spotted fever
Infectious mononucleosis	Streptococcal infections
Legionnaires' disease	Syphilis
Leptospirosis	Toxoplasmosis

3. Primary renal infections
   Bacterial pyelonephritis
   Renal tuberculosis
   Fungal nephritis

4. Immune disorders
   Acute glomerulonephritis associated with anti-tubular basement membrane antibodies and/or secondary interstitial nephritis
   Systemic lupus erythematosus
   Acute rejection of a renal transplant
   Necrotizing vasculitis

5. Other conditions

6. Idiopathic

Table 3.5. Drugs associated with acute interstitial nephritis

Antimicrobial drugs

Cephalosporins	Para-aminosalicylic acid
Chloramphenicol	Penicillins[a]
Colistin	Polymyxin B
Erythromycin	Rifampin[a]
Ethambutol	Sulfonamides[a]
Isoniazid	Tetracyclines
	Vancomycin

Nonsteroidal anti-inflammatory drugs

Allopurinol[a]	Methyldopa
Antipyrine	Phenindione[a]
Azathioprine	Phenylpropanolamine
Bismuth	Phenyloin
Captopril	Probenecid
Cimetidine	Sulfinpyrazone
Clofibrate	Sulfonamide diuretics[a]
Gold	Triamterene

[a] Most frequent or clinically important.

tients with underlying renal disease and in dehydrated patients, is a clinically common cause (BERLYNE and BERLYNE 1962; DAVIDSON et al. 1970). Renal ischemia secondary to shock of any etiology, severe crush injuries or burns, transfusion, or severe allergic reactions can also induce acute tubular necrosis. It is also seen postsurgically in patients having prolonged procedures with hypoperfusion to the kidneys, most commonly cardiovascular surgery, renal transplantation, and aortic surgery where there is actual temporary interruption to renal blood flow. In trauma patients acute tubular necrosis may occur as

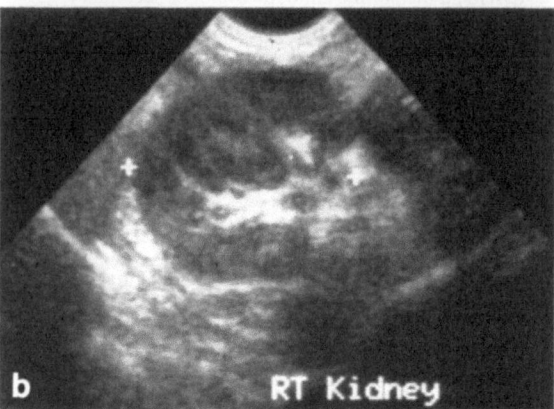

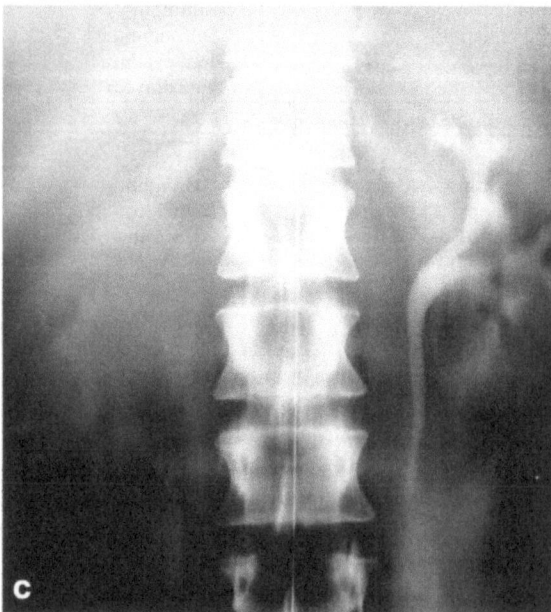

Fig. 3.9 a–c. Diabetic patient with interstitial nephritis complicated by acute bacterial pyelonephritis. Edematous enlarged kidney on ultrasound with decreased excretion on urogram

a consequence of temporary obstruction by circulating myoglobin.

The clinical course is that of oliguria and/or anuria for 10–30 days. The urine is dark, contains protein, casts, and debris, and is isosthenuric. Patients frequently require dialysis for support. Patients then go into a diuretic polyuric phase with large volumes of hypotonic urine which require careful fluid management. There is a progressive drop in blood urea nitrogen and creatinine, with a gradual recovery of tubular function and a return of the ability to concentrate.

Pathology. The main pathologic finding and explanation for this condition is necrosis of the renal tubular epithelium. Tubules are filled with cellular debris and are frequently dilated. These findings are associated with diffuse interstitial edema with an infiltrate of lymphocytes, monocytes, and plasma cells, which produces the renal enlargement. An explanation of the pathogenesis is that renal failure is due to the mechanical obstruction of the tubules. A newer theory is that impaired function is due to preglomerular ischemia and that oliguria is secondary to diminished glomerular filtration and that tubular changes are secondary. Some have proposed changing the name of this condition to "vasomotor nephropathy." No convincing proof has been discovered and both theories have strong proponents. The final conclusion will most likely be that the two mechanisms interact (ANDERSON and SCHRIER 1988).

Radiologic Evaluation. Radiologic findings are dominated by the severely impaired renal function (Fig. 3.9). If acute tubular necrosis is suspected clinically, urographic contrast studies, i.e. intravenous pyelography and angiography, are relatively contraindicated, as the contrast agents may significantly worsen the patient's renal status. Retrograde pyelography may be performed to exclude ureteral abnormality if needed. If urography is done, the classic findings are bilateral enlarged smooth kidneys. The kidneys show an early dense and persistent nephrogram on delayed films, often up to 24 h, with little or no pelvocalyceal visualization. About 25% of patients show a nephrogram which becomes increasingly denser during the examination with no significant pelvocalyceal visualization. Absence of a nephrogram is unusual and suggests possible vascular complications.

Renal arteriography is only useful in the evaluation of arterial complications such as vascular injury or occlusion. If an associated renal vein thrombosis is suspected, renal venography may be necessary if MRI is not readily available to demonstrate patency of the renal veins [also according to DON et al. (1989) color Doppler ultrasound may be the initial procedure of choice today]. Neither renal arteriography nor renal venography has a primary role in evaluating these patients.

Ultrasound is the key diagnostic examination in acute tubular necrosis. It is used to assess overall renal size and contour and most importantly to exclude hydronephrosis as a cause of the impaired function. Loss of corticomedullary definition is a nonspecific finding that is seen with acute tubular necrosis and many other diseases. Abdominal Doppler flow study has been used to evaluate renal blood flow, but has not proven consistently accurate (KOHLER et al. 1986; ALLEN et al. 1988).

Radioisotope blood flow scan and quantitative curve determination is the current method of choice in assessing renal blood flow in patients with impaired renal function. This technique is used to differentiate acute tubular necrosis from early renal transplant rejection. Findings, however, are seldom definitive enough to obviate the need for biopsy.

Computed tomography is really only useful for evaluation of associated problems such as defining abdominal or renal parenchymal injuries in patients with acute tubular necrosis following significant abdominal trauma (LANG 1990).

Magnetic resonance imaging is useful to noninvasively visualize renal arterial and venous patency and current work on MR angiography may someday allow quantitative flow measurement and high resolution anatomic detail. MRI clearly shows loss of normal corticomedullary definition and has also been used to help differentiate acute tubular necrosis from renal transplant rejection (HRICAK et al. 1986). The findings are nonspecific and there is considerable overlap of patterns.

3.6.3 Chronic Interstitial Nephritis

The clinical manifestations are primarily those of renal tubular functional defects or chronic renal failure. Sterile pyuria may be present, but in contrast to AISN, eosinophilia and eosinophiluria are not seen. Table 3.6 outlines the many causes of chronic interstitial nephritis (CISN); some of the major ones will be discussed in the following section.

Pathologically, CISN is characterized by diffuse interstitial fibrosis with atrophy and loss of renal tubules. The glomeruli show only focal loss and contraction. There is usually a patchy infiltration of chronic inflammatory cells. The renal vasculature is

Table 3.6. Causes of chronic interstitial nephritis

1. Persistence or progression of acute interstitial nephritis

2. Chronic urinary tract obstruction

3. Nephrotoxins:
   Drugs: analgesics, nitrosoureas
   Endogenous substances: uric acid, hypercalcemia, hypokalemia
   Metals: cisplatin, copper, lead, lithium, mercury
   Radiation
   Drug abuse

4. Chronic bacterial pyelonephritis or renal tuberculosis

5. Immune disorders:
   AIDS
   Chronic glomerulonephritis with interstitial nephritis
   Chronic rejection of a renal transplant
   Systemic lupus erythematosus
   Sjögren's syndrome

6. Associated with neoplasia or paraproteinemias:
   Leukemia   Waldenström's macroglobulinemia
   Lymphoma   Cryoglobulinemia
   Amyloidosis   Multiple myeloma

7. Cystic diseases:
   Medullary cystic disease
   Polycystic kidney disease

8. Miscellaneous:
   Diabetes mellitus   Advanced renal failure
   Sickle cell hemoglobinopathies Idiopathic
   Vascular diseases

normal, except for associated changes of hypertension and nephrosclerosis. In specific cases, other underlying etiologies may be definable on biopsy such as lymphomatous or leukemic cellular infiltration, amyloidosis, uric acid crystals, or myeloma protein casts obstructing tubules. The clinical history, laboratory findings, and chronic interstitial pattern on biopsy are combined to establish the specific diagnosis.

3.6.3.1 Radiologic Evaluation

Radiologic evalution in these patients is primarily used to determine the presence and extent of obstructive uropathy as either the principal cause or a secondary complication of some conditions such as urolithiasis in hypercalcemia or urate nephropathy. Ultrasound is the procedure of choice for evaluation of the kidneys. CT, nuclear medicine, MRI, and angiography play an ancillary role dictated by clinical circumstances. Contrast examinations (both excretory urography and retrograde pyelography) do play an important role in establishing the diagnosis of an important complicating condition seen with CISN, namely renal papillary necrosis.

3.6.3.2 Papillary Necrosis

Renal papillary necrosis is commonly seen clinically in patients with severe pyelonephritis, diabetes mellitus, sickle cell anemia, gout, analgesic abuse, and chronic obstructive uropathy. The patient usually exhibits severe flank pain, frequently radiating down along the ureter as renal colic. Patients also frequently have hematuria. High fever is common and patients may present with gram-negative bacteremia. Papillary necrosis should be considered in patients who show a rapid deterioration in clinical status during an episode of acute pyelonephritis - especially patients with known underlying conditions such as diabetes or sickle cell anemia.

The renal papilla is less likely to undergo necrosis in the presence of severe active infection when unterlying damage is present from the associated conditions discussed above. Damage to the renal papilla is of major importance in the pathogenesis of CISN in these conditions. The pathogenesis of injury appears to involve two mechanisms: the first is renal vascular injury and ischemia such as is seen in patients with sickle cell disease and in diabetics; the second is a direct toxic effect on the tubules of the high concentrations of medications or metabolic products which are found in the papilla, such as in patients who are analgesic abusers. The presence of infection compounds and potentiates the injury but is not necessarily fundamental to the development of papillary necrosis (SABATINI 1984, EKNOYAN et al. 1982).

The diagnosis of papillary necrosis is definitively made by microscopic demonstration of sloughed papillary tissue in the urine. The diagnosis can also be established by urographic findings in an appropriate clinical setting. The disease almost always involves both kidneys but may be more prominent on one side, especially if there is an associated unilateral obstructive uropathy. The kidneys are usually mildly enlarged and smooth in contour, except when there is an underlying chronic longstanding condition such as analgesic nephropathy. The kidneys have been described as small with a wavy contour. The papillae are enlarged early in the course, but soon show signs of necrosis and slough with central cavity formation or sinus tracts extending from the fornices lateral into the medulla. A completed sloughed papilla will be seen as a filling defect in a dilated and often irregular calyx or within the renal pelvis. The so-called ring sign is pathognomonic for papillary necrosis. In chronic conditions, papillary calcification known as nephrocalcinosis will become apparent at multiple sites throughout the medulla. A chronically sloughed papillary tip may develop ring calcification.

3.6.3.3 Analgesic Abuse

Clinical Background. Chronic interstitial nephritis leading to chronic renal failure secondary to the excessive injection of analgesic drugs, most notably phenacetin or acetaminophen (which is a metabolic conversion product of phenacetin) in combination with aspirin, is a common occurrence. In the United States, 2%–10% of all cases of end-stage renal disease are attributed to analgesic abuse, and in Australia, 20%. Of all such cases due to analgesic abuse, experimental and epidemiologic studies have demonstrated that phenacetin and aspirin either alone or more potently in combination produce permanent and irreversible renal damage, i.e., papillary necrosis and CISN, which leads to renal failure (BUCKALEW and SCHEY 1986).

Analgesic abuse is usually associated with a characteristic grouping of clinical and laboratory findings. It occurs three to five times more commonly in females. There is a direct relationship between the amount of drug ingested and the degree of renal injury. An intake of 1 g phenacetin per day for 3 years or a total of 3 kg in combination with other analgesics, especially aspirin, represents the minimum amount necessary to produce permanent renal damage. Obtaining a history of such abuse is very difficult (KINCAID-SMITH 1980).

Patients frequently do not admit taking analgesics or they may grossly underestimate their actual consumption. The reasons for taking the medication are varied, but the most common complaint is headaches. Many patients demonstrate a strong underlying psychological component and careful investigation of past medical history and family consultation is needed to establish the diagnosis. Urinalysis frequently demonstrates sterile pyuria. Persistence of this finding should raise the clinical index of suspicion for analgesic abuse. These patients may also develop secondary infections, which could complete the clinical picture, and in many such cases a diagnosis of pyelonephritis is made. Analgesic abusers show an inability to concentrate urine maximally an a distal-type renal tubular acidosis, reflecting papillary damage. They usually have mild proteinuria. Hypertension tends to occur late in the course of the disease. An important finding is persistent anemia that is disproportionately severe relative to the renal functional status. This may be aggravated by chronic occult gastrointestinal blood loss or by hemolysis, which these patients are prone to develop. The onset of papillary necrosis in a patient without underlying cause, such as diabetes or sickle cell disease, should raise a strong suspicion of analgesic abuse. Analgesic abusers are also at high risk for the development of urothelial malignancy, especially transitional cell carcinoma of the renal pelvis. Analgesic abusers with onset of hematuria should undergo thorough urologic investigation, including cystoscopy with urine collection for cytology (BLOHME and JOHANSSON 1981).

Pathology. Analgesic abuse is characterized by tubulointerstitial inflammation and papillary necrosis. In the early stages, there is damage to the vasa recta which supply the inner medula. This leads to local interstitial inflammation with necrosis of tubular cells, loops of Henle, and capillaries in the inner medulla. With continued exposure to the drugs there is focal calcification and lipid deposition in the involved areas. There is progression of these changes with fibrosis and ischemia, resulting in papillary necrosis. This usually precedes extension of the disease into the cortex. Renal size and glomerular filtration rate are still normal. As the exposure continues, the cortex becomes involved with resultant loss of renal parenchyma and function, eventually leading to end-stage renal failure (CARVLIN et al. 1987).

Two mechanisms of injury have been suggested in analgesic abuse. The first is a direct toxic effect on tubular cells caused by the very high concentrations of acetaminophen produced by the renal corticomedullary gradient, with the concentration at the tip of the papilla being ten times that in the cortex. A second mechanism of injury is thought to be related to the suppressive effect of aspirin on renal prostaglandin synthesis; this interferes with endogenous hormonal renal vascular blood flow regulation and results in hypoxia in the medulla (COTRAN et al. 1986).

Radiologic Findings. Plain film examinations may demonstrate nephrocalcinosis which should raise the possibility of analgesic abuse in the proper clinical setting. Urographic findings are those of papillary necrosis (discussed in the preceding section). Location of cortical scars between calyces is characteristic for papillary necrosis attendant upon analgesic abuse (HARTMAN et al. 1984). Ultrasound is the basic examination for assessing renal size and evaluating for the presence of obstruction. Other procedures are used as clinical problems dictate.

3.6.4 Nephrophathy of Hematopoietic Disorders

Patients with disorders of the hematopoietic system, be they benign or malignant, develop renal lesions in a significant number of cases. The renal lesion most frequently seen is a tubulointerstitial nephropathy.

3.6.4.1 Sickle Cell Hemoglobinopathies

Renal lesions are most commonly present in patients with a sickle cell hemoglobinopathy. Although tubulointerstitial lesions are most frequent in patients with sickle cell disease, they are also common in those with sickle cell trait, sickle cell hemoglobin C disease, or sickle cell-thalassemia.

The physicochemical properties of hemoglobin predispose toward its polymerization in an environment of low oxygen tension, hypertonicity, and low pH (SARGENT 1974). These conditions are characteristic of renal medulla. The consequent erythrocyte sickling causes the vascular occlusions which underlie the nephropathy that develops in these patients. Histologic study of both autopsy and biopsy material shows alterations in all portions of the kidneys, with vascular engorgement being seen in interlobular arteries, afferent arterioles, and glomeruli. The most striking changes are in the medulla, where dilated vessels and capillaries show extravasation of blood. This also occurs in the renal pelvis and ureter and is the source of frequent hematuria. These acute lesions lead to focal scarring and chronic fibrosis. Scarring in the medulla accounts for these patients' inability to concentrate urine. Occlusion of larger vessels may lead to clinically apparent renal infarctions with perirenal retroperitoneal hemorrhages. Radionuclide scans are the best and least invasive means of demonstrating such infarctions. CT scans or MRI today can be used to best demonstrate the presence and extent of intrarenal and perirenal hemorrhage in these patients (SICKLES and KOROBKIN 1974).

The most common complication in sickle cell hemoglobinopathies is papillary necrosis. The incidence of radiographically demonstrable papillary necrosis has been reported to be as high as 33%–65% (VAAMONDE 1981). The pathophysiology and radiologic findings are described in the preceding section on papillary necrosis. Patients are also highly susceptible to the development of acute and chronic pyelonephritis, which can exacerbate their tubulointerstitial disease and often lead to deterioration in function or papillary necrosis (MAPP et al. 1987).

3.6.4.2 Multiple Myeloma

Disorders of plasma cell function (multiple myeloma) also produce tubulointerstitial disease. The renal complications of multiple myeloma are a major contributing factor in the morbidity and mortality of this neoplastic disorder. Direct infiltration with myeloma cells is infrequent and when it occurs it is patchy and focal in distribution, and therefore usually does not cause functional impairment. The classic lesion seen in the "myeloma kidney" or more accurately "myeloma cast nephropathy" is filling of the distal tubules by precipitation of light chain dimers. Histologically, the affected tubules are surrounded by chronic inflammatory cells, interstitial fibrosis, and numerous multinucleated giant cells. Adjoining tubules show varying degree of atrophy (PIRANI et al. 1983). The propensity of light chains to lead to myeloma cast nephropathy is a function of their high concentration in the tubular fluid, the pH of the tubular fluid, and the intrinsic physicochemical properties of the specific proteins. Increasing the flow rate of urine or alkalinization will prevent or in mild cases reverse protein cast formation. The light chains may in addition cause direct toxicity to the tubules. Another mechanism by which myeloma causes tubulointerstitial disease is by the deposition of paraproteins, either as amyloid fibrils derived from lambda chains or as fragments of light chains derived from kappa chains. The deposition of these substances in the perivascular space and interstitium is called light chain deposition disease (PIRANI 1987).

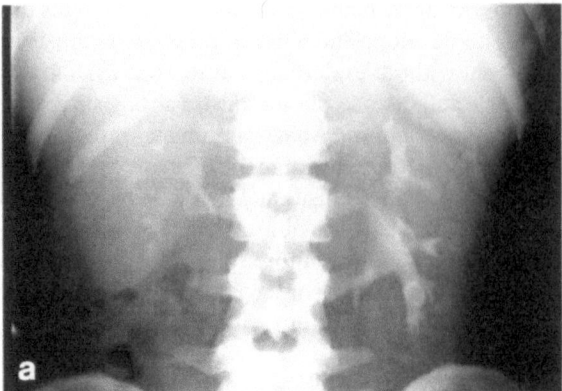
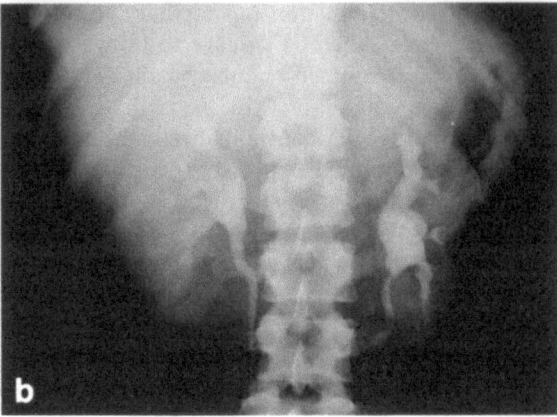

Fig. 3.10. a Intravenous urogram in a patient with leukemia. The enlarged spleen in pushing down on the left kidney. The pelvicalyceal structures are splayed and poorly distended. Both kidneys are enlarged. Thee findings are consistent with diffuse renal infiltration. **b** Same patients 6 months later in clinical remission; the appearance is now normal

3.6.4.3 Lymphoma and Leukemia

At autopsy the kidneys are found to be involved in up to 50% of patients with lymphomas or leukemias (PIRANI et al. 1983). Infiltration of the kidneys is frequent in patients with acute lymphoblastic leukemia and non-Hogdkin's lymphoma. Involvement may be focal in the form of multiple discrete nodules or diffuse with lymphomatous or leukemic infiltration (Fig. 3.10). Diffuse involvement is seen most frequently in non-Hogdkin's lymphoma (GILBOA et al. 1983). The patients may experience flank pain from renal enlargement and sometimes from renal hemorrhage into the retroperitoneum.

The kidneys can also be indirectly involved in leukemias, particularly the monocytic types, by the associated high incidence of hyperuricemia, hypercalcemia, and lysozymuria. The myelogenous leukemias, particularly the monocytic type, may be complicated by functional tubular defects which result in potassium and magnesium wasting.

Radiologic evaluation is used as clinically necessary to manage these patients rather than as a primary diagnostic procedure. Gallium scans may demonstrate renal parenchymal involvement (Fig. 3.11). CT with and without contrast gives the best anatomic delineation (CHILCOTE and BORKOWSKI 1983), especially in looking for hydronephrosis or renal or perirenal hemorrhage (Fig. 3.12) (McMILLIN and GROSS 1985). Patients who need contrast examinations should be well hydrated as iodinated contrast can cause acute renal failure, especially in myeloma patients (MYERS and WITTEN 1971). The use of nonionic contrast should be strongly considered in this patient population. Excretory urography and retrograde pyelography, as discussed earlier, are the best means of diagnosing papillary necrosis.

Fig. 3.11 a, b *(above).* Patient with non-Hodgkin's lymphoma and abnormal urinalysis, but with normal function. **a** Intravenous urogram shows diffuse bilateral renal enlargement. **b** Gallium scan shows diffuse homogeneous uptake in bilaterally enlarged kidneys

Fig. 3.12 *(below).* Decubitus CT examination demonstrating spontaneous retroperitoneal hemorrhage filling the left perirenal fossa in a patient with non-Hodgkin's lymphoma

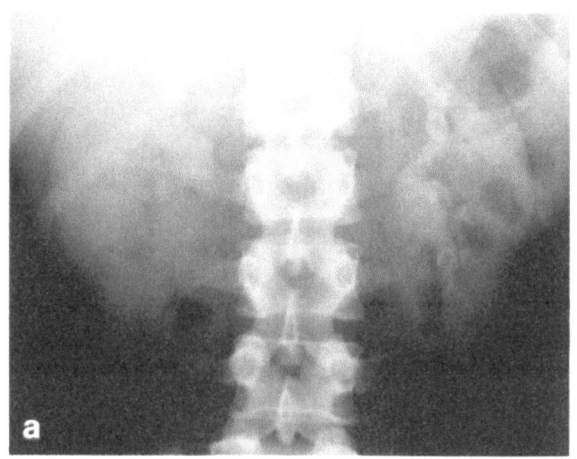

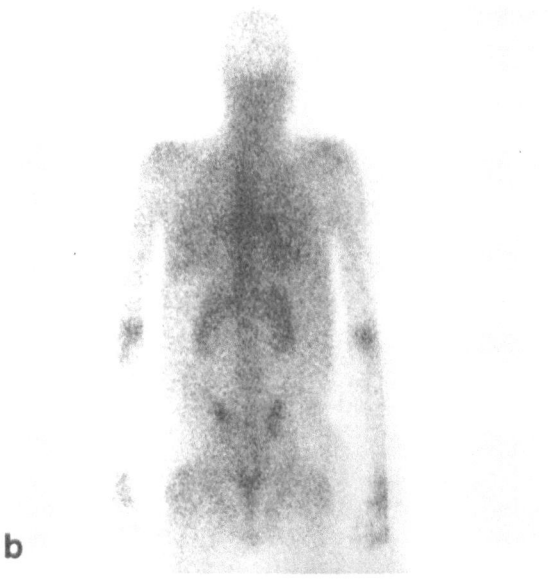

3.6.5 Fanconi's Syndrome

Fanconi's syndrome is the result of diffuse impaired transport in the proximal tubule. These patients exhibit proximal renal tubular acidosis, glycosuria, generalized aminoaciduria, phosphaturia, uricaciduria, and tubular proteinuria (Moss et al. 1980). Fanconi's syndrome is most commonly acquired secondary to diseases such as cystinosis, tyrosinemia, galactosemia, fructose intolerance, glycogen storage disease (type 1), Wilson's disease, familial nephrosis, and hereditary amyloidosis. Lowe's or oculocerebral syndrome is an x-linked recessive form of Fanconi's syndrome associated with ocular and cerebral abnormalities. In adults, acquired Fanconi's syndrome is most often due to dysproteinemias, heavy metal (especially chronic cadmium) or acute lead exposure, or immunologic disease (PASTERNACK and LINDER 1970). An older adult presenting with Fanconi's syndrome should be assumed to have multiple myeloma until proven otherwise. This disease may be seen as an autosomal recessive hereditary disorder called *adult Fanconi's syndrome,* which is not associated with other systemic conditions. Usually recognized in childhood, it is characterized by hypophosphatemic rickets, dwarfism, and the classic laboratory abnormalities of Fanconi's syndrome. These patients rarely develop renal failure (BRENES et al. 1977).

The most prominent clinical finding of Fanconi syndrome is metabolic bone disease – ricketts in children and osteomalacia in adults. Growth retardation and anorexia with nausea and episodic vomiting are frequently seen in children. Polyuria, muscle weakness, and salt wasting are also common. These patients also who disordered reabsorption and secondary decreased serum concentrations of calcium, magnesium, citrate, and low molecular weight proteins. The increased sodium concentrations seen in the distal tubules cause kaliuresis and hypokalemia. The proximal tubule is the principal site of conversion of 25-OH vitamin D to I-25-$(OH)_2$ vitamin D and because of this defect, vitamin D metabolism is impaired in these patients.

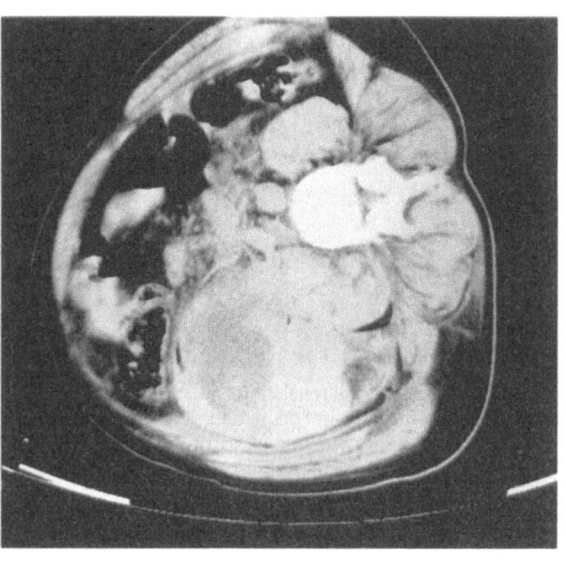

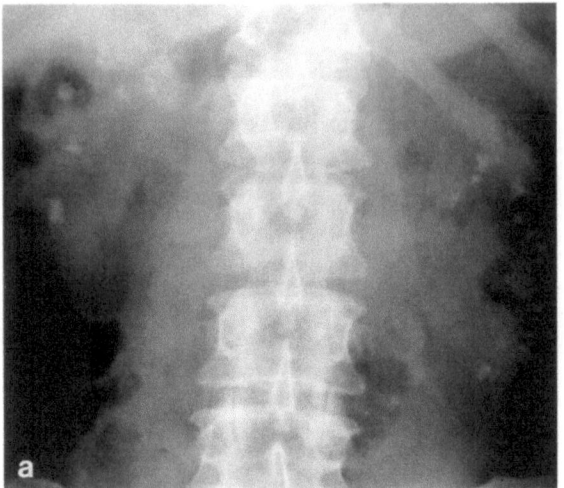

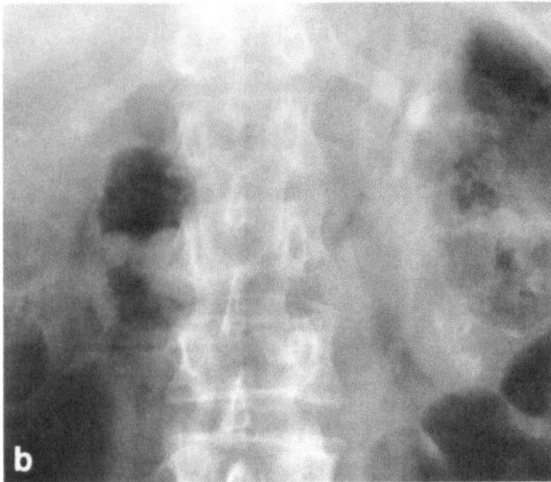

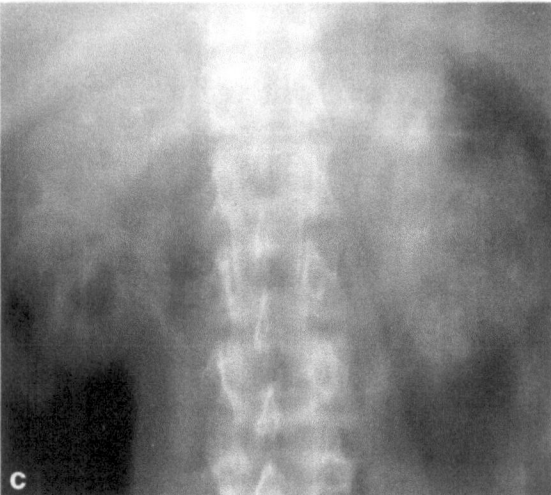

Fig. 3.13. a Patient with renal tubular acidosis and diffuse nephrocalcinosis evident on plain film. **b,c** This patient has diminished excretory function evident on urography, with limited pelvicalyceal visualization early (**b**) and on delayed films (**c**)

The classic pathologic finding in Fanconi's syndrome is "swan neck": deformity of the initial portion of the proximal tubule, with cellular atrophy of the deformed tubular segment. The global functional impairment of the proximal tubular reabsorption of solute is thought to be secondary to altered cell membrane permeability with an abnormal lumen to cell sodium gradient caused by a primary disturbance in cellular ATP and phosphate metabolism.

Radiologic studies are most useful in evaluating bone disease and complications in these patients. Anatomic evaluation of the kidneys is best accomplished by ultrasound. Contrast examinations do not contribute significant clinical information and may be harmful to these functionally impaired kidneys. Patients may develop diffuse nephrocalcinosis as well as nephrolithiasis (Fig. 3.13).

3.6.6 Uric Acid Nephropathy

The kidney is the major organ of uric acid excretion. It is the organ most susceptible to injury from disorders of urate metabolism. The lesions in the kidney are the result of uric acid crystallization in either the urine outflow tract or the renal parenchyma. The principal determinants of uric acid solubility are its concentration and the pH of its surrounding medium. Normal tubular function results in increasing concentrations of uric acid and acidification of urine, conditions which are conducive to the precipitation of uric acid. Birefringent uric acid crystals are formed in tubular fluid, whereas in the more alkaline medium of the renal interstitium amorphous urate salts are deposited (EMMERSON and ROW 1975). Depending upon the load of uric acid placed upon the kidneys, either an acute uric acid nephropathy or a chronic urate nephropathy will be produced. Uric acid urolithiasis may also occur, which can lead to chronic obstructive uropathy.

Acute overproduction of uric acid and extreme hyperuricemia frequently result in rapidly progressive renal insufficiency which is called acute nephropathy. This acute tubulointerstitial nephropathy is most commonly seen in patients given cytotoxic drugs for the treatment of leukemias and lymphomas; however, it can also occur in these disorders without treatment. Intense physical training in hot climates has been associated with acute uric acid nephropathy (KNOCHEL et al. 1974). Massive uricosuria and nephropathy may develop in subjects who resume a normal diet following prolonged starvation for weight reduction (ZUERCHER et al. 1977). Acute uric nephropathy may develop in patients given potent uricosuria agents, most notably sulfinpyrazone (BOELART et al. 1981).

The pathologic changes seen in acute uric acid nephropathy are the result of the deposition of uric acid crystals in the kidneys in the collecting systems, which leads to partial or complete obstruction of the collecting ducts, renal pelvis, or ureter. This produces an acute oliguric renal failure. In the early phases, uric acid crystals are demonstrable in the urine and are usually associated with microscopic or gross hematuria. Radiographic contrast sutdies are relatively contraindicated in these patients. Ultrasound is the best means of demonstrating the anatomic status of the collecting systems in these patients.

Patients with a less severe but more prolonged form of hyperuricemia are predisposed to develop the chronic tubulointerstitial disease known as gouty nephropathy. Other conditions, such as hypertension, pyelonephritis, and lead poisoning, which are associated with hyperuricemia but without clinical gout, may also produce renal injury so that it is sometimes difficult to assess the relative contribution of the hyperuricemia alone. The effect of hyperuricemia alone on renal function is not yet established, although the severity of renal involvement correlates well with the duration and magnitude of the serum uric acid concentration (BRYAN and EMMERSON 1988).

The characteristic pathology feature of the gouty kidney is the presence of acicular urate–uric acid crystals within the renal interstitium. These result in a cellular reaction that forms microtophi with associated changes in the interstitial tissues and renal tubules. There is lymphocytic infiltration, foreign body giant cell reaction, and eventual fibrosis of the medullar and papillary regions of the kidney. Intraluminal obstruction of the distal tubules by crystals of uric acid leads to impaired function and nephron destruction. Many patients with gout also have hypertension and nephrosclerosis and these may produce considerable parenchymal injury which may dominate the pathologic findings and confuse the issue of whether the gout was the primary insult or secondary to an underlying renal injury. These patients also frequently develop the complication of pyelonephritis. Chronic lead poisoning produces a chronic tubulointerstitial nephritis that is associated with a high incidence of hyperuricemia and secondary gout. The diagnosis of chronic lead intoxication should be considered in any patient with slowly progressive renal failure, atrophic kidneys, gout, and hypertension, especially if the renal disease dominates the clinical picture (CRASWELL et al. 1984).

Radiologic studies again only play an ancillary role to assist clinical management of gouty nephropathy patients, with ultrasound being the primary examination for evaluating the kidney.

3.6.7 Radiation Nephritis

The kidney is the most sensitive of the abdominal viscera to clinically significant radiation injury. The threshold dose for renal damage is considered to be 2300 R given over a 5-week period (ARON and SCHLESINGER 1974). The damage depends not only upon the dose given but also upon the type of radiation, its duration, and the amount of renal tissue irradiated. An underlying renal parenchymal disorder would worsen the injurious effects of the radiation. Radiation nephritis has only been seen following clinical radiotherapy. Diagnostic radiation exposure – to either x-rays or radioactive isotopes – has not been shown to produce it, nor has it been seen in people who have experienced atomic exposures. The simultaneous administration of antineoplastic chemotherapeutic agents (notably actinomycin D, vincristine, vinblastine, and bleomycin) with radiation therapy appears to enhance the potential for developing radiation nephropathy (CHURCHILL et al. 1978).

Clinical radiation nephritis may present as an acute or a chronic condition, although usually the chronic changes follow the acute phase. In some cases, no acute stage is recognized and the chronic condition may develop months or years following the exposure. The clinical syndrome is characterized by progressive renal failure, proteinuria, moderate to malignant hypertension, and profound anemia. There are granular and hyaline casts in the urinary sediment.

Radiation nephritis is thought to produce chronic renal failure secondary to interstitial abnormalities. Pathologic examination demonstrated widespread glomerular sclerosis, tubular atrophy, and arteriolar fibrinoid necrosis (GREENBERGER et al. 1982). The basic mechanism is felt to be angiitis of the small renal vessels with secondary ischemic changes in the medulla primarily and in the glomeruli secondarily (MADRAZO et al. 1975). Because of increased awareness of this potentially lethal complication, radiotherapy techniques have been modified to prevent it, and currently it is an uncommon condition.

Radiographic changes are nonspecific and depend upon the overall extent and severity of renal injury. In the acute phase kidneys are normal or slightly swollen but with smooth contours. In the

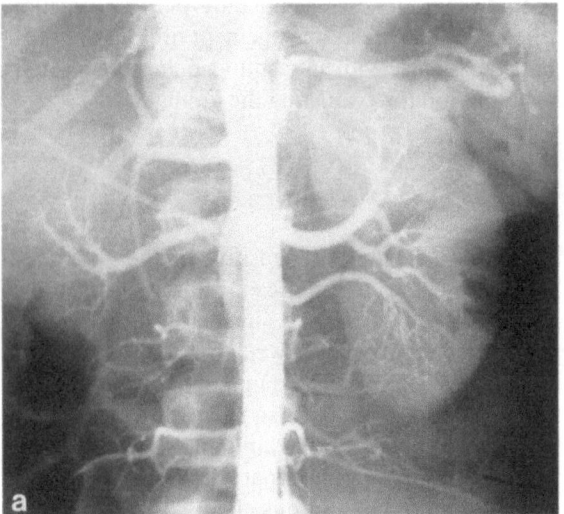

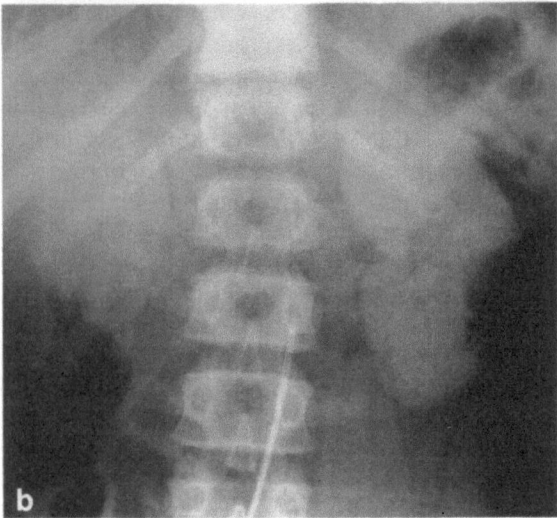

Fig. 3.14 a, b. Unilateral renal atrophy in a patient with prior radiation for a retroperitoneal sarcoma. **a** Arterial phase angiogram. **b** Late postinjection pyelographic film

chronic case, the kidneys may remain normal or can become markedly atrophic (Fig. 3.14). Renal contours and pelvocalyceal structures remain normal. In cases of unilateral injury, especially in children, there may be compensatory hypertrophy of the normal kidney. The radiographic pattern can be identical to that seen with renal ischemia. Hypertension has been cured by nephrectomy in patients with unilateral radiation nephritis (CRUMMY et al. 1965).

3.6.8 Hepatorenal Syndrome

The hepatorenal syndrome is defined as kidney failure in patients with severely compromised liver function in the absence of clinical, laboratory, or anatomic evidence of other known causes of renal failure. This is a functional syndrome that is potentially reversible (PAPPER 1983). Clinically it closely resembles severe hypovolemic prerenal failure, but it does not respond to volume replacement therapy. The cause of death in most patients is hepatic rather than renal failure. The pathogenesis of hepatorenal syndrome is not known, but it has been postulated that it involves a combination of peripheral vasodilatation, pooling of blood in the splanchnic region, and extreme renal vasoconstriction secondary to a complex interaction of multiple mediators including increased adrenergic tone, increased plasma arginine vasopressin, activation of the renin-angiotensin system, and increased renal thromboxin A_2 synthesis coupled with reduced production of renal PGE_2 and kallikrein (BETTER et al. 1988). It has been observed that liver transplantation will reverse hepatorenal syndrome (IWATSUKI et al. 1973). It has also been reported that kidneys from patients who die with hepatorenal syndrome function normally when transplantated into patients with normal livers (KOPPEL et al. 1969).

There is also a pseudohepatorenal syndrome seen in patients with simultaneous injuries to both the liver and kidneys such as with fulminant sepsis toxins, immunologic processes, coagulopathies (LEVENSON et al. 1983), and hepatic and renal ischemic injuries during severe exercise (ROWELL 1974).

Radiographic evaluation is used to exclude other causes of renal insufficiency – primarily obstructive uropathy, but also acute tubular necrosis, to which patients with advanced liver disease are particularly susceptible. Ultrasound and radionuclide scans are the primary methods of investigating these patients. Renal angiography in these patients demonstrates a striking vasoconstrictor pattern similar to that seen in pharmacoangiography following epinephrine injection into the renal artery. This pattern disappears on postmortem angiography (EPSTEIN et al. 1970).

3.7 AIDS and Drug Abuse Nephropathy

The past decade has seen the emergence of a new deadly disease, the acquired immunideficiency syndrome (AIDS). AIDS results in extensive multisystemic involvement with many unusual infectious and neoplastic complications. Acute preterminal renal failure was observed in the early experience with these patients (SIEGAL et al. 1981). The patient population in which the AIDS syndrome is found appears to be fairly stable in the United States. Homosexual and bisexual men constitute 72%–80% of affected patients. The next largest group is intravenous drug abusers, who account for 12%-17% of cases, followed by Haitian immigrants, who account for 5% of cases (FAUCI et al. 1988; CDC 1990). Others at risk are heterosexual partners or children of patients with AIDS and people undergoing transfusions.

The pattern of renal disease which has been described in these patients has been complex. Prerenal ischemia is seen frequently in these severely ill, debilitated, dehydrated patients. Acute tubular necrosis is also a frequent occurrence and pathologic finding. AIDS patients take a large number of potent antimicrobial drugs for their inflammatory complications as well as antineoplastic immune suppression agents in an attempt to control the disease process. Many of these agents are known to produce toxic renal nephropathy of a chronic tubulointerstitial type. Extensive tubulointerstitial changes with fibrosis and tubular dilatation, large intratubular hyaline casts, tubular necrosis, and atrophy, interstitial lymphocytic and plasmocyte cell infiltrations and nephrocalcinosis, are regularly found on an analysis of renal histology of both biopsy and autopsy material (PARDO et al. 1984; GARDENSWARTZ et al. 1984). The kidneys have also been the site of active infection by the many atypical agents seen in these patients, such as mycobacteria, cytomegalovirus, and cryptococcus. The kidneys of AIDS patients have also been involved directly with Kaposi's sarcoma, lymphoma, and renal cell carcinoma (GARDENSWARTZ et al. 1984). Involvement of the bladder or ureters by any of these neoplasms can result in obstructive uropathy.

In 1984 Rao et al. described a series of patients who exhibited a clinical pattern which presented as proteinuria and nephrotic syndrome, but then experienced a very rapid deterioration of renal function with irreversible uremia. These patients all exhibited a glomerular lesion of focal and segmental glomerulosclerosis. They also exhibited some increased mesangial matrix and immune deposits. This pathologic lesion was identical to that seen in patients with heroin nephropathy (RAO et al. 1974), but the clinical course was more severe and unrelenting. GARDENSWARTZ et al. (1984) reviewed 32 cases of AIDS to try and characterize renal involvement and found the wide panoply of lesions described above. They did find that the AIDS patients with renal disease had a higher incidence of oral and esophageal candidiasis, other fungal infections, and infections with *Mycobacterium avium-intracellulare* than their counterparts without renal abnormalities. The renal group also had a higher incidence of ex-

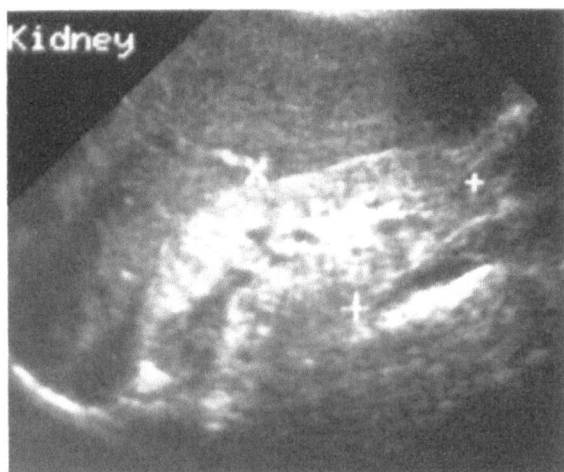

Fig. 3.15. Sonogram of kidneys in patient with AIDS with increased RBC count and protein on urinalysis. The patient had normal function. The scan shows diffuse increase in cortical echoes without any discrete mass. Renal pelvic structures are normal

posure to aminoglycoside antibiotics and amphotericin B and had experienced more clinical shock. The prognosis for the renal group was significantly worse, with 11 or 13 patients dying compared to 5 of 19 patients without demonstrable renal disease.

Given the extensive and varied experience since 1981, it now seems necessary to provide a composite picture of AIDS nephropathy. It is clear that no one pathologic lesion or clinical pattern characterizes AIDS nephropathy. All intrarenal structures are involved in this complex syndrome. Both acute and chronic glomerular and tubulointerstitial disease as well as direct infectious and/or neoplastic involvement are seen. The origins of this involvement appears to be complex and multiple. Immunologic injury, toxic injury from both drug abuse and therapeutic agents, and direct viral involvement (CHANDER et al. 1987) all seem to play a role.

The role of radiologic imaging in AIDS patients is primarily to find and define the extent of inflammatory and neoplastic complications (JEFFREY et al. 1988). This is true for the kidneys, just as it is in the central nervous system, lungs, and gastrointestinal tract (FEDERLE 1988). Renal ultrasound is useful to exclude obstructive uropathy as a cause of functional impairment. Renal ultrasound can also demonstrate changes in echo pattern compatible with parenchymal disease (SCHAFFER et al. 1984), (Fig. 3.15). Recent studies of patients with renal AIDS correlating sonographic patterns of increased echogenicity with histologic analysis concluded that the sonographic pattern largely reflected the exten-

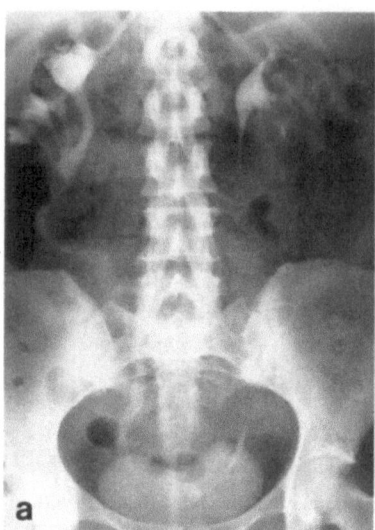 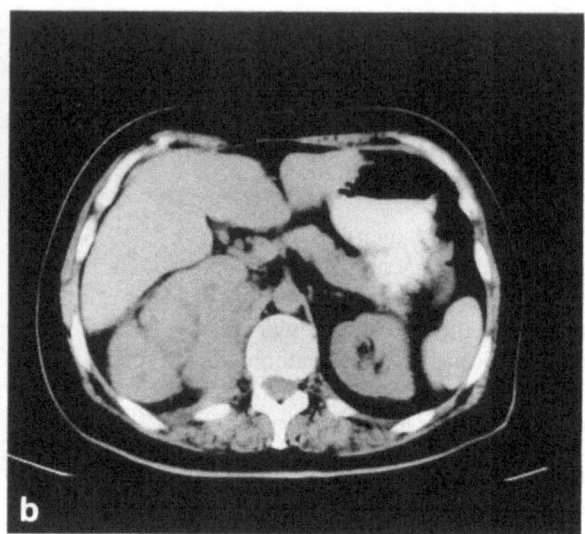

sive tubular abnormalities, with a relatively small contribution from the glomerular changes (HAMPER et al. 1988). Other examinations, primarily CT and MRI, are done as clinically needed to detect neoplastic change in the kidney, primarily lymphomas but also retroperitoneal Kaposi's sarcoma and renal cell carcinomas (Fig. 3.16). Renal and perirenal abscesses secondary to cryptococcus and other atypical infections are not rare (JEFFREY et al. 1986; WEISBERG et al. 1988), (Fig. 3.17).

There is an increasing number (up to 10% of all cases) of young adults with end-stage renal disease with a history of parenteral drug abuse, usually including heroin (ZIELEZNY et al. 1980). These patients exhibit a spectrum of renal pathology similar to AIDS patients. The kidneys show focal glomerulosclerosis or a proliferative glomerulonephritis secondary to bacterial endocarditis (SAVIN 1974) and may exhibit mesangial changes, including hepatitis B associated membranous nephropathy, which is also occasionally seen in AIDS patients. These patients also exhibit interstitial nephritis, including a granulomatous variant, which may be secondary to embolized foreign matter (MCALLISTER et al. 1979). Furthermore they demonstrate a high incidence of renal amyloidosis (SCHOLES et al. 1979; BRUS et al. 1979), and have been subject to toxic renal damage from rhabdomyolysis, which occurs in heroin addicts (RICHTER et al. 1971). The most common clinical entity seen is the combination of hypertension and nephrotic syndrome with a rapidly progressive loss of renal function. With the focal glomerulosclerosis seen on renal histology, this entity is identical to patients with AIDS, as described previously. An interrelationship between these con-

Fig. 3.16. Patient with AIDS and a retroperitoneal tumor, poorly differentiated lymphoma, obstructing and displacing the right kidney and ureter, causing obstruction on **a** the urogram and **b** CT

ditions seems to exist but its nature is not understood (RAO et al. 1974, 1987).

In 1970 Citron et al. described the occurrence of a systemic necrotizing vasculitis in parenteral drug abusers which is clinically the same as classic PAN. They observed a strong relationship between the occurrence of this vasculitis and the intravenous use of amphetamines. An association between classic PAN and hepatitis surface antigen has also been reported (INMAN 1982). Hepatitis surface antigens are also found in patients with parenteral drug abuse and vasculitis and in patients with AIDS (FYE et al. 1977; BENNETT et al. 1977; CITRON and PETERS 1971; HALPERN 1971; RAVENHOLT 1983). It has been postulated that heroin nephropathy is the result of immune response to the hepatitis antigen (KOFF et al. 1973). The relative roles of these two mechanisms in the pathogenesis of this entity is uncertain.

Clinically, these patients exhibit a syndrome similar to PAN, with hypertension, frequently malignant in type, being an important feature. The radiographic and angiographic features of this entity, including microaneurysms, are the same as discussed in the section on PAN (Sect. 3.4.3). Pathologic findings are also similar those for PAN, with vasculitis and glomerulonephritis. Radiological studies are used as clinically needed to evaluate renal anatomic status. Angiography can be used to confirm the clinical diagnosis when tissue is not easily available.

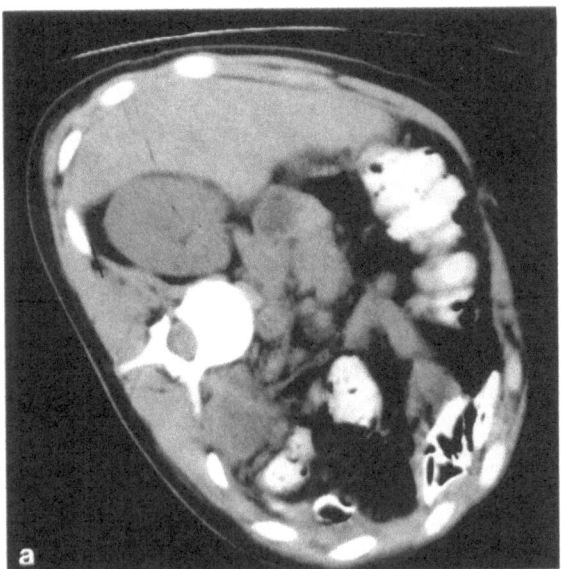

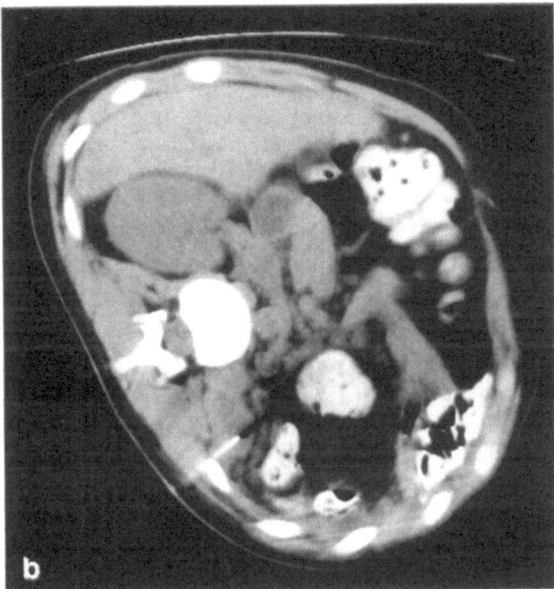

Fig.3.17. a Infrarenal abscess on the left in an AIDS patient. **b** Needle in place for aspiration of the collection

References

Alleman MJ, Janssens AR, Spoelstra P, Kroon HM (1986) Spontaneous intrahepatic hemorrhages in polyarteritis nodosa. Ann Intern Med 105: 712-713

Allen KS, Jorkasky DK, Arger PH et al. (1988) Renal allografts: prospective analysis of Doppler sonography. Radiology 169: 371-376

Allen RC, Petty RE, Lirenman DS, Malleson PN, Laxer RM (1986) Renal papillary necrosis in children with chronic arthritis. Am J Dis Child 140: 20-22

Anderson RJ, Schrier RW (1988) Acute tubular necrosis. In Better OS, Chaimovitz C, Gottschalk CW, Schrier RW (eds) Diseases of the kidney, 4th edn. Little Brown and Co, Boston, pp 1413-1446

Andriole GL, Bahnson RR (1987) Computed tomographic diagnosis of ureteral obstruction caused by a sloughted papilla. Urol Radiol 9: 45-46

Aron BS, Schlesinger A (1974) Complications of radiation therapy: the genitourinary tract. Semin Roentgenol 9: 65-74

Bakir AA, Lopez-Mauano V, Levy PS, Rhee HL, Dunea G (1988) Gallium 67 scintigraphy in glomerular disease. Am J Kidney Dis 12: 481-486

Bakir AA, Lopez-Mauano V, Hryhorczuk DO, Rhee HL, Dunea G (1985) Appraisal of lupus nephritis by renal imaging with gallium-67. Am J Med 79: 175-182

Ballard HA, Eisinger RP, Gallo G (1970) Renal manifestations of the Henoch-Schönlein syndrome in adults. Am J Med 49: 328-335

Bambery P, Katariya S, Sakhuja V, Kaur U, Behera D, Malik SK, Deodhar SD (1988) Wegener's granulomatosis in north India. Radiologic manifestations in eleven patients. Acta Radiol 29: 11-13

Barloon TJ, Zachar CK, Harkens KL, Honda H (1988) Rhabdomyolysis. J Comput Tomogr 12: 193-195

Batuman V, Maesaka JK, Haddad B, Tepper E, Landy E, Wedlen RP (1981) The role of lead in gouty nephropathy. N Engl J Med 304: 520-523

Becker JA (1966) Drip infusion pyelography. AJR 98: 96-101

Becker JA (1967) Nonvisualized kidney - value of nephrotomography. Radiology 89: 676-681

Bender WL, Whelton A, Beschorner WE, Darwich MO, Hall-Craggs M, Solez K (1984) Interstitial nephritis, proteinuria and renal failure caused by nonsteroidal anti-inflammatory drugs. Immunologic characterization of the inflammatory infiltrate. Am J Med 76: 1006-1012

Bennett WM, Plamp C, Porter GA (1977) Drug-related syndromes in clinical nephrology. Ann Intern Med 87: 582-590

Benoit FL, Rulon DB, Theil GB, Doolan PD, Watten RH (1964) Goodpasture's syndrome: a clinicopathologic entity, Am J Med 37: 424-444

Berlyne N, Berlyne GM (1962) Acute renal failure following intravenous pyelography with Hypaque. Acta Med Scand 171: 39-41

Better OS, Chaimovitz C, Gottschalk CW, Schrier RW (1988) Diseases of the kidney, 4th edn. Little Brown and Co, Boston, pp 1489-1500

Blohme I, Johson I (1981) Renal pelvis neoplasms and atypical urothelium in patients with end-stage analgesic nephropathy. Kidney Int 20: 671-675

Blythe WB (1985) Natural history of hypertension in renal parenchymal disease. Am J Kidney Dis 5: 50-56

Blumhardt R, Growcock G, Lahser JL (1983) Cortical necrosis in a renal transplant. AJR 141: 95-96

Boelart J, Meyrier A, Sraer JD (1981) Acute renal failure induced by sulfinpyrazone. Kidney Int 20: 305-312

Bohle A, Christ H, Grund KE, MacKensen S (1979) The role of the interstitium of the renal cortex in renal disease. Contrib Nephrol 16: 109-114

Bonomini V, Vangelista A (1988) Structural and functional renal changes in the elderly. Contrib Nephrol 25: 73-81

Bookstein JJ, Ernst CB (1973) Vasodilatory and vasoconstrictive pharmacoangiographic manipulation of renal collateral flow. Radiology 108: 55-59

Boyce HW, Holdsworth SR (1986) Idiopathic Goodpasture's syndrome. Fatal pulmonary hemorrhage and crescentic glomerulonephritis in the absence of immune-reactant deposition. Nephron 44: 22-25

Brenes LG, Brenes JN, Henandez NM (1977) Familial proximal renal tubular acidosis. Am J Med 52: 244-252

Brus I, Steiner G, Maceda A, Lejano R (1979) Amyloid fibrils in urinary sediment. Heroin addition with renal amyloidosis. NY State J Med 79: 768–771

Buckalew VM Jr, Schey HM (1986) A significant cause of morbidity in the United States. Am J Kidney Dis 7: 164–168

Buckalew VM Jr, Someren A (1974) Renal manifestations of sickle cell disease. Arch Intern Med 133: 660–669

Byrd L, Sherman RL (1974) Radiocontrast-induced acute renal failure: a clinical and pathophysiologic review. Medicine 58: 270–279

Carvlin MJ, Arger PH, Kundel HL, Axel L, Dougherty L, Kassab EA, Moore B (1987) Acute tubular necrosis: use of gadolinium DTPA and fast MR imaging to evaluate renal function in rabbit. JCAT 11: 488–493

CDC (1990) Update: acquired immunodeficiency syndrome - United States, 1989. JAMA 263: 1191–1192

Chander P, Soni A, Suri A, Bhagwat R, Yoo J, Treser J (1987) Renal ultrastructural markers in AIDS-associated nephropathy. Am J Pathol 126: 513–526

Chang VH, Cunningham JJ (1985) Efficacy of sonography as a screening method in renal insufficiency. JCU 13: 415–417

Chilcote WA, Borkowski FP (1983) Computed tomography in renal lymphoma. J Comp Assist Tomogr 7: 439–443

Choyke PL, Pollack HM (1988) The role of MRI in diseases of the kidney. Radiol Clin North Am 26: 617–631

Choyke PL et al. (1989) Dynamic Gd-DTPA enhanced MR imaging of the kidney: experimental results. Radiology 170: 713–717

Churchill DN, Hong K, Gault MH (1978) Radiation nephritis following combined abdominal radiation and chemotherapy (bleomycin-vinblastine). Cancer 41: 2162–2164

Citron BP, Peters RL (1971) Angitis in drug abusers. N Engl J Med 284: 111–113

Citron BP, Halpern M, McCarron M et al. (1970) Necrotizing angitis associated with drug abuse. N Engl J Med 283: 1003–1011

Collins AB, Ghan AK, Dienstag JL, Colvin RB, Haupert JT Jr, Mushahwar IK, McClusky RT (1983) Hepatitis B immune complex glomerulonephritis: simultaneous glomerular deposition of hepatitis B surface and E antigens. Clin Immunol Immunopathol 26: 137–153

Cornfield JZ, Johnson ML, Dolehide J, Fowler JE Jr (1988) Massive renal hemorrhage owing to polyarteritis nodosa. J Urol 140: 808–809

Cotran RS, Rubin RH, Tolkoff-Rubin NE (1986) Tubulo-interstitial disease. The kidney, 3rd edn. WB Saunders, Philadelphia, pp 1085–1142

Cramer GC, Fuglestad JR (1965) Cortical calcification in renal cortical necrosis. AJR 95: 344–348

Craswell PW, Price J, Boyle PD et al. (1984) Chronic renal failure with gout: a marker of chronic lead poisoning. Kidney Int 26: 319–323

Crummy AB, Hellman S, Stansel HR Jr, Hukill PB (1965) Renal hypertension secondary to unilateral radiation damage relieved by nephrectomy. Radiology 84: 108–111

Cunningham EE, Brentjens JR, Zielenzy MA, Andres GA, Venuto RC (1980) Heroin nephropathy: clinicopathologic and epidemiologic study. Am J Med 68: 47–53

Cunningham EE, Zielezny MA, Venuto RC (1983) Heroin-associated nephropathy - a nationwide problem. JAMA 250: 2935–2936

Curry, NS, Gordon L, Gobien RP, Lott M (1984) Renal medullary "rings" possible CT manifestation of hypercalcemia. Urol Radiol 6: 48–50

Cuttino JT Jr, Clark RL (1988) Urothelial microvascular response to chronic renal inflammatory disease. Urol Radiol 10: 68–73

Davidson AJ (1977) Radiologic diagnosis of renal parenchymal disease. WB Saunders, Philadelphia

Davidson AJ (1985) Radiology of the kidney. WB Saunders, Philadelphia

Davidson AJ, Talner LB (1973) Lack of specificity of renal angiography in the diagnosis of parenchymal disease. Invest Radiol 8: 90–95

Davidson AJ, Talner LB, Downs WM III (1969) A study of the angiographic appearance of the kidney in an aging normotensive population. Radiology 92: 975–983

Davidson AJ, Becker J, Rothfield N, Unser G, Ploch DR (1970) An evaluation of the effect of high dose urography on previously impaired renal and hepatic function in man. Radiology 97: 249–254

Dietrich RB, Kangarloo H (1986) Kidneys in infants and children evaluation with MR. Radiology 159: 215–221

Don S, Kopecky KK, Filo RS, Leapman SB, Thomalla JV, Jones JA, Klatte EC (1989) Duplex Doppler US of renal allograft: causes of elevated resistive index. Radiology 171: 709

Duncan DA, Drummon KN, Morach AE, Vernier RL (1965) Pulmonary hemorrhage and glomerulonephritis. Ann Int Med 62: 920–928

Ekelund L, Kaude J, Lindholm T (1973) Angiography in glomerular disease of the kidney. AJR 119: 739–747

Eknoyan G (1984) Analgesic nephrotoxicity and renal papillary necrosis. Semin Nephrol (4:65) pp 67–71

Eknoyan G, Qunibi WY, Grissom RT, Tuma SN, Ayus JC (1982) Renal papillary necrosis: an update. Medicine 61: 55–73

Elliott C, Reger M (1988) Acute renal failure following low osmolality radiocontrast dye. Clin Cardiol 11: 420–422

Emmerson BR, Row PG (1975) An evaluation of the pathogenesis of the gouty kidney. Kidney Int 8: 65–71

Emmerson BT (1988) Hyperuricemia, gout and the kidney, 4th edn. Little Brown & Co, Boston, pp 2481–2510

Epstein FH, Pigeon G (1964) Experimental urate nephropathy. Studies of the distribution of urate in renal disease. Nephron 1: 144–157

Epstein M, Berk DP, Hollenberg NK, Adams DF, Chalmers TC, Abrams HL, Merrill JP (1970) Renal failure in the patient with cirrhosis. The role of active vasconstriction. Am J Med 49: 175–185

Essinger A, Bonard M (1971) Periarteritis nodosa: an angiographic entity - presentation of two cases. Br J Radiol 44: 184–188

Ewald EH, Griffin D, McCune WJ (1987) Correlation of angiographic abnormalities with disease manifestations and disease severity in polyarteritis nodosa. J Rheumatol (Oct: 145): 952–956

Falkhoff GE, Rigsby CM, Rosenfield AT (1987) Partial, combined cortical and medullary nephrocalcinosis: US and CT patterns in AIDS-associated MAI infection. Radiology 162: 343–344

Fauci AS, Masur H, Gelmann EP, Markham PD, Hahn BH, Lane HL (1985) The acquired immunodeficiency syndrome: an update. Ann Intern Med 102: 800–813

Federle MP (1988) A radiologist looks at AIDS: imaging evaluation based on symptom complexes. Radiology 166: 553–562

Foley RJ, Winman EJ (1984) Urate nephropathy. Am J Med Sci 208–211

Friedenberg MJ, Eisen S, Kissane J (1965) Renal angiography

in pyelonephritis, glomerulonephritis, and arteriolar nephrosclerosis. AJR 95: 349-363

Fye KH, Becker MJ, Theofilopoulos AN, Moutsopoulos H, Feldman JL, Talal N (1977) Immune complexes in hepatitis B antigen associated periarteritis nodosa; detection by antibody dependent cell-mediated cytotoxicity and the raj cell assay. Am J Med 62: 783-791

Gardenswartz MH, Lerner CW, Seligson GR et al. (1984) Renal disease in patients with AIDS: a clinicopathologic study. Clin Nephrol 21: 197-204

Gilboa N, Lum GN, Urizar RE (1983) Early renal involvement in acute lymphoblastic leukemia and non-Hogdkin's lymphoma in children. J Urol 129: 364-367

Gill WM Jr, Pudvan WR (1970) The arteriographic diagnosis of renal parenchymal disease. Radiology 96: 81-84

Glazer GM (1988) MR imaging of the liver, kidneys and adrenal glands. Radiology 66: pp 303-312

Glazer GM, Francis IR, Gross BH, Amendola MA (1984) Computed tomography of renal vein thrombosis. J Comput Assist Tomogr 2: 288-293

Gold RP, McClennon BL, Rottenberg RR (1983) CT appearance of acute inflammatory disease of the renal interstitium. AJR 141: 343-349

Goodman GC, Chuurg J (1954) Wegener's granulomatosis; pathology and review of the literature. Arch Pathol Lab Med 58: 533-547

Greenberger JS, Weichselbaum RC, Cassady JR (1982) Radiation nephropathy. In Kieslbach KE, Garneck MR (eds) Cancer in the kidney. Lea & Febiger, Philadelphia

Greene ER, Avasthi PS, Hodges JW (1982) Noninvasive Doppler assessment of renal artery stenosis and hemodynamics. JCU 15: 653-659

Halpern M (1971) Angitis in drug abusers. N Engl J Med 284: 111-113

Halpern M, Citron BP (1971) Necrotizing angiitis associated with drug abuse. AJR 111: 663-671

Hamper VM, Goldblum LE, Hutchin GM, Sheth S, Dahnert WF, Bartlett JR, Sanders RG (1988) Renal involvement in AIDS: sonographic-histologic correlation. AJR 150: 1321-1325

Hartman DS, Davidson AJ, Davis CJ Jr, Goldman SM (1988) AJR 150: 1061-1064

Hartman GW, Torres VE, Leago GF, Williamson B Jr, Hattery RR (1984) Analgesic-associated nephropathy. Pathophysiological and radiological correlation. JAMA 251: 1734-1738

Hattery RR, Hartman GW, Williamson B (1986) General case of the day. Analgesic nephropathy with bilateral transitional cell carcinomas. Radiographics 6: 1091-1095

Heiberg E, Wolverson MI, Sunderman M, Shields JB (1988) Body computed tomography findings in systemic lupus erythematosus. J Comput Tomogr 12: 168-174

Hekali PE, Pajari RI, Kivisaari ML, Haapanem EJ, Leirisalo M (1984) Bilateral renal artery dissections: unusual complication of polyarteritis nodosa. Eur J Radiol 4: 6-8

Hekali PE, Kivisaari L, Standerskjold-Nordenstrm CG, Pajari R, Turto H (1985) Renal complications or polyarteritis nodosa: CT findings. J Comput Assist Tomogr 9: 333-338

Heptinstall RH (1983 a) Pathology of the kidney. Little Brown and Co, Boston, pp 676-696

Heptinstall RH (1983 b) Renal complications of therapeutic and diagnostic agents, analgesic abuse and addition to narcotics. Pathology of the kidney. Little Brown and Co, pp 1195-1256

Herschman A, Blum R, Lee YC (1970) Angiography findings in polyarteritis nodosa. Radiology 94: 147-148

Hillman BJ (1985) Digital radiology of the kidney. Radiol Clin North Am 23: 211-226

Hodson CJ (1972) The lobar structure of the kidney. Br J Urol 44: 246-262

Honda H, Yuh WT, Lu CC (1988) Magnetic resonance imaging of renal vein and inferior vena cava thrombosis in a patient with glomerulonephritis: a case report. J Comput Tomogr 12: 147-149

Horner BA, Hunt JC, Kincaid OW, DeWeerd JH (1966) Perirenal hematoma secondary to intrarenal microaneurysms of periarteritis nodosa demonstrated radiographically. Mayo Clin Proc 41: 169-178

Hricak H, Cruz C, Romanski R et al. (1982) Renal parenchymal disease: sonographic-histologic correlation. Radiology 144: 141-147

Hricak H, Crooks L, Sheldon P, Kauman L (1983) Nuclear magnetic resonance imaging of the kidneys. Radiology 146: 425-432

Hricak H, Terrir F, Demas B (1986) Renal allografts: evaluation by MR imaging. Radiology 159: 435-441

Humes HD, Weinberg JM (1986) Toxic nephropathies. The kidney, 3rd end. WB Saunders, Philadelphia, pp 1491-1532

Inman RD (1982) Rheumatic manifestations of hepatitis B virus infection. Semin Arthritis Rheum May 11 (4): 406-420

Iwatsuki S, Popovtzer MM, Corman JL, Ishikawa M, Putnam CW, Katz FH, Starzl TE (1973) Recovery from "hepatorenal syndrome" after orthotopic liver transplantation. N Engl J Med 289: 1155-1159

Jacques PF, Parker LA, Mauro MA (1988) Fulminant systemic necrotizing arteritis: CT findings. J Comput Assist Tomogr 12: 104-108

Jeffrey RB Jr, Nyberg DA, Bottles K et al. (1986) Abdominal CT in acquired immunodeficiency syndrome. AJR 146: 7-13

Jeffrey RB Jr, Goodman PC, Olsen WL, Wall SD (1988) Radiologic imaging of AIDS. Curr Probl Diagn Radiol 17: 73-117

Kikinis R, von Schluthess GK, Jager P, Durr R, Bino M, Kuoni W, Kubler O (1987) Normal and hydronephritic kidney: evaluation of renal function with contrast-enhanced MR imaging. Radiology 165: 837-842

Kincaid-Smith P (1980) Analgesic abuse and the kidney. Kidney Int 17: 250-277

Knochel JP, Dotin LL, Hamburger RS (1974) Heat stress, exercise and muscle injury effect on urate metabolism and renal function. Ann Intern Med 81: 321-344

Koff RS, Widrich WC, Robbins AH (1973) Necrotizing angiitis in a methamphetamine user with hepatitis B-angiographic diagnosis, five month follow-up results and localization of bleeding site. N Engl J Med 288: 946

Kohler TR, Zierler RE, Martin RL et al. (1986) Noninvasive diagnosis of renal artery stenosis by ultrasonic duplex scanning. J Vasc Surg 4: 450-456

Koppel MH, Coburn JW, Mims MM, Goldstein H, Boyle JD, Rubin ME (1969) Transplantation of cadaveric kidneys from patients with hepatorenal syndrome. Evidence for functional nature of renal failure in advanced liver disease. N Engl J Med 280: 1367-1371

Kreusser W, Herrmann R, Tschope W, Ritz E (1982) Nephrology complications of cancer therapy. Contrib Nephrol 33: 223-238

Lang EK (1971) Superselective arterial catheterization as a vehicle for delivering radioactive infarct particles to tumors. Radiology 98: 391-399

Lang EK (1983) Assessment of renal trauma by dynamic computed tomography. Radiographics 3: 566-584

Lang EK (1984) Angio-computed tomography and dynamic computed tomography in staging of renal cell carcinoma. Radiology 151: 149-155

Lang EK (1990) Intra-abdominal and retroperitoneal organ injuries diagnosed on dynamic computed tomograms obtained for assessment of renal trauma. J Trauma (in print)

Laupacis A, Ulan RH, Rankin RN, Stiller CR, Keown PA (1983) CT findings in postpartum renal cortical necrosis. J Can Assoc Radiol 34: 53-55

Lester PD, Koehler PR (1971) The renal angiographic changes in scleroderma. Radiology 99: 517-521

Leung AW, Bydder FM, Steiner RE, Bryant DJ, Young IR (1984) Magnetic resonance imaging of the kidneys. AJR 143: 1215-1227

Levenson DJ, Skorecki KL, Narins RG (1983) Acute renal failure associated with hepatobiliary disease. In: Brenner BM, Lazarus UJM (eds) Acute renal failure. Saunders, Philadelphia, pp 467-498

Lignelli GH, Buchheit WA (1971) Angiitis in drug abusers. N Engl J Med 284: 111-113

Linton HL, Richmond JM, Clark WF, Lindsay RM, Driedger AA, Lamki LM (1985) Gallium 67 scintigraphy in the diagnosis of acute renal disease. Clin Nephrol 24: 84-87

Longsstreth PL, Korobkin M, Palubinskas AJ (1974) Renal microaneurysms in a patient with systemic lupus erythematosus. Radiology 113: 65-66

Love L et al. (1989) Persistent CT nephrogramm: significance in diagnosis of contrast nephropathy. Radiology 172: 125-131

Lovett I, Douse B, Orr N (1988) The role of ultrasound in the diagnosis of parenchymal disease in transplanted kidneys. Australas Radiol 32: 104-106

MacPherson RI (1974) The radiologic manifestations of Henoch-Schönlein purpura. J Can Assoc Radiol 25: 275-281

Madrazo A, Schwarz G, Churg J (1975) Radiation nephritis: a review. J Urol 114: 822-237

Mapp E, Karasick S, Pollack M, Wechsler RJ, Karasick D (1987) Uroradiological manifestations of S-hemoglobinopathy. Semin Roentgenol 22: 186-194

Marchal G, Veroeken E, Oyen R, Moerman F, Baert AL, Lauweryne J (1986) Ultrasound of the normal kidneys, a sonographic, anatomic and histologic correlation. Ultrasound Med Biol 12: 999-1009

Marotti M, Hricak H, Terrier F, McAninch JW, Thuroff JW (1987) MR in renal disease, importance of cortical-medullary distinction. Magn Reson Med 5: 160-172

Marrocco FS, Leekam RN, Matzinger M, Gray RR (1986) Displaced calcium as a sign of transitional cell carcinoma in analgesic nephropathy. J Can Assoc Radiol 37: 1122-1124

McAllister CH, Horn R, Havron S, Abramson JM (1979) Granulomatous interstitial nephritis: a complication of heroin abuse. South Med J 72: 162-165

McCluskey RF (1982) Immunologically mediated tubulo-interstitial nephritis. In: Contran RS (guest ed), Brenner B, Stein JH (eds) Tubulointerstitial nephropathy, Churchill Livingstone, New York (Contemporary issues in nephrology 10, p 121)

McDonald MI, Hamilton JS, Durach DT (1983) Hepatitis B antigen could harbour the infective agent of AIDS. Lancet I: 882-884

McKinney TD (1986) Renal complications of neoplasia. Prager, New York

McMillin KI, Gross BH (1985) CR demonstration of peripelvic and periureteral non-Hodgkin lymphoma. AJR 144: 945-946

Mean E, Bookstien JJ, Gikas PW (1973) Angiographic diagnosis of renal parenchymal disease; chronic glomerulonephritis, chronic pyelonephritis, and arteriolonephrosclerosis. Radiology 108: 523-532

Mendez G, Ilikoff MB, Morillo G (1980) The role of computer tomography in the diagnosis of renal and perirenal abscesses. J Urol 122: 582-591

Moore L, Curry NS, Jenrette JM (1986) 3D computed tomography of acute radiation nephritis. Urol Radiol 8: 89-91

Moss AH, Gabow PA, Kehny WD, Goodman SI, Haut LL (1980) Fanconi's syndrome and distal renal tubular acidosis after glue sniffing. Ann Intern Med 92: 69-70

Moulin B, Sahall D, Baud LG, Toussaint P, Michel C, Ronco P, Mignon F (1988) Gallium 67 scintigraphy in the diagnosis of glomerulonephritis. Clin Nephrol 30: 128-133

Muehrcke RC, Kark PM, Pirani CL, Pollack VE (1957) Lupus nephritis: a clinical and pathologic study based on renal biopsies. Medicine 36: 1-56

Murray TG, Stolley PD, Anthony JC, Schinnar R, Hepler-Smith E, Jeffreys JL (1983) Epidemiologic study of regular analgesic use and end-stage renal disease. Arch Intern Med 143: 1687-1693

Myers GH Jr, Witten DM (1971) Acute renal failure after excretory urography in multiple myeloma. AJR 113: 583-588

O'Dell JR, Hays RC, Guggenheim SJ, Steigerwald JC (1985) Tubulointerstitial renal disease in systemic lupus erythematosus. Arch Intern Med 145: 1996-1999

Odita JC, Ugbodaga CL, Dkafir LA, Ojofwu LI, Osisi OA (1982) Urographic changes in nonzygous sickle cell disease. Diagn Imaging 52: 259-263

Padovani J, Kasbarian M, Pollini J, Faure F, Leynaud D (1974) Value of renal angiography in periarteritis nodosa. Ann Radiol 17: 135-140

Papo J, Peer G, Aviram A, Paizer R (1985) Acute renal cortical necrosis as revealed by computerized tomography. Isr J Med Sci 21: 862-863

Papper S (1983) The hepatorenal syndrome. In: Epstein M (ed) The kidney in liver disease (2). Elsevier Biomedical, New York, pp 87-106

Pardo V, Aldana M, Colton RM (1984) Glomerular lesions in the acquired immunodeficiency syndrome. Ann Intern Med 101: 429-434

Pasternack A, Linder E (1970) Renal tubular acidosis: an immunological study on four patients. Clin Exp Immunol 7: 115-123

Patel PG (1986) Renal parenchymal disease: histopathologic-sonographic correlation. Urol Int 41: 289-291

Pear BL (1981) Radiologic recognition of extrahepatic manifestations of hepatitis B antigenemia. AJR 137: 135-140

Pennes DR, Martel W (1986) Hyperuricemia and gout. Semin Roentgenol 21: 245-255

Piccirillo M, Rigsby CM, Rosenfield AT (1987) Sonography of renal inflammatory disease. Urol Radiol 9: 66-78

Pirani CL, Silva FG, Appel GB (1983) Tubulo-interstitial disease in multiple myeloma and other non-renal neoplasias. Contemp Issues Nephrol 10: 287-293

Platt JF, Rubin JM, Bowerman PA, Marn CS (1988) The inability to detect kidney disease on the basis of echogenicity. AJR 151: 317-319

Pollack HM, Banner MP (1985) Current status of excretory urography. Urol Clin North Am 12: 585-601

Poynter JD, Hare WSC (1974) Necrosis-in-situ: a form of papillary necrosis seen in analgesic nephropathy. Radiology 111: 69-76

Puvaneswary M, Segasathy M (1988) Analgesic nephropathy: ultrasonic features. Australas Radiol 32: 247-252

Rao TK, Nicastri AD, Friedman EA (1974) Natural history of heroin-associated nephropathy. N Engl J Med 290: 19-23

Rao TK, Filippone EJ, Nicastri AD, Landesman SH, Frank E, Chen CK, Friedman EA (1984) Associated focal and segmental glomerulosclerosis in the acquired immunodeficiency syndrome. N Engl J Med 310: 669-673

Rao TK, Friedman EA, Nicastri AD (1987) The types of renal disease in the acquired immunodeficiency syndrome. N Engl J Med 316: 1062-1068

Ravenholt RT (1983) Role of hepatitis B virus in acquired immunodeficiency syndrome. Lancet I: 885-886

Richter RW, Challenor YB, Pearson J, Kagen LJ, Hamilton LL, Ramsey WH (1971) Acute myoglobinuria associated with heroin addiction. JAMA 216: 1172-1176

Ritchie WW, Vick CW, Glocheski SK, Cook DE (1988) Evaluation of azotemic patients: diagnostic yield of initial US examination. Radiology 167: 245-247

Robertson R, Murphy H, Nubbins PA (1988) Renal artery stenosis: the use of duplex ultrasound as a screening technique. Br J Radiol 61: 196-201

Rosenfield AT (1982) Ultrasound evaluation of renal parenchymal disease and hydronephrosis. Urol Radiol 4: 125-133

Rosenfield AT, Stegel NJ (1981) Renal parenchymal disease: histopathologic-sonographic correlation. AJR 137: 793-798

Ross B, Freeman D, Chan L (1986) Contributions of nuclear magnetic resonance to renal biochemistry. Kidney Int 29: 131-141

Rowell LB (1974) Human cardiovascular adjustment to exercise and thermal stress. Physiol Rev 54: 75-159

Sabatini S (1984) The pathophysiology of experimentally induced papillary necrosis. Semin Nephrol 4: 27-39

Sahn DJ, Schwartz AD (1972) Schönlein-Henoch syndrome: observations of some atypical clinical presentations. Pediatrics 49: 614-616

Sandler CM, Raval B, David CL (1985) Computed tomography of the kidney. Urol Clin North Am 12: 657-675

Sargent GT (1974) The clinical features of sickle cell disease. New York American, Elsevier

Sasaki T, Kojima S, Kubodera A (1985) Renal gallium accumulation in mice with acute immune complex glomerulonephritis. Int J Nucl Med Biol 12: 103-110

Savin V (1974) Glomerulonephritis in acute bacterial endocarditis in addicts. Clin Res 22: 208-219

Schaffer RM, Schwartz GE, Becker JA, Rao TKS, Shih YH (1984) Renal ultrasound in acquired immune deficiency syndrome. Radiology 153: 511-513

Schapira HE, Kapner J, Szporn AH (1986) Wegener granulomatosis presenting as renal mass. Urology 28: 307-309

Scholes J, Derosena R, Appel GB, Jao W, Boyd MT, Pirani CL (1979) Amyloidosis in chronic heroin addicts with the nephrotic syndrome. Ann Intern Med 91: 26-29

Schrier RW, Gottschalk CW (eds) (1988) Diseases of the kidney, 4th edn. Little Brown & Co, Boston

Sickles EA, Korobkin M (1974) Perirenal hematoma as a complication of renal infarction in sickle cell trait: a case report. AJR 122: 800-803

Siegal FP, Lopez C, Hammer GS et al. (1981) Severe acquired immunodeficiency in male homosexuals, manifested by chronic perianal ulcerative herpes simplex lesions. N Engl J Med 305: 1439-1444

Simmons JT, Leavitt R, Kornblut AD, Cauci HS (1987) CT of the paranasal sinuses and orbits in patients with Wegener's granulomatosis. Ear Nose Throat J 66: 134-140

Strake L, Schultze Kool LJ, Paul LC et al. (1988) Magnet resonance imaging of renal transplants: its value in the differentiation of acute rejection and cyclosporin A nephrotoxicity. Clin Radiol 39: 220-228

Streiter ML, Bosniak MA (1983) The radiology of drug addiction: urinary tract complications. Semin Roentgenol 18: 221-226

Sze G, Zimmerman RD (1988) The magnetic resonance imaging of infectious and inflammatory diseases. Radiol Clin North Am 26: 839-859

Taliercio CP, Burnett JC (1988) Contrast nephropathy, cardiology and the newer radiocontrast agents. Int J Cardiol 19: 145-151

Tasdemir I, Turgan C, Emri S et al. (1988) Spontaneous perirenal haematoma secondary to polyarteritis nodosa. Br J Urol 62: 219-222

Templeton PA, Pais SD (1985) Renal artery occlusion in PAN. Radiology 156: 308

Terrier F, Hricak H, Justich E, Dooms GC, Grodd W (1986) The diagnostic value of renal cortex to medulla contrast on magnetic resonance images. Eur J Radiol 6: 121-126

Thal A (1955) Selected renal vasospam and ischemic renal necrosis produced experimentally with staphylococcal toxin. Observations on the pathogenesis of bilateral cortical necrosis. Am J Pathol 31: 233-259

Thornburn GD, Kopald HH, Mollenberg M, Ormorchoe CC, Barger A (1963) Intrarenal distribution of nutrient blood flow determined with kryton 85 in the unanesthetized dog. Circ Res 13: 290-299

Tuffanelli DL, Winkelmann RK (1961) Systemic scleroderma. A clinical study of 727 cases. Arch Dermatol 84: 359-371

Vaamonde CA (1984) Renal papillary necrosis in sickle cell hemoglobinopathies. Semin Nephrol 4: 48-54

Varizi ND, Barbari A, Licorish K, Cesario T, Gupta S (1985) Spectrum of renal abnormalities in acquired immune-deficiency syndrome. J Natl Med Assoc 77: 369-375

Weiner MW, Adam WR (1985) Magnetic resonance spectroscopy for evaluation of renal function. Semin Urol 3: 34-42

Weisberg LA, Garcia C, Stazio A (1988) Computerized tomographic diagnostic aspects of acquired immunodeficiency syndrome. Comput Med Imaging Graph 12: 225-236

Whelan JC Jr, Ling JT, Davis LA (1967) Antemortem roentgen manifestations of bilateral renal cortical necrosis. Radiology 89: 682-689

Wilms G, Dyer K, Waer M, Baert AL, Michielsen P (1986) CT demonstration of aneurysms in polyarteritis nodosa. J Comput Assist Tomogr 10: 513-515

Winkler P, Hitrogge H (1985) Sonographic signs of nephritis in children. A comparison of renal echography with clinical evaluation, laboratory data and biopsy. Pediatr Radiol 15: 231-237

Winsett MZ, Amparo EG, Fawcett HD, Kumar R, Johnson RF Jr, Bedi DG, Winsett DE (1988) AJR 150: 319-323

Yousefzadeh DK, Chow DC, Benson CA (1981) Polyarteritis nodosa: regression of arterial aneurysms following immunosuppressive and corticosteroid therapy. Pediatr Radiol 10: 139-421

Zielezny MA, Cunningham EE, Venuta RC (1980) The impact of heroin abuse on a regional end-stage renal disease program. Am J Public Health 70: 829-831

Zuercher HV, Meier HR, Huber M et al. (1977) Acute renal failure complicating starvation for weight reduction. Schweiz Med Wochenschr 107: 1025-1028

4 Inflammatory Renal Disease

STANFORD M. GOLDMAN

CONTENTS

4.1   Introduction 103
4.2   Acute Pyelonephritis
         (Acute Pyelitis, Acute Interstitial Nephritis) . . . 104
4.2.1   Radiologic Findings 105
4.3   Acute Bacterial Nephritis (Acute Suppurative
         Nephritis, Severe Acute Pyelonephritis) 107
4.4   Acute Focal Pyelonephritis
         (Focal Lobar Nephronia, Focal Bacterial
         Nephritis, the Preabscess State) 108
4.4.1   Radiologic Findings 108
4.5   Emphysematous Pyelonephritis 109
4.5.1   Radiologic Findings 110
4.6   Chronic Pyelonephritis (Chronic Atrophic
         Pyelonephritis, Reflux Nephropathy,
         Chronic Infection, Abacterial Nephritis) 111
4.6.1   Radiologic Findings 112
4.7   Granulomatous, Fungal, and the Rare
         Inflammatory Processes 116
4.7.1   Tuberculosis 116
4.7.1.1 Radiologic Findings 117
4.7.1.2 The Differential Diagnosis 120
4.7.2   Schistosomiasis 120
4.7.2.1 Radiologic Findings 121
4.7.3   Xanthogranulomatous Pyelonephritis 121
4.7.3.1 Radiologic Findings 122
4.7.4   Echinococcosis 125
4.7.4.1 Radiologic Findings 125
4.7.5   Candidiasis 126
4.7.5.1 Radiologic Findings 126
4.7.6   Brucellosis 127
4.7.6.1 Radiologic Findings 127
4.7.7   Malacoplakia 127
4.7.7.1 Radiologic Findings 128
4.7.8   Actinomycosis 128
4.7.8.1 Radiologic Findings 128
4.7.9   Amebiasis 129
4.7.10   Cryptococcal Infections 129
4.7.11   Coccidioidomycosis 130
4.7.12   Blastomycosis 130
4.7.12.1 Radiologic Findings 130
4.7.13   Aspergillosis 130
4.7.14   Histoplasmosis 130
4.7.15   Dioctophyma Renale 131
4.7.16   Chronic Granulomatous Disease of Infancy . . 131
4.8   Intrarenal Abscess 131
4.8.1   Radiologic Findings 131

4.9   Perinephric and Pararenal Abscesses 133
4.9.1   Radiologic Findings 134
4.10   Pancreatitis 136
4.11   Acute and Chronic Pyonephrosis 136
4.12   Pyelitis Cystica 138
4.13   Renal Papillary Necrosis 138
4.13.1   Radiologic Findings 140
4.14   Septic Emboli and Mycotic Aneurysms 141
4.15   Cholesteatoma 142
4.16   Leukoplakia and Squamous Metaplasia 142
4.17   Urinary Tract Infection During Pregnancy ... 142
4.18   Infected Cysts 143
         References 143

STANFORD M. GOLDMAN, M.D., Professor of Radiology and
Urology; Johns Hopkins School of Medicine, Radiologist-in-
Chief, Department of Radiology, Francis Scott Key Medical
Center, 4940 Eastern Avenue, Baltimore, MD 21224, USA

4.1 Introduction

A disparity in terminology for inflammatory renal conditions has caused increasing difficulty in comparing observations reported in the radiologic vs urologic vs pathologic literature in the last two decades. The definitions of such terms as *focal bacterial nephritis, lobar nephronia,* and *reflux nephropathy* appear to vary by specialty, or the terms may be avoided altogether (WALSH et al. 1986; GILLENWATER et al. 1987). The fact that many of these new terms are not recognized by the pathologist is also disconcerting. This feature carries over into the radiologic literature and has caused disagreement among radiologists as to the precise definition for each term. *Focal bacterial nephritis* and *focal lobar nephronia* have been used synonymously to indicate focal acute pyelonephritis by some radiologists, whereas others have used the latter term only if parenchymal destruction has occurred, but not a frank abscess.

A second example is *acute bacterial nephritis,* which originally denoted an acute severe renal infection that presented radiographically with a nonfunctioning or poorly functioning kidney on intravenous urograms, but more recently has been used more widely to describe almost any acute severe pyelonephritis without reference to the state of function.

One other pertinent example is *chronic atrophic pyelonephritis,* which according to Hodson's description (HODSON et al. 1975b) consisted of renal scarring caused by reflux. Although originally only reflux was identified as the noxious cause, it had been recognized that urinary infection may often be present. This resulted, once again, in blurring of the borders for this term. Some radiologists use it interchangeably with *chronic pyelonephritis, atropic pyelonephritis,* and *reflux nephropathy.* Others feel that purity in concept based on pathologic definition demands that only in the presence of renal infection, irregardless of whether reflux is present or not, the term *chronic pyelonephritis* be used.

Some radiologists have used *interstitial nephritis* synonymously with *acute pyelonephritis* (WICKS and THORNBURY 1979; GIKAS 1976), while urologists tend to use it synonymously with *chronic pyelonephritis* (DAIRIKI-SHORTLIFFE and STAMEY 1986a). Nephrologists reserve the term for noninfectious pyelonephritis. In this chapter an attempt will be made to indicate some of the discordant views, perhaps permitting the reader to exercise his own judgment as to how the prevailing classifications fit the known radiologic and pathologic findings described herein.

Some basic pathologic principles may be of special use to the reader in achieving a cohesive approach to infection. In any acute infection, the polymorphic leukocyte is the primary defense mechanism. This stage of the process is termed pathologically *acute pyelonephritis.* If the primary defense mechanism fails to contain the infection, the process becomes chronic and indolent. At this point in time, lymphocyte, histiocyte, and/or giant cell macrophages attempt to curtail and demarcate the process. Formation of a fibrous capsule is a further attempt to isolate the process. In pathologic terms, this leads to granuloma formation. Generally, infections caused by *Escherichia coli,* proteus, or streptococcus will present with a pattern of acute pyelonephritis. Conversely, infections due to *Mycobacterium tuberculosis* or *Brucella abortus* will often present as chronic infections in various stages of the granulomatous phase of the disease.

4.2 Acute Pyelonephritis
(Acute Pyelitis, Acute Interstitial Nephritis)

Although urinary infection is common in childhood (STY et al. 1987), in many instances, particularly in little girls, one may be dealing with asymptomatic bacteriuria [2% of females below the age of 2 years (KUNIN et al. 1964)]. Spread of the infection is thought to be (a) via reflux, i.e., ascending from the bladder, (b) hematogenous, or (c) lymphatic. The lymphatic route is probably quite rare. Gram-positive organisms such as streptococcus and staphylococcus, in particular, tend to spread to the kidney during uncontrolled bacteremia (LAPIDES 1978; EVANS et al. 1971; ROBERTS 1983a). While the advent of antibiotics has reduced the incidence of hematogenous spread, unrecognized dental infections still tend to lead to gram-positive urinary tract infections in adults. Drug addicts are particularly prone to this type of infection since bacteria may be introduced through unsterile needles and lead to hematogenous seeding.

In general, however, most renal infections today occur via the ascending route secondary to ureteral vesical reflux. Gram-negative organisms such as *E. coli,* proteus, klebsiella, and pseudomonas are the most commonly encountered offending organisms. Female patients are particularly susceptible since the short female urethra offers little resistance to bacterial invasion. Moreover, vaginal epithelial cells of infected females seem to have a greater avidity for pathogenic bacteria to adhere to them (FOWLER and STAMEY 1977). Once they reach the bladder, gram-negative bacteria can attach themselves to the bladder mucosa by means of mannose-resistant fimbriae, which prevents their being flushed from the bladder during micturition. Furthermore, overdistention of the bladder, particularly in combination with decreased host resistance, may lead to proliferation of bacteria in the bladder (LAPIDES 1978).

Reflux may exist in many children without sequelae. An immaturity of the ureterovesical sphincter mechanism is incriminated for reflux in young children. While reflux tends to predate the onset of urinary infection, the presence of reflux facilitates passage of bacteria from the bladder into the upper urinary tract (ROBERTS 1983a, b). Once again, bacteria may attach themselves to the ureter by means of fimbriae and thus prevent their elimination by normal flushing (FUSSEL 1984). Moreover, P blood group antigen receptors as well as ureteral endotoxins may cause atony of the ureter and promote stasis (LOMBERG et al. 1983).

From that point on, entry of bacteria into the kidney is unopposed. Reflux into the renal parenchyma occurs particularly via the compound calyces of the upper and lower poles since the alignment of their collecting tubules facilitates reflux of bacteria-laden urine into the renal parenchyma. Conversely, most other calyces are protected against reflux into the papillae by the alignment of the terminal tubules (CREMIN 1979). Alternately and coincidentally, however, increased retrograde pressure attendant upon stasis in the ureters will cause reflux into these papillae and pyramids as well. If unchecked by the host's defenses, the process tends to proceed to a focal suppurative coagulation necrosis presenting as multiple microabscesses. In general, the cortex is more involved than the medulla and one can appreciate purulent material filling the collecting tubules. The state of coalescing cortical microabscesses is termed by some as *focal bacterial nephritis*.

The clinical presentation of this state of the disease comprises acute flank pain, dysuria, frequency, pyuria, bacteriuria, and hematuria. Infants often present with failure to thrive of unkown orgin and/or with enuresis. In children, renal damage can occur after a single acute infection. Laboratory findings, specifically white cells and white cell casts as well as red cells and bacterial rods and cocci in the urine, support the diagnosis.

Pregnant women are also particularly prone to urinary tract infection. This may, in part, be due to the obstruction of the ureter by either pregnancy or the atonic hormonal effects upon the ureter.

In male children, in particular, aggressive radiographic evalutation is mandatory on the first such infection (BURBIGE et al. 1984; LEBOWITZ and MANDELL 1987). In many instances, an anatomic abnormality responsible in part for such infection may be uncovered. Conversely, in female children workup may be delayed until the second documented urinary tract infection. Acute uncomplicated pyelonephritis in adults, in general, does not require a comprehensive radiographic workup (DAIRIKI-SHORTLIFFE and STAMEY 1986b).

If possible, the radiologic workup should be delayed until response to appropriate treatment has occurred. The radiologic workup is initiated by a voiding cystourethrogram, followed by intravenous urography. To minimize radiation effect, intravenous urography can be tailored to consist of only three films (i.e., scout, 6 min, and 12 min) or can be reserved only for children in whom reflux is noted on the cystourethrogram (REDMAN and SEIBERT 1984; LAHDE et al. 1981). Since some of the more important anatomic variants can be identified by ultrasonography and radionuclide scans, there are those who strongly advocate their substitution for intravenous pyelography (IVP) (KANGARLOO et al. 1985; JAQUIER et al. 1985). The radionuclide cystogram, in particular, is sensitive in demonstrating reflux. However, if anatomic detail is necessary to establish the diagnosis, such as with papillary or medullary necrosis or pyelitis cystica, one has to resort to the intravenous urogram. For a detailed assessment of progressive disease such as abscesses, computed tomography (CT) is the procedure of choice in both children and adults (MONTGOMERY et al. 1987; LANG 1990).

We advocate the use of ultrasound and nuclear medicine studies in follow-up of these children on a periodic basis in order to reduce radiation exposure. Since renal malfunction and scar formation may not be apparent until years after the initial insult, continued documentation of renal growth and development is a sine qua non to detect incipient changes and progressive disease.

4.2.1 Radiologic Findings

In a large number of patients, the intravenous urogram tends to be normal (FAIR et al. 1979; WICKS and THORNBURY 1979). However, in 25%–40% of the patients, distinct urographic abnormalities may be discernible on high quality detailed studies (SILVER et al. 1976). Acute pyelonephritis presents as an enlarged kidney. Cloudy swelling and cortical vasoconstriction result in both compression of the calyces and a decrease in glomerular filtration. This, in turn, often causes poor opacification of the calyces (Fig. 4.1). Edema of the pelvic mucosa and ureter may result in longitudinal striations along the axis of the ureter and in the kidney pelvis (Fig. 4.2). However, the striation pattern can be seen after relief of obstruction and collapse of a previously dilated ureter (BERLINER and BOSNIAK 1982; GWINN and BARNES 1964; RICHIE et al. 1978; SILVER et al. 1976). Opacification of the pelvis and calyceal walls may reflect a capillary blush of inflammatory tissues (BARBARIC 1977; OLDER et al. 1978). The nephrogram is frequently delayed and patchy, and diffuse areas of decrease density may also be appreciated. This irregular parenchymal opacification may persevere for hours. At times, one can appreciate cortical and medullary striation. This probably correlates to fluid and purulent material-filled tubules.

The ureters may be either dilated due to paralyzing bacterial toxins (Fig. 4.3) or narrowed and constricted attendant upon decreased contrast excretion (Figs. 4.1–4.3).

A swollen kidney with hypoechoic cortex is often seen on ultrasonograms (Figs. 4.4, 4.5). Occasionally, scattered low density echoes may be present, indicating microabscesses (EDELL and BONAVITA 1979). Increased fluid content may result in increased transmission (Fig. 4.5) (FIEGLER 1983). Dilated pyelocalyceal structures are present only with obstruction (EDELL and BONAVITA 1979; DINKEL et al. 1986; PICCIRILLO et al. 1987).

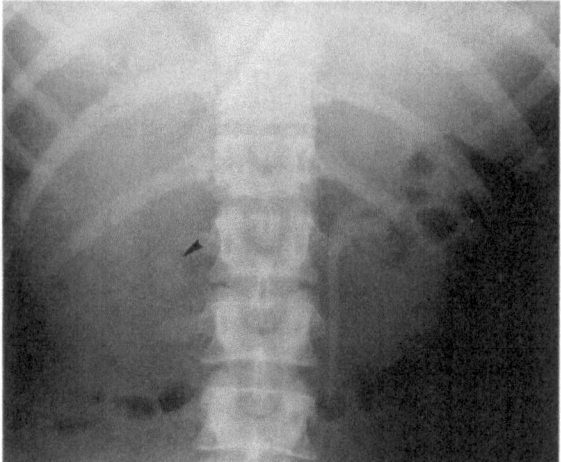

Fig. 4.1. Right-sided acute pyelonephritis. Enlarged kidney with excretion so poor that only the renal pelvis is seen *(arrow)*

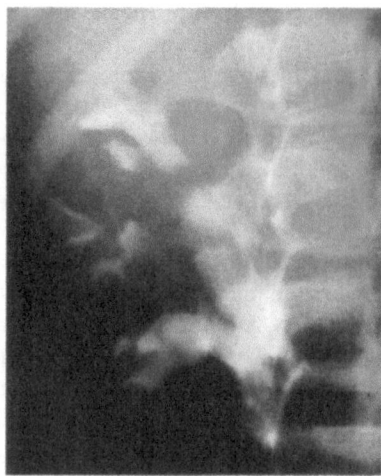

Fig. 4.2. Acute pyelonephritis. Striated pattern of the major calyces, infundibula, and renal pelvis secondary to submucosal edema

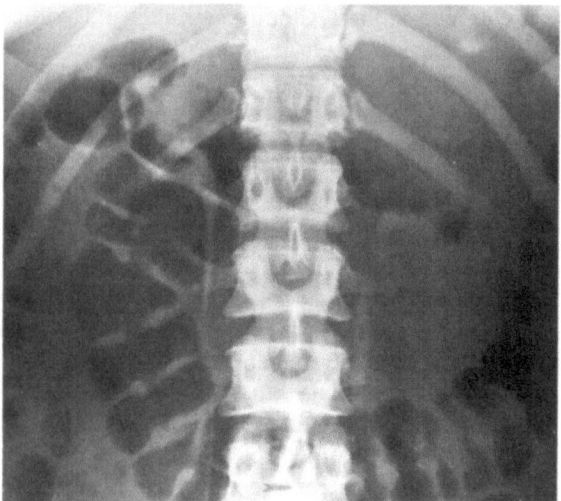

Fig. 4.3. Left-sided acute pyelonephritis. IVP: Note the poor excretion and the enlarged kidney. The ureter is also dilated, possibly secondary to the limited peristalsis caused by bacterial endotoxins

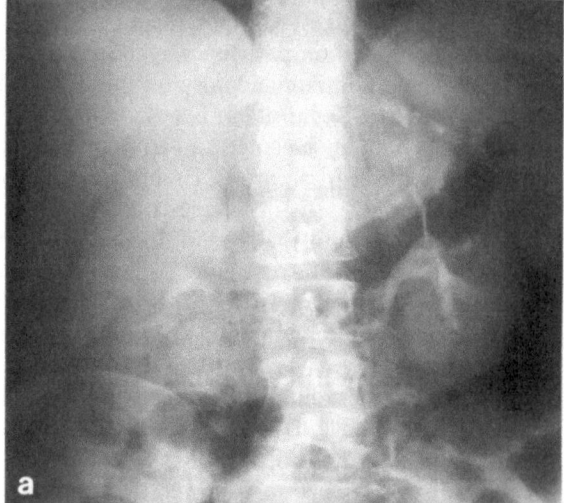

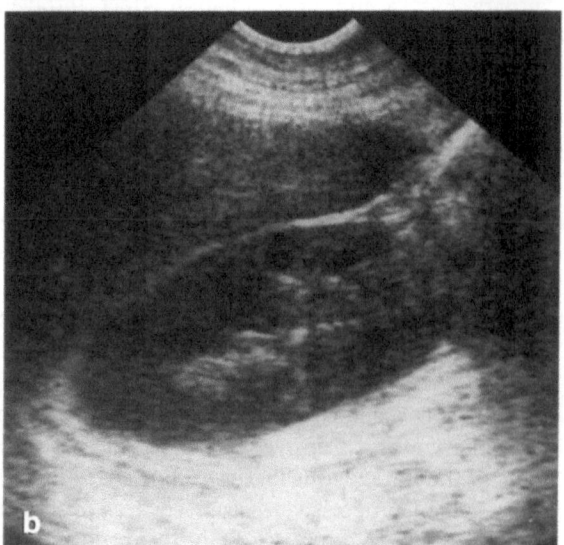

▷

Fig. 4.4 a, b. Right-sided acute pyelonephritis in a 65-year-old female. **a** IVP shows denser nephrogram on right, with slight swelling. **b** Ultrasound shows kidney to be slightly enlarged with some decrease in echogenicity, especially on the dorsal surface. Note good through transmission due to the edema

The presence of a striated nephrogram is a classical CT finding (GOLD et al. 1983) (Fig. 4.6). Most likely, this pattern reflects unopacified fluid between tubules or unopacified urine within dilated tubules. Occasionally, a delay in excretion is demonstrated on contrast-enhanced CT scans (SENN et al. 1982). If wedge-shaped areas of heterogeneous enhancement are present on the initial postenhancement CT scan, follow-up CT may show these as hyperdense (ISHIKAWA et al. 1985), which permits differentiation from renal infarcts (BANKOFF et al. 1984).

Technetium 99 m glucoheptonate scans tend to show absent or poor uptake in affected segments. Technetium 99 m 2,3-dimercaptosuccinic acid (DMSA) scans similarly demonstrate poor uptake in affected areas (STOLLER and KOGAN 1986; STY et al. 1987) Indium-labeled white blood cells (WBCs) or gallium can rarely localize in an area of demarcation by an abscess membrane or concentrate in a wall of an abscess (BRUGH et al. 1979; FROELICH and SWANSON 1984; HANDMAKER 1982; McDOUGALL et al. 1979; GARCIA et al. 1984).

Increased accumulation of edema fluid results in a high signal intensity on T2-weighted magnetic resonance imaging (MRI) scans. Corticomedullary differentiation tends to be lost due to edema.

Arteriograms may demonstrate attenuation of intralobar vessels or stretching of the intralobular or arcuate arteries. An inhomogeneous nephrogram and occasionally a striated pattern is appreciated on late phase nephrographic films. These changes appear to reflect the presence of renal microabscesses. Akin to CT (striate and feathery pattern), amputation of vessels may be demonstrated correlating to the pathologic findings of endarteritis obliterans (LANG 1973).

The epinephrine renal venogram may demonstrate marked distortion of the normal intraparenchymal venous architecture. Linear streaks of contrast medium extending from the segmental or interlobar veins to the periphery of the kidney are encountered (GOLDMAN ML et al. 1978).

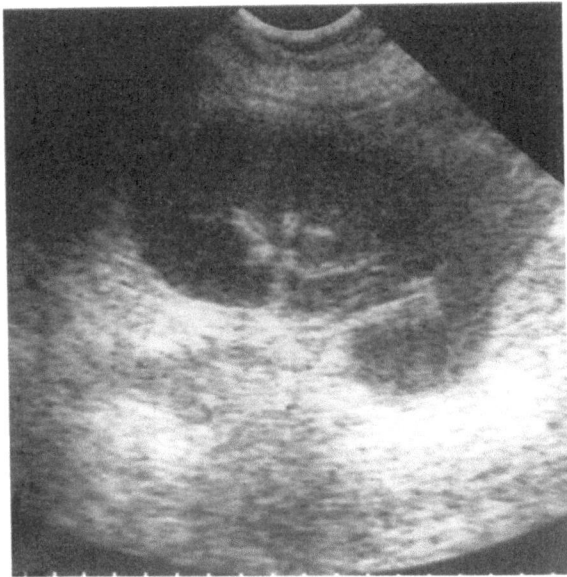

Fig. 4.5. Acute pyelonephritis. Ultrasound shows slightly enlarged kidney with good through transmission. (LANG 1986 c)

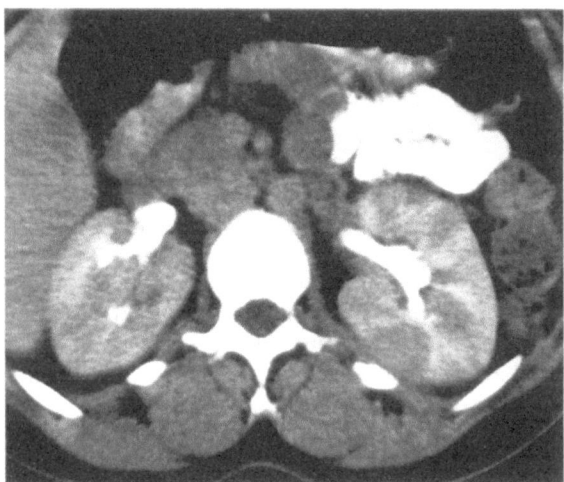

Fig. 4.6. Bilateral acute pyelonephritis. Note both the striated nephrogram in some areas and the wedge-shaped defects found in other affected portions clearly involving both kidneys

4.3 Acute Bacterial Nephritis (Acute Suppurative Nephritis, Severe Acute Pyelonephritis)

Acute bacterial nephritis is not defined pathologically. The term is often used interchangeably with *acute pyelonephritis* and even *pyonephrosis* (DAVIDSON and TALNER 1973; MOREAU 1982). This has resulted in an overlap of radiologic findings attributed to this entity. In all probability, this group represents a subset of diabetic female patients with severe acute pyelonephritis.

On intravenous urography, the kidney is enlarged, the nephrogram decreased or absent. Arteriograms tend to show poor cortical flow resultant from shunting of blood into the medulla (Trueta phenomenon). Late phase films show a striated nephrogram (Fig. 4.7). On ultrasound, the kidneys may be swollen with a diffuse echo pattern not dissimilar to that seen with rejected transplant kidneys (WICKS and THORNBURY 1979).

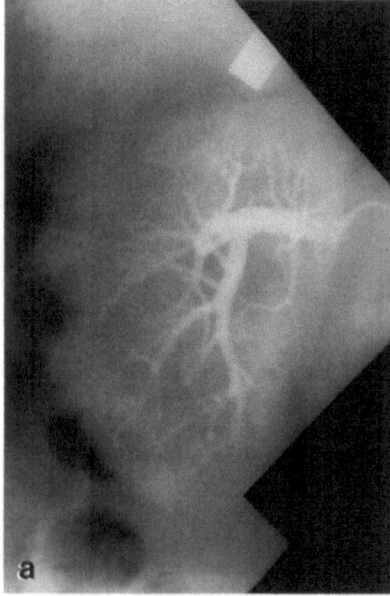
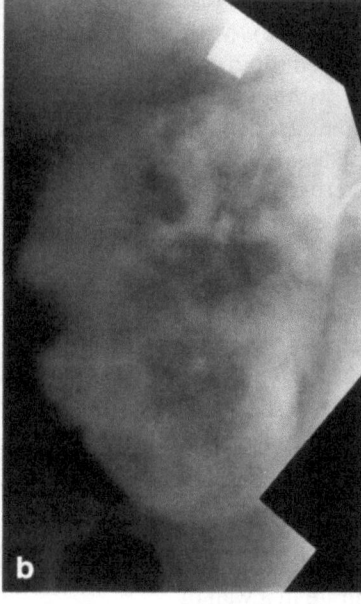

Fig. 4.7 a, b. Acute bacterial nephritis in diabetic female. On IVP, no function was present. Angiography shows extremely poor flow characteristic of this entity. (LANG 1986 c)

4.4 Acute Focal Pyelonephritis (Focal Lobar Nephronia, Focal Bacterial Nephritis, the Preabscess State)

The site of focal pyelonephritis probably represents the portal for infection of the kidney by the hematogenous or retrograde route. The term denotes a process that is still localized to a lobar distribution. To some, the term also implies a preabscess state with parenchymal destruction but as yet without liquefaction necrosis. Since the upper and lower pole calyces represent a locus of lesser resistance to reflux for bacteria, acute focal pyelonephritis is often found in this distribution (SIEGEL and GLASIER 1981).

Clinically, most patients present with fever, flank pain, and pyuria. *E. coli* and proteus are the most common organisms (ROSENFIELD et al. 1979).

4.4.1 Radiologic Findings

Nephrotomograms demonstrate a pertinent focal deformity of the renal outline attendant upon a poorly defined mass of a density lower than that of adjacent parenchyma. Otherwise, the intravenous urogram may be normal (Fig. 4.8).

Technetium 99 m glucoheptonate scans show decreased accumulation of the radiotracer in the involved area. Conversely, indium-labeled WBC or gallium scans show increased focal uptake (Fig. 4.9 b).

Arteriograms may occasionally show an area of increased vascularity attendant upon the inflamma-

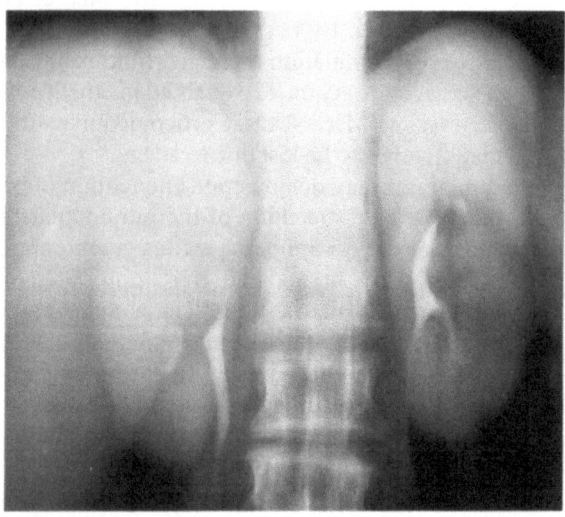

Fig. 4.8. Focal acute pyelonephritis. Tomogram shows an enlarged right upper pole. Its density is indistinguishable from that of normal parenchyma

tory neovascularity. Differentiation from a neoplasm can be difficult. Characteristic narrowing of veins in the afflicted area on renal venography is, unfortunately, nonspecific.

A hypoechoic area with reduced through transmission is the most common pattern of this entity seen on ultrasonograms (ROSENFIELD et al. 1979). Hyperechogenicity attendant upon hemorrhage into the lesion is the other form of presentation (PICCIRILLO et al. 1987; RIGSBY et al. 1986). However, in some

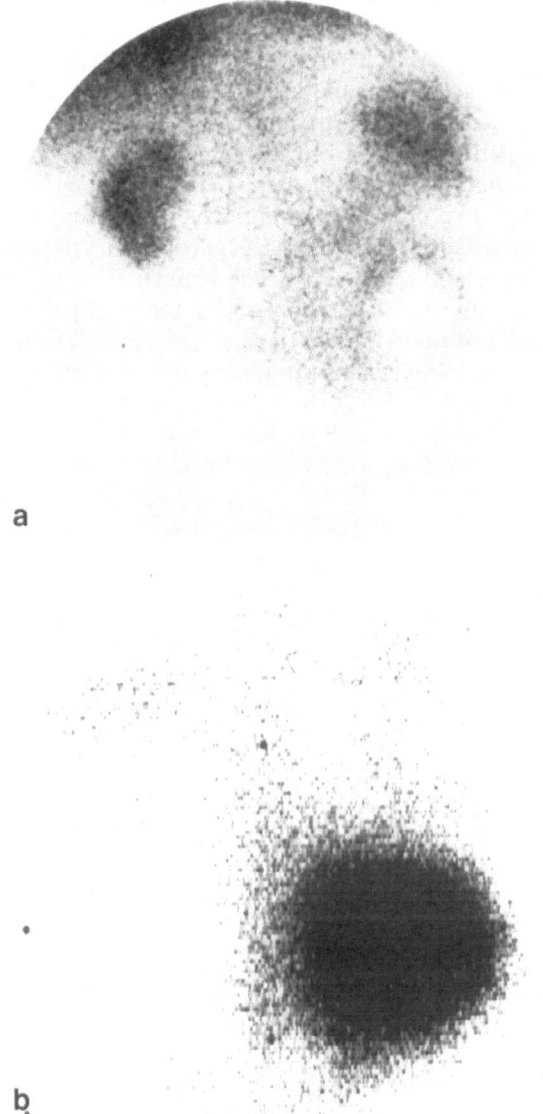

a

b

Fig. 4.9 a, b. Acute focal pyelonephritis in an 82-year-old. **a** Technetium scan showing no uptake in lower pole of left kidney. **b** Gallium scan shows increased uptake in this area. It is impossible to differentiate this pattern from an infected cyst, abscess, etc. (LANG 1986 c)

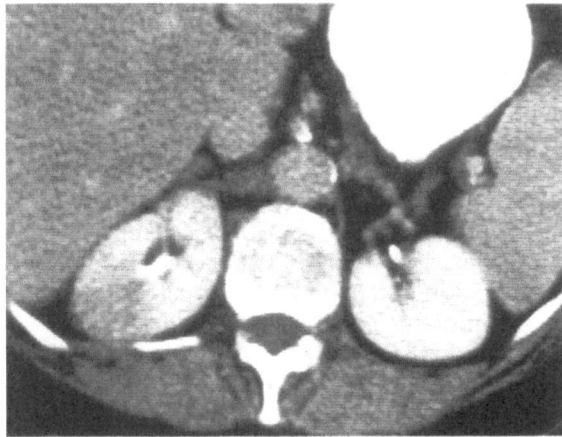

Fig. 4.10. Right-sided acute pyelonephritis. CT shows typical wedge-shaped defect. Density too high for fluid. On another scan, a small low density area (CT number clearly near that of water) was seen, possibly representing early breakdown. Patient treated successfully with intravenous antibiotics

instances the area is isoechoic, reflecting only the presence of mild edema.

Computed tomography tends to provide the most conclusive criteria constellation. Single or multiple wedge-shaped or rounded and often poorly marginated defects are demonstrated on both pre- and particularly post-contrast enhancement scans. The density on preenhancement scans tends to be equivalent to that of water or very slightly above it (Figs. 4.10, 4.12, 4.13) (GOLD et al. 1983; HOFFMAN EP et al. 1980; LEE et al. 1980; SOULEN et al. 1989).

At times, the low density areas tend to increase in density on delayed scans (ISHIKAWA et al. 1985). An exception is the hemorrhagic form, as these lesions may present with increased density on nonenhanced CT scans (RIGSBY et al. 1986). Sometimes a focal striated pattern may also be appreciated and afflict larger areas of the same kidney.

On MRI, these segmental areas will have low signals on T1- and high signals on T2-weighted images. Cortical medullary discrimination will be lost.

4.5 Emphysematous Pyelonephritis

Emphysematous pyelonephritis is a suppurative infection, usually of mixed flora, producing intrarenal gas (SPAGNOLA 1968). The most common organisms are *E. coli,* klebsiella, *Aerobacter aerogenes,* proteus, and pseudomonas (LANGSTON and PFISTER 1970).

In its classic form, emphysematous pyelonephritis is a severe, life-threatening situation usually seen in diabetics, often with an obstructive uropathy (MICHAELI et al. 1984). In nondiabetics, obstructive uropathy, neoplasms, calyceal or pelvic stenosis, or other infectious processes are found to be the underlying etiology (OLZABAL et al. 1987). Prompt recognition is of importance because of the high morbidity.

It has been felt that carbon dioxide and hydrogen are produced by the organism using the substrate of necrotic tissue and a high glucose concentration (OLZABAL et al. 1987).

Pathologically, a nonspecific necrotizing pyelonephritis is present (50%) with multiple cortical abscesses (38%). Renal papillary necrosis (21%), intravascular thrombi (19%), and an entirely sloughed kidney are other associated findings.

Clinically, signs consistent with severe acute pyelonephritis, of refractory infection, may be the presenting symptom. Most patients are diabetic, with an average age of 54 (19–81). Fevers above 101○F (56%), nausea and vomiting, flank pain (49%), localized flank tenderness, lethargy and confusion may be present (MICHAELI et al. 1984; ALLEN et al. 1984). A crepitant mass is palpable in many cases, most often on the left (MICHAELI et al. 1984). Laboratory studies will variously reveal hyperglycemia, leukocytosis, and/or azotemia.

Surgical management combined with aggressive antibiotic therapy has been considered mandatory in the past, but a few nontoxic and very select patients have been successfully treated with aggressive antibiotic therapy alone (MOGLE et al. 1984). HALL et al. (1988) has reported successful treatment of an 82-year-old diabetic with extensive pyelonephritis using antibiotics and percutaneous drainage. Mortality can approach 40%–50%.

4.5.1 Radiologic Findings

Gas dissecting through the parenchyma in a tubular pattern is the diagnostic finding on plain radiographs (Fig. 4.11). Gas may also be identified in the perinephric space, in the calyces, in pockets of intrarenal abscesses, and as crescents subcapsularly.

Such gas collections need to be differentiated from gas within the urinary tract of other origin. Diagnostically or traumatically introduced atmospheric air must be considered. Air in the calyces can be normal post ileal loop. Gas can also be introduced secondary to an intrarenal fistula and lastly bacterially produced gas can gravitate into the renal pelvis and calyces from the bladder (CARRIS and SCHMIDT 1977). Gas confined to the renal pelvis or calyces should be designated as emphysematous pyelitis. Intravenous urography does not offer fur-

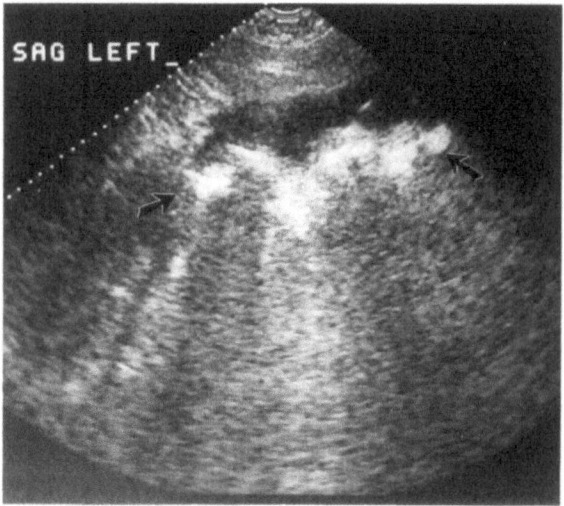

Fig. 4.12. Emphysematous pyelonephritis. Note highly echogenic intraparenchymal air *(arrows)* with dirty shadowing

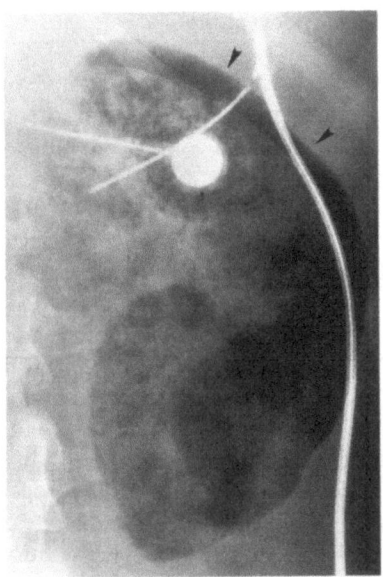

Fig. 4.11. Emphysematous pyelonephritis on left. Coned down film of the left kidney shows classic finding of intraparenchymal air. Note subcapsular air as well *(arrow)*. (GOLDMAN and GATEWOOD 1989)

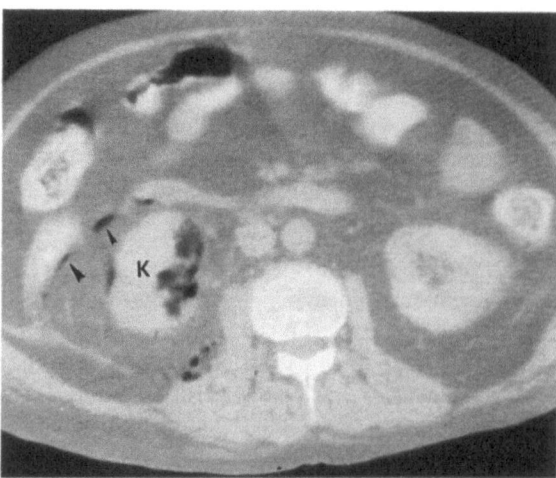

Fig. 4.13. Emphysematous pyelonephritis. CT shows intraparenchymal and subcapsular air within the kidney *(K)*. Note air below Gerota's fascia *(arrows)*

ther diagnostic information since absent or extremely poor function on the affected side precludes further detailed assessment. Acoustic shadowing from intrarenal gas may be appreciated on ultrasonograms (VAS et al. 1985; ALLEN et al. 1984). The characteristically multiple and low echoes ("dirty shadows") allow differentiation against the shadowing caused by a calculus (Fig. 4.12). Moreover, a "ring down" artifact indicating resonance of fluid trapped between adjacent gas bubbles may present as one other characteristic ultrasonographic finding (PICCIRILLO et al. 1987). Gas bubbles in the perirenal space may result in similar hyperechogenicity (OLZABAL et al. 1987). A plain film is often of value to differentiate stone from gas.

Computed tomography provides the most sensitive criteria for diagnosing intracalyceal or intraparenchymal air (Fig. 4.13) (KIM et al. 1979; VAS et al. 1985; OLZABAL et al. 1987; ALLEN et al. 1984; GRAHAM et al. 1986; LEEKAM et al. 1987; LACHANCE et al. 1985; LAUTIN et al. 1979). Perinephric and pararenal extension can be ideally categorized (GRAHAM et al. 1986; LANG et al. 1986). The ability to demonstrate minimal amounts of gas permits aggressive treatment at an early stage. This may increase the use of interventional radiologic techniques and medical therapy in such patients.

Technetium 99 m DTPA studies may simply show lack of accumulation of the radiotracer in the emphysematous portions of the enlarged kidney, a nonspecific finding (LEEKAM et al. 1987).

4.6 Chronic Pyelonephritis (Chronic Atrophic Pyelonephritis, Reflux Nephropathy, Chronic Infection, Abacterial Nephritis)

The plethora of terms employed for this condition reflects the confusion existing in our specialty literature. Most often, chronic pyelonephritis develops in childhood after vesicoureteral reflux with bacteria-laden urine. The term *reflux nephropathy* connotes renal damage secondary to reflux. It has therefore also been called *abacterial nephritis,* suggesting that no bacteria but only bacterial antigens are present in the upper tract and cause the changes (DAIRIKI-SHORTLIFFE and STAMEY 1986a; AOKI et al. 1969). Most commonly, however, bacteria are present in the urine and the effect is due to a combination of reflux and bacteria-laden urine (HODSON et al. 1975a; RANSLEY and RISDON 1979). The designation *chronic atrophic pyelonephritis* or *reflux nephropathy* is based on an elegant experiment in pigs by HODSON (HODSON and SMITH 1979; RANSLEY and RISDON 1975). In

this animal model, HODSON caused ureteral reflux to occur experimentally and demonstrated pyelonephritic, end-stage kidneys identical to human chronic pyelonephritis. HODSON believed that this mechanism alone could cause scarring in human kidneys. However, HODSON, himself, showed that the presence of an infection in patients with reflux causes more serious renal damage than reflux alone. This is particularly true as a result of childhood infection and reflux since progressive renal damage from primary adult-onset pyelonephritis is uncommon (DAVIDSON 1985). We, however, have see de novo focal scar formation develop on CT studies in adults (SOULEN et al. 1989).

The gross pathologic findings are a generalized loss of renal parenchyma with varying amounts of focal scarring or fibrosis, especially at the poles. In advanced cases, the kidneys are small and shrunken, due to extensive scar formation. The scars tend to overlie calyces with fibrosis causing puckering of the cortex. Calyceal blunting or cupping may underlie the area and full thickness fibrosis may extend from cortex through medulla to the underlying calyx. This leads to the classical cortical depression or pitting seen on the surface of such kidneys. Microscopically, there is evidence of fibrosis around glomeruli and atrophy and dilatation of the tubules, and chronic leukocytic infiltrates are present. Between the involved areas, the kidney may be normal, and, in fact, there may be compensatory hypertrophy.

The precise reason for development of scars is controversial. In general, children who have had symptomatic bacteriuria tend to develop chronic changes and scars more frequently (KUNIN 1964). There also appears to be a significant relationship between a degree of reflux and scarring (Cardiff-Oxford Study Group 1979). However, there are patients with asymptomatic bacteriuria, reflux, and as yet unscarred kidneys and normal growth (CLAESSON and LINDBERG 1977). The major theories proposed to explain the renal scarring focus around the following possibilities:

1. Severe edema leads to ischemic changes.
2. Inflammatory changes may lead to endarteritis obliterans or vascular thrombosis and hence renal scarring.
3. Bacterial antigens cause scarring (ROBERTS 1983a). This postulates an autoimmune response as a result of Tamm-Horsfall protein entering the kidney intraarterially by reflux or attendant upon nephrolithiasis. Immunoautoradiographs have demonstrated protein containing subunits of *E.coli* that can cross-react with anti-Tamm-Hors-

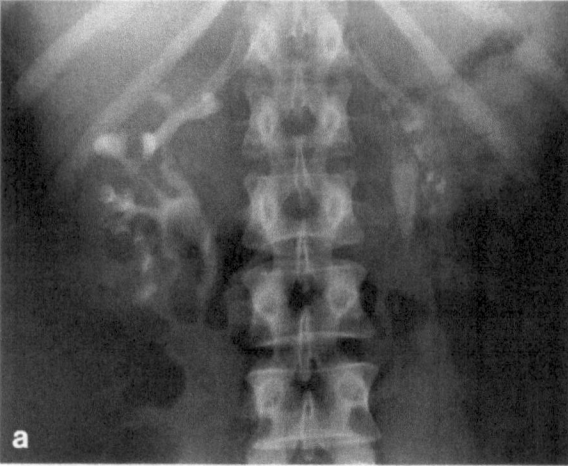
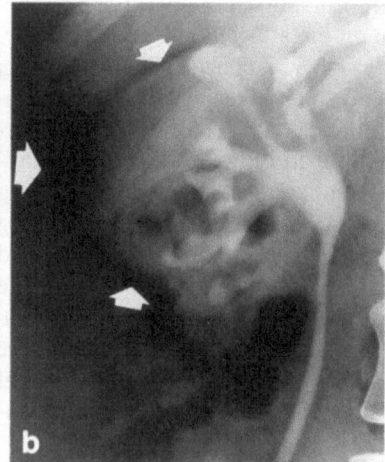

Fig. 4.14. a Bilateral chronic pyelonephritis with right lower pole pseudotumor and end-stage small left kidney. **b** Coned down, oblique film of right kidney. Note blunt upper pole calyces with loss of overlying cortical tissue. Note "pseudotumor" *(arrows)* secondary to compensatory hypertrophy

fall protein antibody (MAYER et al. 1983; DAIRIKI-SHORTLIFFE 1986a).

4. Scarring occurs attendant upon a granulocytic response initiated by bacterial destruction releasing superoxide, hydrogen peroxide, or hydroxyl radicals with resultant autotoxicity (ROBERTS 1983a).

The fact that aggressive, early antibiotic therapy may prevent scarring in symptomatic patients may partly support the last supposition (ROBERTS 1983a). It is felt that children with reflux should be kept on prophylactic antibiotics until maturation of the ureterovesical junction and cessation of reflux (HULAND and BUSCH 1984). Surgery is now reserved for those patients in whom conservative treatment has failed. Since scarring occurs often after a latent period of 2 or 3 years following the initial insult, all corrective measures may only prevent scarring developing from new infections and not be effective against the damage that has already resulted or been initiated.

4.6.1 Radiologic Findings

Plain films may indicate contour alterations and global or focal shrinkage of the afflicted kidney. The irrefutable criterion by which pyelonephritis is diagnosed on intravenous urograms is the documentation of a renal scar directly over a blunted calyx (Fig. 4.15). Most often, such scars are seen at the

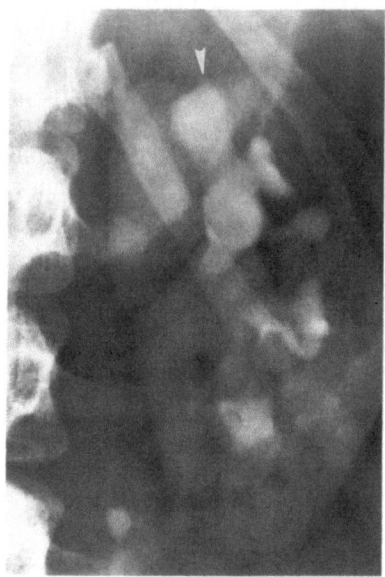

Fig. 4.15. Chronic pyelonephritis in a 27-year-old. Note scar with underlying blunt calyx *(arrow)*

poles of the kidneys (Fig. 4.15). They must be differentiated from isolated parenchymal scars occurring in nephrosclerosis or attendant upon infarction. With progression of the disease, the kidney may shrink focally or diffusely (Fig. 4.14). At the same time, compensatory hypertrophy simulating a tumor may be present (Fig. 4.14b). Rarely, there may be thickening of the renal pelvis and calyces attendant upon fibrosis, resulting in changes similar to those encountered with tuberculosis. A nonfunctioning kidney may result as the end-stage of this disease.

Cortical scars present as linear hyperechoic areas on ultrasound (Fig. 4.16). Focal or diffuse cortical tissue loss is appreciated as cortical thinning

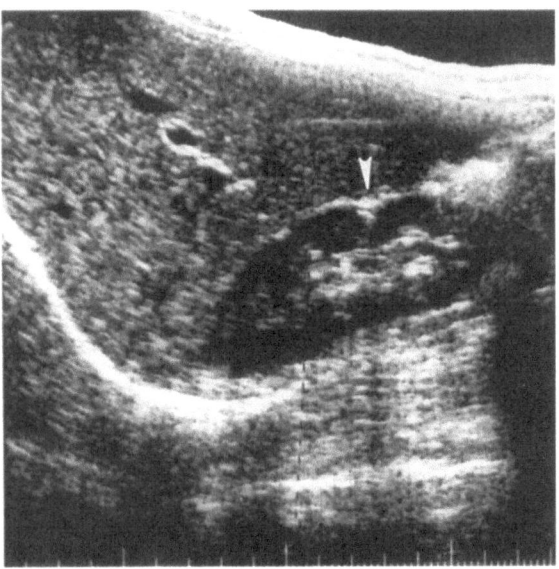

Fig. 4.16. Chronic pyelonephritis with hyperechoic scar on ultrasound *(arrow)*

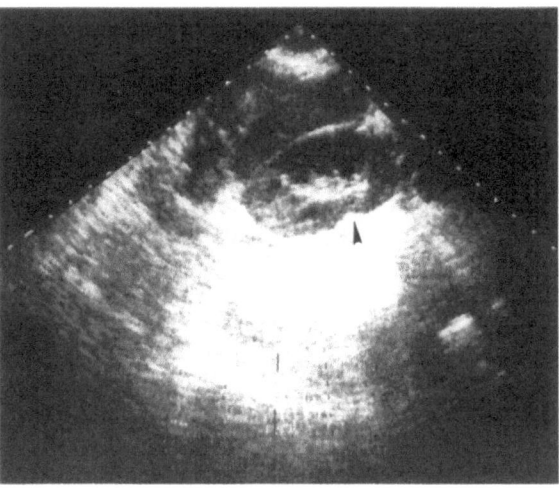

Fig. 4.17. Chronic pyelonephritis with ultrasound evidence of focal parenchymal loss with diffuse renal shrinkage

(Fig. 4.17). Chronic intraparenchymal changes may result in scattered increased echogenicity (KAY et al. 1979) (Fig. 4.18). Loss of tissue resulting in replacement sinus fat causes an increase in the central echo pattern.

Some of the morphologic changes, the size and presence of scars, are documented on technetium 99 m DTPA or DMSA scans (STOLLER and KOGAN 1986). However, radionuclide studies are particularly useful to assess relative renal function and renal plasma flow rates and thus help to determine the therapeutic course (SCHLEGEL and LANG 1980).

Focal and global shrinkage of renal cortex attendant upon chronic pyelonephritis is often discovered serendipitously on studies performed for other reasons (Figs. 4.19, 4.20).

The angiographic appearance is often confusing and inflammatory neovascularity may mimic tumor neovascularity (GOLDMAN et al. 1977a; LANG 1971; LEVIN et al. 1976). At times, one may even observe encasement of vessels simulating the findings of transitional or squamous cell carcinoma. A characteristic tortuosity of relatively large interlobar arteries which appear crowded by the loss of parenchyma is perhaps the most typical arteriographic manifestation of chronic pyelonephritis. Loss of cortical tissue results in a "pruned" tree appearance of the vessels (Fig. 4.21). Early opacification of veins may be seen with inflammation, although, in general, premature opacification of draining veins is prominently encountered with tumors featuring arteriovenous shunts (Fig. 4.22) (FRIMANN-DAHL

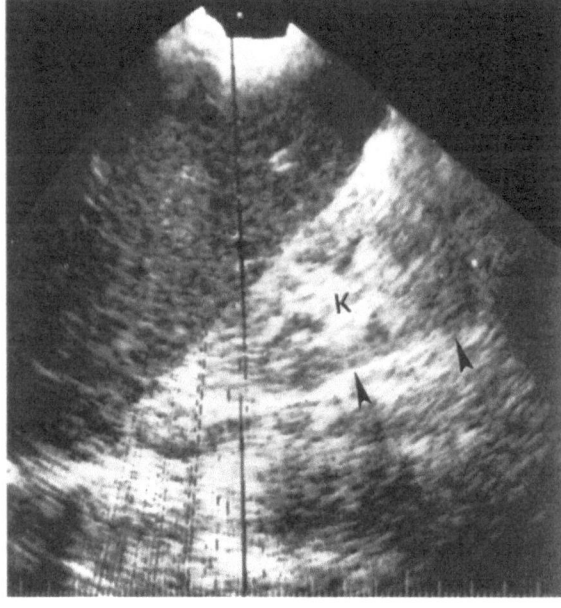

Fig. 4.18. Chronic pyelonephritis. Note small hyperechoic kidney *(K) (arrows)*. Compare this echogenicity with that of liver

1966). Follow-up of patients and particularly of children is important. This is accomplished by the intravenous urogram, voiding cystourethrogram, radionuclide urogram, nuclear cystogram, and ultrasonograms. Technetium 99 m glucoheptonate is perhaps the optimal scanning agent for assessment of progressive changes and alterations for functional

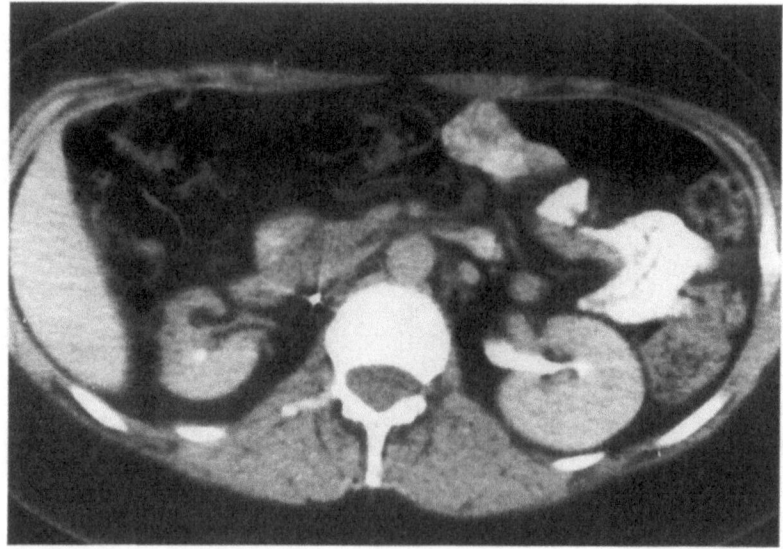

Fig. 4.19. Chronic pyelonephritis. CT shows loss of cortex on lateral aspect of right kidney. Incidental finding as CT was performed for other reasons

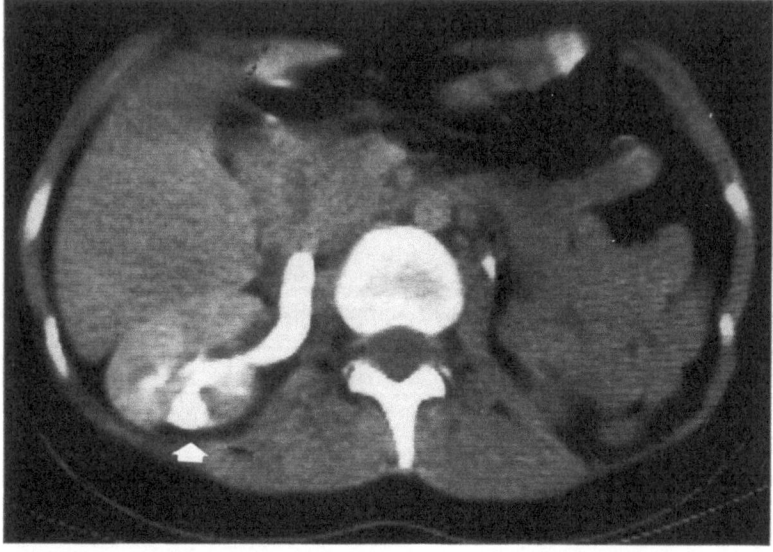

Fig. 4.20. Chronic pyelonephritis. Note blunt calyx and overlying scar. (GOLD-MAN 1988)

parameters, renal plasma flow rate etc. (SCHLEGEL and LANG 1980; SHAPIRO et al. 1988). Radionuclide studies are lauded for a lower dose rate, which advocates their use particularly in children. Careful analysis of growth rate on the basis of measurement from the intrapapillary line to the renal pole is indicated in the follow-up of children (Fig. 4.23 a–c). Disassociation of parenchymal volumes in the upper and lower poles must be viewed with suspicion and as a potential indicator of renal damage (HODSON 1967, 1981).

The severity of reflux must be graded. One classification establishes the following grades:

1. Reflux into ureter only
2. Reflux into pelvis but not into the parenchyma
3. Evidence of intralobular reflux

Others grade on the degree of decompensation of the ureter and whether reflux occurs during the filling phase of the bladder or only during the high pressure voiding phase. Many pediatric radiologists now divide reflux into five grades. It is, however, generally conceded that intrarenal reflux in patients under the age of 5 years results in a significant incidence of subsequent scarring (ROLLESTON et al. 1970; HULAND and BUSCH 1984; GINALSKI et al. 1985).

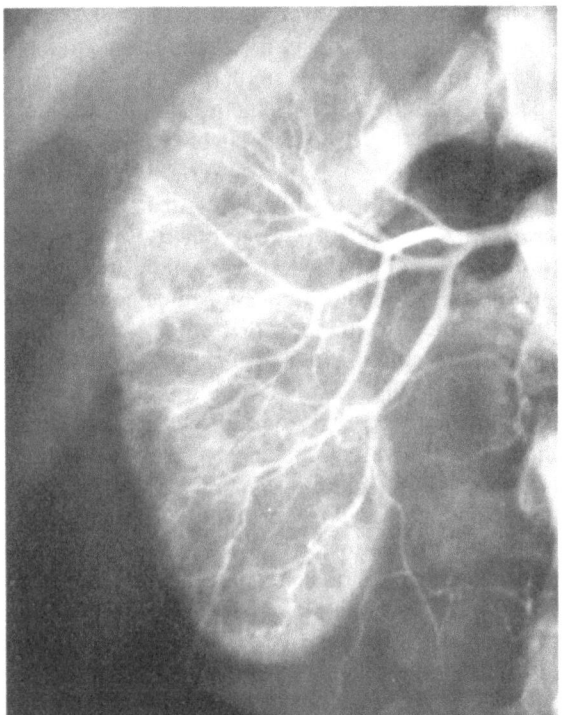

Fig. 4.21. Chronic pyelonephritis. Arterial phase showing small kidney with narrow corkscrew distal arterial vessels. (LANG 1986c)

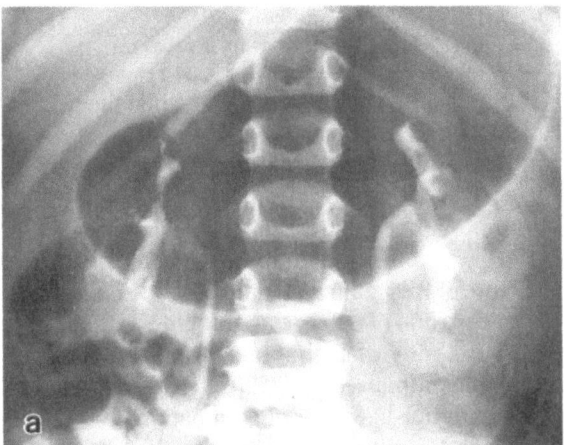

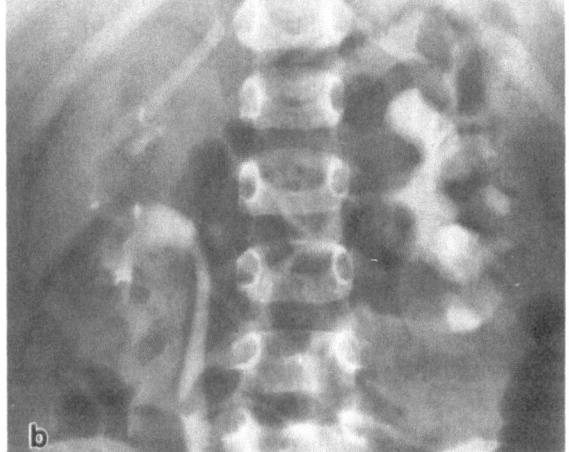

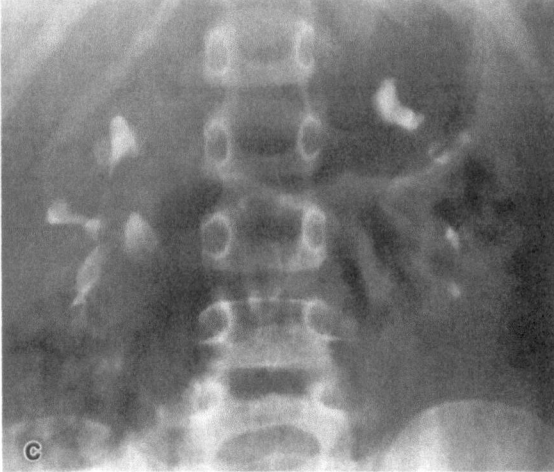

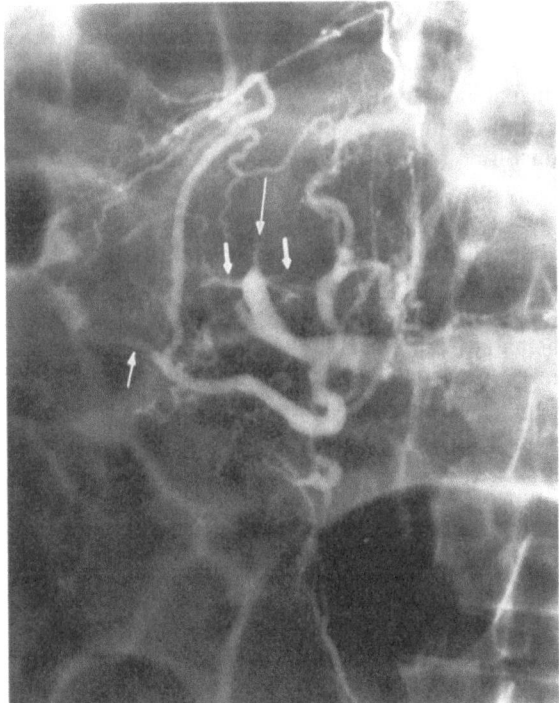

Fig. 4.22. Chronic pyelonephritis. Renal vein study shows encasement of intrarenal veins *(arrows)*. This finding is non-specific and can be seen in both inflammation and neoplasm. (GOLDMAN 1977a)

Fig. 4.23 a–c. Chronic pyelonephritis progressing over several years. Damage to right side initially unsuspected and confirmed only on later studies. **a** Initial study at 2 years. Note scar in lateral superior aspect of left kidney. Right looks normal. **b** Study 1 year later. Note marked progression on left. Right side, although looking normal, has not shown any growth from previous study. **c** Study at 5 years of age. Note significant scarring on right with blunt calyces. This progressive scarring occurred despite only one confirmed incident of infection

4.7 Granulomatous, Fungal, and the Rare Inflammatory Processes

Granulomatous diseases develop when the primary or acute defense mechanism is insufficient due to the virulence of the infecting organism or a deficiency in the host or a combination thereof. It is a failure of degradation of the bacteria by the scavenger cells (polymorphonuclear leukocytes). Because of this failure, the human body marshals its secondary line of defense. A granuloma is the result, which is a somewhat abnormal response to a variety of noxious stimuli (BOYD 1970). The granuloma produces a tumor-like mass of granulation tissue, fibroblasts, and capillaries. Microscopically, one notes a focal area of vascularity with a multiplicity of histiocytes, macrophages, and/or giant cells (i.e., the phagocytic or scavenger cells) surrounded by fibroblasts which tend to engulf the insulting organism. Under ideal circumstances, the macrophages or histiocytes (varyingly called xanthoma cells, etc.) engulf the infecting organism, ingest it, isolate it, and destroy it. In certain situations, the ingested organism cannot be destroyed by the host white cells (e.g., the Michaelis-Gutmann body in malacoplakia).

4.7.1 Tuberculosis

Tuberculosis (TB) has been recognized in human skeletal remains estimated to be at least 7000 years old (GOW 1986). Hippocrates discussed the existence of phthisis, as did Galen. Periodic epidemics have occurred, and about a quarter of the deaths in England during the eighteenth century were due to TB. In 1882, KOCH described the etiology of TB, having grown the organism outside the body and reproduced the disease in an appropriate host. In 1908 EKEHORN suggested the mechanism of its spread to the kidney, and in 1962 MEDLAR correctly described its pathogenesis (GOW 1986).

Tuberculosis represents the classic example of a granulomatous disease and is caused by *Mycobacterium tuberculosis*. Bovine TB, usually acquired by drinking unpasteurized milk, is rarely encountered today. The lung is the most common site involved. While the incidence of pulmonary TB has been decreasing in the United States and Europe, it should be noted that the kidney is the most frequently involved organ after the lung (LOWE et al. 1983). Between 4% and 8% of patients with pulmonary TB were recognized by LATTIMER and KOHEN (1954) as ultimately developing renal TB. Yet, renal TB remains a diagnostic dilemma unappreciated by the patients's physician for long periods of time.

Urinary TB invariably arises from hematogenous spread from a pulmonary focus, the latter often appearing inconsequential in nature, even in retrospect. A secondary defense parameter, the granuloma, develops. First, the tubercle bacillus localizes in the glomerular and cortical arteries. In some patients, multiple bilateral small cortical granulomas develop that remain asymptomatic and stable (GOLDMAN et al. 1985). Parenchymal destruction results when the bacillus first enters the nephrons and then advances to the loop of Henle. A necrotizing papillitis results and is one of the first identifiable radiologic findings. A reactive fibrosis may develop next, leading to cicatrization at the infundibula, at the renal pelvis, along the ureter, and/or at the ureteropelvic junction. Subsequent destruction and breakdown may lead to cavitation, ulcerocavernous lesions, and caseation.

The end result is quite variable, leading to the appellation of "great imitators." The kidney may be small, nonfunctioning, and often calcified (the tuberculous autonephrectomized kidney) or large and nonfunctioning, suggesting a pyonephrosis. Renal calculi, single or multiple masses (tuberculomas), parenchymal calcifications, focal scarring, abscesses, obstructed calyces, and renal parenchymal scars are all seen to variable degrees.

Clinical involvement of the kidney occurs many years after the initial pulmonary exposure, with a higher incidence in males in their twenties to forties (SIMON et al. 1977; FERRI and RUNDLE 1985). Thus, the patient may be asymptomatic for years followed by mild complaints such as frequency, mild dysuria, nocturia, and pain. With advanced progression, there may be fever, weight loss, sweating (especially at night), hematuria, and anemia. Physical examination may reveal only a tender kidney unless there is active disease in the lungs, prostate, epididymis, seminal vesicles, etc. Urinalysis will generally reveal hematuria and pyuria, but with negative routine cultures (i.e., sterile pyuria). However, in 20% of patients, pyuria may not be present (GOW 1986). In 20%, secondary infections are present, causing further confusion (GOW 1986). Special and multiple cultures and techniques looking for the acid fast bacillus must be instituted in order to make the diagnosis; these may require 6–8 weeks.

Treatment consists of the use of appropriate antituberculous drugs such as isoniazid, ethambutol, pyrazinamide, paraaminosalicylic acid, streptomycin, and rifampicin.

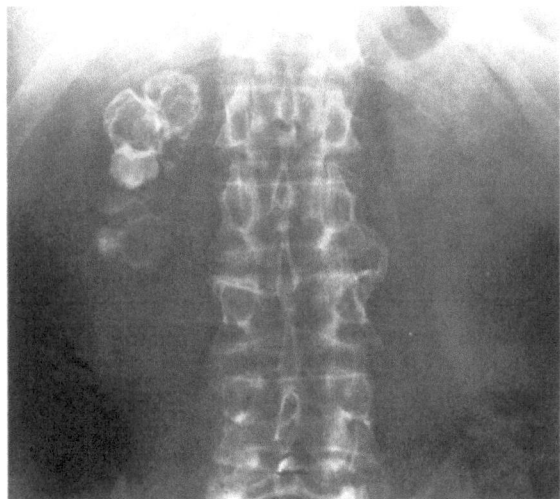

Fig. 4.24. Tuberculosis. Plain film showing autonephrectomized calcified kidney. Ring-like calcifications suggest the outlines of the calyces

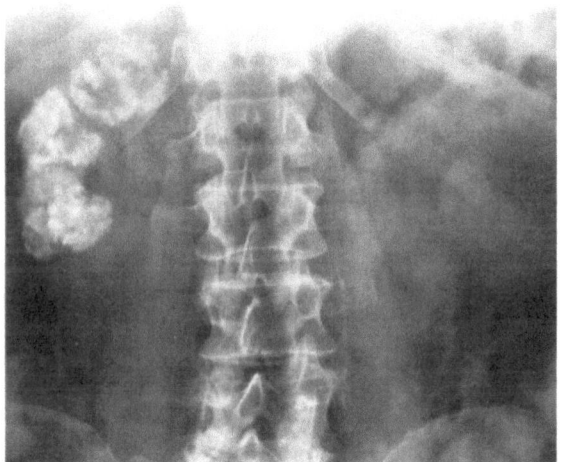

Fig. 4.25. Tuberculosis. Plain film shows the right kidney replaced with "putty-like" calcifications

4.7.1.1 Radiologic Findings

Plain films (KOLLINS et al. 1974) may demonstrate a small kidney. Rarely, an enlarged kidney is found when acute or subacute infection is present. On occasion, a focal mass with or without caseous material will be identified, simulating a tumor. Calcification, when present, is a helpful diagnostic finding and can be variously described as irregular, granular, indistinct, mottled, indefinite, putty-like, faint, ground glass, etc. It may be curvilinear, lobular, or ring-like as well (Figs. 4.24, 4.25). There is a significant prevalence of renal calculi (DOLEV et al. 1985)

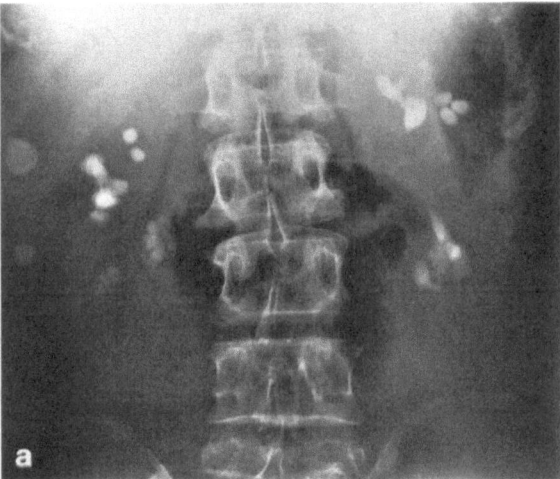

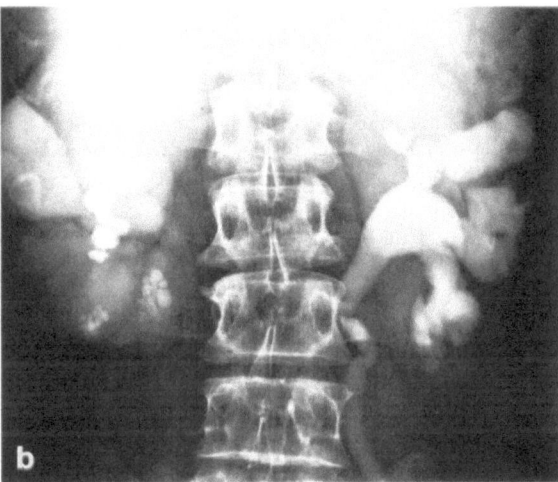

Fig. 4.26a, b. Tuberculosis. Unusual case. **a** Plain film shows multiple bilateral renal calculi. **b** IVP shows bilateral pyonephrosis

(Fig. 4.26). Enlargement of the psoas muscle ("cold" abscess), destruction of the spine, or inflammatory changes of the hip are ancillary findings which aid in the diagnosis when present.

Calcification of the seminal vesicles may be present but is more commonly found in diabetics. Calcification may occasionally be noted in the prostate, and, very rarely, in the bladder and ureter. The latter location is much more common in patients with schistosomiasis. Splenic granulomas should also be looked for, along with calcified mesenteric lymph nodes.

Early renal involvement will present on IVP with an enlarged kidney and poor function. One of the earliest radiologically visible manifestations of TB is an ulcerating papillitis with a focal erosion of the papilla presenting as an irregular amorphous, fuzzy,

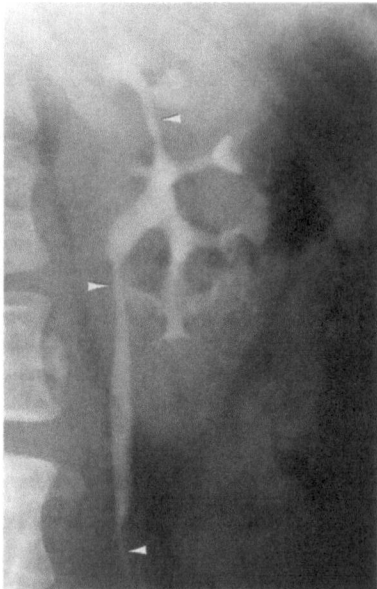

Fig. 4.27. Tuberculosis – somewhat more advanced case showing infundibular, ureteropelvic, and ureteric stenosis secondary to fibrosis *(arrows)*

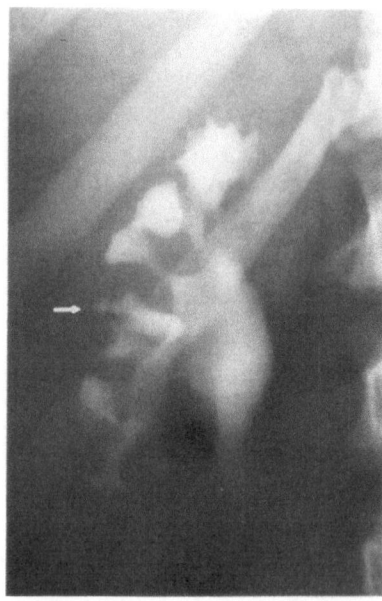

Fig. 4.28. Tuberculosis in a 21-year-old black male. Example of medullary form of renal papillary necrosis *(arrow)*

smudged, feathery calyx (BRUCE et al. 1969). Infundibular fibrosis (Fig. 4.27) leads to a stricture with ultimate blunting of the involved calyx or calyces secondary to either obstruction or a sloughed papilla from renal papillary necrosis (Fig. 4.28). Cortical abscesses, i.e., cavitations, often filled with caseous material may be recognized by IVP or tomography. This may lead to a focal "tumor" which may or may not communicate with the collecting system. Thus, a focal tuberculous mass, a tuberculoma, is formed which is indistinguishable from a neoplasm. Tuberculomas may be smooth-walled or irregular. Involvement of the renal pelvis leads to narrowing, and, if the ureteropelvic junction is affected, obstructive pyonephrosis may be noted (Fig. 4.26 b). Scar formation, loss of cortical tissue, and other changes consistent with pyelonephritis are seen. If the disease is unchecked, nonfunction will develop, leading to an enlarged kidney totally replaced by tuberculous abscesses or an end-stage small autonephrectomized kidney (Figs. 4.24, 4.25). Fistulization to the large bowel and skin is occasionally noted. There are typical changes of TB in the ureter and bladder (Fig. 4.29). These include ureteritis cystica or a striated pattern early in the disease. With fibrosis; a corkscrew, pipe stem or string of bead ureter will be noted. Bladder involvement with fibrosis leads to a contracted bladder with vesicoureteral reflux.

Retrograde pyelography will demonstrate a variety of patterns. The study may be normal or show

an occluded individual calyx. There may be total occlusion at the ureteropelvic junction. Finally, contrast will enter a contracted renal pelvis (Fig. 4.30). In this form, the calyces and pelvis are often lined with extensive tuberculous granulomas giving a nodular appearance to the collecting system.

The angiographic pattern (GIUSTRA et al. 1971) is variable, suggesting a solid mass, a "cystic tumor" or pyonephrosis. Vascularity is variable, making it impossible to differentiate inflammation from tumor (Fig. 4.31). Radionuclide techniques have been advocated to evaluate functional status during and after treatment.

Ultrasonically, two patterns have been observed (SCHAEFER et al. 1983): (a) hydro- or pyonephrosis (Fig. 4.32) and (b) an infiltrating pattern. The second pattern is much more common with masses that show definite echogenicity reflecting the presence of calcification, infected debris, and/or abscesses. Ultrasound, of course, is inferior to CT in determining the presence of calcification and the changes in the distal ureter (PREMKUMAR et al. 1987).

There is also a spectrum of CT patterns (GOLDMAN et al. 1985; PREMKUMAR et al. 1987). At one end is the small calcified, nonfunctioning kidney (advanced findings). At the other, one may see one or more obstructed calyces due to infundibular stenosis (an early finding) (Fig. 4.33). Still another pattern is that of a hydronephrotic kidney with a narrowed obstructed pelvis secondary to peripelvic

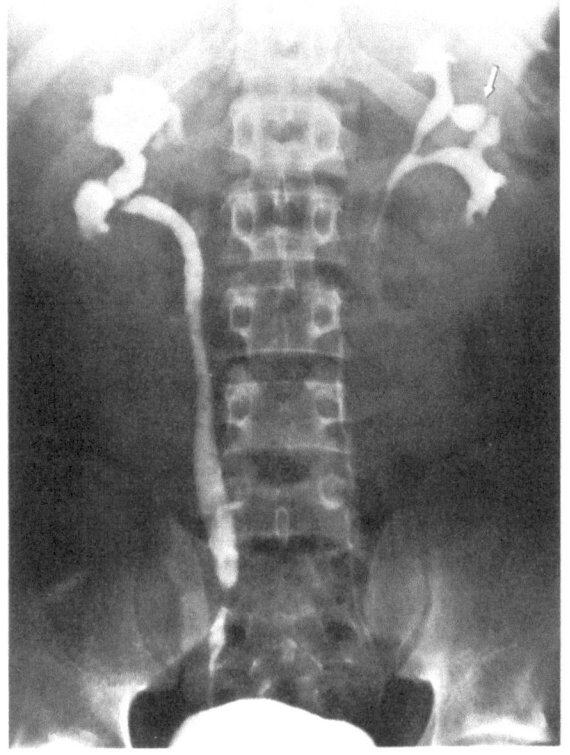

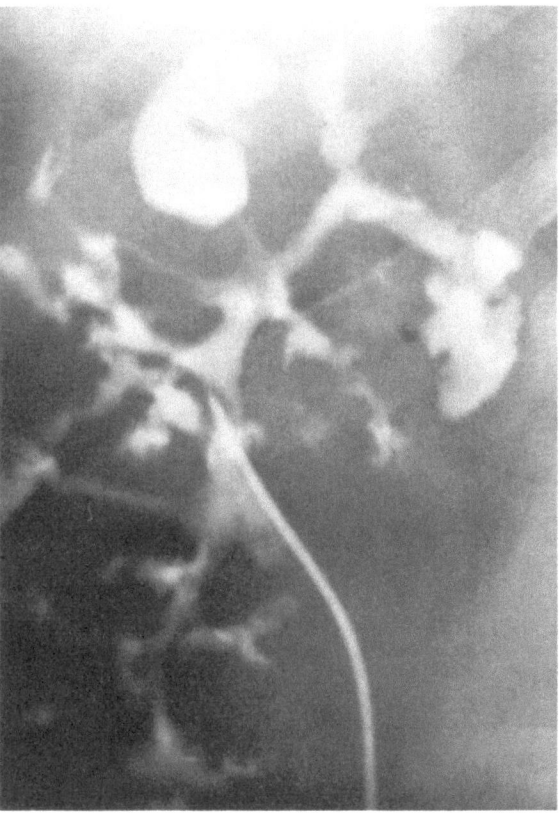

Fig. 4.29. Advanced tuberculosis. On right side, note hydrone-phrosis with renal pelvic scarring. Ureter is dilated with narrowed distal ureter. Note single blunt calyx on the left side *(arrow)*. The cause of the asymmetry of renal TB, which occurs in spite of its hematogenous origin, is unknown

Fig. 4.30. Advanced tuberculosis. Retrograde studies show renal pelvis to be almost occluded, as are the major infundibula. Calyces irregular with extensive fistulae into the cortex from multiple calyces. (GOLDMAN 1989)

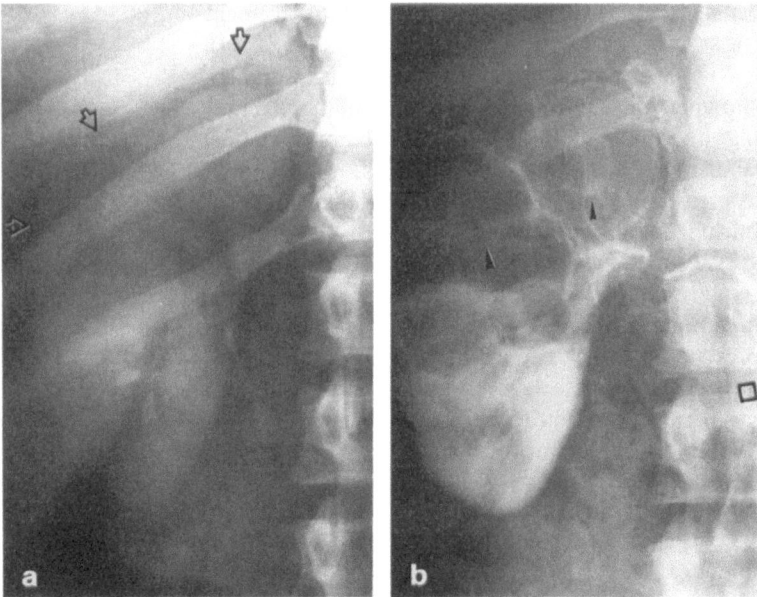

Fig. 4.31 a, b. Tuberculosis involving right upper pole of kidney in a black male with weight loss. Clinical impression was that of a tumor. **a** IVP shows nonfunctioning right upper pole *(arrows)*. **b** Angiogram shows relatively normal lower pole. Upper pole shows what really is an inflammatory pyonephrosis with some areas of hypervascularity *(arrowhead)*

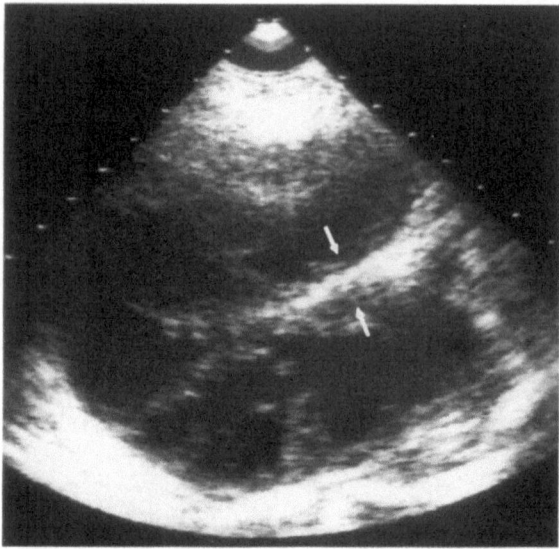

Fig. 4.32. Tuberculosis. Ultrasound shows a pyonephrotic pattern. The findings are nonspecific. Note some internal echoes representing debris within the calyces. Scarred renal pelvis present *(arrows)*

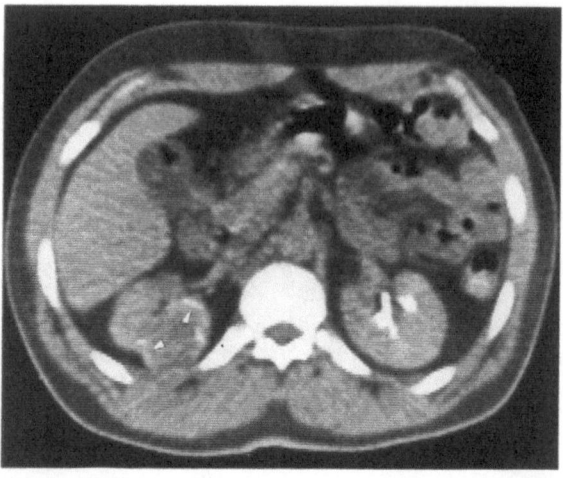

Fig. 4.33. Tuberculosis. CT revealing focal upper pole lesion on right. This enhanced study shows some focal uptake *(arrows)* corresponding to the increased vascularity seen on angiography (see angiogram in the same case, shown in Fig. 4.28)

fibrosis. The cortex may be thinned and fluid-fluid levels representing debris within obstructed calyces, pelvis, or abscesses may be identified. This picture may resemble xanthogranulomatous pyelonephritis except there are usually no obstructing stones or renal enlargement. Intrapelvic or intracalyceal stones are not unusual. In addition, throughout the cortex and medulla, scattered focal calcification (40%) is also readily identifiable. CT is best suited for identifying perirenal and psoas involvement (BERGNER et al. 1982; LANG et al. 1982) (Fig. 4.34). CT is felt to be superior to IVP and ultrasound in showing renal morphologic abnormalities, including hydronephrosis and extrarenal abnormalities (PREMKUMAR et al. 1987). Finally, CT plays an extremely important role in following these patients during and after treatment.

Nuclear medicine may also be used for quantifying renal function. Nonfunction does not always mean progression of disease: it may reflect the presence of an obstruction by fibrotic stricture. Fortunately, most cases are responsive to therapy and radiographs will show arrest of the disease or, in early cases, actual improvement.

4.7.1.2 The Differential Diagnosis

Tuberculosis is a great imitator and may mimic pyelonephritis, xanthogranulomatous pyelonephritis, pyonephrosis, tumor and tumor-like lesions

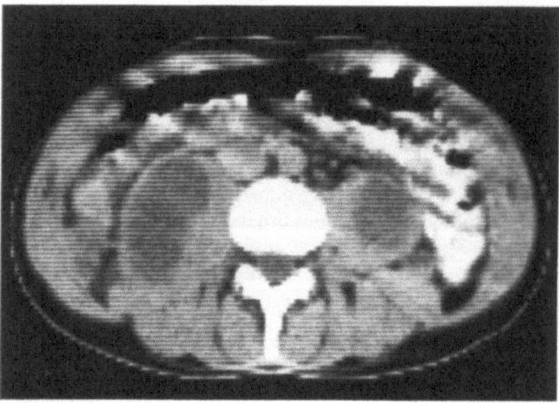

Fig. 4.34. Bilateral psoas abscesses are shown. (LANG et al. 1982)

(leukoplakia, cholesteatoma), calculus disease, renal papillary necrosis and all its etiologies, transitional cell carcinomas, medullary sponge kidney, etc.

4.7.2 Schistosomiasis

Schistosoma haematobium is indigenous to the Near East, parts of Africa, and southwest Asia. It is one of the oldest known infections in man, having been discovered in the kidneys of Egyptian mummies (VON LICHTENBERG and LEHMAN 1986; HANNA 1977). Between 2 and 300 million individuals may be presently infected with this parasite. We have recently seen a young black male from Chicago who contracted the disease as a child in Africa.

Renal involvement by *Schistosoma haematobium,* a digenetic blood fluke, occurs secondarily by reflux from the bladder. Most cases affect the bladder and to a lesser extent the ureter. Stone formation and the development of squamous cell carcinoma are associated complications if reflux develops.

The disease is more commonly found in males since they are more likely to be exposed to the parasite through swimming, bathing, and occupational exposure (such as being fisherman, boatyard workers, etc.) (VON LICHTENBERG and LEHMAN 1986). Children, especially, and young adults under 30 are most commonly affected, with the exposure having occurred between 5 and 10 years earlier.

Schistosoma haematobium is a parasite carried in a snail in sporocyst form which then changes into cercariae. The latter are discharged into a watery environment (e.g., the Nile river), where they invade their human host. The infecting organisms are picked up by the veins and lymphatics, carried to the heart and then to the lung, ultimately becoming lodged in the portal vein. There, they mature into the adult worm, and ultimately travel against the blood flow in the inferior and superior mesenteric veins and enter the vesical, pelvic, and ureteral plexus. In the vesical plexus, the smaller female deposits her eggs beneath the bladder mucous membrane. The ova ultimately enter the bladder, where they are voided in the urine into the snail-infested water and become miracidium. From here, the cycle begins again.

Pathologically, as with the other granulomatous diseases, granulomas (schistosomomas) consisting of macrophages, foreign body giant cells, and lymphocytes with varying amounts of fibrosis develop which may coalesce into bilharziamata. The may or may not ulcerate. Careful analysis to exclude the secondary development of squamous cell carcinoma is extremely important. The diagnosis is made upon the demonstration of terminally spined eggs in the voided urine. The skin and immunologic tests confirm the presence of past infections but are unable to determine the presence of active disease.

Treatment consists of drugs like metrifonate (Bilhareil), hycanthone mesylate (Etrenol), praziguantel (Biltricide), niridazole (Ambilhar), and oltipraz (VON LICHTENBERG and LEHMAN 1986).

4.7.2.1 Radiologic Findings

Radiographically, the diagnosis can be suggested if the characteristic calcification of the bladder and ureter is appreciated (HANNA 1977; AL-GHORAB 1968). A renal calculus (staghorn or otherwise) may also be present on plain film as the result of reflux. Nephrocalcinosis may develop as well as obstructive hydro- or pyonephrosis. A large tumefactive process representing a schistosomoma or squamous cell carcinoma is often present. These often cannot be differentiated radiographically. One of the commonest findings is that of a striated pelvis (HUGOSSON 1987) secondary to the reflux und/or infection. Other important findings include mucosal abnormalities (ureteritis cystica), calcifications (linear or punctate), ureteral stenosis, and polyps (HUGOSSON 1987).

4.7.3 Xanthogranulomatous Pyelonephritis

Xanthogranulomatous pyelonephritis (XGP) is a granulomatous inflammation of the kidney whose hallmark is the xanthoma cell, an eponym for a lipid-laden macrophage. Just as in TB, the host's secondary defense mechanism is evoked, with use of fibroblasts, histiocytes or macrophages, lymphocytes, plasma cells, etc. and the formation of granulomas to excapsulate the offending organism. XGP is usually the result of a severe, chronic obstruction of the renal pelvis or calyx with resultant parenchymal inflammation and destruction.

The process classically begins within the obstructed calyx or pelvis and extends to the medulla and cortex as the xanthoma cells creep along the transitional mucosa with consequent destruction, cavitation, and/or abscess formation. The kidney is usually markedly enlarged. Extension into the perinephric and pararenal spaces is an important and frequent finding (GOLDMAN et al. 1984). An obstructing staghorn or calyceal stone is often present. Scattered calcific flecks may be present elsewhere within the parenchyma and probably represent the initiating event. The renal pelvis is usually obliterated and the affected kidney parenchyma is replaced by yellowish-orange (xanthomatous) tissue, with obstructed calyces with abscesses of varying size and numbers scattered throughout the parenchyma.

In the focal or tumefactive form, one or two calyces are obstructed (GOLDMAN et al. 1984; ELDER and MARSHALL 1980).

Xanthogranulomatous pyelonephritis is much more common in middle-aged females (ROSI et al.

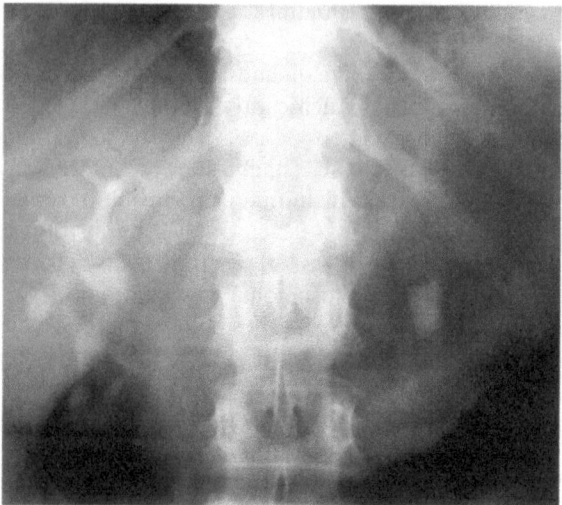

Fig. 4.35. Xanthogranulomatous pyelonephritis. IVP shows nonfunctioning left kidney. Several blunt calyces of unknown etiology are seen on right

1986; GRAINGER et al. 1982). However, the entity can be seen at any age, including childhood (GOLDMAN et al. 1984). Complaints are often nonspecific, with low grade fevers, back or flank pain, weight loss, chills, and/or dysuria. Diabetes is a common associated finding. Urinalysis will demonstrate pyuria with possible proteinuria and/or microhematuria. Urine cultures reveal *E. coli, Proteus, Pseudomonas,* and/or *Aerobacter*. However, the organism cultured from the urine may not be the same as that found in the operative specimen because of the presence of an obstructed collecting system (MALEK and ELDER 1978). For unexplained reasons, liver function tests may be initially elevated only to return to normal ranges following nephrectomy (ELDER and MARSHALL 1980; ROSI et al. 1986). The ESR is invariably elevated. Leukocytosis is present in 65% and anemia in 47%. Similarly, there is often an increase in alpha and gamma globulins as well as serum IgA, IgG, and IgM (ROSI et al. 1986).

The exact immunologic defect is unknown but there seems to be a failure of the primary (acute) defense mechanism which necessitates the marshaling of the secondary protective system (HARTMAN et al. 1984), consisting of the lymphocyte, macrophage, fibroblast, etc.

4.7.3.1 Radiologic Findings

Obstruction is the hallmark of XGP. As such, a pelvic (diffuse XGP) or calyceal (focal XGP) stone is identified in at least a third of cases on plain film

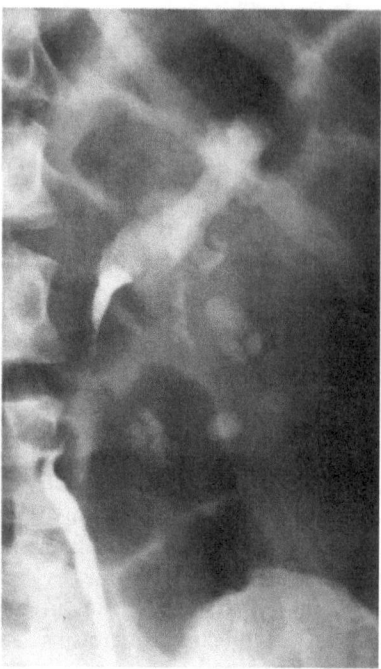

Fig. 4.36. Xanthogranulomatous pyelonephritis. Retrograde pyelogram shows staghorn calculi obstructing flow into large kidney

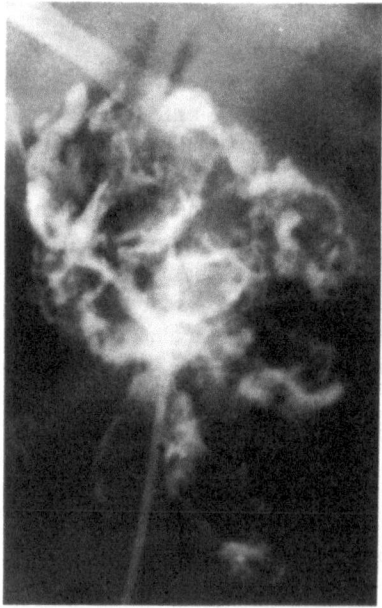

Fig. 4.37. Xanthogranulomatous pyelonephritis. Retrograde pyelogram demonstrates contrast medium entering calyces which are lined by multiple xanthogranulomatous lesions. The renal pelvis is narrowed

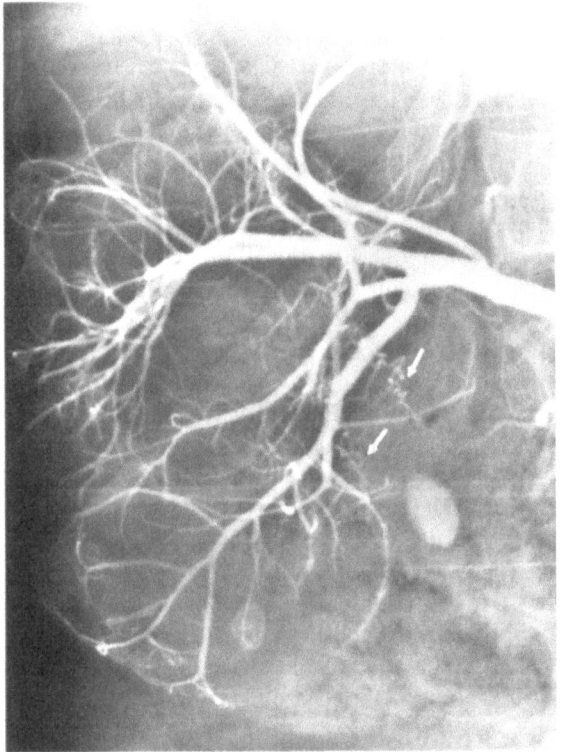

Fig. 4.38. Xanthogranulomatous pyelonephritis. Characteristic angiographic appearance of an obstructive pyonephrosis. Note abnormal neovascularity in arteriographic phase *(arrows)* with intracalyceal blush in nephrographic phase. (LANG 1986c)

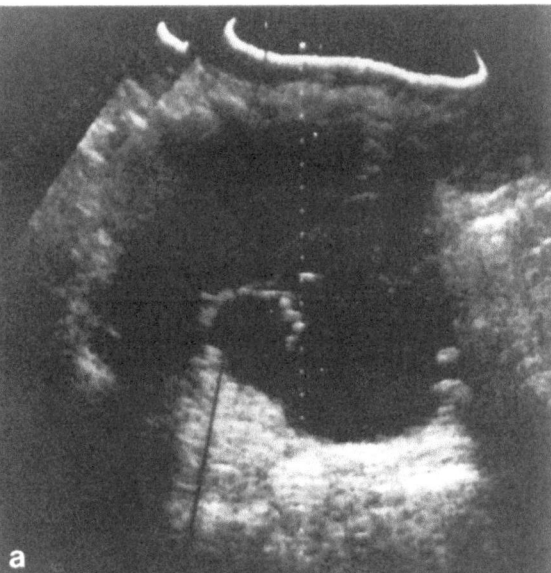

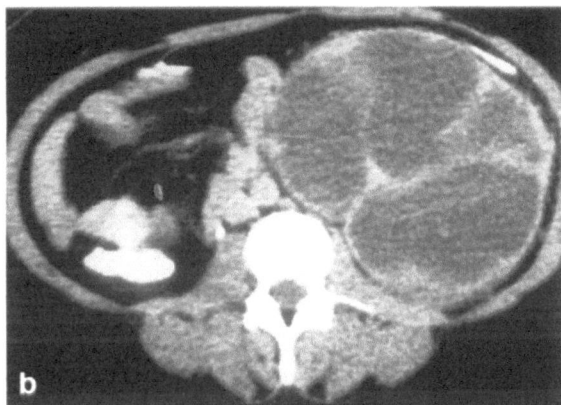

Fig. 4.39 a, b. Xanthogranulomatous pyelonephritis. **a** An ultrasonic study shows similar findings. The pelvis is small and is surrounded by larger sonolucent areas representing dilated calyces and abscesses with some internal echoes representing debris. **b** CT study without contrast and with contrast shows enhancement of the remaining parenchyma that is present between the low density, nonenhancing calyces or abscess. (GOLDMAN 1989)

(BEACKLEY et al. 1974). Since the kidney is usually enlarged secondary to obstruction and infection, either a focal mass or a globally enlarged kidney is recognized on plain film.

On intravenous urography, the affected kidney fails to opacify in the majority of cases (Fig. 4.35). If function is maintained, the calyces may be displaced by an inflammatory "mass" which may be solid or necrotic. Without the presence of a stone, focal XGP can be impossible to differentiate from a carcinoma.

On retrograde pyelography, the contrast material may not enter the obstructed renal pelvis (Figs. 4.36, 4.37) or, if it does, only a small, narrowed renal pelvis is identified. Sometimes, contrast material enters the constricted pelvis, the calyces, and even the communicating abscesses. These are lined with granulomatous tissue giving a diffuse, nodular, or "hobnail" appearance.

The arteriographic pattern (Fig. 4.38) is that of an enlarged kidney with stretching of the vessels around both dilated calyces and varying sized abscesses. There is inflammatory neovascularity. In the nephrographic phase, multiple low density areas representing abscesses and/or distended calyces will be recognized.

The ultrasonographic pattern correlates with the gross pathologic findings (Fig. 4.39 a). The kidney is enlarged with focal hypoechoic areas scattered throughout, representing dilated calyces and/or abscesses. The renal pelvis is small. The obstructing renal stones, if present, may not shadow, possibly because of the presence of peripelvic fibrosis. In rare instances, fine needle aspiration will give a definitive diagnosis (SEASE and ELYADERANI 1987; VAN KIRK et al. 1980).

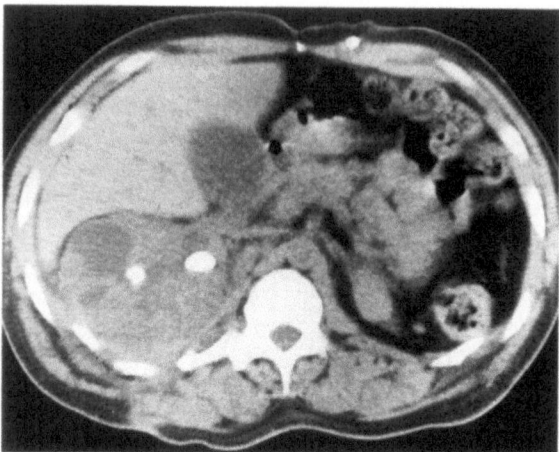

Fig. 4.40. Xanthogranulomatous pyelonephritis. CT demonstrates an enlarged kidney with several scattered stones. The low density areas represent abscesses and/or dilated obstructed calyces

The CT examination is extremely important in the diagnosis and management of these patients (GOLD-MAN et al. 1984; LANG 1984; SUBRAMANYAM et al. 1982). As with the other studies, the kidney is usually enlarged and there are multiple rounded low attenuation areas corresponding to the dilated calyces and abscesses (Figs. 4.39 b, 4.40). It has been found that the CT numbers of xanthoma cells do not correspond to fat, but, usually, approach those of water. The renal calculi, including the obstructing stone if present, are readily identifiable, as are any other parenchymal calcifications. With contrast enhancement, the cortical rim will usually enhance, corresponding to the inflammatory hypervascularity seen on angiography (GOLDMAN et al. 1984; CLAES et al. 1987) (Fig. 4.39 B). Most significantly, CT readily identifies the extrarenal spread of the XGP (GOLD-MAN et al. 1984; CLAES et al. 1987). This spread is not confined to the perirenal space but may progress down the psoas muscle into the pelvis or spread superiorly into the chest via the often involved posterior pararenal space (PARSONS et al. 1986) (Fig. 4.41). Fistulization to the gastrointestinal tract can occur

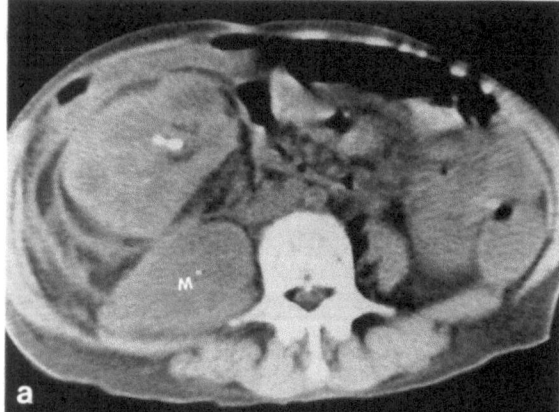

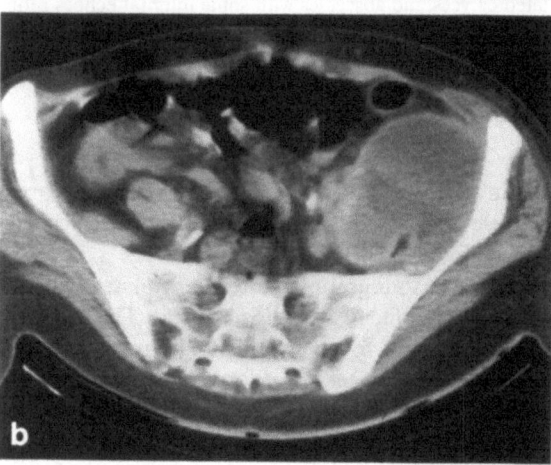

Fig. 4.41 a, b. Xanthogranulomatous pyelonephritis. An example of extrarenal spread. Note low density inflammatory masses. Involvement of the psoas muscle *(M)*. (GOLDMAN 1984)

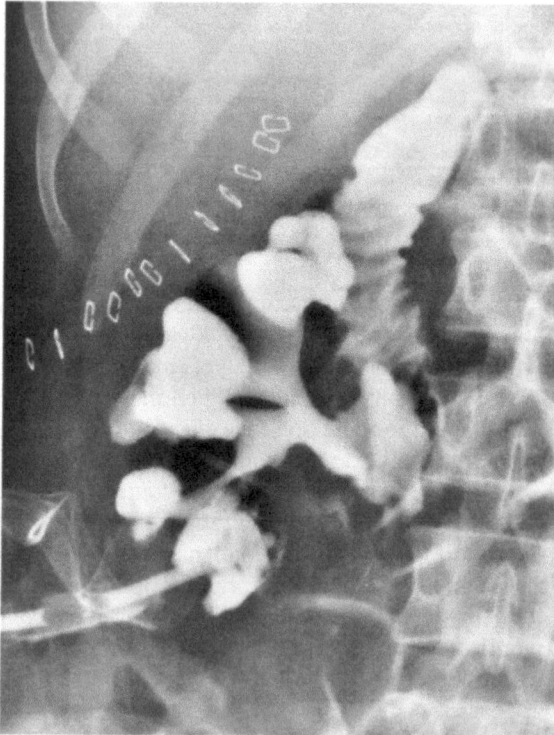

Fig. 4.42. Xanthogranulomatous pyelonephritis with renal duodenal fistula. (LANG 1986 c)

(PARSONS et al. 1986; CHEATLE et al. 1985; SUSSMAN et al. 1987). We have seen a right-sided XGP fistulize to the duodenum (Fig. 4.42). Thrombosis of the renal vein and inferior vena cava has been reported (MITCHELL et al. 1985).

On MRI (LiPUMA 1984; MULOPULOS et al. 1986) (Fig. 4.43), an enlarged multiloculated mass is demonstrated. The abscesses and/or calyces have an intermediate signal intensity on T1-weighted images with a very high intensity on the T2 sequences (less than hemorrhage). The calcifications and the central stones are not readily identified by this modality. Involvement of posterior pararenal structures, psoas, and spleen may be better appreciated as high intensity areas on T2-weighted images (FELDBERG et al. 1988).

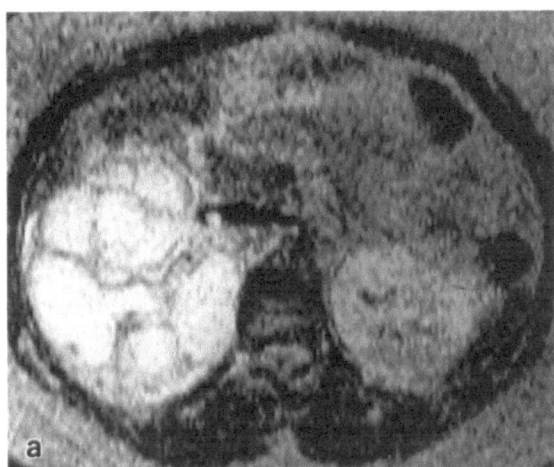
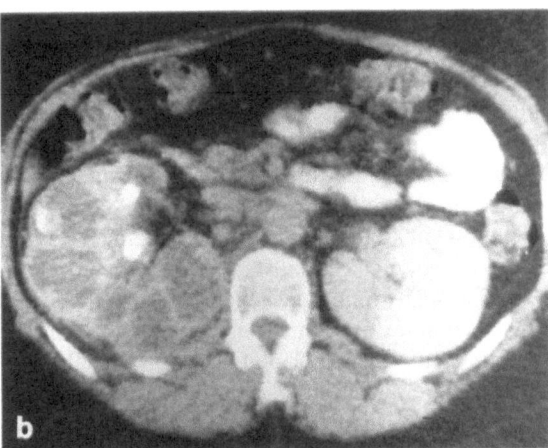

Fig. 4.43a, b. Xanthogranulomatous pyelonephritis - MRI study. T2w images (**a**) demonstrate an enlarged kidney with multiple high intensity structures representing obstructed calyces and/or abscesses. The CT (**b**) better demonstrates the renal calculi. (MULOPULOS et al. 1986)

4.7.4 Echinococcosis

Hydatid disease (causes by *Echinococcus granulosus*) is a parasitic infestation secondary to the larvae of the dog tapeworm *(Taenia echinococcus)*. Related parasites include *E. multilocularis* (Alaska, Siberia, Europe) and *E. vogeli* (Central America) (HERTZ et al. 1984).

The liver and lungs are target organs in the human (accidental host) as well as in sheep and cattle (intermediary hosts). These two organs act as filters so that the kidneys are rarely involved. Kidney involvement is usually hematogenous (primary) or by spread from adjacent organs. Intrarenal growth is slow for years and asymptomatic.

Classically, the unruptured or *closed* echinococcal cyst is composed of three layers (endocyst, ectocyst, pericyst). In the *exposed* cyst, the third layer (adventitia or pericyst) or the lining of the cyst is lost. An *open* or *communicating* cyst is present when all three layers have ruptured, leading to free communication with the calyces and pelvis.

Clinical involvement of the urinary tract is suggested by the presence of an abdominal mass, flank pain, and burning on urination (HERTZ et al. 1984). Acute colic may result if the cyst ruptures into the collecting system. It is commonly seen in patients of 30–50 years (ARAGONA et al. 1984; VON LICHTENBERG and LEHMAN 1986).

This reflects the slow growth of the cysts over years, as infection usually occurs in childhood. The rare identification of grape-like daughter cysts and scoleces in the urine is diagnostic. Serologic and intradermal studies (CASSONI and WEINBERG) are helpful but often unfortunately negative.

4.7.4.1 Radiologic Findings

Abdominal plain films may demonstrate rim-like calcifications in the kidney. These may be single or multiple. When multiple, they may mimic adult polycystic kidney. They may also be located in other organs, especially the liver.

Intravenous urography will demonstrate one or more masses. The cysts compress the adjacent calyces, giving them a cresentic contour (GILSANZ et al. 1980). With communication to "closed" or "exposed" cysts, a "goblet" or "crescent" sign is appreciated (SURRACCO 1939). On nephrotomography, these masses are noted to be thick walled. They may invade the calyces and/or renal pelvis (GILSANZ et al. 1980). A "bunch of grapes" appearance may thus be recognized (ARAGONA et al. 1984). An air-fluid level may be present.

At angiography, the lesions are usually avascular, sometimes with a vascular rim (GILSANZ et al. 1980; HAINES et al. 1977; HERTZ et al. 1984). The cyst should not be punctured for diagnostic purposes since spillage of cyst content can lead to the formation of intraperitoneal daughter cysts. However, in select cases and with experienced personnel, diagnostic punctures have been successfully accomplished under the strictest of aseptic techniques.

On CT, thick-walled cystic disease with calcification is readily discernible. The air and layered debris can be recognized. Characteristic septae are often present, simulating a multilocular cyst, and PETRILLO et al. (1981) and KALOVIDOURIS et al. (1986) have reported the CT density of viable daughter cysts to be invariably lower (0–15 HU) than that of the mother cysts (15–40 HU). Type A lesions are cysts with small round daughter cysts in the periphery along the mother cysts' germinal membrane. In type B lesions, the daughter cysts encompass the entire maternal cyst except for a small amount of fluid in the middle. Type C lesions are calcified lesions, with a few peripheral daughter cysts.

The ultrasonographic appearance (BABCOCK et al. 1978; HERTZ et al. 1984; GILSANZ et al. 1980) is variable, with a mixed or cystic pattern. There may be layering of debris in cysts. The calcification may cause acoustic shadowing (HERTZ et al. 1984). A multiseptated mass on ultrasound is also highly suggestive in the appropriate setting (LEWALL et al. 1986).

CT and ultrasound are useful to determine the extent of the disease, particularly in the liver and chest, and hence to determine treatment.

4.7.5 Candidiasis

Candida albicans is a saprophytic fungus but can occasion granulomas. In the immune-compromised patient, this saprophyte may become invasive (KIRPKEKAR et al. 1986). Host resistance is affected adversely by diabetes, indwelling catheters, chemotherapy, antibiotic or steroid therapy, and/or chronic debilitating situations (CLARK et al. 1971). The kidney can be affected hematogenously (COHEN et al. 1986; PATRIQUIN et al. 1980; KINTANAR et al. 1986; SCHMITT and HSU 1985; KIRPKEKAR et al. 1986). Involvement of the kidney may also occur via reflux from the bladder. In the hematogenously spread disease, the yeast cells are filtered by the glomeruli. Once inside the renal tubules, the fungus prolif-

erates, forming cortical and medullary abscesses. Breakthrough into the calyces (or retrograde involvement from the bladder) leads to intrapelvic and intracalyceal mycelial clump development resulting in flank pain but only rarely hematuria. Diagnosis may be made by smear, urine or blood culture.

Treatment consists of amphotericin and 5-flucytosine.

4.7.5.1 Radiologic Findings

Several radiographic patterns have been described. If the bladder is involved, air envelops the strand-like mycelia. Occasionally, air may be seen surrounding the intrarenal pelvic mycetomas as well. Rarely, calcification is present (PATRIQUIN et al. 1980).

The IVP may show swollen kidneys associated with acute pyelonephritis, an enlarged kidney with multiple abscesses, a scarred kidney secondary to chronic pyelonephritis, nonfunction secondary to renal failure, or renal papillary necrosis (SCHMITT and HSU 1985; COHEN et al. 1986).

Most significant is the recognition of a filling defect(s) in the renal pelvis or calyces on IVP or retrograde pyelogram. The mobile fungus balls behave radiographically similar to blood clot (BIGGERS and EDWARDS 1980; GERLE 1973; KOZINN et al. 1978; CLARK et al. 1971) or debris. In addition, there may be mucosal irregularity. On ultrasound, the mycetoma is usually echogenic without shadowing (KINTANAR et al. 1986; SCHMITT and HSU 1985; COHEN et al. 1986; STUCK et al. 1981). A variable amount of hydronephrosis/pyonephrosis may be present. A hypoechoic zone between the mucosa and the renal sinus echoes reflects submucosal edema/infections (BICK and BRYAN 1987). SCHMITT and HSU (1985) reported the use of percutaneous antegrade pyelography to show the fungus balls and to perform a brush biopsy for definitive diagnosis in a neonate in renal failure, while LANG and PRICE (1983) used the technique in adults. Percutaneous drainage also can be utilized occasionally (COHEN et al. 1986) (Fig. 4.44). The fungus ball may be fragmented using this technique and direct irrigation with amphotericin B can be performed (BARTONE et al. 1988; LANG 1986a). Candidiasis is becoming a serious problem in neonates and early diagnosis and treatment are necessary (PATRIQUIN et al. 1980); KINTANAR et al. 1986). CT will demonstrate perinephric spread (Fig. 4.45) as well as the presence of filling defects within the collecting system (COHEN et al. 1986; MILLER et al. 1982). With treatment, scattered calcifications form (SHIRKHODA 1987). WHITE and SPENCER (1983) reported inceased uptake of gallium in the affected kidney with a return to normal after treatment. Unfortunately, there seems to be only a poor correlation between activity of the disease and the radiographic findings in the neonates.

4.7.6 Brucellosis

Brucellosis is an amicrobic urinary tract infection caused by a nonmotile, non-spore-forming gram-negative rod, *Brucella abortus*. Most infections are obtained by direct contact with infected meat. In affected patients, the organism can be found in 50% of cases. Renal and bladder infestation, however, is unusual.

Common complaints include dysuria, nocturia, and frequency. Chills, sweats, and fever are common. Anorexia and weight loss are also common. An agglutination test is available. Cystoscopy demonstrates an ulcerating cystitis similar to TB. Urinalysis will reveal pyuria but no organism on gram stain. Special culture techniques of the urine (blood agar plates in carbon dioxide environment) are necessary to identify the organism.

Initially called Malta fever or undulant fever, it affects almost every organ of the body. The testes, prostate, and epididymis are the most commonly affected organs of the genitourinary system. The urine is not always positive for the organism in affected individuals.

Brucellosis mimics TB. Brucellomas, sometimes with extensive calcification, calicectasis with infundibular strictures, and cold abscesses, can be seen in involved kidneys. Treatment consists of combined streptomycin–tetracycline therapy (BUCHANAN 1982).

4.7.6.1 Radiologic Findings

As with any granulomatous disease, calcifications may be present on abdominal film. These have a characteristic "paint-brush" or "bull's eye" appearance and may be noted scattered throughout the kidney or spleen, apparently not confined to the calyces as in TB. On IVU, cicatricial narrowing of calyces and pelvis (KELALIS et al. 1962) is recognized, as with other granulomatous diseases. As the disease advances, infundibular narrowing progresses with focal areas of nonfunction. In general, the amount of calcification is far out of proportion to the amount of renal involvement when compared to TB.

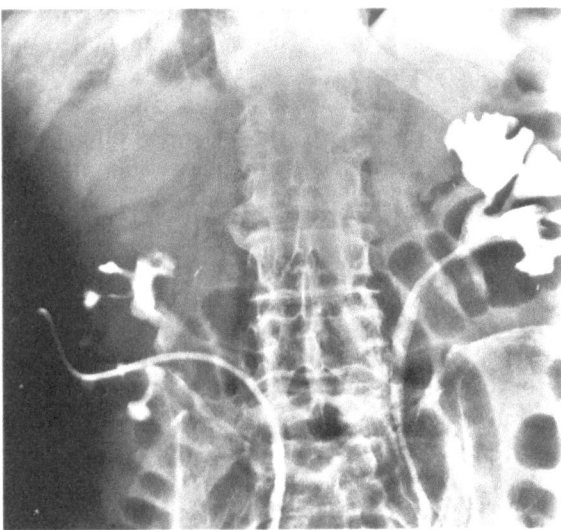

Fig. 4.44. Bilateral candidiasis being treated with percutaneous nephrostomies

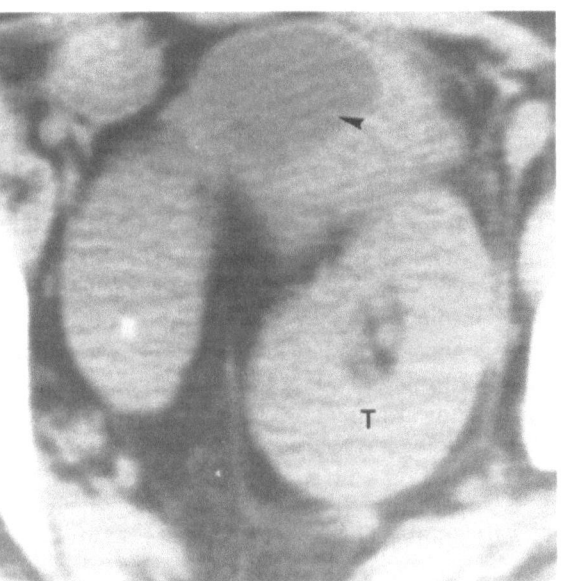

Fig. 4.45. Candida abscess next to a transplant kidney *(T)*. Note low density area in abscess

4.7.7 Malacoplakia

Malacoplakia was first reported by MICHAELIS and GUTMANN in 1902 ans was better described by VON HANSEMANN (HILL and SEEDAT 1972). It, too, is a granulomatous disease in which the lysosome of the macrophage is capable of engulfing but not destroying the various infecting organims. The resultant inclusion body is called the Michaelis-Gutmann body. We believe that "megacystic interstitial nephritis" is, in fact, the same entity. The disease may be a milder form of chronic granulomatous disease of childhood.

Malacoplakia is commonly seen in females (STANTON and MAXTED 1981) with recurrent urinary tract infections. There is flank pain, dysuria, fever, hematuria, pyuria, bacilluria, and leukocytosis. Diabetes, transplanted kidneys, hemolytic uremic syndrome, rheumatoid arthritis, lymphocyte-depleted thymus, lymphoma, carcinoma, or any form of immune suppression predispose to its development (HARTMAN et al. 1980). The infecting organism is usually *E. coli*. The bladder is the most common site of involvement, with prostate, testes, ureter, renal pelvis, kidney, epididymis, and adrenal being involved less often.

Two patterns are recognized: unifocal and multifocal. In the multifocal pattern, the kidney is enlarged with multiple masses which vary from multiple, miniscule, sharply defined, yellowish lesions to ones several centimeters in size. There may be foci of hemorrhage or suppuration. Sometimes, multiple small lesions may coalesce to form larger nodules which can distort the renal outline. Lesions may be found in the cortex and/or medulla. In the latter, they may mimic necrotizing papillitis. In the unifocal form, the sharply defined masses range from 2.5 to 8 cm and may show central necrosis or "cyst" formation (HARTMAN et al. 1980). Lesions may extend into the perirenal space (TRILLO et al. 1977). IVC thrombosis is an important complication. In those cases confined to the papilla or with pelvic obstruction, malacoplakia is probably derived from ascending infection. Treatment is directed toward treating the infection. However, nephrectomy is often the ultimate outcome.

4.7.7.1 Radiologic Findings

Radiologically, the findings correspond to the pathologic pattern.

Multifocal malacoplakia presents as a "tumor" including the presence of neovascularity on angiography, indistinguishable from a renal cell carcinoma (HARTMAN et al. 1980). Thrombosis of the IVC or renal vein may occur (CLARK et al. 1979). This can be demonstrated on MRI, ultrasound, CT, or cavography.

In cases of multifocal malacoplakia the kidney is globally enlarged without hydronephrosis. Ocassionally, individual lesions may be identified on nephrotomography. With medullary involvement, an obstructive uropathy with nonfunction may be present. Multiple, irregular mural lesions can be identified if function is present, or on retrograde pyelography. Ultrasonically, hypoechoic masses may be present which distort the calyces. There may be disassociation of the central echo complex. Other patterns include those of hydronephrosis or pyonephrosis (PICCIRILLO et al. 1987). On angiography, the pattern varies from normal to an avascular mass with arterial stretching, to a patchy nephrogram, to neovascularity (SCULLIN and HARDY 1972; DERIDDER et al. 1977). Renal vein thrombosis can occur (CLARK et al. 1979).

An important clue is the identification of the more common bladder malacoplakia. A renal biopsy can be used to diagnose the latter (HILL and SEEDAT 1972).

4.7.8 Actinomycosis

The pathophysiology of actinomycosis is that of a noncontagious saprophytic infection caused by a gram-positive, filamentous anaerobe (usually *Actinomyces israelii*) normally found in the mouth, tonsils, and gastrointestinal tract. Cultures must be performed under anaerobic conditions. However, sulfur granules may be seen on smears from the wound.

Most often, actinomycosis involves the head and neck region. This process spreads to adjacent tissue without regard to facial planes. There is a marked tendency toward sinus formation (DENTON 1985; YU et al. 1978) and spread via contiguity (or less commonly via the bloodstream) to the lung, intestine, brain, spine, kidney, etc.

Renal involvement is rare, secondary to hematogenous spread. Penicillin is the antibiotic of choice.

4.7.8.1 Radiologic Findings

A variety of radiographic patterns have been reported, including (a) diffuse pyelonephritis, (b) pyonephrosis, and (c) chronic suppuration with cortical abscess (PATEL et al. 1983; ELLIS et al. 1979; ANHALT and SCOTT 1970; DENTON 1985).

Actinomycosis can resemble a carbuncle, abscess, or cancer. Any fistulous connection to the kidney without known etiology should suggest this rare inflammatory process. A connection to the gastrointestinal tract or above the diaphragm to the lung or pleura is especially suggestive of this entity. A smear from the tract looking for sulfur granules should be

Fig. 4.46 a–c. Retroperitoneal actinomycosis invading right renal pelvis. **a** CT shows large retroperitoneal inflammatory mass *(R)* with multiple low density areas. **b** CT at level of kidney shows infection to be invading the kidney pelvis *(arrows)*. **c** IVP shows similar invasion of right renal pelvis. (Case courtesy of Dr. JACK SCATARIGE, Richmond, Virginia). (GOLDMAN 1989)

performed. CT may be of special value in delineating the extent of disease both below and above the diaphragm (DENTON 1985; ALLEN et al. 1987) (Fig. 4.46).

4.7.9 Amebiasis

The kidney is the fifth most common location of amebic abscesses (BRANDT and PEREZ-TAMAYO 1970) but kidney involvement invariably is associated with liver abscesses. *Entamoeba histolytica* is a species of protozoa which affects humans in both its cystic and trophozoite forms (KROGSTAD 1982). Hematuria is the most common complaint and the right kidney is most often involved. Prognosis is poor. Chemotherapy is mandatory (metronidazole, emetine, chloroquine) with surgery sometimes being required as well (GRIGSBY 1969).

4.7.10 Cryptococcal Infections

Cryptococcosis (caused by *Cryptococcus neoformans,* formerly called *Torula histolytica*) may variously present as chronic pyelonephritis, multiple abscesses, and/or renal papillary necrosis.

Torulopsis glabrata is a yeast-like organism much like candida. This rare fungal infection is seen in patients who are varyingly diabetics, on immunosuppression therapy, on prolonged antibiotics, or have urinary tract obstruction. Primary renal involvement is rare, with only about a dozen cases of pyelonephritis having been reported (VORDERMARK et al. 1980; KAUFFMAN and TAN 1974). Most patients are women, with most being in their sixties. Clinically, the patients present with symptoms of pyelonephritis. Diagnosis is made by urine culture. Treatment is with amphotericin B. The radiographic pattern is that of pyelonephritis, possibly with superimposed renal papillary necrosis (VORDERMARK et al. 1980).

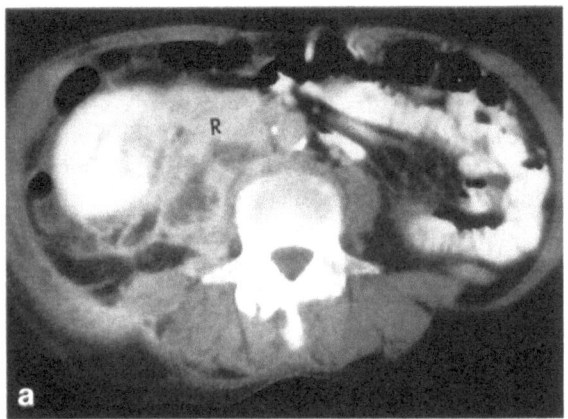

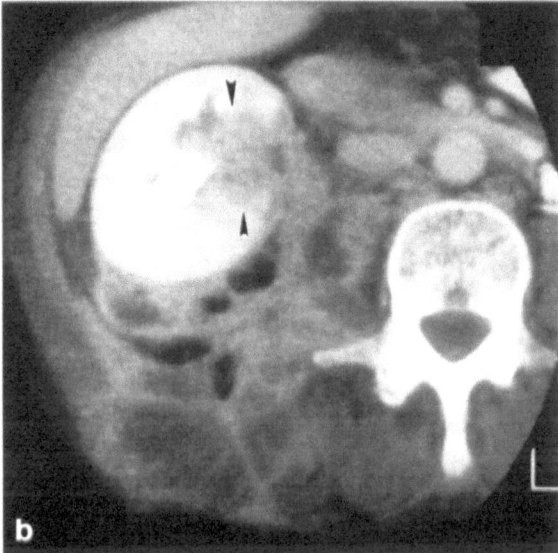

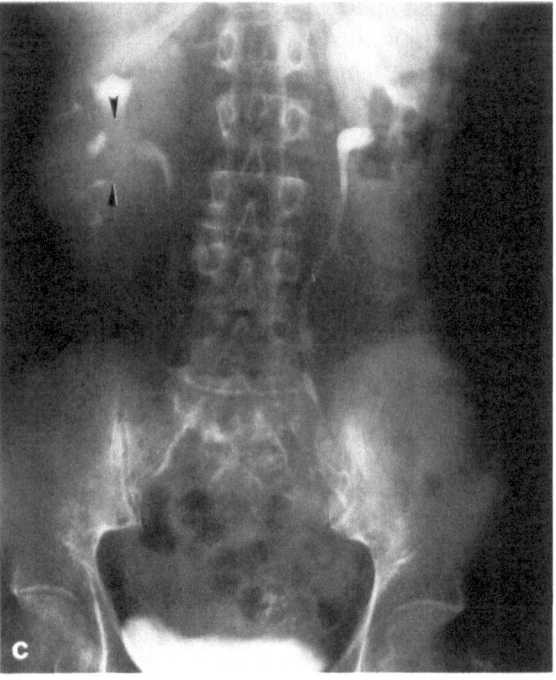

4.7.11 Coccidioidomycosis

Coccidioidomycosis involving the urinary tract is usually seen as disseminated disease (CONNER et al. 1975). It is found in the lower Sonoran life zone (i.e., southern California, Arizona, Mexico, etc.). Coccidioidomycosis can present with an acute or chronic renal abscess. Miliary granulomas and/or microabscesses may be seen (HUNTINGTON 1971). Parenchymal cavitation, moth-eaten calyces, chronic scarring, infundibular and pelvic narrowing with consequent calyceal clubbing, and calcifications as seen with tuberculosis and other granulomatous diseases have reported (CONNER et al. 1975). A colovesical fistula has recently been reported (KUNTZE et al. 1988). In transplantation patients on immunosuppression, reactivation of prior "healed" coccidioidomycosis may occur (YOSHINO et al. 1987). On IVP, pyelocalyceal changes indistinguishable from tuberculosis and other granulomatous diseases can be seen in the orthoptic kidney.

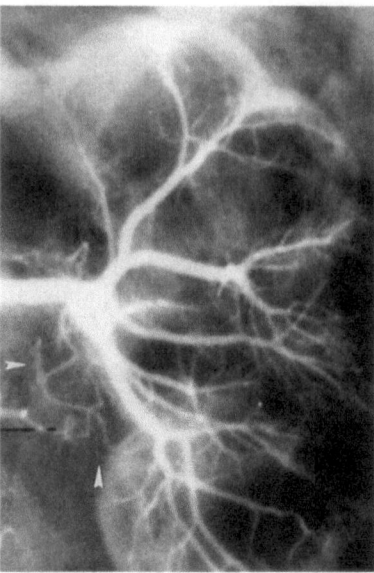

Fig. 4.47. Blastomycosis. Angiogram demonstrates large kidney with obstructing pyonephrosis. Note enlarged inflammatory parapelvic vessels *(arrows)*. (GOLDMAN et al. 1977 a)

4.7.12 Blastomycosis

Blastomycosis is found predominantly in the southeastern United States, such as the Mississippi valley, and in the Great Lakes region.

The lungs are the primary site of entrance, with the bones and the genitourinary system (20%–30%) affected secondarily (EICKENBERG et al. 1975).

To make the diagnosis in the urinary tract, the following methods can be used: (a) positive culture from the urine, abscess, or prostate, (b) identification of the actual organism in the urine or secretions, and (c) histologic examinations of tissue specimens (EICKENBERG et al. 1975). Pathologic examination reveals granulomas with many giant cells being present. Treatment consists of the use of amphotericin B and 2-hydroxystilbamidine.

4.7.12.1 Radiologic Findings

In a retrospective analysis of 51 cases of systemic blastomycosis, 11 patients had genitourinary tract involvement, mostly of the prostate and the epididymis (EICKENBERG et al. 1975) (Fig. 4.47).

4.7.13 Aspergillosis

Aspergillar infection of the kidney is usually associated with secondary disseminated aspergillosis in patients with malignancy, steroid therapy, and/or diabetes. However, it can rarely affect the kidney via the ascending route (FLECHNER and MCANICH 1981). The lesions can present as an abscess or a fungus ball. Pathologically, granulomatous masses or abscesses attesting to the hematogenous origins are also seen (EISENBERG et al. 1977). Treatment is with amphotericin B.

The radiographic pattern is nonspecific, with varying patterns including renal enlargement, a localized mass, or a filling defect in a collecting system with or without obstruction (ZIRINSKY et al. 1987). An intrapelvic fungus ball may also be identified. In one confirmed case (ZIRINSKY et al. 1987), a multiseptated cystic mass (i.e., multilocular) with focal calcification on ultrasound and enlarged paraaortic lymph nodes on CT was reported.

4.7.14 Histoplasmosis

Renal involvement by the dimorphic intracellular organism *Histoplasma capsulatum* is found in patients with systemic involvement (KEDAR et al. 1988). It may even be the presenting symptom although most cases present similarly to pulmonary TB. Urinary symptoms are usually nonspecific and include an elevated serum BUN and creatinine with albumin, blood cells, and casts in the urine. The renal manifestations will probably be indistinguishable from TB. Renal calcifications, absence of function, and evidence of a pyelocutaneous fistula have been reported (KEDAR et al. 1988).

4.7.15 Dioctophyma Renale

Dioctophyma renale is the largest of the parasitic nematodes. According to HALLBERG (1953), occasionally man's kidneys are invaded from the duodenum. The worms then enter the renal pelvis where they destroy the kidney and block the ureter. The kidney is literally tunneled through and excavated with most of the parenchyma being destroyed. The eggs and even the worms can be found in the urine on occasion. It is a rare process with only a few cases having been reported (HANJANI et al. 1968).

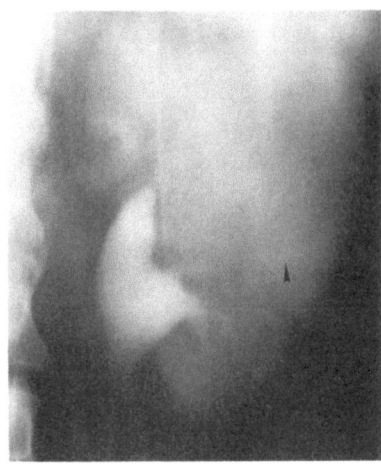

Fig. 4.48. Renal abscess. Nephrotomogram shows low density mass focally enlarging the renal outline *(arrow)*. Note thick rim to mass. Clearly not a simple cyst

4.7.16 Chronic Granulomatous Disease of Infancy

Chronic granulomatous disease of infancy is a rare hereditary disease which appears sex-linked in the male and is recessive in the female. There is a metabolic defect in the peripheral blood granulocytes (as demonstrated by the nitro blue tetrazolium test) which leads to an inability to destroy peroxidase-negative organisms.

Plain films may demonstrate calcified lymph nodes, hepatosplenomegaly, and calcified liver and spleen granulomas. Mostly noted for involvement of the bladder (YOUNG and MIDDLETON 1980; HASSEL et al. 1987), vesicourinary reflux can lead to calyceal clubbing, hydronephrosis, renal abscesses, and focal scarring (YOUNG and MIDDLETON 1980).

4.8 Intrarenal Abscess

An intrarenal abscess is a fluid- or pus-filled cavity containing no functioning renal parenchyma. It appears to be the consequence of suppuration and liquefaction necrosis of an area of focal lobar nephronia. Abscesses may be single or multiple. Small abscesses often coalesce into a single larger cavity. Most often, intrarenal abscesses are due to gram-negative organisms. They tend to spread by the hematogenous route from furuncles, infected teeth, etc. Nonetheless, obstruction of the urinary tract is often present. Men are said to be affected twice as often as females (DAVIDSON 1985). Most recently, a shift to female predominance has been reported (MORGAN and NYBERG 1985).

Although the classical presentation is that of an acutely ill patient with fever, flank pain, chills, and septicemia, at times the disease is insidious, vague, and even nonspecific. Patients may be misdiagnosed and nondefinable symptomatology is ascribed to many nonrenal causes.

Diabetes and staghorn calculi are commonly associated with renal abscess. Other factors predisposing to renal abscess are malignancy, trauma, alcoholism, steroid abuse, prostatitis, hemodialysis, and intravenous drug abuse (MORGAN and NYBERG 1985).

The gross specimen tends to show a well-defined mass with a softer liquefied core and a thickened rim or capsule. Microscopically, necrotic debris, white cells, and fluid are found in the center, surrounded by a rim or capsule of granulation tissue and fibrosis.

4.8.1 Radiologic Findings

Plain radiographs, in particular tomograms, of the kidneys may demonstrate displacement of the fat pad, indicating the presence of a bulging tumor mass. A scoliosis with a convexity to the contralateral side reflects muscle spasm attendant upon pain and tends to be particularly prominent in the presence of involvement of the perirenal space. Ancient abscesses may demonstrate dystrophic calcifications as well as shell-like curvilinear calcifications.

On intravenous urograms, function may vary from normal to none. Depending on the location of the abscess, deformity of contour, deformity of calyces, or displacement of calyces may result. In the

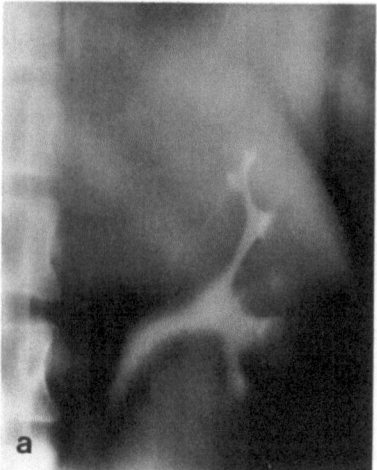
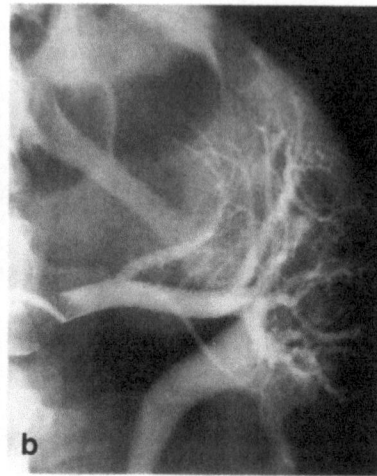
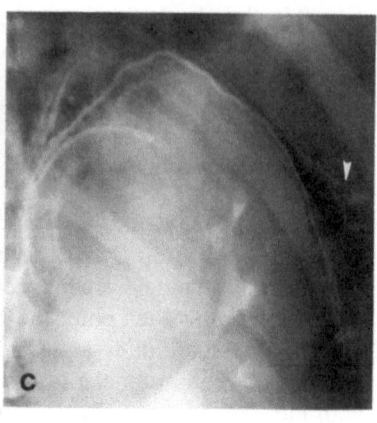

early stages of abscess formation, phlegmon, and beginning liquefaction necrosis, nephrotomograms tend to show a solid-looking mass (Fig. 4.48). However, as liquefaction necrosis progresses, a cyst-like mass with irregular thick walls is generally appreciated on nephrotomograms. The thick, irregular, and staining wall is a major differential point against the presence of a simple, benign cyst (Fig. 4.49a). Communication to the collecting system may exist if an abscess fistulizes into the collecting system and drains via this route. Under these circumstances, the cavity will tend to opacify on both intravenous urograms and retrograde pyelograms. This may, in fact, be one etiology of the so-called pyelocalyceal diverticulum (SOULEN et al. 1989). Debris is frequently demonstrated within the cavity.

In the early stages, an abscess may present merely as a space-occupying lesion resulting in stretching of interlobar arteries on arteriograms (KOEHLER 1978; FRIMMANN-DAHL 1966; LANG 1973) (Fig. 4.49b, c). With progressive liquefaction necrosis, the center tends to be hypovascular, the rim hypervascular (Fig. 4.50). Neovasularity on the rim of the lesion often does not respond to epinephrine (GOLDMAN et al. 1977b). Draining veins in the parameter of the mass may be prominent and remain opacified for a prolonged period (i.e., inflammatory venous hyperemia) (LANG 1986b). In the terminal phases of the inflammatory disease, arteritis obliterans occurs which, in fact, the development of liquefaction necrosis.

Gallium or indium-labeled WBC scans demonstrate increased uptake in the membrane of such abscesses, which is occasionally helpful in some cases but can be seen in necrotic renal tumors as well.

On ultrasonograms, abscesses tend to present predominantly as an anechoic mass. Occasionally, a

Fig. 4.49a–c. Renal abscess in 25-year-old male initially treated with antibiotics for left flank pain and chills only to recur a few weeks later. After workup, patient admitted to use of intrevenous drugs. **a** Nephrotomogram shows low density mass involving upper pole of the kidney. No sharp border is seen to suggest simple cyst. **b** Selective renal arteriogram shows mass not to be simple cyst. **c** Selective injection of capsular vessels shows abnormal, focal vessels in the perinephric phase *(arrow)*. (GOLDMAN 1977b)

few internal echoes are elicited from debris layering within the abscess (Fig. 4.51) (GOLDMAN et al. 1977b). Refraction of the beam at the fluid-soft tissue junction is one other characteristic finding, being caused by the difference between the speed of sound within fluid and adjacent soft tissue. The result is an acoustic shadow at their junction (PICCIRILLO et al. 1987).

Computed tomograms complemented by dynamic phase recording are the gold standard for diagnosis and categorization of abscesses. On the unenhanced study, the abscess content tends to be less than tissue density (Fig. 4.52). Following enhancement during both the dynamic and the postenhancement phase, the abscess content fails to enhance. Conversely, the membrane demarcating the abscess tends to show prominent enhancement during the phase of capillary transit of contrast medium (LANG and SRINGER 1986; BALFE et al. 1984; MOREHOUSE et al. 1984). The rim-like enhancement on both dynamic and postenhancement computed tomograms is a characteristic finding. This thick rim differentiates the abscess membrane from the slightly thickened wall of an infected or hemorrhagic cyst. Moreover, layering of debris may be identified within the abscess on preenhancement computed tomograms. Septation within the abscess or formation of daughter abscesses is likewise readily appreciated on computed tomograms. Daughter abscesses frequently occur in the perinephric space (MENDEZ et al. 1979; KUNIN 1986; LANG 1984) (Fig. 4.58). The mere thickening of septae in the perinephric space, however, is not an unequivocal indication of infection but may merely reflect edema of septae attendant upon the inflammatory process.

In recent years, percutaneous abscess drainage under CT or ultrasound control has gained increased acceptance (GOLDMAN et al. 1977 b; FINN et al. 1982; GERZOF and GALE 1982; BERNARDINO and BAUMGARTNER 1986; SACKS et al. 1988; LANG and SPRINGER 1986, 1990) (Fig. 4.53). Entry into the abscess cavity from a dependent point and advancement to the cephalad extension of the abscess via an extraperitoneal route is the proper method for percutaneous drainage. Follow-up computed tomograms and ultrasonographic examinations are mandatory to monitor the shrinkage of the abscess. Finally, diffusion studies, i.e., injection of contrast medium into the abscess cavity and documentation of computed tomograms, may be necessary to identify subseptation and formation of loculated abscess components which demand separate additional drainage (LANG 1990) (Fig. 4.58). This can be accomplished by adjustment of the existing drainage catheters or addition of further catheters. In addition to defervescence usually attained within 48 h after establishing drainage, cessation of drainage and disappearance of the abscess space must be observed before discontinuing drainage and pronouncing the abscess cured (Fig. 4.53). Surgery should be resorted to only if percutaneous drainage has proven unsuccessful after an adequate trial. Successfully treated kidneys with abscesses will return to normal, develop scars, or demonstrate communication to the calyceal system on follow-up studies (SOULEN et al. 1989 b).

On MRI scans, abscesses are similar to those elsewhere in the body. The signal intensity on T1-weighted scans is low and inhomogeneous (LIPUMA 1984); on T2-weighted scans, signal intensity increases yet inhomogeneity perseveres. The signal intensity is influenced by the amount of debris within the abscess and also the amount of protein.

4.9 Perinephric and Pararenal Abscesses

Perinephric abscesses most commonly occur as a consequence of an extension of a primary intrarenal process (70%); however, such extrarenal processes as diverticulitis, pancreatitis, and cholecystitis can

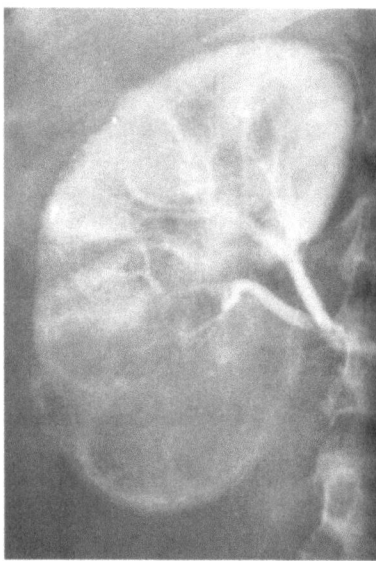

Fig. 4.50. Renal abscess. Angiogram shows hypervascular rim with hypovascular mass

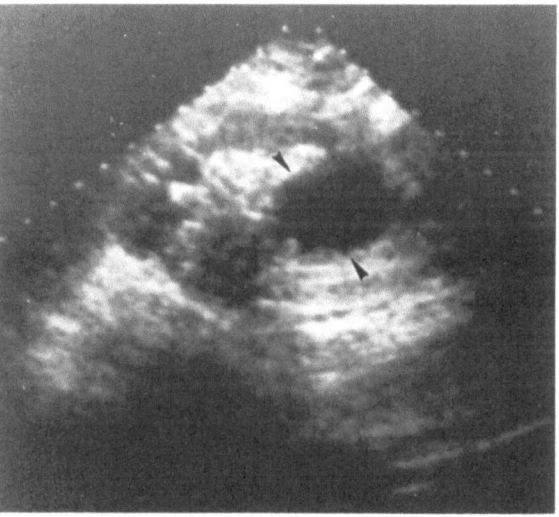

Fig. 4.51. Renal abscess. Ultrasound shows hypoechoic mass *(arrows)* in patient with chronic pyelonephritis. (LANG 1986 c)

extend into the perirenal space (MYERS 1976; LOVE et al. 1981; PARIENTY and PRADEL 1980). Conversely, the pararenal space is more often affected from extrarenal sources such as pancreas, bowel, spine, and chest.

Symptoms of a perirenal abscess are similar to those of an intarenal abscess, i.e., fever, flank pain, chills, septicemia, and sometimes a bulging flank mass. Limitation of motion of the hip implies extension of the process along the psoas muscles. Similarly, supradiaphragmatic pain may indicate sub-

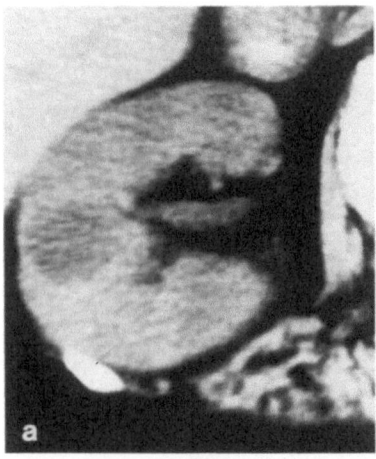
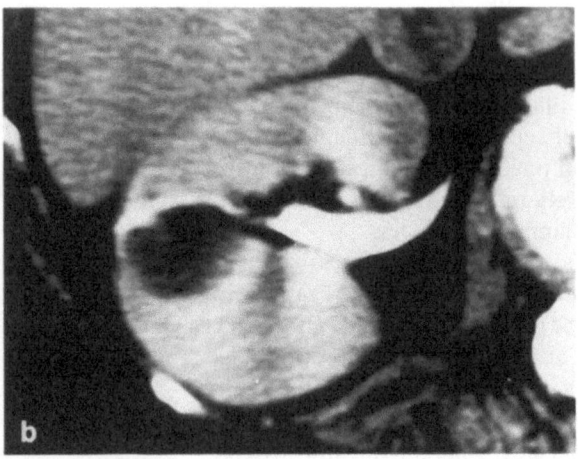

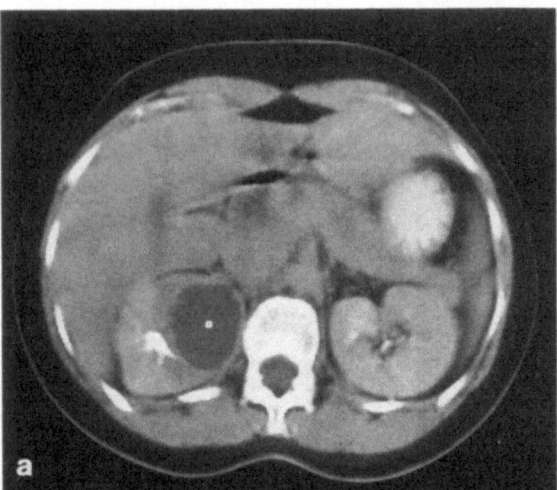

△

Fig. 4.52 a, b. Renal abscess in a 71-year-old female with septicemia and enhancing mass. a Unenhanced CT shows well-
circumscribed, low density mass with CT numbers above
water. b Enhanced CT better delineates mass, which does not
enhance

phrenic or even intrathoracic extension (MORGAN
and NYBERG 1985). Often, perinephric abscesses are
misdiagnosed as appendicitis or cholecystitis (MOR-
GAN and NYBERG 1985). Diabetes and calculi appear
to be presdisposing causes of perirenal abscesses.
The mortality in cases of perirenal abscess may be as
high as 50%.

4.9.1 Radiologic Findings

A scoliosis with a convexity to the contralateral side
is seen almost uniformly. On nephrotomograms, a
soft tissue mass may occasionally be noted. Air bubbles within Gerota's fascia or in the pararenal space
are highly suggestive of peri- or paranephric emphysema secondary to an abscess in the peri- or
paranephric space (Figs. 4.54–4.57).

On intravenous urograms, the function is decreased and sometimes absent (RABINOWITZ et al.
1972). Frequently, the kidney is displaced and the
normal perinephric fat pad obscured. MYERS (1976)
described perinephric collections as classically causing the kidney to be displaced anteriorly, medially,
and superiorly with acute collections and superiorly
and laterally with chronic collections. Obscuration
of the lower psoas shadow, medial deviation of the
upper ureter, and superior displacement of the
lower pole of the kidney were other findings
suggesting the presence of a perirenal abscess of
fluid collection. At times, a black rim of fat parallel-

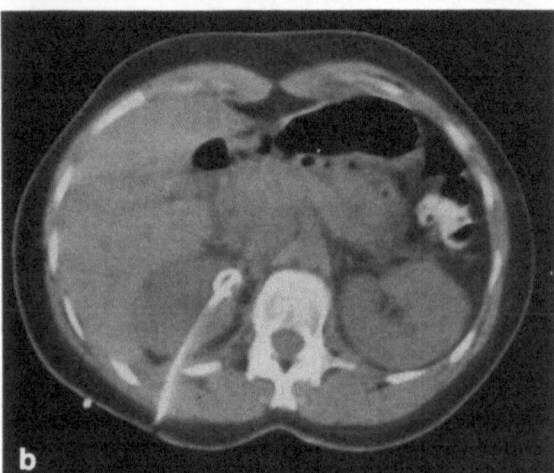

Fig. 4.53 a, b. Intrarenal abscess with thick wall completely
drained by percutaneous CT guided drainage. (LANG 1990)

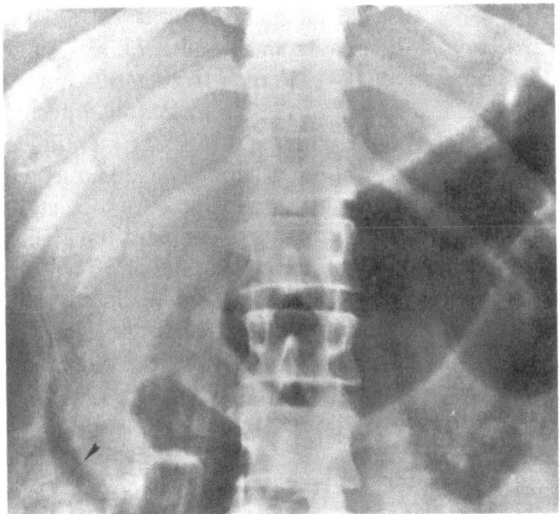

Fig. 4.54. Perinephric abscess and emphysema *(arrow)* secondary to ruptured duodenum

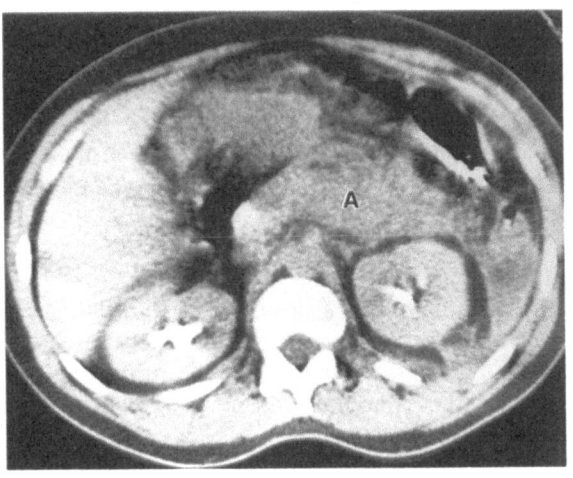

Fig. 4.56. Classic anterior pararenal abscess *(A)* secondary to pancreatitis clearly surrounding the fat-filled left perinephric space

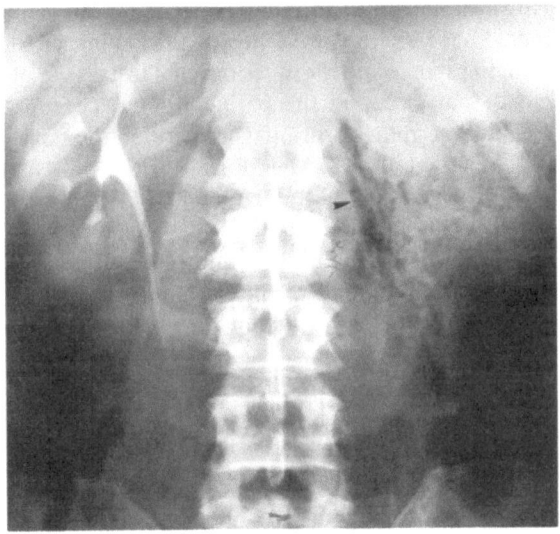

Fig. 4.55. Left-sided perinephric emphysema. IVP shows non-function. Air clearly outlines medial aspect of Gerota's fascia (arrow). Care should be taken not to confuse this air with intracolonic air. If there is ever a question, a colonic contrast study or CT should be performed

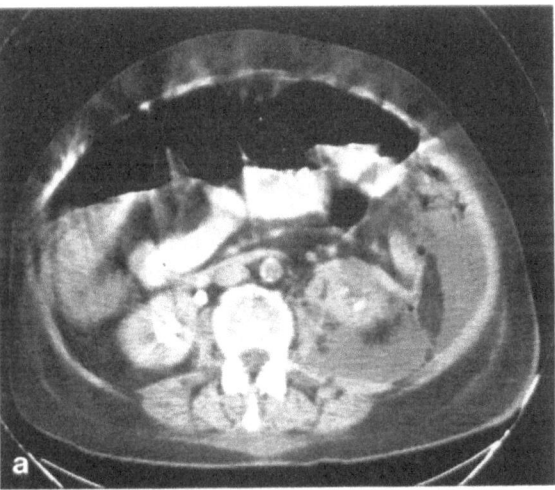

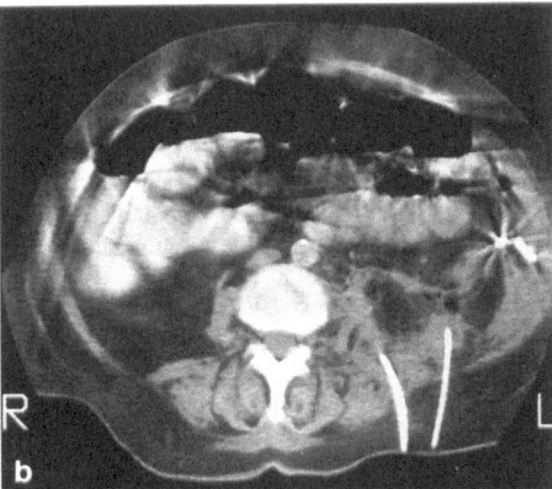

▷

Fig. 4.57 a, b. An abscess in the perirenal and posterior pararenal space is drained with multiple catheters introduced under CT guidance. (LANG 1982)

ing the renal capsule results from compression of the perinephric fat by the abscess accumulating in the perimeter (FRITZCHE et al. 1979). Respirograms, i.e., superimposed inspiratory and expiratory double exposures, indicate an abscess based on lack of motion due to the kidney floating in "a lake of pus". At times, the morphology of a fluid can indicate its location, i.e., the crescentic collection in the subcapsular space (MYERS 1976).

The inflammatory neovascularity in the rim of such abscesses can be shown on arteriograms (KOEHLER 1978). Hypertrophy of capsular and peripelvic arteries occurs in response to collateral demand flow.

Ultrasonograms identify perirenal abscesses as a relatively anechoic collection. At times, layering may be identified and echoes may be elicited from debris (SCHNEIDER et al. 1975). The variability and the echogenicity of retroperitoneal fat, however, pose a problem and may obscure abscesses (PICCIRILLO et al. 1987). Moreover, often associated, adynamic ileus may cast "dirty shadows" further confusing the usually accepted criteria.

Computed tomography, particularly the combination of dynamic recordings and postenhancement CT, is currently the method of choice for demonstrating and defining the extent of perirenal involvement (PARIENTY and PRADEL 1980; MENDEZ et al. 1979; LOVE et al. 1981; LANG 1984). In the acute and subacute stage, bulging of Gerota's fascia is a characteristic finding. This serves to differentiate the process from an intrarenal or subcapsular abscess (MYERS 1976). The presence and location of any air collections is best demonstrated on CT (BALFE et al. 1984).

The dynamic computed tomogram often readily demonstrates the inflammatory membrane delineating a chronic abscess. The ensuing fibrotic changes between renal capsule and Gerota's fascia may in fact act as a conduit of infection into the pararenal space (SAKSOUK et al. 1984). Thickening of the septae in the perinephric space is often an early finding merely indicating edema; however, the same septae are a conduit for the renal infection extending to Gerota's fascia and beyond. Percutaneous techniques may be used both for aspiration and bacteriologic categorization (GOLDMAN et al. 1977a; CONRAD et al. 1977; LANG 1986a; BERNARDINO and BAUMGARTNER 1986) and for drainage (LANG 1983; BERNARDINO and BAUMGARTNER 1986; SACKS et al. 1988). Drainage can be performed under both ultrasonic and CT guidance. Once again, entry from a dependent point and preferably via the posterior perirenal space is recommended. Drainage must be

carried out with an adequate number of, as well carried out with an adequate number of, as well as adequately sized (14–16 French), catheters to ensure complete evacuation of the highly viscous infected material (Fig. 4.57). Drainage must be continued until there is cessation of drainage, documented evacuation of the abscess, and absence of loculation or subseptation (LANG 1990). In critically ill patients, drainage may be instituted as a temporizing measure to precede definitive, surgical eradication of the process (LANG 1986c). Severe blood dyscrasias are one contraindication to percutaneous drainage of an abscess (BERNARDINO and BAUMGARTNER 1986).

4.10 Pancreatitis

By definition, pancreatitis involves the anterior pararenal space. Involvement on the left side is more common than on the right (NICHOLSON 1981). Fluid enters in the anterior pararenal space toward the lateral conal ligament and tends to collect in that space. However, in addition to fluid collection in the pararenal space, there is evidence of thickening of the bridging septae and the anterior renal fascia. Fat necrosis may occur in the perinephric space and a pseudocyst may form in the perinephric space (FELDBERG et al. 1987; NICHOLSON 1981; BAKER et al. 1983; LANG 1990). In fact, the kidney parenchyma itself can be involved. CT is capable of making the diagnosis on the basis of morphologic criteria, though confirmation by aspiration and analysis for amylase content is recommended (BAKER et al. 1983).

4.11 Acute and Chronic Pyonephrosis

The term *pyonephrosis* connotes an infected hydronephrosis. The infection may have occurred after the obstruction (i.e., secondarily) or may have been the primary event leading to the hydronephrosis. A staghorn calculus can be a related cause. Percutaneous or retrograde procedures (or both) may inoculate a hydronephrosis with bacteria. Pathologically, one observes dilated renal calyces and pelvis with cortical thinning secondary to the obstruction or the infection or both. *E. coli* is the most common organism. Extension into the perinephric space is an important complication to look for.

The abdominal radiographic findings may vary, demonstrating a small, normal, or enlarged kidney. Obstructing stones may be present. At urography, using appropriate nephrotomographic technique, the typical finding of hydronephrosis will be ob-

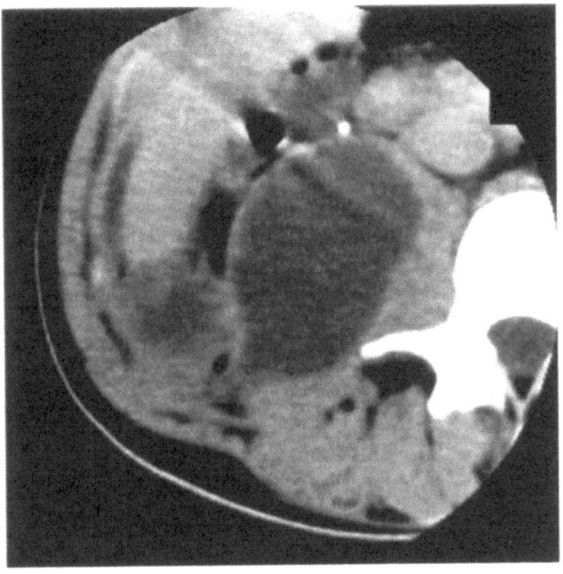

Fig. 4.58. Note the daughter abscess in the posterior pararenal space *(arrows)*. (LANG 1990)

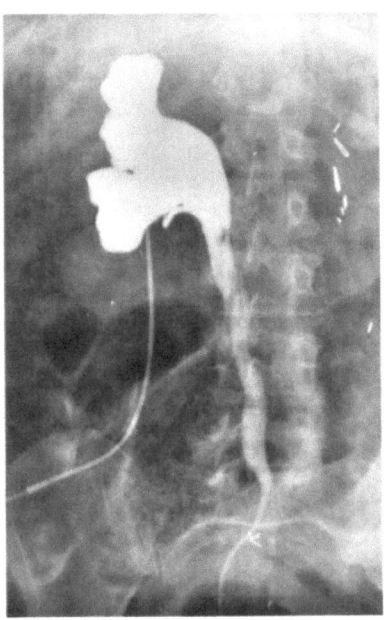

Fig. 4.60. Pyonephrosis. Antegrade study showing dilated collecting system with infected debris. Stent placed into bladder

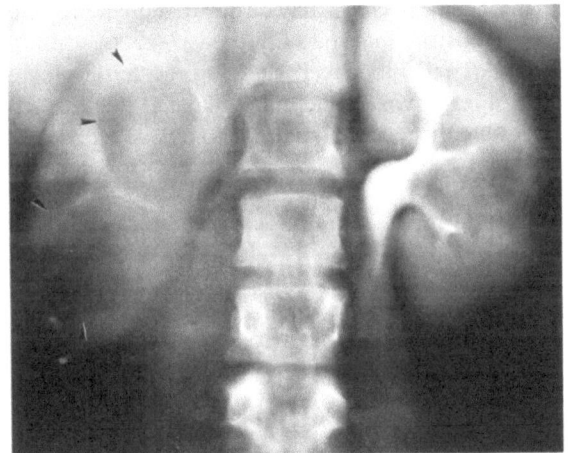

Fig. 4.59. Pyonephrosis. IVP shows cortical function surrounding dilated fluid-filled calyces (rim sign) *(arrows)*. No excretion into the calyces was seen in spite of delayed films.

served (Fig. 4.59). If any degree of function is preserved, one will usually note a mild to severe cortical tissue loss as well as dilated renal calyces and pelvis with possible ureterectasis. Antegrade pyelography will commonly demonstrate the site of obstruction (Fig. 4.60). Moreover, filling defects within the collecting system may suggest the presence of infected material. Retrograde pyelography will show a similar pattern if the obstruction is incomplete or the renal pelvis may fail to fill if total obstruction is present (Figs. 4.61 a, 4.63).

Angiography shows splaying of vessels bowed over dilated calyces and renal pelvis with thinning of the renal cortex and varying degrees of inflammatory neovascularity.

The ultrasonogram will demonstrate changes consistent with hydronephrosis, although rarely transmission may be reduced compared to a simple hydronephrosis. One notes multiple areas of low echogenicity (i.e., the calyces) with a larger central hypoechoic area representing the renal pelvis. In the decubitus position intracalyceal pelvic fluid–fluid levels as well as scattered echoes representing debris and infected material can be visualized. In many cases, however, only a pattern of hydronephrosis may be appreciated (Fig. 4.61 b).

The CT findings are also characteristic of an obstructive hydronephrosis except the CT numbers are usually slightly higher. In addition, the infected debris may be recognized, if present (Figs. 4.62, 4.64 a).

In rare instances, direct coronal and sagittal images of MRI may be of value. However, CT is usually the preferred modality because of cost. On T1-weighted images, the dilated calyces and ureter will appear black, and on T2-weighted images, they will be noted to be white (Fig. 4.64 b). Occasionally, the debris can be recognized. Direct coronal and sagittal images are the main advantages of this modality. However, secondary peri- and paranephric involvement is less clearly identified than with CT because of motion artifacts, etc.

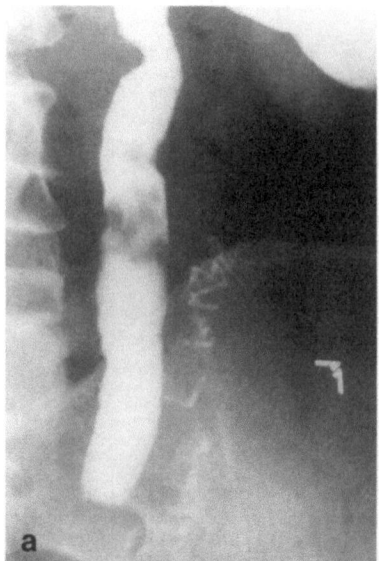

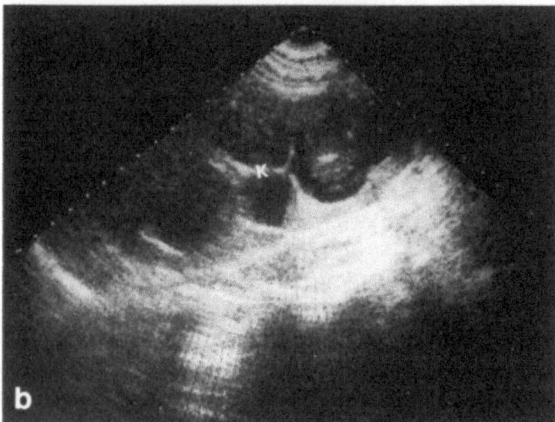

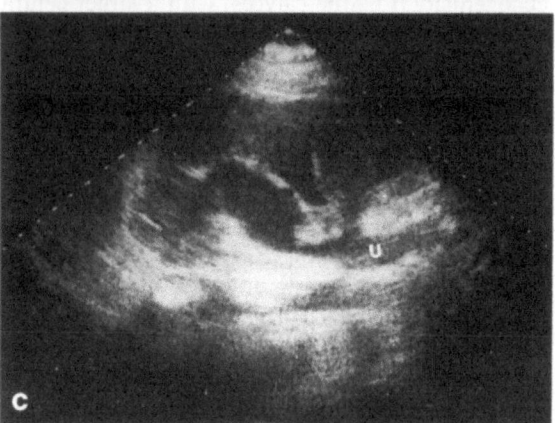

Percutaneous drainage may replace surgical intervention (LANG 1986c).

4.12 Pyelitis Cystica

Pyelitis cystica and its ureteral and bladder counterpart represent mucosal and submucosal inflammatory processes usually secondary to infection, often due to *E. coli* (McNULTY 1957). The cystic changes in von Brunn's glands comprise solid buds of displaced uroepithelium which fill with fluid. These cysts lift the transitional mucosa as they fill with fluid.

Radiographically, one notes multiple discrete smooth, sharply defined, well-circumscribed, small filling defects or "cysts" in the pelvis and ureter on intravenous or retrograde pyelography (Fig. 4.65).

4.13 Renal Papillary Necrosis

The etiology of renal papillary necrosis (RPN) is ischemic necrosis of one or more of the renal pyramids. This necrosis may be due to damage secondary to obstruction, spasm of the vasa recta, or intravascular red blood cell sludging. Many etiologies have been invoked, including diabetes mellitus, analgesic (phenacetin) abuse (MURPHY 1968; COVE-

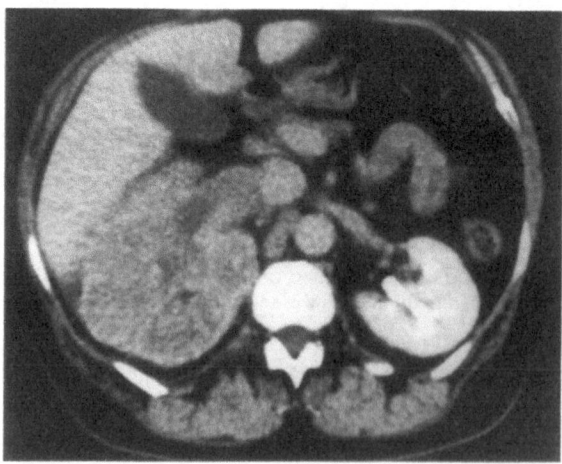

Fig. 4.61 a, b. Pyonephrosis. **a** Antegrade pyelogram shows debris-filled obstructed ureter (GOLDMAN 1989). **b** Ultrasonogram of the kidney *(K)* demonstrates the enlarged calyces filled with debris (GOLDMAN 1989). **c** Sagittal sonogram demonstrates the dilated ureter *(U)*. Again, note the debris-filled dilated calyces

Fig. 4.62. Pyonephrosis. CT shows enlarged right kidney with thin filled rim of cortical tissue. The calyces and pelvis are filled with material (debris) that is clearly above water density

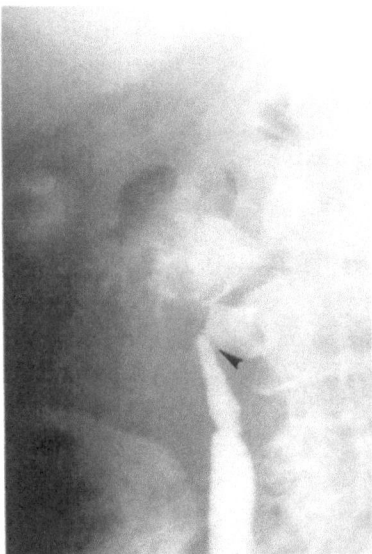

Fig. 4.63. Pyonephrosis with upper ureteric obstruction. Retrograde pyelogram shows narrowing of ureter *(arrow)* with debris in dilated renal pelvis

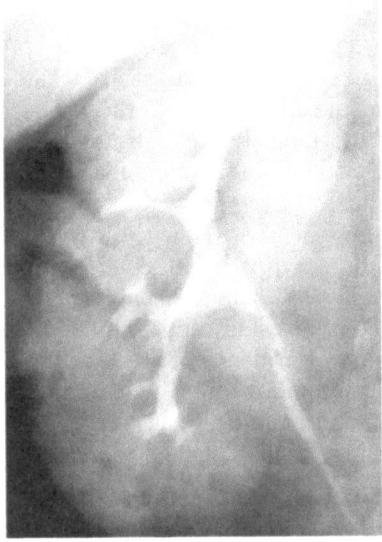

Fig. 4.65. Pyelitis cystica. Note extensive cyst-like filling defects lining the walls of the calyces and renal pelvis. (LANG 1986c)

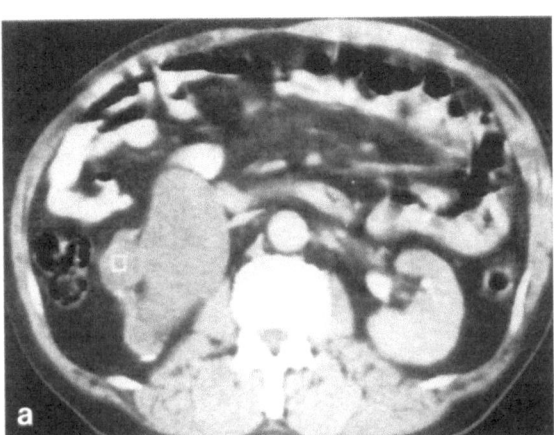

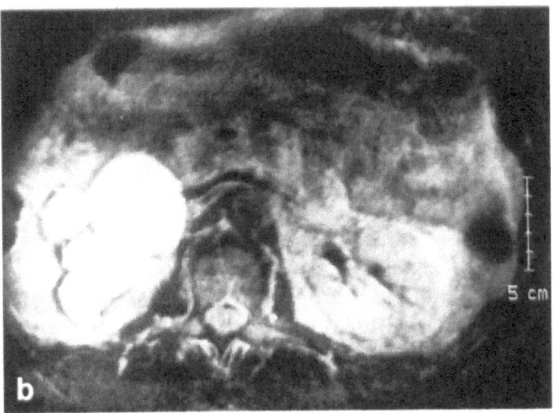

Fig. 4.64 a. Pyonephrosis. CT shows dilated right calyces and renal pelvis. **b** T2-weighted MRI image shows exactly the same findings and gives no new insight

SMITH and KNAPP 1970; EISINGER 1981), sickle cell anemia (ECKERT et al. 1976), tuberculosis, obstruction (DHOLAKIA and HOWARTH 1979), pyelonephritis, renal vein thrombosis, renal transplantation (KAUDE et al. 1976), hemophilia, Christmas disease (ROBERTS GM et al. 1983; DHOLAKIA and HOWARTH 1979), cirrhosis, ankylosis spondylitis (rheumatoid arthritis), and thyroid carcinoma (MITAS et al. 1981), to mention just a few. One commonly used mnemonic is POSTCARD (pyelonephritis, obstruction, sickle cell disease, tuberculosis, cirrhosis, analgesic abuse, renal vein thrombosis, diabetes). Of these, analgesic abuse is an extremely common but often overlooked cause, especially in women. Only careful history taking will reveal improper use of analgesics. Phenacetin was the main culprit in the past, but most analgesics, if abused, can cause similar severe damage.

Pathologically, RPN can be divided into two forms: medullary and papillary. Both forms can be seen simultaneously in the same kidney. In the medullary form, the ischemic changes affect the tip of the papilla. Focal necrosis and sloughing lead to irregular streaklike or clublike cavities that ultimately enter the affected calyx. Occasionally, one or two streaklike calcifications radiating into the papilla may develop (MURPHY 1968). In the papillary form, the ischemia leads to fistulization developing from each of the fornices of the involved papilla. In time, these fistulae undercut the papilla, resulting in a floating papilla in situ. This sloughed papilla may remain there and calcify. The sloughed papilla may obstruct or be excreted in the urine. Finally, it may liquefy and disappear. The disease may be progressive, leading to an end-stage, scarred kidney with absent or moth-eaten papilla. Cortical changes in these end-stage kidneys are indistinguishable from chronic interstitial fibrosis although glomerular changes are rare.

Clinical features include frequency, hematuria, nocturia, polydipsia, hypertension, colic, and progressive renal failure with hyposthenuria and inability to perform urine acidification. Urinalysis reveals sterile pyuria or evidence of active infection, proteinuria, microscopic or gross hematuria, and urinary casts. Careful straining of the patient's urine may reveal fragments of the sloughed papilla.

4.13.1 Radiologic Findings

On plain film, papillary calcifications (medullary nephrocalcinosis) can be seen. These calcifications may radiate from the renal pyramids (MURPHY 1968). They can be quite dense, and may be ring shaped (HARROW 1965), with the center representing the non-calcified papilla.

The IVP is relatively insensitive with as few as 26% of histologically proven cases with RPN being abnormal (COVE-SMITH and KNAPP 1970). Early on, the findings are nonspecific and include loss of sharpness or fuzziness of the affected calyx as well as a diminution or absence of excretion in the involved pyramid. The medullary form, also called partial papillary sloughing (PPS) (HARE and POYNTER 1974), presents as irregular linear to club-shaped cavities communicating with the draining calyx. These may be found in one or more calyces (Figs. 4.66, 4.67). As compared to medullary sponge kidney, only one or two streaks are seen per renal pyramid. Multiple linear streaks are not usually seen with RPN but commonly represent opacification of numerous dilated tubules in medullary sponge kidney. In the papillary form of RPN, also called total papillary sloughing (TPS; HARE and POYNTER 1974), fistulous tracts are noted slowly extending from the fornix of one side of the papilla to the opposite fornix (Fig. 4.68). If complete fistulization between the fornices develops, the unopacified sloughed papilla is sorrounded by a white ring of contrast. This sloughed papilla may then be excreted from its calyx, leaving a blunted calyx. Initially, the resulting cavity is irregular, but, with time, it becomes smooth and indistinguishable from the hydrocalyx of obstruction, reflux, or infection. The

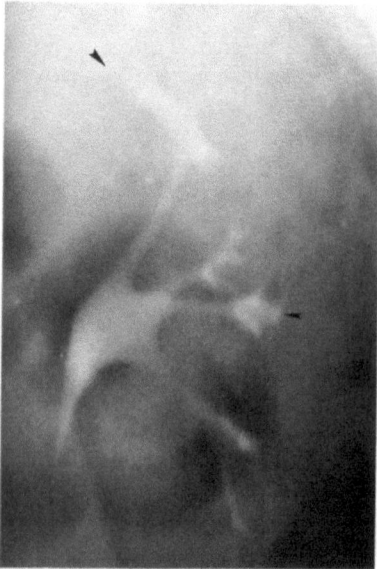

Fig. 4.66. Renal papillary necrosis, medullary type. Note small club-shaped medullary cavities communicating with underlying calyces *(arrows)*

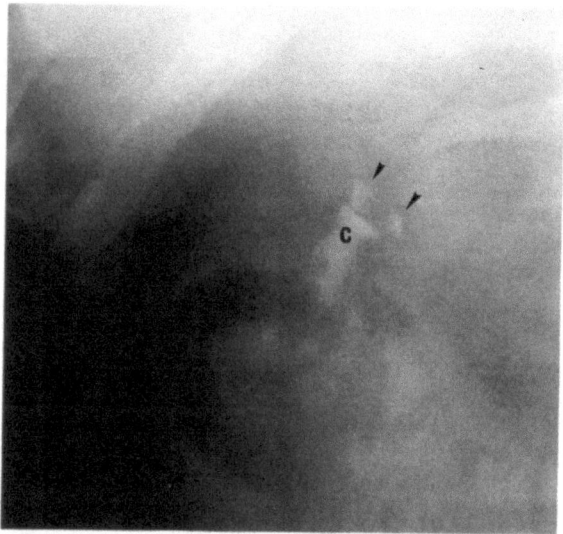

Fig. 4.67. Renal papillary necrosis, medullary type in a 67-year-old male. Coned-down view shows a single calyx *(C)* with two cavities communicating with it *(arrows)*

sloughed papilla may or may not calcify. It also may or may not obstruct the renal pelvis or the ureter. Occasionally, the papilla undergoes necrosis in situ (NIS) (HARE and POYNTER 1974) and does not detach from the cortex but does shrink. In this situation, the IVP may be normal. Later the sloughed papilla may calcify and be indistinguishable from other causes of medullary nephrocalcinosis.

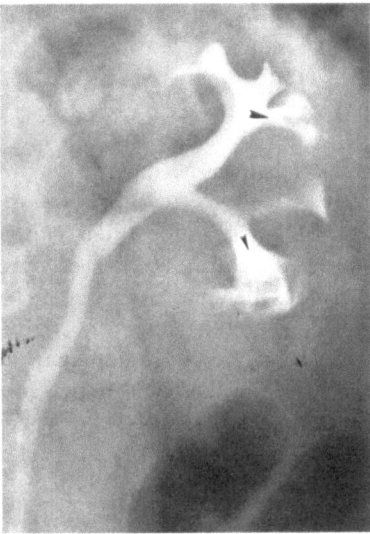

Fig. 4.68. Renal papillary necrosis, papillary type. Note sloughed papilla within calyces *(arrows)*

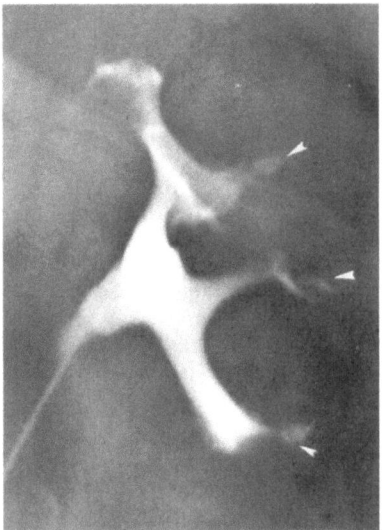

Fig. 4.69. Renal papillary necrosis in a 65-year-old diabetic female, medullary type, seen on retrograde pyelography. *Arrows* point to the medullary cavities.

Usually, the etiology is not obvious. However, one should look for the spinous changes of sickle cell disease or the presence of an obstructing stone.

Retrograde pyelography is indicated in patients with nonfunction on intravenous urography and (ANDRIOLE and BAHNSON 1987) shows similar findings (Figs. 4.69, 4.70). In similar situations, an antegrade study can demonstrate the obstructing sloughed papilla as well (ANDRIOLE and BAHNSON 1987). In the latter case, stents were used to relieve the obstruction.

On ultrasound, the sloughed papilla may be identified as a filling defect, usually with little shadowing unless calcification and stone formation have developed. If the papilla has been excreted, one notes single or multiple echopenic areas representing the combined fluid-filled space of the missing pyramid and its underlying calyx (HOFFMAN et al. 1982).

On CT, the sloughed papilla may be recognized surrounded by a thin rim of contrast. Any calcification that is present can be readily identified on a non-contrast-enhanced scan. ANDRIOLE and BAHNSON (1987) report demonstrating a sloughed papilla obstructing the ureter. The latter was of soft tissue density with punctate central calcifications.

4.14 Septic Emboli and Mycotic Aneurysms

Septic emboli most commonly originate from verrucae on the mitral valve in patients with rheumatic heart disease and other valvular abnormalities of the

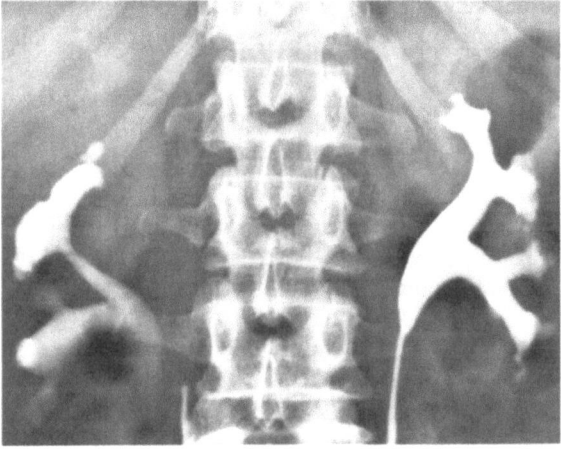

Fig. 4.70. Renal papillary necrosis, medullary type, seen on bilateral retrograde pyelography performed in a patient in renal failure

mitral valve. Multifocal renal scars and/or abscesses develop, as may intrarenal mycotic aneurysms (Du-BROW and PATEL 1981). The latter develop at branch points, sites of rapid tapering or bending. Contiguous spread from local inflammatory areas and trauma are other causes of septic emboli (DuBROW and PATEL 1981).

The plain film may demonstrate a focal enlargement due to an abscess or there may be evidence of multifocal scars. This will be even more obvious with nephrotomography. Nuclear medicine scans performed with agents such as Tc99 DMSA will identify focal filling defects, while gallium or in-

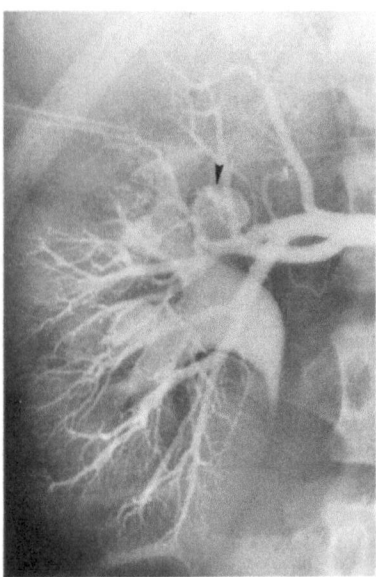

Fig. 4.71. Angiogram of right kidney showing intrarenal mycotic aneurysm *(arrow)*. (LANG 1986 c)

dium-labeled WBCs may occasionally be avidly taken up by the membrane delineating the inflammatory process.

Angiography reveals clots in the branch vessels of the renal artery as well as single or multiple, intra- or extrarenal aneurysms (Fig. 4.71) (KAUFMAN et al. 1975). Ultrasound will demonstrate the low echo abscesses and some of the cortical scars, as will CT. However, dynamic CT may possibly yield the definitive diagnosis if clots or the mycotic aneurysms are identified (although the resolution of CT is somewhat doubtful in this regard).

4.15 Cholesteatoma

Cholesteatoma is a nonmalignant, inflammatory process. Pathologically, it represents a desquamative form of keratinizing squamous metaplasia. Conversely, proliferation of squamous cells is felt to indicate squamous metaplasia, which some believe to be a premalignant entity (MOLINA et al. 1988). There appears to be a relationship with chronic infection, obstruction, stones, and possibly vitamin A deficiency.

Radiographically, there is irregularity of the affected calyx or pelvis (FREEDBERG et al. 1977; WILLS et al. 1981). The cholesteatoma may be intraluminal or submucosal in location. Occasionally, there may be one or two intraluminal masses. Papillarly lesions may be present. On retrograde pyelography a mass may be seen. The tumor may mimic the goblet sign

of a transitional cell tumor. On ultrasound, the intraluminal mass is believed not to shadow. On CT, the lesions have high CT numbers (WILLS et al. 1981).

4.16 Leukoplakia and Squamous Metaplasia

Classically, leukoplakia has been identified as premalignant (ARMSTRONG et al. 1950; REECE and KOONTZ 1975). Squamous metaplasia would then be a replacement of the normal transitional cell epithelium with squamous cells. Keratinization may or may not be present. Various texts seems to disagree on this point, some regarding leukoplakia, which means "white plaque", as a cystoscopic and not a pathologic entity. The lesions may be sharply defined with well-demonstrated edges but can be irregular or wrinkled or moth-eaten. The sloughed material may obstruct and ureteral calculi are frequently present. The lesions are more common in the middle aged and elderly, and there is usually a long history of urinary infections, colic, and fever.

4.17 Urinary Tract Infection During Pregnancy

Urinary tract infections during pregnancy are far from uncommon. Bacteriuria is present in at least 4% of pregnant women. In part this reflects the hormonal atony (progesterone effect) of the ureters and in part the obstructive effect of the enlarged uterus and the bladder hypertrophy secondary to the increased estrogen secretion. Because of the possible effects of radiation, radiologic workup should be deferred unless the patient fails to respond to antibiotic therapy.

If workup is indicated, one might start with ultrasonography. This will give some anatomic information. However, dilatation is a normal phenomenon in these patients. Shadowing from a ureteral stone should be looked for. In our experience, this technique has rarely been helpful but is worth trying.

If an IVU is done, a scout film and then a followup at 30 min are suggested. Subsequent delayed films should be used sparingly and only as indicated (Figs. 4.72, 4.73).

We have used a percutaneous nephrostomy in a patient with an obstructing stone who failed to respond to initial treatment. Not only did this control the infection, but the stone subsequently passed. We have used a similar approach in a pregnant female with a renal transplant. This technique has been reported by others (VAN SONNENBERG et al. 1988; QUINN et al. 1988). Similarly, percutaneous aspira-

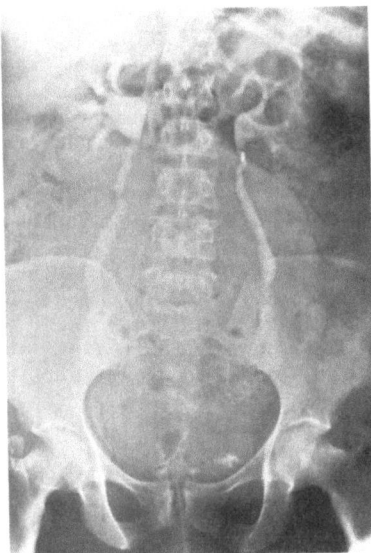

Fig. 4.72. IVP in a pregnant female with suspicion of a stone. As is often the case, the study is nondiagnostic as bilateral hydronephrosis is present secondary to pregnancy. Only a scout film and this delayed film were obtained

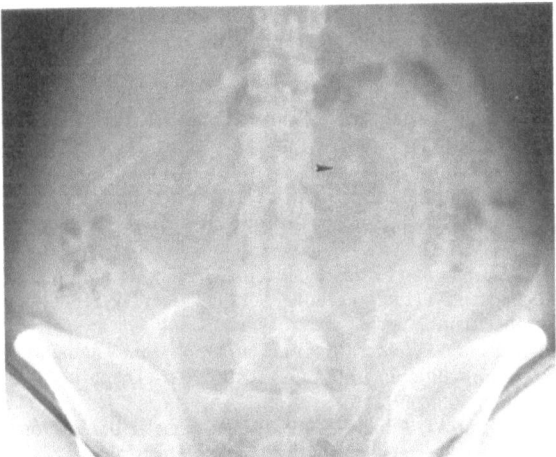

Fig. 4.73. Pregnancy and stone successfully treated with percutaneous nephrostomy. Scout film shows left ureteral calculus *(arrow)*

tion of renal abscesses in pregnancy can be an ideal way of managing these patients (COSTELLO et al. 1983). Difficulties with transplants in the pregnant female also can be amenable to percutaneous techniques.

4.18 Infected Cysts

Infected cysts and abscesses are difficult to differentiate on the basis of symptomatology or radiologic criteria. Nephrotomograms and particularly the dynamic phase of computed tomograms often demonstrate a thickened wall in both infected cysts and abscesses. In general, the wall thickness and irregularity is greater in abscesses than in infected cysts. Moreover, the degree of layering observed on computed tomograms is likewise greater in abscesses though debris in infected cysts may present in a similar fashion. Gallium scans and indium-labeled WBC scans are identical. However, nuclear medicine scans have occasionally been of value in localizing information in patients with polycystic kidneys (BRETAN et al. 1988). Likewise, shell-like calcifications occur both in ancient abscesses and in infected or hemorrhagic cysts. There are no criteria that allow echoic differentiation of such calcifications. Evidence of a previously unaffected cyst on old studies is the only unequivocable method of differentiating an infected cyst from an abscess.

References

Al-Ghorab MM (1968) Radiological manifestations of genitourinary bilharziasis. Clin Radiol 19: 100–111

Allen III HA, Walsh JW, Brewer WH, Vick CW, Haynes JW (1984) Sonography of emphysematous pyelonephritis. J Ultrasound Med 3: 533–537

Allen III HA, Scatarige JC, Kim MH (1987) Actinomycosis: CT findings in six patients. AJR 149: 1255–1258

Alvi AA, Goel TG, Dubey PC (1973) Reno-broncho-pyelocutaneous fistula. Br J Urol 45: 233

Andriole GL, Bahnson RR (1987) Computed tomographic diagnosis of ureteral obstruction caused by a sloughed papilla. Urol Radiol 9: 45–46

Angel JR, Smith TW Jr, Roberts JA (1979) The hydrodynamics of pyelorenal reflux. J Urol 122: 20–26

Anhalt M, Scott R Jr (1970) Primary unilateral renal actinomycosis: case report. J Urol 103: 126–129

Aoki S, Imamura S, Aoki M, McCabe WR (1969) "Abacterial" and bacterial pyelonephritis. N Engl J Med 281: 1375–1382

Appel R, Musmanni MC, Knight JG (1988) Nephrocolic fistula complicating percutaneous nephrostolithotomy. J Urol 140: 1007–1008

Aragona F, DiCandio G, Serretta V, Fiorentini L (1984) Renal hydatid disease: report of 9 cases and discussion of urologic diagnostic procedures. Urol Radiol 6: 182–186

Armstrong CP Jr, Harlin HC, Fort CA (1950) Leukoplakia of the renal pelvis. J Urol 63: 208–213

Babcock DS, Kaufman L, Cosnow I (1978) Ultrasonic diagnosis of hydatid disease (echinococcosis) in two cases. AJR 131: 895–897

Bahn DK, Brown RKJ, Reidinger AA, Dahamel PA, Shei KY, Gontina H (1988) Renal stone ileus. AJR 150: 145–146

Baker MK, Kopecky KK, Wass JL (1983) Perirenal pancreatic pseudocysts: diagnostic management. AJR 140: 729–732

Balfe DM, Stanley RJ, McClennan BL (1984) The CT spectrum of renal inflammatory disease. In: Siegelamn SS, Gatewood OMB, Goldman SM (eds) Computed tomography of the kidneys and adrenals. Churchill Livingstone, New York, pp 167–188

Bankoff MS, Sarno RC, Mitcheson HD (1984) Computed tomography differentiation of pyelonephritis and renal infarction. Comput Tomogr 8: 239–243

Barbaric ZL (1977) Pelvocalyceal wall opacification: a new radiological sign. Radiology 123: 587–589

Bartone FF, Hurwitz RS, Rojas EL, Steinberg E, Franceschini R (1988) The role of percutaneous nephrostomy in the management of obstructing candidiasis of the urinary tract in infants. J Urol 140: 338–359

Beackley MC, Ranniger K, Roth FJ (1974) Xanthogranulomatous pyelonephritis. AJR 121: 500–507

Bergner DM, Roth JK Jr, Lang EK (1982) The role of computerized tomography in the management of bilateral tuberculous psoas abscess. J Urol 124: 1020–1022

Berliner L, Bosniak MA (1982) The striated nephrogram in acute pyelonephritis. Urol Radiol 4: 41–44

Bernardino ME, Baumgartner BR (1986) Abscess drainage in the genitourinary tract. Radiol Clin North Am 24: 539–549

Bick RJ, Bryan PJ (1987) Sonographic demonstration of thickened renal pelvic mucosa/submucosa in mixed candida infection. J Clin Ultrasound 15: 333–336

Biggers R, Edwards J (1980) Anuria secondary to bilateral ureteropelvic fungus balls. Urology 15: 161–163

Bissada NK, Cole AT, Fried FA (1973) Reno-alimentary fistula: an unusual urological problem. J Urol 110: 273–276

Bourne HH, Condon VR, Hoyt TS, Nixon GW (1976) Intrarenal reflux renal damage. J Urol 115: 304–306

Boyd W (1970) Textbook of pathology, 8th edn. Lea & Febiger, Philadelphia, pp 111–113

Brandt H, Perez-Tamayo RP (1970) Pathology of human amebiasis. Human Pathol 1: 351–385

Bretan PN Jr, Price DC, McClure RD (1988) Localization of abscess in adult polycystic kidney by indium-111 leukocyte scan. Urology 32: 169–179

Bruce AW, Awad SA, Challs TW (1969) The recognition and treatment of tuberculous pyocalyx of the kidney. J Urol 101: 127–131

Brugh R III, Gooneratne NS, Rous SN (1979) Gallium-67 scanning and conservative treatment in acute inflammatory lesions of the renal cortex. J Urol 121: 232–235

Buchanan TM (1982) Brucellosis. In: Wyndaarden JB, Smith LH Jr (eds) Cecil textbook of medicine, 16th edn. W. B. Saunders, Philadelphia, pp 1535–1537

Burbige KA, Retik AK, Colodny AH, Bauer SB, Lebowitz R (1984) Urinary tract infections in boys. J Urol 132: 541–542

Caberwal D, Katz J, Reid R et al. (1977) A case of nephrobronchial and colonobronchial fistula presenting as lung abscess. J Urol 117: 371–373

Caplan LH, Siegelman SS, Bosniak MA (1967) Angiography in inflammatory space occupancy lesions of the kidney. Radiology 88: 14–23

Cardiff-Oxford Study Group (1979) Long term effects of bacteriuria on the urinary tract in schoolgirls. Radiology 132: 343–350

Carris CK, Schmidt JE (1977) Emphysematous pyelonephritis. J Urol 118: 457–459

Chandeysson PL, Varma VM (1982) Renal scan in papillary necrosis. J Clin Nucl Med 7: 294

Cheatle TR, Waldron RP, Arkell DG (1985) Xanthogranulomatous pyelonephritis associated with pyeloduodenal fistula. Br J Surg 72: 764 ·

Claes H, Vereeken R, Oyen R, Van Damme B (1987) Xanthogranulomatous pyelonephritis with emphasis on computerized tomographic scan. Urology 29: 389–393

Claesson I, Lindberg U (1977) Asymptomatic bacteriuria in schoolgirls. Radiology 124: 179–183

Clark RA, Weiss MA, Colley DP, Wyatt GM (1979) Renal malakoplakia with renal vein thrombosis. AJR 133: 1170–1173

Clark RE, Minagi H, Palubinskas AJ (1971) Renal candidiasis. Radiology 101: 567–572

Cohen EL, Greenstein AJ, Katz SE (1983) Nephrocolocutaneous fistula: use of CT to aid diagnosis. Comput Radiol 7: 291–294

Cohen HL, Haller JO, Schechter S, Slovis T, Merola R, Eaton DH (1986) Renal candidiasis of the infarct: ultrasound evaluation. Urol Radiol 8: 17–21

Coleman BG, Arger PH, Mulhern CB Jr, Pollack HM, Banner MP (1981) Pyonephrosis: sonography in the diagnosis and managment. AJR 137: 939–943

Conner WT, Drach GW, Bucher WC Jr (1975) Genitourinary aspects of disseminated coccidioidomycosis. J Urol 113: 82–88

Conrad MR, Sanders RC, Mascardo AD (1977) Perinephric abscess aspiration using ultrasound guidance. AJR 128: 459–466

Costello AJ, Blandy JP, Hately W (1983) Percutaneous aspiration of renal cortical abscesses. Urology 21: 201–204

Cove-Smith JR, Knapp MS (1970) Analgesic nephropathy: an important cause of chronic renal failure. J Med 47: 49–69

Cremin BJ (1979) Observations of vesico-ureteric reflux and intrarenal reflux: a review and survey of material. Clin Radiol 30: 607–621

Dairiki-Shortliffe LM, Stamey TA (1986a) Infections of the urinary tract: introduction and general principles. In: Walsh PC, Gittes RF, Perlmutter AD, Stamey TA (eds) Campbell's urology, 5th edn. W. B. Saunders, Philadelphia, pp 738–796

Dairiki-Shortliffe LM, Stamey TA (1986b) Urinary infections in adult women. In: Walsh PC, Gittes RF, Perlmutter AD, Stamey TA (eds) Campbell's urology, 5th edn. W. B. Saunders, Philadelphia, pp 797–830

Dairiki-Shortliffe LM, Stamey TA (1986c) Urinary tract infections during pregnancy. In: Walsh PC, Gittes RF, Perlmutter AD, Stamey TA (eds) Campbell's urology, 5th edn. W. B. Saunders, Philadelphia, pp 802–808

Davidson AJ (1985) Radiology of the kidney. W. B. Saunders, Philadelphia, p 282

Davidson AJ, Talner LB (1973) Urographic and angiographic abnormalities in adult-onset acute bacterial nephritis. Radiology 106: 249–256

Davidson AJ, Talner LB (1978) Late sequelae of adult-onset acute bacterial nephritis. Radiology 127: 367–371

Denton AE III (1985) Computed tomographic findings in thoracic and renal actinomycosis: case report and review of the literature. J Am Osteopath Assoc 85: 57–60

Deridder PA, Koff SA, Gikas PW, Heidelberger KP (1977) Renal malakoplakia. J Urol 117: 428–432

Dholakia AM, Howarth FH (1979) The urinary tract in haemophilia. Clin Radiol 30: 533–538

Dinkel E, Orth S, Dittrich M, Schulte-Wissermann H (1986) Renal sonography in the differentiation of upper from lower urinary tract infection. AJR 146: 775–780

Doemeny JM, Banner MP, Shapiro MJ, Amendola MA, Pollack HM (1988) Percutaneous extraction of renal fungus ball. AJR 150: 1331–1332

Dolev E, Bass A, Nussinowitz N (1985) Frequent occurrence of renal calculi in tuberculous kidney in Israel. Urology 26: 544–545

Doughney KB, Dineen MK, Venable DD (1986) Nephrobronchial colonic fistula complicating perinephric abscess. J Urol 35: 765–767

Drutz DJ (1982) Candidiasis. In: Wyngaarden JM, Smith LH Jr (eds) Cecil textbook of medicine, 16th edn. W.B.Saunders, Philadelphia, pp 1706–1708

DuBrow RA, Patel SK (1981) Mycotic aneurysm of the renal artery. Radiology 138: 577–582

Eckert DE, Jonutis AJ, Davidson AJ (1976) The incidence of manifestations of urographic papillary abnormalities in patients with S hemoglobinopathy. Radiology 113: 59–63

Edell SL, Bonavita JA (1979) The sonographic appearance of acute pyelonephritis. Radiology 132: 683–685

Eickenberg H, Amin M, Lich R Jr (1975) Blastomycosis of the genitourinary tract. J Urol 143: 650–652

Eisenberg RL, Hedgcock MW, Shanser JD (1977) Aspergillus mycetoma of the renal pelvis associated with ureteropelvic junction obstruction. J Urol 118: 466–467

Eisinger AJ (1981) Analgesic nephropathy. Br J Hosp Med 25: 265–268

Elder JS, Marshall FF (1980) Focal xanthogranulomatous pyelonephritis in adulthood. Johns Hopkins Med Bull 146: 141–147

Ellis LR, Kenny GM, Nellans RE (1979) Urogenital aspects of actinomycosis. J Urol 122: 132–133

Elo J, Tallgren LG, Alfthan O, Sarna S (1983) Character of urinary tract infections and pyelonephritis renal scanning after anti-reflux surgery. J Urol 129: 343–346

Emmett JL, Witten DM (1971) Clinical urography, 3rd edn. W.B.Saunders, Philadelphia

Evans JA, Myers MA, Bosniak MA (1971) Acute renal and perirenal infections. Semin Roentgenol 6: 274–291

Fair WR, McClennan BL, Jost RG (1979) Are excretory urograms necessary in evaluating women with urinary tract infection? J Urol 121: 313–315

Feldberg AM, Hendricks MJ, van Waes PGFM, Sung KJ (1987) Pancreatic lesions and transfascial perirenal spread: computed tomographic demonstration. Gastrointest Radiol 12: 121–127

Feldberg MAM, Driessen KP, Witkamp TD, Leeuwen MS, van Waes PFGM (1988) Xanthogranulomatous Pyelonephritis: Comparision of extent using computed tomography and magnetic resonance imaging in one case. Urol Radiol 10: 92–94

Fernandez JA, Miles BJ, Buck AS, Gibbons RP (1988) Renal carbuncle: comparison between open drainage and closed percutaneous drainage. Urology 25: 142–144

Ferrie BG, Rundle JSH (1985) Genitourinary tuberculosis in patients under twenty-five years of age. Urology 25: 576–578

Fiegler W (1983) Ultrasound in acute renal inflammatory lesions. Eur J Radiol 3: 354–357

Filly R, Friedland GW, Goven DE, Fair WR (1974) Development and progression of clubbing and scarring in children with recurrent urinary infection. Radiology 113: 145–153

Finn DJ, Palestrant AM, DeWolf WC (1982) Successful percutaneous management of renal abscess. J Urol 127: 425–426

Flechner SM, McAninch JW (1981) Aspergillosis of the urinary tract: ascending route of infection and evolving patterns of disease. J Urol 125: 598–601

Fowler JE Jr, Stamey TA (1988) Studies of introital colonization in women with recurrent urinary infection. VII. The role of bacterial adherence. J Urol 117: 472–476

Freedberg LE, Stables DP, Blousten PA, Donoh R (1977) Cholesteatoma of renal pelvis. Urology 10: 263–265

Friedland GW (1977) Long term effects of urinary tract infections. Radiology 124: 263–264

Frimann-Dahl J (1966) Angiography in renal inflammatory disease. Kincaid OW, David GD (eds) Renal angiography. Yearbook Medical, Chicago, pp 230–252

Fritzsche P, Toomey FB, Ta HN (1979) Alteration of perirenal fat secondary to diffuse retroperitoneal infiltration. Radiology 131: 27–29

Froelich JW, Swanson D (1984) Imaging of inflammatory processes with labelled cells. Semin Nucl Med 14: 128–139

Fussel EN, Roberts JA (1984) The ultrastructure of acute pyelonephritis in the monkey. J Urol 133: 179–183

Garcia JE, Van Nostrand D, Howard WH III, Kyle RW (1984) The spectrum of gallium-67 renal activity in patients with no evidence of renal disease. J Nucl Med 25: 575–580

Gerle RD (1973) Roentgenographic features of primary renal candidiasis. AJR 119: 731–738

Gerzof SG, Gale ME (1982) Computed tomography and ultrasonography for diagnosis and treatment of renal and retroperitoneal abscess. Urol Clin North Am 9: 185–193

Gikas PW (1976) Uropathology. In: Lapides J (ed) Fundamentals of urology. W.B.Saunders, Philadelphia, pp 110–165

Gilbert PG, Shirley SW (1973) The use of angiography in the diagnosis of space occupying renal and perirenal inflammation. J Urol 110: 11–15

Gillenwater SY, Grayhack JT, Howards SS, Duckett JE (1987) Adult and pediatric urology. Yearbook Medical, Chicago

Gilsanz V, Lasano F, Jiminez J (1980) Renal hydated cysts: communicating with collecting system. AJR 135: 357–361

Ginalski M, Michaud A, Genton N (1985) Renal growth retardation in children: Sign suggestive of vesicoureteral reflux? Am J Radiol 145: 617–619

Guistra PE, Watson RC, Shulman H (1971) Arteriographic findings in the various stages of renal tuberculosis. Radiology 100: 587–602

Gold RP, McClennan BL, Rottenberg RR (1983) CT appearance of acute inflammatory disease of the renal interstitium. AJR 141: 343–349

Goldman ML, Gorelkin L, Rude JC III, Sybers RG, O'Brien DD (1978) Epinephrine renal venography in severe inflammatory disease of the kidney. Radiology 127: 93–101

Goldman SM (1988) Acute and chronic urinary infection: present concepts and controversies. Urol Radiol 10: 17–24

Goldman SM (1989) Simple renal cyst. In: Hartman DS, Davidson AJ (eds) Renal cystic disease, fascicle I. AFIP atlas of radiologic pathologic correlation, Chap 2. W.B.Saunders, Philadelphia, pp 6–37

Goldman SM, Gatewood OMB (1989) Inflammatory Renal Disease. Problems in Urology 3: 607–668

Goldman SM (to be published) Benign renal cysts. In: Pollack H (ed) Clinical urography, 5th edn. W.B.Saunders, Philadelphia

Goldman SM, Meng CH, White RI, Siegelman SS (1977a) Transitional cell tumors of the kidney: How diagnostic is the angiogram? AJR 129: 99–105

Goldman SM, Minkin SD, Naraval DC et al. (1977b) Renal carbuncle: the use of ultrasound in its diagnosis and treatment. J Urol 118: 525–528

Goldman SM, Hartman DS, Fishman EK, Finizio JP, Gatewood OMB, Siegelman SS (1984) CT of xanthogranulomatous pyelonephritis: radiological-pathological correlation. AJR 141: 963–969

Goldman SM, Fishman EK, Hartman DS, Kim YC, Siegelman SS (1985) Computed tomography of renal tuberculosis and its pathological correlates. J Comput Assist Tomogr 9: 771–776

Gow JG (1986) Genitourinary tuberculosis. In: Walsh PC, Gittes RF, Perlmutter AD (eds) Campbell's urology, 5th edn. W. B. Saunders, Philadelphia, pp 1037-1069

Graham JN, Berlin BB, Graydon RG (1986) Case profile: computed tomography in emphysematous pyelonephritis. Urology 27: 277

Grainger RG, Longstaff AJ, Parsons MA (1982) Xanthogranulomatous pyelonephritis: a reapparaisal. Lancet I: 1398-1401

Grigsby WP (1969) Surgical treatment of amebiasis. Surg Gynecol Obstet 128: 609-627

Gwinn JL, Barnes GR Jr (1964) Striated ureters and renal pelvis. AJR 91: 666-668

Haines JG, Mayo ME, Allan NA, Ansell JS (1977) Echinococcal cyst of the kidney. J Urol 117: 788-789

Hall JRW, Choa RG, Wells IP (1988) Percutaneous drainage in emphysematous pyelonephritis - an alternative to major surgery. Clin Radiol 39: 622-624

Hallberg CW (1953) Dioctophyma renale (Goaze 1782) A study of the migration routes to the kidneys of mammals and resultant pathology. Trans Am Microsc Soc 721: 351-363

Hanafy HM (1984) Renoenteric fistula. Urology 23: 394-395

Handmaker H (1982) Nuclear renal imaging in acute pyelonephritis. Semin Nucl Med 12: 246-263

Hanjani A, Sadighian A, Nikakhtar B, Arfaa F (1968) The first report of human infection with Dioctophyma renale in Iran. Trans R Soc Trop Med Hyg 62: 647-648

Hanna AAZ (1977) Genitourinal bilharziasis. In: Witten DM, Myers HJ Jr, Uta DC (eds) Emmett's clinical urography, 4th edn. W. B. Saunders, Philadelphia, pp 921-940

Hare WSC, Poynter JD (1974) The radiology of renal papillary necrosis as seen in analgesic nephropathy. Clin Radiol 25: 423-443

Harrow BR (1965) Early forms of renal papillary necrosis. AJR 93: 335-343

Hartman DS, Davis CJ Jr, Lichtenstein JE, Goldman SM (1980) Renal parenchymal malakoplakia, Radiology 136: 33-42

Hartman DS, Davis CJ Jr, Goldman SM, Isbister SS, Sanders RC (1984) Xanthogranulomatous pyelonephritis: sonographic-pathologic correlation of 16 cases. J Ultrasound Med 3: 481-488

Hartman GW (1971) Nontuberculous infections of the genitourinary tract. In: Emmett JL, Witten DM (eds) Clinical urography, 3rd edn. W. B. Saunders, Philadelphia, pp 749-854

Hassel DR, Glasier CM, McConnel JR (1987) Granulomatous cystitis in chronic granulomatous disease: ultrasound diagnosis. Pediatr Radiol 17: 254-255

Hertz M, Zissin R, Dresnik Z, Morag B, Itzchak Y, Jonas P (1984) Echinococcus of the urinary tract: radiologic findings. Urol Radiol 6: 175-181

Hill JW, Seedat YK (1972) The diagnosis of malakoplakia of the kidney by percutaneous renal biopsy. S Afr Med J 46: 953-956

Hodson CJ (1967) The radiological contribution towards the diagnosis of chronic pyelonephritis. Radiology 88: 857-871

Hodson CJ (1970) Chronic pyelonephritis. In: Progressive pediatric radiology, vol 3. Yearbook Medical, Chicago, pp 231-251

Hodson CJ (1981) Reflux nephropathy: a personal historical review (Neuhauser Lecture). AJR 137: 451-462

Hodson CJ, Smith PK (eds) (1979) Reflux nephropathy. Masson, New York

Hodson CJ, Davies Z, Prescod A (1975a) Renal parenchymal radiographic measurements in infants and children. Pediatr Radiol 3: 16-19

Hodson CJ, Maling TM, McManamon JJ, Lewis MG (1975b) The pathogenesis of reflux nephropathy (chronic atrophic pyelonephritis). Br J Radiol [Suppl] 48: 1-26

Hoffman EP, Mindelzun RE, Anderson RU (1980) Computed tomography in acute pyelonephritis associated with diabetes. Radiology 135: 691-695

Hoffman JC, Schnur MJ, Koenigsberg M (1982) Demonstration of renal papillary necrosis by sonography. Radiology 145: 785-787

Hopkins GB, Hall RL, Mende CW (1976) Gallium-67 scintigraphy for the diagnosis and localization of perinephric abscess. J Urol 115: 126-128

Hugosson C (1987) Striation of the renal pelvis and ureter in bilharziasis. Clin Radiol 19: 100-111

Huland H, Busch R (1984) Pyelonephritis scarring in 213 patients with upper and lower urinary tract infections: long term followup. J Urol 132: 936-939

Huntington RW Jr (1971) Coccidioidomycosis. In: Baker RD (ed) The pathologic anatomy of mycoses. Springer, Berlin, pp 147-210

Ishikawa I, Saito Y, Onouchi Z, Matsuura H, Saito T, Suzuki M, Futyu Y (1985) Delayed contrast enhancement in acute focal bacterial nephritis: CT features. J Comput Assist Tomogr 9: 894-897

Israel J (1878) Neue Beobachtungen auf dem Gebiete der Mykosen des Menschen. Virchow's Arch Path Anat Physiol 74: 15-53

Jacobson SH, Kallenius G, Lars-Eric L, Svenson SB (1988) P. fimbriae receptors in patients with chronic pyelonephritis. J Urol 139: 900-902

Jaquier S, Forbes PA, Nogrady MB (1985) The value of ultrasonography as a screening procedure in a first documented urinary tract infection in children. J Ultrasound Med 4: 393-400

Jeffrey RB, Laing FC, Wing WV, Hoddock W (1985) Sensitivity of sonography in pyonephrosis: a re-evaluation. AJR 144: 71-73

Jimenez F, Lopez Pacios MA, Llamazeres G, Conejero J, Sole-Balcells F (1978) Treatment of pyonephrosis. J Urol 120: 287-289

Kahn PC, Wise HM Jr (1967) Simulation of renal tumor response to epinephrine by inflammation disease. Radiology 89: 1062-1064

Kalovidouris A, Pissiotis C, Pontifex A, Gouliamos A (1986) CT characterization of multivesicular hydated cysts. J Comput Assist Tomogr 10: 428-431

Kangarloo H, Gold RH, Fine RN, Diament MJ, Boechat MI (1985) Urinary tract infection in infants and children evaluated by ultrasound. Radiology 154: 367-373

Karamchandani MC, Riether R, Sheets J, Stasik J (1986) Nephrocolic fistula. Dis Colon Rectum 29: 747-749

Kass EJ, Silver TM, Konnak JW, Thornbury JR, Wolfman MG (1976) The urographic findings in acute pyelonephritis: nonobstructive hydronephrosis. J Urol 116: 544-546

Kaude JV, Stone M, Fuller TJ, Cade R, Tarrant DG, Juncos LI (1976) Papillary necrosis in kidney transplant patients. Radiology 120: 69-74

Kauffman CA, Tan JS (1974) Torulopsis glabrata renal infection. Am J Med 57: 217-224

Kaufman SL, White RI Jr, Harrington DP, Barth KH, Siegelman SS (1975) Protean manifestations of mycotic aneurysms. AJR 131: 1019-1025

Kay CJ, Rosenfield AT, Taylor KJW, Rosenberg MA (1979) Ultrasonic characteristics of chronic atrophic pyelonephritis. AJR 132: 47-49

Kedar SS, Eldar S, Abrahamson J, Boss J (1988) Histoplasmosis of kidneys presenting as chronic recurrent renal disease. Urology 31: 490-494

Kelalis PP, Greene LF, Weed LA (1962) Brucellosis of the urogenital tract: mimic of tuberculosis. J Urol 88: 347-353

Kim DS, Woesner ME, Howard TF, Olson LK (1979) Emphysematous pyelonephritis demonstrated by computed tomography. AJR 132: 287-288

Kintanar C, Cramer BC, Reid WD, Andrews WL (1986) Neonatal renal candidiasis: sonographic diagnosis. AJR 147: 801-805

Kirpekar M, Abiri MM, Hilfer C, Enerson R (1986) Ultrasound in the diagnosis of systemic candidiasis (renal and cranial) in very low birth weight premature infants. Pediatr Radiol 16: 17-20

Kneeland JB, Auh YH, Rubenstein WA, Zirinsky K, Morrison H, Whalen JP, Kazam E (1987) Perirenal spaces. CT evidence for communication across the midline. Radiology 164: 657-664

Koehler PR (1978) The roentgen diagnosis of renal inflammatory masses, special emphasis on angiographic changes. Radiology 112: 257-266

Kollins SA, Hartman GW, Carr CT, Segura JW, Hattery RR (1974) Roentgenologic finding in urinary tract tuberculosis: a 10 year investigation. AJR 121: 487-500

Kozinn PJ, Taschdjian CL, Goldberg PK, Wise GJ, Toni EF, Seelig MS (1978) Advances in the diagnosis of renal candidiasis. J Urol 119: 184-187

Krogstad DJ (1982) Amebiasis. In: Wyndaaden JB, Smith LH Jr (eds) Cecil textbook of medicine, 16th edn. W. B. Saunders, Philadelphia, pp 1736-1739

Kunin CM, Deutcher R, Paquin AJ (1964) Urinary tract infection in school children: an epidemiological, clinical laboratory study. Medicine 43: 91-130

Kunin M (1986) Bridging septa of the perinephric space: anatomic, pathologic, and diagnostic consideration. Radiology 158: 361-365

Kuntze JR, Herman MH, Evans SG (1988) Genitourinary coccidioidomycosis. J Urol 140: 370-374

Lachance S, Wicklund R, Carey T, Totonchi M (1985) Emphysematous pyelonephritis complicated by hemorrhage diagnosed by computed tomography Scans. J Urol 134: 940-941

Lahde S, Standertskjold-Nordenstam C, Suornta H, Pyhtinen J (1981) Two-picture urography in urinary tract infection. J Urol 125: 820-821

Lang EK (1971) Arteriographic Assessment and Staging of Renal cell Carcinoma. Analysis of a series of 120 patients. Radiology 101: 17-27

Lang EK (1973) Roentgenographic assessment of asymptomatic renal lesions: An analysis of the confidence level of diagnosis established by segmental roentgenographic investigation. Radiology 109: 257-269

Lang EK (1977a) Renal cyst puncture and aspiration: survey of complications. AJR 128: 723-727

Lang EK (1977b) Asymptomatic space-occupying lesions of kidney: a programmed sequential approach and its impact on quality and cost of health care. South Med J 70: 277-285

Lang EK (1980) Roentgenologic approach to the diagnosis and managment cystic lesions of the kidney: Is cyst exploration mandatory? Urol Clin North Am 7: 677-688

Lang EK (1984) The effect of percutaneous nephrostomy drainage upon renal plasma flow rate in the partially obstructed kidney. AJR 142: 236

Lang EK (1986a) Estratto da Progressi in Radiologia, Radiourologia Nefrostomia Percutanea Nel Trattamento Delle

Infezioni Renali. Ludovico Dalla Palma, Edizioni, Lint Trieste, pp 193-198

Lang EK (1986b) Current cost effective diagnosis of asymptomatic renal mass lesions in tumors of the kidney. In: De Kernion JB (ed) Tumors of the kidney, Williams & Wilkins, Baltimore, pp 11-33

Lang EK (1986c) Percutaneous and interventional urology and radiology. Springer, Berlin Heidelberg New York

Lang EK (1987) Renal cyst puncture studies. Urol Clin North Am 14: 91-102

Lang EK (1990) Renal, perirenal and pararenal abscesses: percutaneous drainage. Radiology 174: 109-113

Lang EK, Glorioso LW (1986) Management of urinomas by percutaneous drainage procedures. Radiol Clin North Am 24: 551-559

Lang EK, Price EW (1983) Redefinition of indication for percutaneous nephrostomy. Radiology 147: 419-426

Lang EK, Redetzki JE, Brown RL (1972) Lymphangiographic demonstration of lymphaticocalyceal fistulas causing chyluria (filariasis). J Urol 108: 321-324

Lang EK, Bellina PV Jr, Norman S (1980) Ultrasonography echinococcus granulosus cyst of the liver. J La State Med Soc 132(3): 40-41

Lang EK, Bergner BM, Both JK Jr (1982) The role of computerized tomography in the management of bilateral tuberculous psoas abscess. J Urol 128: 1020-1022

Langston CS, Pfister RC (1970) Renal emphysema. A case report and review of the literature. AJR 110: 778-786

Lapides J (1978) Mechanism of urinary tract infection. Urology 14: 217-225

Lattimer JK, Kohen RJ (1954) Renal tuberculosis. Am J Med 17: 533-539

Lautin EM, Gordon PM, Friedman AC, Dourmashkin L, Fromowitz F (1979) Emphysematous pyelonephritis: optimal diagnosis and treatment. Urol Radiol 1: 93-96

Lebowitz RL, Mandell J (1987) Urinary tract infection in children putting radiology in its place. Radiology 165: 1-9

Lee JKT, McClennan BL, Nelson GL, Stanley RJ (1980) Acute bacterial nephritis. AJR 135: 87-92

Leekam RN, Shankar L, Bayley TA (1987) Emphysematous pyelonephritis as seen on technetium 99m DTPA renal imaging. Clin Nucl Med 12: 140-141

Levin DC, Gordin D, Kinkhabwala M, Becker JA (1976) Reticular neovascularity in malignant and inflammatory renal masses. Radiology 120: 61-68

Lewall DB, Bailer TM, McCorkell SJ (1986) Echinococcal matrix: computed tomography, sonographic and patholic correlation. J Ultrasound Med 5: 33-35

LiPuma JP (1984) Magnetic resonance imaging of the kidney. Radiol Clin North Am 22: 925-941

Lomberg H, Hanson LA, Jacobsson B, Jodal U, Leffler H, Svanborg Eden C (1983) Correlation of P blood group, vesicoureter reflux and bacterial attachement in patients with recurrent pyelonephritis. N Engl J Med 308: 1189-1192

Love L, Myers MA, Churchill RH (1981) Computed tomography of extraperitoneal spaces. AJR 136: 781-789

Lowe J, Pfau A, Stein H (1983) Reactivated musculoskeletal tuberculosis with concomitant asymptomatic genitourinary infections. Isr J Med Sci 19: 262-266

Malek RS, Elder JS (1978) Xanthogranulomatous pyelonephritis: a critical analysis of 26 cases and the literature. J Urol 119: 589-593

Mayer AR, Miniter P, Andriole VT (1983) Immunopathogenesis of chronic pyelonephritis. Am J Med 74: 59-70

McDougall IR, Baumert JE, Lanteri RL (1979) Evaluation of

indium 111 in leukocyte whole body scanning. AJR 133: 849–854

McNulty M (1957) Pyeloureteritis cystica. Br J Radiol 30: 648–652

Mendez G Jr, Isikoff MB, Morillo G (1979) The role of computed tomography in the diagnosis of renal and perirenal abscess. J Urol 122: 582–586

Michaeli J, Mogle P, Perlberg S, Heiman S, Caine M (1984) Emphysematous pyelonephritis, review article. J Urol 131: 203–208

Miller JH, Greenfield LD, Wald BR (1982) Candidiasis of the liver and spleen in childhood. Radiology 142: 375–380

Mitas JA II, Higgenbottom PA, Handler J, Vesquez M, Stone RA (1981) Renal papillary necrosis in thyroid carcinoma. Urology 17: 177–180

Mitchell DG, Friedman AC, Druy EM, Swanberg LE, Philipps M (1985) Xanthogranulomatous pyelonephritis: unusual case of renal vein and renal caval thrombosis. Urology 7: 35–38

Mogle JM, Perlberg S, Heiman S, Caine M (1984) Emphysematous pyelonephritis. J Urol 131: 203–208

Molina RP, Dulabon DA, Roth RB (1988) Renal cholestaetoma. Urology 31: 153–155

Montgomery P, Kuhn JP, Afshani E (1987) CT evaluation of severe renal inflammatory disease. Pediatr Radiol 17: 216–222

Mooreville M, Ekloyss GC, Schuster A, Pearch AE, Rosen J (1988) Spontaneous renocolic fistula secondary to calculous pyonephrosis. Urology 31: 147–150

Moreau JF (1982) Acute renal infections in adults. Fourth Annual Uroradiological Course, Society of Uroradiology. Palm Beach, Florida, p 44

Morehouse HT, Weiner SN, Hoffman JC (1984) Imaging in inflammatory disease of the kidney. AJR 143: 135–141

Morgan WR, Nyberg LM Jr (1985) Perinephric and intrarenal abscesses: a review article. Urology 26: 529–536

Mulopulos GP, Patel SK, Pessis D (1986) MR imaging of xanthogranulomatous pyelonephritis. J Comput Assist Tomogr 10: 154–156

Murphy KJ (1968) Calcification of the renal papillae as a sign of analgesic nephropathy. Clin Radiol 19: 394–399

Myers MA (1976) Dynamic radiology of the abdomen: normal and pathological anatomy. Springer, Heidelberg Berlin New York, pp 113–194

Neerhut G, Politis G, Alpert L, Griffith DP (1988) Cholesteatoma of the renal pelvis: endoscopic management. J Urol 139: 1032–1034

Newcastle Asymptomatic Bacteriuria Research Group (1975) Asymptomatic bacteriuria in school children in Newcastle-upon-Tyne. Arch Dis Child 50: 90–102

Nicholson RC (1981) Abnormalities of the perinephric fascia and fat in pancreatitis. Radiology 139: 125–127

Nino-Murcia M, Friedland GW (1988) Obliterative pyelitis. Urol Radiol 10: 100–102

Older RA, Cleeve DM, McLelland R (1978) The nonspecifity of some radiological signs in excretory urography. Radiology 127: 553–554

Olzabal A, Velasco M, Martinez A, Villavicencio H, Codina M (1987) Emphysematous pyelonephritis. Urology 29: 95–98

Owen JP, Ramos JM, Keir MJ et al. (1985) Urographic findings in adults with chronic pyelonephritis. Clin Radiol 36: 81–87

Parienty RA, Pradel J (1980) Radiological evaluation of the perirenal and pararenal spaces by computed tomography. CRC Crit Rev Diagn Imaging 20: 1–26

Parsons MA, Harris SC, Grainger RG, Ross B, Smith JAR, Williams JL (1986) Fistula and sinus formation in xantho-granulomatous pyelonephritis. A clinico-pathological review and report of four cases. Br J Urol 58: 488–493

Patel BJ, Moskowitz H, Hashma TA (1983) Unilateral renal actinomycosis. Urology 21: 172–174

Patriquin H, Lebowitz R, Perreault G, Yousefzzdeh D (1980) Neonatal candidiasis: renal and pulmonary manifestations. AJR 135: 1205–1210

Petrillo G, Tomaselli S, Greco S (1981) Renal echinococcosis, Case report. J Comput Assist Tomogr 5: 912–913

Piccirillo M, Rigsby CM, Rosenfield AT (1987) Sonography of renal inflammatory disease. Urol Radiol 9: 66–78

Premkumar A, Lattimer J, Newhouse JH (1987) CT and sonography of advanced urinary tract tuberculosis. AJR 148: 5–69

Quinn AD, Kusuda L, Amar AD, Das S (1988) Percutaneous nephrostomy for treatment of hydronephrosis of pregnancy. J Urol 139: 1037–1038

Rabinowitz JG, Kinkhabwala MN, Robinson T, Spyropoulos E, Becker JA (1972) Acute renal carbuncle, the roentgenographic clarification of a medical enigma. AJR 116: 740–748

Ransley PG (1976) The renal papilla and intrarenal reflux. In: Williams DI, Chrishoms GD (eds) Scientific foundations of urology, vol 1. Heinemann, London, pp 79–87

Ransley PG (1978) Vesicoureteric reflux: continuing surgical dilemma. Urology 12: 246–255

Ransley PG, Risdon RA (1975) Renal papillary morphology and intrarenal reflux in the young pig. Urol Res 3: 105–109

Ransley PG, Risdon RA (1979) The renal papilla intrarenal reflux and chronic pyelonephritis. In: Hodson CJ, Smith PK (eds), Reflux nephropathy. Masson, New York, pp 126–133

Rauch RF, Korobkin M, Silverman PM, Dunnick NR (1983) Subcapsular pancreatic pseudocyst of the kidney. J Comput Assist Tomogr 7: 536–538

Redman JF, Seibert JJ (1984) The role of excretory urography in the evaluation of girls with urinary tract infection. J Urol 132: 953–955

Reece RW, Koontz WW Jr (1975) Leukoplakia of the urinary tract: a review. J Urol 114: 165–171

Richie JP, Nicholson TC, Hunting D, Brosman SA (1978) Radiographic abnormalities in acute pyelonephritis. J Urol 119: 832–835

Rigsby CM, Rosenfield AT, Glickman MG, Hodson J (1986) Hemorrhagic focal bacterial nephritis: findings on gray-scale sonography and CT. AJR 146: 1171–1177

Roberts GM, Evans KT, Bloom AL, Al-Gailani F (1983) Renal papillary necrosis in hemophilia and Christmas disease. Clin Radiol 34: 201–206

Roberts JA (1983a) Pathogenesis of pyelonephritis. J Urol 129: 1102–1106

Roberts JA (1983b) Vesicoureteral reflux in the monkey: a review. Urol Radiol 5: 211–217

Rolleston GL, Shannon FT, Utley WF (1970) Relations of the infantile vesicoureteric reflux of renal damage. Br Med J I: 460–463

Rosenfield AJ, Glickman MG, Taylor KJW, Crade M, Hodson J (1979) Acute focal bacterial nephritis (acute lobar nephronia). Radiology 132: 553–561

Rosi P, Selli C, Carin M, Rosi MD, Mottola A (1986) Xanthogranulomatous pyelonephritis: clinical experience with 62 cases. Eur Urol 12: 96–100

Rushton HG, Majd M, Chandra R, Yim R (1988) Evaluation of 99 m technetium-dimercapto-succinic acid renal scans in acute pyelonephritis in piglets. J Urol (part 2) 140: 1169–1174

Sacks D, Banner MP, Meranze SG, Burke DR, Robinson M, McLean GK (1988) Renal and related retroperitoneal abscesses: percutaneous drainage. Radiology 167: 447–451

Saksouk FA, Tipton-Donovan A, Amis ES Jr, Goldman SM (1984) Computed tomography of perirenal and pararenal inflammatory disease complicating renal calculi. Urology 24: 200–204

Schaefer R, Becker JA, Goodman J (1983) Sonography of tuberculous kidney. Urology 21: 209–211

Schlagenhaufer F (1916) Über eigentümliche Staphylomykosen der Nieren und des paranalen Bindegewebes. Frankfurt Z Pathol 19: 139–148

Schlegel JU, Lang EK (1980) Computed Radionuclide Urogram for assessing acute renal failure. AJR 124: 1029–1034

Schmitt GH, Hsu AS (1985) Renal fungus balls: diagnosis by ultrasound and percutaneous antegrade pyelography and brush biopsy in a premature infant. J Ultrasound Med 4: 155–156

Schneider M, Becker JA, Staiano S, Campos E (1975) Sonographic-radiographic correlation of renal and perirenal infections. AJR 127: 1007–1014

Scullin DR, Hardy R (1972) Malakoplakia of the urinary tract with spread to the abdominal wall. J Urol 107: 908–910

Sease WC, Elyaderani MK (1987) Ultrasonography and needle aspiration in diagnosis of xanthogranulomatous pyelonephritis. Urology 29: 231–235

Senn E, Zaunbauer W, Bandhauer K, Haertel M (1982) Computed tomography in acute pyelonephritis. Br J Urol 59: 118–121

Shapiro E, Slovis TL, Perlmuter AD, Kuhns LR (1988) Optimal use of 99 m technetium-glucoheptonate scintigraphy in the detection of pyelonephritis scarring in children. A preliminary report. J Urol (part 2) 140: 1175–1177

Shirkhoda A (1987) CT findings in hepatosplenic and renal candidiasis. J Comput Assist Tomogr 11: 795–798

Siegel MJ, Glasier CM (1981) Acute focal bacterial nephritis in children: significance of ureteral reflux. AJR 137: 257–260

Silver TM, Kass EJ, Thornbury JR (1976) The radiological spectrum of acute pyelonephritis in adults and adolescents. Radiology 118: 67–71

Simon HB, Weinstein AJ, Pasternak MS, Swartz MN, Kunz LJ (1977) Genitourinary tuberculosis: clinical features in a general hospital population. Am J Med 63: 410–420

Soulen M, Fishman EK, Goldman SM, Gatewood OMB (1989a) Bacterial renal infection: role of computed tomography. Radiology 171: 703–707

Soulen M, Fishman EK, Goldman SM, Gatewood OMB (1989b) Sequelae of acute renal infections: CT evaluation. Radiology 173: 423–426

Spagnola AM, Maxted W (1981) Malacoplakia: a study of the literature and current concepts of pathogenesis, diagnosis, and treatment. J Urol 125: 139–146

Stanton MJ, Maxted W (1981) Malakoplakia: a study of the literature and current concepts of pathogenesis, diagnosis, and treatment. J Urol 125: 139–146

Stoller ML, Kogan BA (1986) Sensitivity of 99 m technetium-dimercaptosuccinic acid for the diagnosis of chronic pyelonephritis: clinical and theoretical considerations. J Urol 135: 977–980

Stuck KJ, Silver TM, Jaffe MH, Boweman RA (1981) Sonographic demonstration of renal fungus ball. Radiology 142: 473–474

Sty JR, Wells RG, Starshak RJ, Schroeder BA (1987) Imaging in acute renal infection in children. AJR 148: 471–477

Subramanyam BR, Megibow AJ, Raghavendra BN, Bosniak MA (1982) Diffuse xanthogranulomatous pyelonephritis: a analysis by computed tomography and sonography. Urol Radiol 4: 5–9

Subramanyam BR, Raghavendra BN, Bosniak MA, Lefleur RS, Rosen RJ, Horii SC (1983) Sonography of pyonephrosis: a prospective study. AJR 140: 991–993

Surraco LA (1939) Renal hydatidosis. AM J Surg 44: 581–586

Sussman SK, Gallmann WH, Cohan RH, Saeed M, Lawton JS (1987) CT findings in xanthogranulomatous pyelonephritis with coexistent renocolic fistula. J Comput Assist Tomogr 11: 1088–1090

Talner LB (1982) Radiology in adults with acute urinary infection. Society of Uroradiology 3rd Annual Postgraduate Course. San Diego, California, pp 43–44

Talner LB (1985) Diagnostic strategies in imaging patients with urinary infection. Uroradiological Course, Society of Uroradiology Scientific Meeting, St. Thomas, U.S. Virgin Islands, p 116

Thornbury JR (1979) Perirenal anatomy: normal and abnormal. Radiol Clin North Am 17: 321–331

Trillo A, Lorentz WB, Whitley NO (1977) Malakoplakia of kidney simulating renal neoplasm. Urology 10: 472–477

Van Kirk OC, Go RT, Wedel VJ (1980) Sonographic features of xanthogranulomatous pyelonephritis. AJR 134: 1035–1039

van Sonnenberg E, Casola G, Talner LB, Varney R, Wittich GR, Christensen R (1988) Us-guided percutaneous nephrostomy for urinary obstruction during pregnancy. Presented at the 88th Meeting of the American Roentgen Ray Society Meeting, San Francisco, California, p 127

van Waes PFGM, Feldberg MAM, Mali WPTM et al. (1983) Management of loculated abscesses that are difficult to drain: a new approach. Radiology 147: 57–63

Vas W, Carlin B, Salimi Z, Tang-Barton P, Tucker D (1985) CT diagnosis of emphysematous pyelonephritis. Comput Radiol 9: 37–39

von Lichtenberg F, Lehman JS (1986) Parasitic diseases of the genitourinary system. In: Walsh PC, Gittes RF, Perlmutter AD, Stamey TA (eds) Campbell's urology, 5th edn. W. B. Saunders, Philadelphia, pp 983–1024

Vordermark JS, Modarelli RO, Buck AS (1980) Torulopsis pyelonephritis associated with papillary necrosis: a case report. J Urol 128: 96–99

Walsh PC, Gittes RE, Perlmutter AD, Stamey TA (1986) Campbell's urology, 5th edn. W. B. Saunders, Philadelphia

Wechsler H (1977) Recurrence of renal tuberculosis 29 years after therapy. J Urol 118: 102

White WB, Spencer RP (1983) Radiogallium imaging in primary candidiasis. J Clin Nucl Med 8: 445

Whyte KM, Abbott GD, Kennedy JC, Maling TMJ (1988) A protocol for the investigation of infants and children with urinary tract infection. Clin Radiol 39: 278–280

Wicks JD, Thornbury JR (1979) Acute renal infections in adults. Radiol Clin North Am 17: 245–260

Wills JS, Pollack HM, Curtis JA (1981) Cholesteatoma of the upper urinary tract. AJR 136: 941–944

Yoder IC, Lindfors KK, Pfister RC (1984) Diagnosis and treatment of pyonephrosis. Radiol Clin North AmK 2: 407–414

Yoshino MT, Hillman BJ, Galgiani JN (1987) Coccidioidomycosis in renal dialysis and transplant patients: radiologic findings in 30 pts. AJR 149: 989–992

Young AK, Middleton GR (1980) Urologic manifestations of chronic granulomatous disease of infancy. J Urol 123: 119–120

Yu HHY, Yim CM, Leong CH (1978) Primary actinomycosis of kidney presenting with reno-colic fistula. Br J Urol 50: 140

Zirinsky K, Auh Y, Hartman BJ, Rubinstein WA, Morrison HS, Sherman SJ, Kazam E (1987) Computed tomography of renal aspergillosis. J Comput Assist Tomogr 11: 177–178

5 Urinary Obstruction

NICHOLAS PAPANICOLAOU and RICHARD C. PFISTER

CONTENTS

5.1 Introduction 151
5.2 Pathophysiology 151
5.3 Radiologic Imaging 153
5.3.1 Introduction 153
5.3.2 Intravenous Urography 153
5.3.3 Retrograde Pyelography 159
5.3.4 Sonography 159
5.3.5 Computed Tomography 161
5.3.6 Angiography 162
5.3.7 Radionuclide Renography 163
5.3.8 Magnetic Resonance Imaging 166
5.3.9 Antegrade Pyelography and Pressure-Flow
      Study (Whitaker Test) 167
5.4 Percutaneous Interventions 169
5.4.1 Introduction 169
5.4.2 Patient Selection and Preparation 170
5.4.3 Percutaneous Nephrostomy Placement 171
5.4.4 Percutaneous Ureteral Stenting 172
5.4.5 Percutaneous Drainage of Fluid Collections .. 173
      References 173

5.1 Introduction

Urinary tract obstruction is a common urologic problem occurring at all ages. If left untreated, obstruction invariably results in loss of renal tissue and function, the extent of which depends on duration and severity of the obstruction, unilateral or bilateral renal involvement, and the presence of preexisting renal disease. Furthermore, obstructive uropathy enhances the progress of superimposed infection, often leading to pyonephrosis, sepsis, and rapid renal and systemic failure.

Basic animal research and clinical observations have made substantial contributions to our understanding of the anatomic and pathophysiologic changes that occur during and following obstructive uropathy. One cannot overemphasize the importance of early diagnosis, leading to correction of the

NICHOLAS PAPANICOLAOU, M.D., Associate Professor of Radiology, Harvard Medical School, Rockville, MD 20850, USA; RICHARD PFISTER, M.D., Professor of Radiology; University Medical Center, University of South Alabama, 2451 Fillingim Street, Mobile, AL 36617, USA

cause of urinary obstruction. The literature has ample documentation of complete or significant recovery of renal function, when diagnosis and treatment have been prompt. Radiologic imaging of and percutaneous interventions in the management of urinary obstruction have been well established. For the purposes of this chapter, obstruction at or proximal to the level of the ureterovesical junction will be discussed.

5.2 Pathophysiology

Shortly, within minutes to hours, after severe or complete acute ureteral obstruction, the pressure within the urinary tract proximal to the obstructing lesion increases manyfold its normal level. The increased urine pressure is accompanied by elevated pressures within the proximal and distal renal tubules and a decrease in the glomerular filtration (GFR) and tubular reabsorption (WILSON 1977). The diminished GFR along with the eventual decrease in renal blood flow (RBF) have been attributed to constriction of afferent arterioles of individual nephrons (JAENICKE 1970). Urine production continues within the acutely obstructed kidney, but at a very low rate. Continued water reabsorption by the tubules and pyelorenal backflow with leakage of urine into the renal interstitium, veins, and lymphatics are the main factors responsible for maintaining the formation of urine (SALOMON and LANZA 1962; GILLENWATER 1986). In chronic hydronephrosis, most urine exits into the veins. Obviously, if the obstruction is incomplete, the drainage of urine around the obstructing lesion promotes ongoing urine formation. Urine may leak into and around the kidney following the rupture of a calyceal fornix, resulting in the formation of a urinoma. If the obstruction persists for days or longer, the calyces, renal pelvis, and ureter begin to dilate and the kidney becomes enlarged owing to edema. Nephron damage and parenchymal atrophy have been observed microscopically as early as a few days to 2 weeks following the obstruction. Within several weeks, macroscopic renal atrophy is evident, as the kidney appears darker with scattered areas of ischemia or infarcts (GILLENWATER 1986).

The duration and severity of the obstruction, unilateral or bilateral urinary involvement, and the presence or absence of preexisting renal and vascular disease or superimposed infection are the major factors in determining the degree of impending irreversible renal parenchymal damage. Animal experiments indicate that following release of unilateral ureteral obstruction, there is partial recovery of renal function, which depends on the duration of the process and the presence of a normal contralateral kidney (HINMAN 1934; KERR 1954; VAUGHAN et al. 1973). The obstructed kidney will recover more function if the obstruction lasts less than 2 or 3 weeks and the contralateral kidney is removed after relief of the obstruction, instead of simultaneously with the ureteral ligation. Furthermore, the longer the duration of the obstruction, the longer it takes the affected kidney to recover its function, albeit partially. Human studies documenting the degree of retrieval of renal function after relief of obstruction are incomplete. It is probable that complete or near complete recovery is likely if the obstruction is less than 3 weeks in duration (EARLAM 1967). No return of renal function could be documented after 7.5 months of obstruction, and a 20% of normal return of function was shown after a 3-month duration of complete unilateral ureteral occlusion was relieved (BETTER et al. 1973).

Postobstructive diuresis, namely the profound excretion of water and sodium, is observed following reversal of complete or severe bilateral ureteral obstruction or obstruction of a solitary kidney. The mechanisms proposed for this interesting clinical event are the inhibition of tubular fluid reabsorption by urea and other natriuretic factors that appear in uremia and the decrease in water an sodium reabsorption secondary to increased intrapelvic pressures from the obstruction (WILSON and HOWRATH 1976; WILSON 1977). The role of inappropriate antidiuretic hormone activity has also been implicated.

Chronic, complete, or severe unilateral obstruction results in decreased GFR and RBF (WILSON 1977). Further experimental data indicate that functional impairment mainly affects the distal tubule and collecting ducts and deeper parenchymal or juxtamedullary nephrons, whereas surface nephrons and the proximal tubules function normally or are less severely affected (WILSON 1975). Prolonged obstruction eventually leads to decreased nephron mass and permanent renal dysfunction. Urine concentrating ability is impaired during obstruction as well as after its relief. This defect is in part attributed to depressed renal ATPase activity that regulates sodium reabsorption and the capacity to concentrate the glomerular filtrate (WILSON et al. 1974). Additional factors include the elevated intrapelvic pressure, passive diffusion of interstitial solute out of the papilla, or removal of such solute by increased lymph flow.

There is a sudden increase in the intrapelvic pressure following acute urinary obstruction. Levels as high as 70 mmHg have been recorded after surgically induced acute urinary obstruction in animals undergoing diuresis. The elevated pressures persist for several days to a few weeks and gradually return toward normal levels if the obstruction is not relieved.

Peristalsis is the main force normally propelling urine from the kidney to the bladder. In the normal, low pressure urinary tract contraction waves can be seen passing down the ureter at a rate of 2–7 times per minute. The amplitude of these waves usually produces pressures ranging from 3 cm H_2O in the renal pelvis to 25–70 cm H_2O in the lower ureter, depending on the pressure measuring system used (WEISS 1976). These contraction waves do not propel urine toward the bladder until they reach the pyeloureteral junction level, at which point the pelvis has a definite funnel shape, and continue throughout the ureter. According to Whitaker's concept, a bolus of urine is formed at the ureteropelvic junction by apposition of the funnel shaped renal pelvic walls (WHITAKER 1975). This bolus then triggers a peristaltic wave, which is a combination of coordinated, successive circular muscle contractions that collapse the ureteral lumen on top of the bolus and longitudinal muscle contractions and relaxation ahead of the bolus. A presumed pacemaker, located in either a calyx or the renal pelvis, is thought to initiate the electric stimulation that causes the smooth muscles of the pyeloureteral wall to contract (WEISS et al. 1967). Nerves do not participate in the propagation of the peristaltic waves in the urinary tract. Experiments indicate that there is no specific unidirectional conductivity of these waves, since reversal of a ureteral segment does not alter the direction of peristalsis and stimulation of the lower ureter may produce a reversed peristaltic direction.

The frequence and force of the ureteral contractions increase with increased volume of urine, until, at very high urine flow rates (e. g., diabetes insipidus, postobstructive diuresis), peristalsis ceases and urine flows continuously through the ureter. The main forces, then, of urine propagation are the hydrostatic pressure of the formed urine on the calyces and renal pelvis and gravity. Conversely, anuria from renal parenchymal disease and experimental renal artery occlusion have been shown to severely depress ureteral peristaltic activity.

In acute urinary obstruction, ureteral peristalsis initially increases, as the urinary tract attempts to counterbalance the increased ureteral resistance by forcing urine through the occluding lesion under high pressure. Eventually, within days, the peristaltic activity is exhausted and either ceases completely or is markedly diminished, unless the obstruction is relieved. The obstructed ureter begins to dilate and stretch within several days to a few weeks from the onset of the obstruction. In chronic obstruction, peristalsis and ureteral caliber and length are influenced by the severity of the occlusion and its effect on renal function and urine formation, Continuous urine production may maintain some peristaltic activity and result in ureteral dilatation and tortuosity (PFISTER and NEWHOUSE 1978).

Following relief of obstruction, the dilatation of the pyelocalyceal system and ureter may return to normal; in other cases it improves and peristaltic activity reappears. Sometimes, following longstanding obstruction or with superimposition of bladder outlet obstruction, the ureter cannot generate a high bolus pressure to effectively transport urine into the bladder, although some peristalsis exists. Such a urinary tract can only empty when the bladder pressure is low, otherwise the renal parenchyma is subjected to ongoing hydronephrotic damage. Surgical reduction in ureteral caliber (tapering) has been employed in assisting ureteral emptying.

Failure of localized ureteral segments to transmit the peristaltic wave is encountered in congenital ureteropelvic junction obstruction and obstructed primary megaureter (PFISTER and NEWHOUSE 1978). Several theories have been proposed but have not been adequately validated to date; developmental deficiency of the musculature, excessive inelastic collagen, and deficiency of transmitter substance have been implicated among others. Whitaker introduced the concept of functional ureteropelvic junction obstruction, when the renal pelvic walls do not appose at the ureteropelvic junction area because of the lack of funnel shaped pelvis. Urine bolus formation is affected and urine flow across the junction is impaired. Similarly, this thesis has been thought to be responsible for the persistence of many hydroureters once obstruction has been relieved. Last, but not least, is the ureteral and pyelocalyceal dilatation and depression of peristalsis secondary to significant vesicoureteral reflux. Renal damage resulting from reflux is well documented, particularly in the pediatric age patient.

5.3 Radiologic Imaging

5.3.1 Introduction

The primary goal of radiologic imaging for assessing suspected obstructive uropathy is to confirm or exclude the clinical diagnosis. In the presence of urinary obstruction, the level, degree, and cause can usually be determined by imaging techniques, thus enabling the physician to recommend or institute appropriate treatment. Emphasis should always be placed on early diagnosis if permanent renal parenchym damage is to be avoided.

For many years radiologists relied exclusively on intravenous urography or retrograde pyelography to make the diagnosis of urinary obstruction. Despite the current addition of many more imaging modalities, intravenous urography remains the procedure of choice for many patients evaluated for obstructive uropathy. Sonography, computed tomography, radionuclide renography, antegrade percutaneous pyelography, and magnetic resonance imaging are being utilized with increased frequency, as the indications for diagnosis and intervention are further defined or expanded. The ideal imaging study would be safe and reproducible and provide both anatomic and urodynamic physiologic data, since dilatation of the urinary tract is not synonymous with obstruction. In clinical practice, a combination of imaging modalities is often required for evaluating the patient with suspected urinary obstruction. An understanding of the yield and limitations of each technique is necessary for optimal individual patient care.

5.3.2 Intravenous Urography

All urography contrast media are freely filtered at the glomerulus and concentrated by tubular reabsorption of water. No reabsorption or secretion of these agents by the tubules is observed. Physiologic parameters responsible for the handling of contrast media by the kidney include blood pressure (systolic), RBF, GFR, and water reabsorption and urine concentrating ability (NEWHOUSE and PFISTER 1979).

The nephrogram represents the radiographic image of the renal parenchyma, as it becomes opacified following intravascular injection of a contrast agent. In recent years, high dose urography and/or nephrotomography achieve adequate visualization of the nephrogram in the vast majority of patients studied. Contrast material usually is administered intravenously either as a bolus or as a drip infusion.

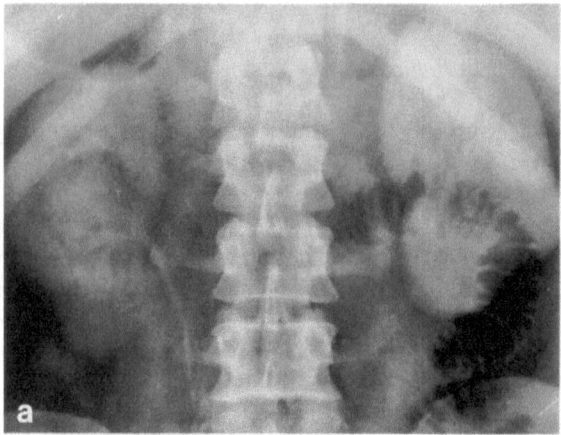

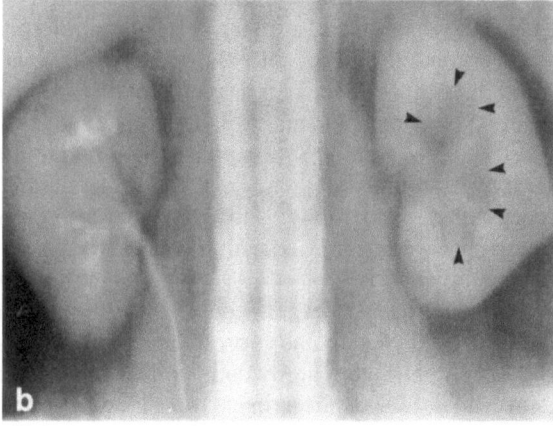

Fig. 5.1a, b. Intravenous urography in acute urinary obstruction secondary to ureteral stone. **a** Fifteen-minute film from high dose drip infusion urogram shows a normal density right nephrogram and prompt opacification of a nondilated collecting system. The left nephrogram is distinctly denser and there is no visualization of the calyces. **b** Nephrotomography shows the absent (delayed) left pyelogram to a better advantage. There is some widening of the renal sinus space, indicative of minimal to mild pyelocaliectasis *(arrowheads)*

degree, the renal intravascular and interstitial spaces. The amount of contrast material in the tubules depends on water reabsorption. Hydration affects water reabsorption in the distal tubules and collecting ducts, whereas reabsorption in the proximal tubule varies very little. Hydration, though, does not significantly affect nephrogram density, as the overall volume of proximal tubule is greater than the volume of the remaining nephron and the osmotic diuresis, caused by the contrast material, limits water reabsorption from the collecting ducts.

Within the first 1–2 min after a bolus injection, the normal nephrogram reflects more opacification of the cortex over the medulla, as filtered contrast agent enters the proximal tubules. Corticomedullary differentiation rapidly fades as the filtrate moves into the distal segments of the nephron. Over the next 2 or 3 min, calyceal opacification begins as the fully formed, opacified urine reaches the collecting system (NEWHOUSE and PFISTER 1979).

In acute urinary obstruction, the typical radiographic findings is that of an increasingly dense nephrogram (ELKIN 1963; ELKIN et al. 1964) (Fig. 5.1). Depending on the severity and duration of the obstruction and the preexisting renal function, the peak density may not occur until several hours into the study. If the obstruction is postrenal, further typical radiographic features include delayed opacification of the pyelocalyceal system (pyelogram), slow transport of opaque urine to the level ob obstruction, and variable, usually slight to mild, dilatation of the collecting system proximal to the occlusion. In a smaller percentage of patients (5%–25%) intra- or perirenal extravasation secondary to forniceal rupture (pyelorenal backflow) may be observed.

The mechanism proposed for the production of the obstructive nephrogram is a combination of elevated renal pelvic pressure, reduced effective filtration pressure and glomerular filtration, slow flow of fluid along the renal tubules, and increased reabsorption of water proximally, resulting in increased concentrating of contrast material in the forming urine (NEWHOUSE and PFISTER 1979). Striations extending from the medulla to the outer cortex (medullary rays) may be seen in addition to the overall increased nephrogram density (BIGONGIARI et al. 1977). These striations presumably are produced by dilated collecting ducts containing opaque urine although alternative explanations exist. The appearance of striations has also been observed in infantile polycystic kidney disease and medullary sponge kidney or tubular ectasia, the latter two limited to the renal medulla. There is no difficulty separating these entities from acute urinary obstruction when

The former technique results in rapid peak plasma concentration, followed by a biphasic time–concentration curve of the intravascular contrast agent, with an initial rapid decline caused by intravascular mixing and extravascular diffusion of the agent (CATTELL et al. 1967). The latter technique results in a slower peak plasma concentration, followed by an elongated equilibrium phase, where infusion and clearance rates are similar, and ending with a decline curve when the infusion is finished that closely resembles the second phase of the bolus injection curve (CATTELL 1970). Total dose and rate of administration, therefore, affect the time–concentration curves.

Nephrogram density is produced by contrast material in the intratubular space and, to a much lesser

other radiologic and clinical features are considered. Peak density of the obstructive nephrogram in complete, acute obstruction is usually seen 3–6 h into the study. The density gradually fades subsequently, but a nephrogram often can remain 1–2 days later. The differential diagnosis of the increasingly dense nephrogram with slow onset includes systemic hypotension, sometimes induced by the contrast agent, renal vein thrombosis, partial renal artery occlusion, and acute renal failure, besides acute urinary obstruction. One can usually arrive at the correct diagnosis when one takes into consideration additional radiologic and clinical findings.

Sometimes, heterotopic liver excretion of contrast material into the gallbladder can be seen in acute obstruction, even if the opposite kidney functions normally (Sokoloff 1973). It should be noted that generation of the dense, obstructive nephrogram depends on the existence of normal nephrons and adequate blood supply to the kidney. Severe renal parenchymal diseases or renal infection coexisting with acute urinary obstruction may preclude the development of the obstructive nephrogram.

The delay in opacification of the pyelocalyceal system is quite variable, from several minutes to several hours or a day after the injection. This delay depends mainly on the degree of obstruction. Identifying the site of obstruction is always desirable, but may not always be accomplished, even on delayed radiographs. Sometimes, placing the patient in the prone or upright position enhances mixing of opaque with nonopaque urine and helps define the level of obstruction (Davidson 1985). The density of the opacified urine within the collecting system and ureter depends on the degree and duration of the obstruction. Not infrequently, this density is quite faint to allow precise visualization of the urinary tract. Small ureteral calculi may pass spontaneously during an intravenous urogram. For several hours after such an event, the density of urine in the collecting system and ureter remains decreased, an indication of the time required before renal function and concentrating ability are fully restored.

Dilatation of the calyces, renal pelvis, and ureter following acute urinary obstruction ranges from nonexisting to slight to mild for a period of a few days. Normally, visualization of the entire ureter on one or more radiographs during high dose urography is not uncommon. Ureteral fullness not due to obstruction usually disappears on the postvoid radiograph, on a prone or erect film, or by simply waiting for several minutes before repeating an exposure. This fullness should not be confused with obstruction. Measurements of ureteral size are not always conclusive and absolute ureteral diameters for normal and dilated urinary tracts have not been determined. In general, we consider a ureter exceeding 8 mm in diameter to be dilated (Pfister and Newhouse 1978). Recognition of calyceal dilatation, likewise, may not be easy early on during obstruction or in the presence of partial or low grade obstruction. Calyces and ureter become more dilated if the obstruction persists. Ureteral tortuosity is not a feature of acute urinary tract obstruction, as it requires several days to weeks before the ureter becomes elongated and tortuous. It usually implies a chronic process, such as sustained obstruction or reflux (Pfister and Newhouse 1978). Simple ureteral meandering or kinks should not be misinterpreted as indicating obstruction.

The recognition of urothelial striations in the renal pelvis and ureter has been reported in nephrolithiasis, obstruction, infection, or reflux, the latter usually in children (Hyde and Wastie 1971; Cremin and Stables 1971). The etiology of these striations is attributed to the common denominator of dilatation or intermittent stretching of normal urothelial folds. In the presence of infection, these folds may become more pronounced, possibly because of the edema.

An additional radiographic finding, indicative of elevated intrapelvic pressure and, therefore, seen in acute urinary obstruction is extravasation of opacified urine. Urine escapes the pyelocalyceal system either through a ruptured calyceal fornix or by papillary reflux or backflow (Rabinowitz et al. 1966; Cooke and Bartucz 1974). Regardless of the route of the urine leak, the cause is a sudden significant increase in the renal pelvis pressure that may result either from acute ureteral obstruction or a rapid direct injection of contrast material in an antegrade or retrograde fashion.

Backflow in acute obstruction decompresses the pyelocalyceal system, compensating for the abnormally high pressures that reduce GFR, and allows for continuing urine formation. Renal backflow has been conveniently classified into pyelosinus, pyelovenous, pyelolymphatic, pyelointerstitial, and pyelotubular to describe the different pathways followed during extravasation of opacified urine. It should be noted that use of abdominal compression during intravenous urography may result in urine extravasation in a very small number of nonobstructed patients. Pyelotubular or pyelovenous backflow cannot be diagnosed on intravenous urography (Talner 1990). Visualization of collecting ducts in the papillary regions in young adults is a relatively common uroradiologic phenomenon and

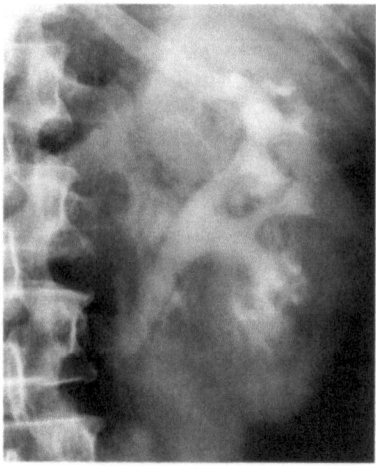

Fig. 5.2. Rupture of calyceal fornices secondary to acute ureteral obstruction by stone. Extension pyelosinus and pyelointerstitial extravasation are noted around the mildly distended left pyelocalyceal system

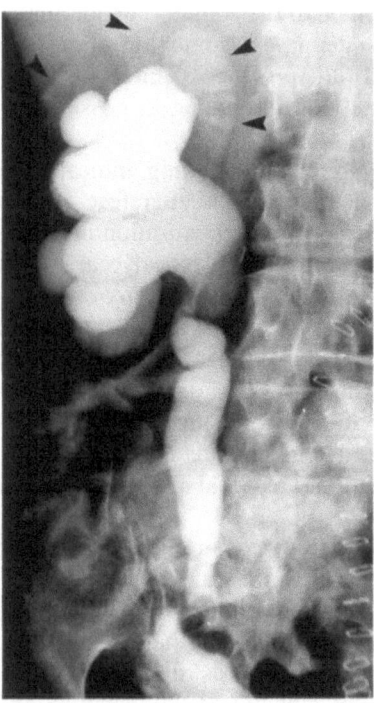

Fig. 5.3. Pyelotubular backflow observed during cystography, following right ureteroneocystostomy (psoas hitch operation) for malignancy. The free reflux of contrast material from the bladder into the right urinary tract raised the pressure sufficiently to result in renal backflow, best seen around the upper pole calyces *(arrowheads)*

should not be considered as a sign of obstruction or elevated intrapelvic pressure. Presumably it occurs because of the high concentration of contrast medium in the urine after water reabsorption although other possibilities exist. Benign tubular ectasia may have a similar appearance on excretory urography, as it appears as discrete linear densities in one or more papillary regions of one or both kidneys. It represents the innocuous end of the medullary sponge kidney spectrum of clinical and radiologic features. The linear striations are wider than normal collecting ducts and, in more advanced forms of the process, they may have a Lacunar appearance, as the ducts are more dilated. Again, in the absence of corollary findings this entity should not be mistaken as urinary obstruction.

Pyelosinus backflow is the most common type of extravasation observed during excretory urography of an acutely obstructed urinary tract (Fig. 5.2). It results from the rupture of calyceal fornix. Sometimes, the extravasation of opacified urine can be substantial, extending into the perinephric space and along the ureter and psoas muscle. This sometimes impressive radiographic appearance quickly resolves following relief of the obstruction. If the obstruction persists, on the other hand, a urinoma may be formed around the kidney and caudally, within Gerota's fascia. The typical large urinoma displaces the kidney anteriorly and laterally and is usually located inferior and posterior to the lower renal pole, with a medial direction as it extends towards the pelvis. On rare occasions a urinothorax has been described with acute and chronic obstruction (FRIEDLAND et al. 1971). In the pediatric age group, urinary ascites can occur secondary to urinary obstruction, regardless of the level and etiology of the obstructing lesion (MONCADA et al. 1968; WELLER and MILLER 1973). Small to moderately sized urinomas usually resolve spontaneously, provided that the obstruction is relieved. Larger collections may require percutaneous drainage. Retroperitoneal urine extravasation incites a fibrotic reaction and may lead to periureteral fibrosis and ureteral obstruction, if left undrained over a period of time.

Renal backflow can be further observed in situations where there is a sudden increase in intrapelvic pressure, often in nonobstructed systems (Fig. 5.3). The most common examples are iatrogenic and occur during antegrade or retrograde injection of contrast material via a stent or nephrostomy tube or when performing ileal loopograms. Intermittent monitoring of the pressures with a water manometer helps prevent excessive pressure levels within the collecting system during these radiographic procedures.

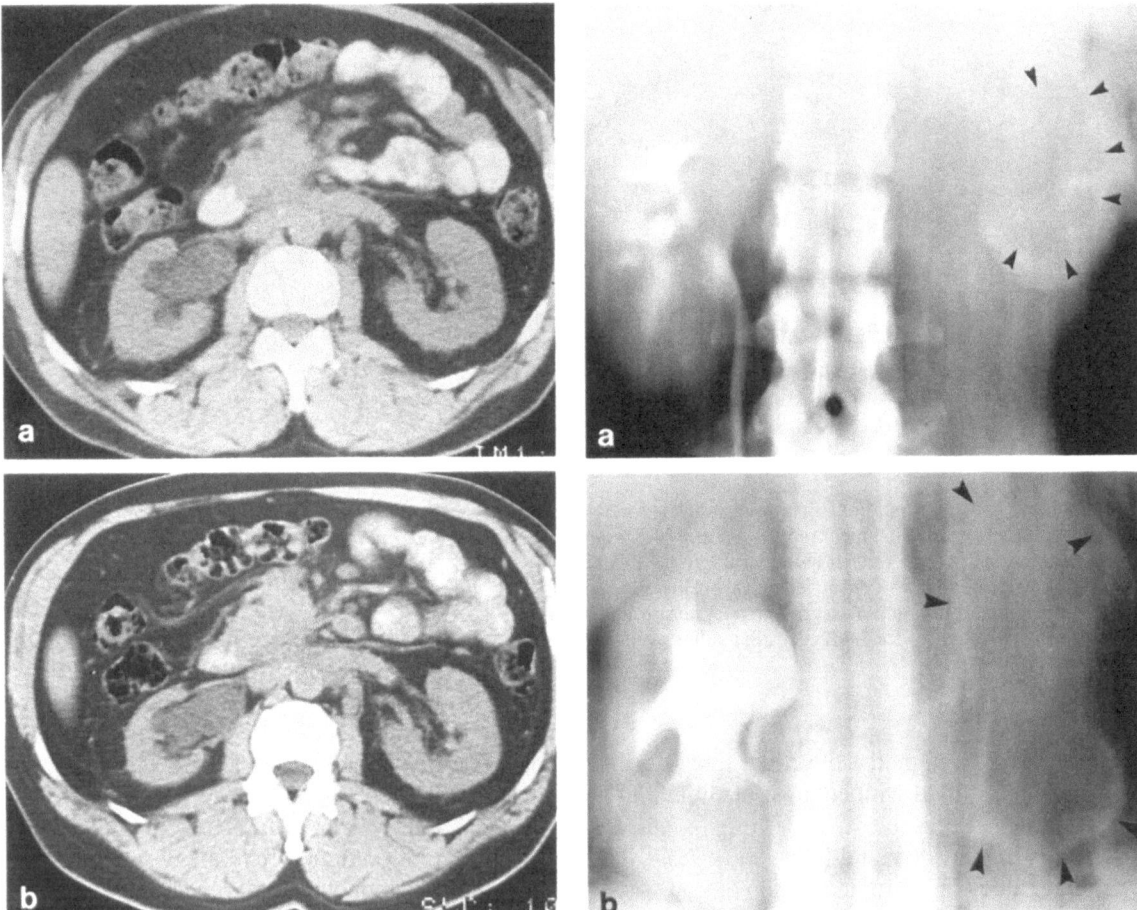

Fig. 5.4 a, b. Obstructive atrophy of right kidney secondary to extrinsic compression of the ureter by lymphoma. **a** Non-enhanced CT shows mild right pyelocaliectasis with slight decrease in renal size compared to the nonobstructed, normal left kidney. **b** Six months later there is significant reduction of the right renal unit with persistent hydronephrosis. A percutaneous nephrostomy tube was placed after this CT examination for relief of the obstruction

Fig. 5.5 a, b. Nephrotomography in the evaluation of chronic urinary tract obstruction. **a** There is considerable thinning of the left renal parenchyma, accompanied by marked pyelocaliectasis and delayed excretion. The dilated collecting system is easily seen, because the uniform, low attenuation density of the unopacified urine it contains contrasts with the relatively normal nephrogram density *(arrowheads)*. **b** Shell nephrogram, left kidney, after longstanding ureteropelvic junction obstruction resulting in irreversible total loss of renal function *(arrowheads)*

Chronic urinary obstruction produces characteristics anatomic and pathophysiologic alterations in the kidney, collecting system, and ureter (DAVIDSON 1985; TALNER 1990). Renal size varies from normal in mild cases to small in obstructive or postobstructive atrophy to large in giant hydronephrosis (Fig. 5.4). Renal function also is compromised. The extent of renal damage depends on the degree and duration of the obstruction. The dense and sometimes striated nephrogram of acute urinary obstruction is not seen in the chronic form, since several contributing physiologic parameters, such as GFR, tubular reabsorption, and RBF, are impaired, Consequently, the chronic obstructive nephrogram often

is of near normal to decreased density, with a faint nephrogram obtained in severe obstruction. Nephrotomography often is necessary to demonstrate opacification of the thinned parenchyma of a poorly functioning, chronically obstructed kidney (Fig. 5.5a). In advanced obstruction, parenchymal thickness is reduced to 1 cm or less, a "shell" nephrogram is obtained, indicating severe pyelocaliectasis and irreversible parenchymal damage and renal dysfunction (HODSON and CRAVEN 1966; NEWHOUSE and PFISTER 1979) (Fig. 5.5 b). In moderate obstruction and parenchymal thinning, often one sees curvilinear renal medullary opacities, paralleling the margins of the dilated calyces. They represent com-

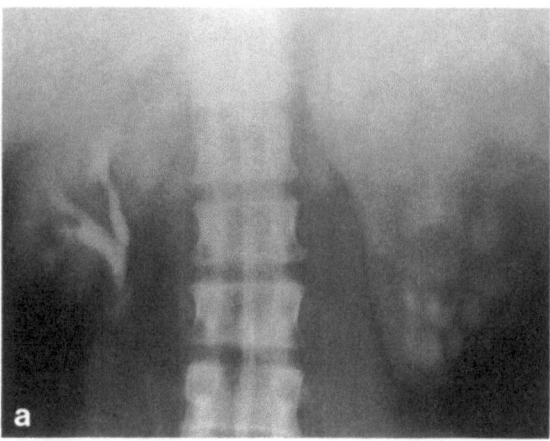 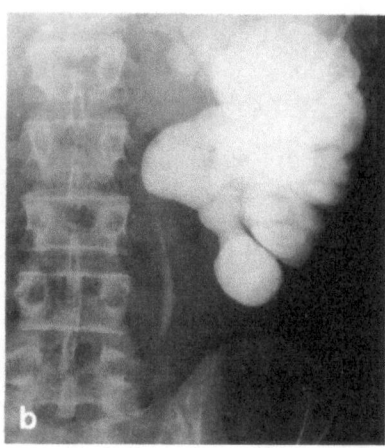

Fig. 5.6. a, b. Giant hydronephrosis in a young adult secondary to congenital ureteropelvic junction obstruction. **a** Nephrotomography shows an enlarged left kidney with grossly dilated, slowly opacifying calyceal system. There is considerable global parenchymal thinning. **b** Antegrade pyelogram results in optimal opacification of the markedly dilated left pyelocalyceal system

pressed and realigned collecting and papillary (Bellini) ducts filled with contrast medium and are known as calyceal crescents (DUNBAR and NOGRADY 1970; GRISCOM and KROEKER 1973). Dilated papillary ducts in chronic incomplete obstruction often appear on urography as dots or short lines surrounding the dilated calyces. The markedly lobulated renal contour of the end-stage obstructive rim nephrogram is easily differentiated from the smooth contour "rim" nephrogram which may be encountered in acute renal artery occlusion, renal vein thrombosis, and acute renal failure (HANN and PFISTER 1982).

Measurements of parenchymal waisting in chronic obstruction have been correlated with residual or reversible renal function following relief of obstruction (BERDON et al. 1970). These measurements sometimes over- or underestimate the ability of the kidney to recover its function and are not as accurate as radionuclide quantitative renography or split creatinine clearance obtained via a stent or nephrostomy tube (DE MAEYER et al. 1982; NIMMO et al. 1987; THOMSEN et al. 1987). However, evaluation of the opacified renal parenchyma on nephrotomography may provide a rough or reasonable estimate of the function expected to return several weeks after decompression of the urinary tract (Fig. 5.5).

Delayed opacification of the pyelocalyceal system in chronic obstruction varies, depending on the degree of renal impairment. Initial imaging most often

results in the so-called absent or negative pyelogram, in that there is parenchymal opacification only, while the urine in the collecting system remains unopacified. The diagnosis of hydronephrosis can, therefore, be made indirectly with confidence. If the remaining renal function is sufficient, calyceal opacification takes place over a period of several hours. In addition, there is definite widening of the pyelocalyceal system and/or ureter, depending on the level of the obstructing lesion. This dilatation as well as the appearance of the nephrogram help separate acute from chronic obstruction when history or additional radiographic findings are equivocal. The degree of pyelocalyceal dilatation varies from mild to marked; in extreme cases the kidney in children but not in adults enlarges manyfold its normal size and presents as a palpable abdominal mass. The term giant hydronephrosis usually refers to the marked pyelocaliectasis and parenchymal thinning that result from longstanding obstruction, often congenital, and frequently from ureteropelvic junction obstruction (USON et al. 1969; BROCK et al. 1979) (Fig. 5.6). Lower ureteral obstruction may cause massive hydroureter and hydronephrosis and may involve commonly the obstructed upper moiety of a duplicated collecting system. The differential diagnosis mainly involves ureteral reflux and a variety of nonobstructing megaureter conditions. Significant ureteral tortuosity is often seen in patients with chronic obstruction, especially the longstanding partial type. Sometimes, moderately severe hydronephrosis and hydroureter may return to normal or improve substantially after decompression; most often, though, some dilatation of the urinary tract or mild blunting of the calyces is permanent (PFISTER and NEWHOUSE 1978).

Since the renal pelvic pressure may be normal or decreased in chronic obstruction, most patients are asymptomatic and, therefore, at risk of sustaining irreversible renal damage unless diagnosis and treatment are promptly instituted. Anatomic and functional recovery following relief of chronic obstruction in children often occurs over a period of several weeks to months. The severity and duration of the obstruction and age of the patient dictate the changes seen in renal size and function and pyelocalyceal widening.

5.3.3 Retrograde Pyelography

Cystoscopic retrograde opacification of the upper urinary tract used to be the most reliable technique for demonstration of ureteral or pyelocalyceal pathology, prior to the introduction of effective and safe contrast media. Today, retrograde pyelography is reserved mainly for patients in whom adequate opacification of the urinary tract by excretory urography is either contraindicated (e.g., poor renal function) or impossible (e.g., obstruction). In the case of urinary tract obstruction diagnosed by a modality other than intravenous urography, the retrograde ureteropyelogram can provide valuable anatomic information up to the level of the obstruction and helps evaluate its etiology, such as calculus, neoplasm or ureteropelvic junction obstruction, among many potential causes (Fig. 5.7). Sometimes, contrast material may flow around the lesion and proximal to it, allowing visualization of the pyelocalyceal system, although usually in a limited fashion. Retrograde pyelography also is routinely employed prior to ureteroscopic manipulations and placement of retrograde ureteral stents for relief of obstruction.

5.3.4 Sonography

Sonography currently is an important and commonly used imaging modality in urinary obstruction (Amis and Hartman 1984). In general, the information provided is mainly anatomic rather than physiologic; therefore, caution is indicated in interpreting the findings. In pregnant women sonography can be used to screen for both maternal and fetal hydronephrosis, which, if found, usually implies chronic urinary obstruction. Furthermore, it can be routinely used in the diagnosis and follow-up of suspected, known, or treated chronic obstruction in children and adults alike. However, the etiology of hydronephrosis detected by sonography usually is uncertain and the presence of obstruction, although possible, is by no means certain (Morin and Baker 1979;

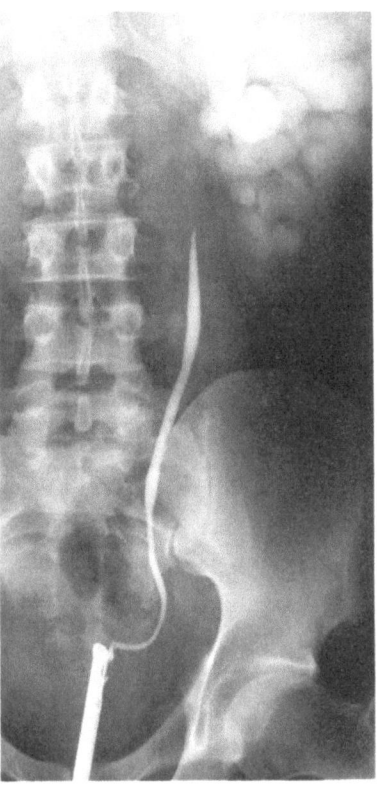

Fig. 5.7. Retrograde pyelography in the young adult patient with giant hydronephrosis. Following cystoscopic retrograde cannulation of the left ureter and injection of contrast material, a normal ureter tapers to a narrow ureteropelvic junction with partial filling of the markedly dilated calyces. The findings are consistent with ureteropelvic junction obstruction

Amis et al. 1982a). Thus, in addition to obstruction, dilatation of the urinary tract may be due to permanent postobstructive hydronephrosis, ureteral reflux, and a high urine flow state, especially in solitary kidneys or during diuresis. The use of sonography in acute urinary obstruction may be particularly misleading, since pyelocaliectasis often is minimal or absent (Rascoff et al. 1983; Maillet et al. 1986). Several hours to 2 days are usually required before hydronephrosis in acute obstruction can be reliably shown sonographically. The demonstration of a perinephric urinoma, although not common, helps suggest the diagnosis of acute urinary obstruction with higher confidence.

In hydronephrosis, the fluid filled pyelocalyceal system is widened, separating the middle portion of the echogenic renal sinus fat (Fig. 5.8). Numerous studies have documented the ability of sonography to correctly diagnose hydronephrosis. It befalls the radiologist to be aware of the limitations of the technique and to remember that hydronephrosis is not always synonymous with obstruction.

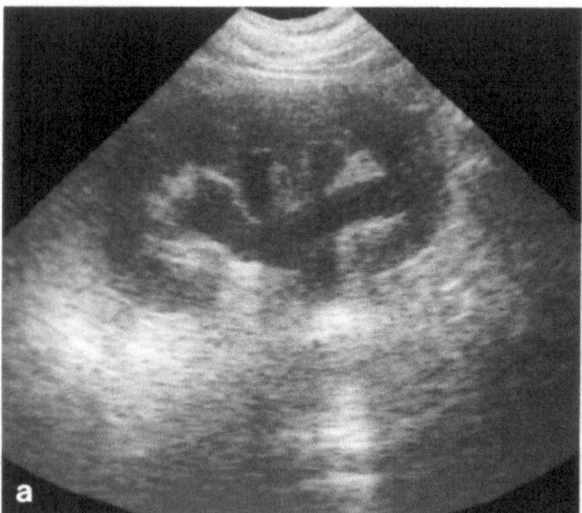

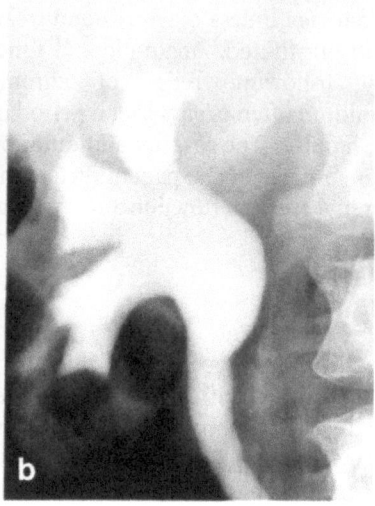

△

Fig. 5.8 a, b. Sonographic detection of hydronephrosis secondary to ureteral obstruction by stone. **a** There is widening and separation of the echogenic right renal sinus fat, caused by dilated urine containing calyes. **b** The intravenous urogram confirms the mild dilatation of the right collecting system and upper ureter

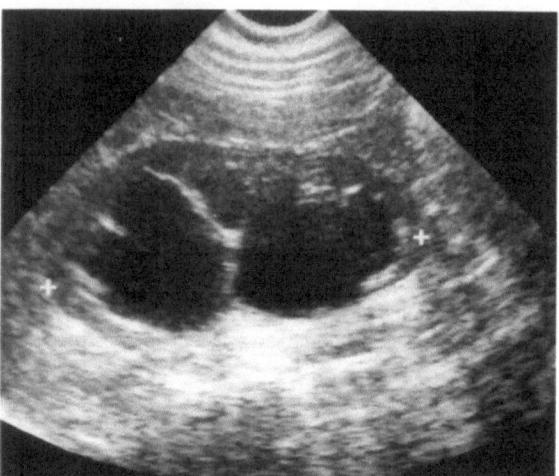

Fig. 5.9. Sonography of marked hydronephrosis, the result of longstanding urinary obstruction. The degree of calyceal dilatation is severe and the thickness of the renal parenchyma has been considerably diminished

Considering acute urinary obstruction, the most significant potential sonographic pitfall is missing the diagnosis, because of the lack of obvious pyelocalyceal dilatation early on. It is generally agreed that such pyelocaliectasis can be identified within a day or two after the obstruction. Therefore, sonography alone may not suffice in the early evaluation of the patient and excretory urography may be necessary, because of its ability to demonstrate the pathophysiologic changes that occur before the anatomic alterations of the collecting system.

However, in chronic urinary obstruction, sonography accurately demonstrates the anatomic consequences of the process, namely hydronephrosis of varying severity, thinning of the renal parenchyma, and in the adult often a decrease in renal size (Fig. 5.9). Again, one should exercise caution when confronted with these findings since they are not specific for chronic obstruction. Ureteral reflux and permanent postobstructive changes are two common entities that share the same sonographic features with chronic obstruction. Additional history, radiologic, and clinical data are then required for the establishment of the correct diagnosis.

A variety of conditions may mask or, more often, imitate hydronephrosis on sonography (Amis and Hartman 1984). The acoustic shadowing of branched or staghorn calculi usually obscures hydronephrosis. A wide extrarenal pelvis, peripelvic cysts, a high urine flow state, a fully distended bladder, inflammatory disease (chronic pyelonephritis, tuberculosis), renal cystic disease (multicystic dysplastic kidney, autosomal dominant adult type polycystic disease, medullary cystic disease), and congenital megacalyces are among a long list of entities that mimic hydronephrosis and obstruction on sonography (Fig. 5.10). Recent reports recommend the use of Doppler flow sonography to distinguish the renal vascular pedicle from the renal pelvis when the suspicion for minimal or mild pyelectasis is raised (Platt et al. 1989; Scola et al. 1989).

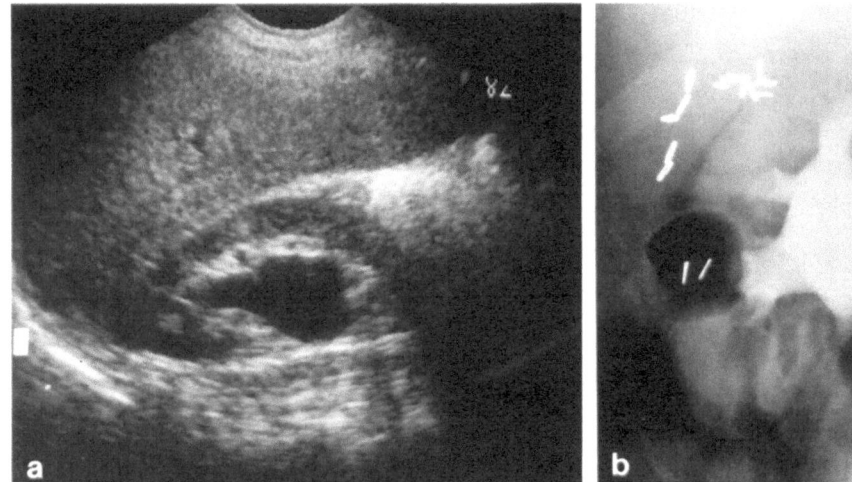

Fig. 5.10 a, b. False-positive diagnosis of hydronephrosis and urinary obstruction by sonography. **a** Sagittal right renal sonogram shows dilatation of the renal pelvis and calyceal infundibula. **b** Intravenous urogram shows a fairly large right extrarenal pelvis and wide infundibula, but normal appearing calyces and no evidence for urinary obstruction

Localization of the obstructing process often is limited or impossible with sonography. In infants and young children, the dilated ureter usually can be demonstrated in its entirety, whereas in the adult patient it may be visible in the proximity of the ureteropelvic or ureterovesical junctions only. Therefore, ureteral obstruction in the adult is best investigated by urography or pyelography, either antegrade or retrograde.

In summary, the detailed anatomic information provided by sonography usually allows one to adequately evaluate the kidney. However, the lack of pathophysiologic data is a limitation that should be considered in certain patients suspect for obstruction and compensated for by other functional or urodynamic studies. In the presence of renal failure or a history of severe reaction to contrast media, sonography invariably is the initial imaging modality of the urinary tract.

5.3.5 Computed Tomography

Computed tomography (CT) in the evaluation of suspected urinary obstruction usually is reserved for patients in whom intravenous urography, retrograde pyelography, and/or sonography fail to determine the presence, level, and nature of an obstructing lesion (TALNER 1990). This is often the case with pathologic processes extraneous to the urinary tract which cannot be directly imaged because of the nature and limitations of the imaging technique or when the renal function or extent of the obstruction is such that urography is not indicated and a retrograde study may not be helpful.

Minimal or mild hydronephrosis is not always easily detected on a nonenhanced CT study. As with sonography, blunted calyces. megacalyces, a capacious extrarenal pelvis, and peripelvic cysts may mimic hydronephrosis, leading one to the incorrect diagnosis of obstruction (AMIS et al. 1982b). Furthermore, distinguishing nonobstructive from obstructive hydronephrosis often is difficult on the nonenhanced study. The demonstration of parenchymal atrophy does not necessarily imply active chronic obstruction, since it is commonly seen in postobstructive kidneys or as the result of ureteral reflux. Nonenhanced CT is capable of detecting small to moderately sized perinephric urinomas, which usually result from the obstruction. If the obstruction is distal to the ureteropelvic junction, the dilated ureter often can be readily seen on nonenhanced CT images, because the water density urine filling the ureteral lumens is significantly different from the soft tissue density of adjacent structures (Fig. 5.11). Sometimes, a transition from water density to soft tissue density of structures within the ureteral lumen can be observed, indicative of a mural or intraluminal lesion, such as a ureteral neoplasm. The ureter distal to the lesion usually returns to a normal caliber and may not be identifiable. Ureteral calculi are readily demonstrable on a nonenhanced CT study; however, imaging of the entire ureteral length at 5- or 10-mm contiguous slices is not the most practical and appropriate

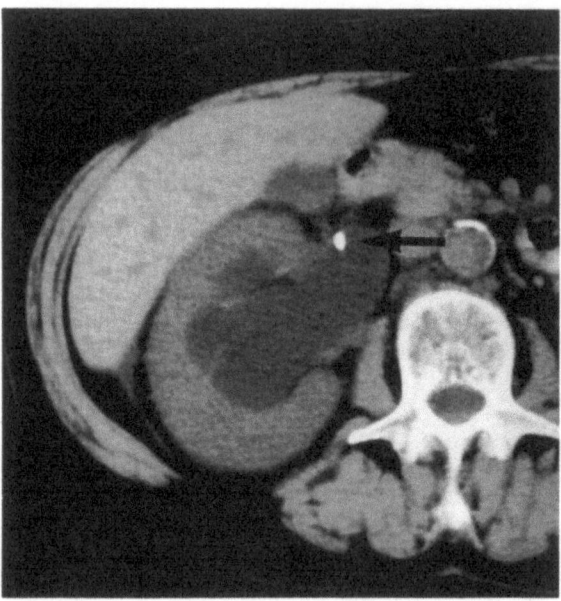

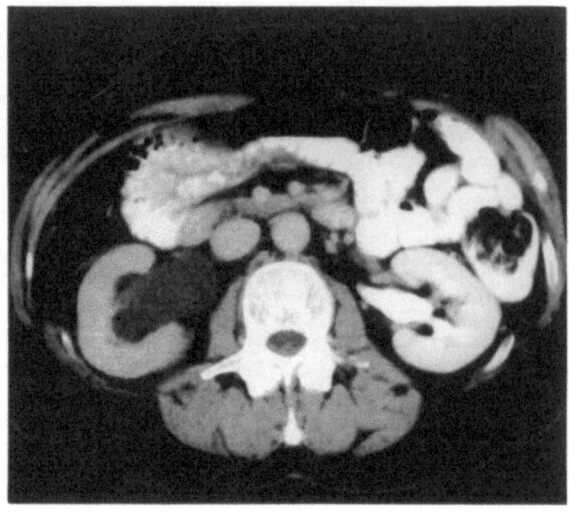

Fig. 5.11. Nonenhanced CT imaging of obstructive hydrone-phrosis. The moderately distended right collecting system is easily seen surrounded by the higher density renal parenchyma. The patient's stent *(arrow)* was clogged and had to be replaced

Fig. 5.12. Contrast enhanced CT study in patient with right ureteral obstruction secondary to colon carcinoma. The obstruction resulted in mild to moderate pyelocaliectasis and delayed pyelogram effect; however, the thickness of the renal parenchyma is near normal, suggestive of recent or incomplete obstruction

method of searching for ureteral calculi, even the radiolucent ones.

As in intravenous urography, but with greater detail, a dense nephrogram can be seen on CT in acute or subacute obstruction, following the intravenous administration of contrast medium. The visualized obstructive nephrogram is a composite of cortical and medullary opacification, the former occurring early on, the latter being somewhat delayed. The differential-time opacification of the cortical and medullary tissues can be easily demonstrated on serial CT images. The pyelocalyceal system often is minimally to markedly dilated, the latter in prolonged chronic urinary obstruction. The pyelogram effect is delayed from several minutes to many hours after the injection, depending on the severity and duration of the obstruction (Fig. 5.12). Since the patient usually is examined in the supine position, opaque urine is seen settling in the most dependent parts of the pyelocalyceal system, with "urine-contrast" levels being formed. An extrarenal pelvis undergoes considerable dilatation before the calyces begin to dilate, as opposed to an intrarenal pelvis, which undergoes dilatation simultaneous with and proportional to calyceal dilatation. It may be necessary to place the patient prone to hasten uniform opacification of the urine within the ureter proximal to the obstruction and determine the exact level of the le-

sion. If calculus disease is suspected, a nonenhanced CT study is indicated prior to any contrasted CT examination.

In summary, CT can be a useful diagnostic modality in the evaluation of urinary obstruction primarily in patients who cannot undergo urography or when the nature and extent of the obstructing lesion (neoplasm, retroperitoneal adenopathy or fibrosis) cannot be otherwise imaged or requires staging and, possibly, guidance for needle biopsy. Unusual cases of obstruction, such as complicated duplex collecting system or unilateral horseshoe kidney obstructions, infiltrating intrarenal disease obstructing one or more calyces selectively, and inflammatory abdominal disease extending to the retroperitoneum (pancreatitis, regional enteritis, appendicitis) may benefit from CT imaging (DALLA-PALMA et al. 1981; CRONAN et al. 1986). Another relative indication may be the search for radiolucent stones, which may or may not be associated with obstruction, when other modalities have failed or cannot be applied (Fig. 5.13).

5.3.6 Angiography

Several years ago, prior to the widespread use of cross-sectional imaging techniques, radionuclide

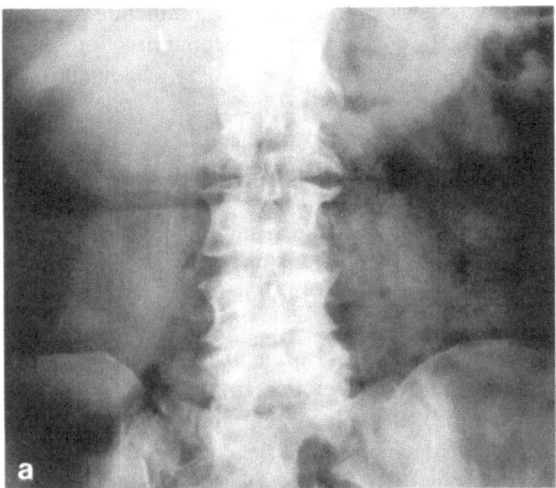

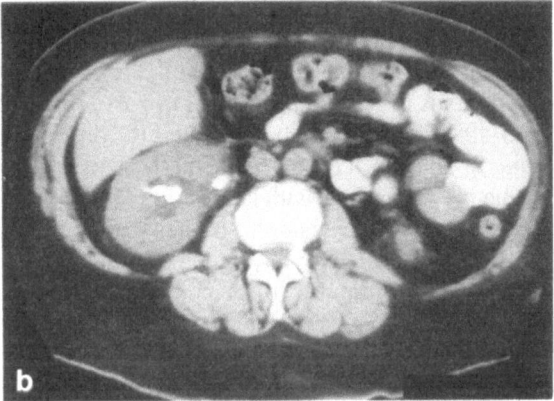

Fig. 5.13 a, b. Nonenhanced CT imaging of radiolucent (cystine) renal stones. **a** CT scan shows three radiodense stones in the right collecting system, one of them near or at the ureteropelvic junction. Mild caliectasis is present. The patient was post left nephrectomy and had a history of severe reaction to intravenous contrast material. **b** The plain film shows no opaque right renal stones. The right upper quadrant surgical clip is from previous cholecystectomy

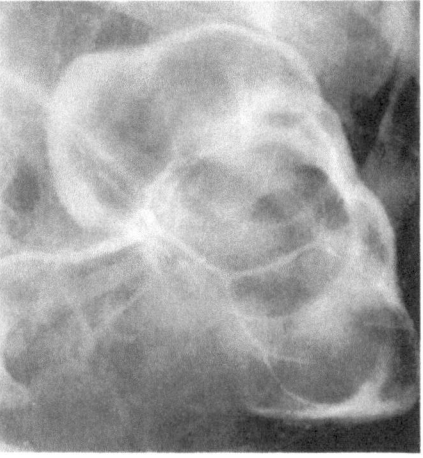

Fig. 5.14. Angiographic demonstration of advanced chronic obstruction secondary to left ureteral neoplasm. In addition to the marked parenchymal atrophy seen, the segmental renal arteries are splayed by the dilated pyelocalyceal system

monly reduced in caliber and number (Fig. 5.14). The segmental branches of the main renal artery are splayed by the dilated renal pelvis, while the more peripheral interlobar and arcuate branches are attenuated by the dilated calyces. In many patients with congenital or intermittent ureteropelvic junction obstruction, an accessory artery to the lower renal pole may be encountered. However, this supernumerary vessel, even when present, is not always the cause for such obstruction.

5.3.7 Radionuclide Renography

Radionuclide imaging in suspected or known urinary obstruction yields a wealth of information on renal function and urine drainage, but has serious limitations regarding the anatomy, morphology, and collecting system of the kidney. An exception to the latter fact may be static renal cortical imaging, which is equivalent or superior to nephrotomography and sonography in detecting parenchymal scarring (SMELLIE et al. 1985). The advantage of radionuclide renography over other radiologic modalities providing a similar type of physiologic and functional information lies with its ability to quantify differential renal function during the evolution of a disease process and monitor the results of treatment on serial studies. Additionally, radionuclide renography is widely used to estimate residual or recoverable renal function following relief of obstruction (CHIBBER et al. 1981; LANG and PRICE 1983; LANG 1984). Finally, the value of the modality is enhanced by induced diuresis to screen for suspected urinary obstruction

renography, and the radiologist's becoming familiar with antegrade pyelography, angiography was often used to evaluate a poorly functioning kidney secondary to vascular disease, infection, neoplasms, or obstruction. Today, the role of angiography in the evaluation of patients with obstructed kidneys is limited to the few indications where obstruction either coexists with or is caused by a pathologic process that requires preoperative or therapeutic angiographic investigation.

Angiographic examination in acute obstruction often shows normal vasculature and nephrogram with delayed pyelogram effect. In chronic obstruction there is reduced renal blood flow and parenchymal atrophy (SIEGELMAN and BOSNIAK 1965). The parenchymal branches of the renal artery are comin equivocal cases, mostly situations where the urinary tract is dilated but obstruction cannot be firmly established on clinical, urographic, or sonographic ground (O'REILLY et al. 1978, 1979; KOFF et al. 1979). It should be noted, however, that radionuclide renography also has certain limitations, as will become evident in the ensuing discussion.

The radionuclide renogram is a time versus radioactivity curve derived from the aorta and the kidney(s) following the intravenous bolus injection of the tracer. Continuous monitoring of the radionuclide from the time it appears in the cardiac blood pool to the time when most radioactivity has been washed out of the renal parenchyma and collecting system is provided by a gamma camera coupled with a computer. The radionuclide agent usually is a technetium-99m labeled substance, most often diethylenetriamine pentaacetic acid (DTPA) or glucoheptonate (GH). In the earlier years of radionuclide renography, iodine labeled agents were widely used for renal imaging (orthoiodohippurate). A limited use still exists for these agents, mostly labeled with I 123. DTPA is handled by glomerular filtration only, whereas the other agents undergo a more complex renal metabolism that involes glomerular filtration, tubular secretion, and binding to proteins. For the diuretic study, furosemide (Lasix) is given intravenously at an approximate dose of 0.5 mg/kg body weight, usually 15 min after the injection of the radionuclide.

The major clinical applications of radionuclide renal studies are in the evaluation of urinary obstruction and quantification/imaging of individual kidney function/parenchyma. Individual quantification usually is carried out in an effort to estimate existing or recovered (posttreatment) individual renal function in a noninvasive manner.

Many physiologic, anatomic, and technical factors may interfere with the performance and interpretation of the diuretic renogram. Adequate renal function is an essential requirement for obtaining a reliable response to the diuretic. It is estimated that an absolute GFR measurement below 20 ml/min usually renders the diuretic renogram uninterpretable (HJORTSO et al. 1988; UPSDELL et al. 1988). Poor radionuclide renal uptake and a relatively flat renogram curve, indicators of poor perfusion and/or function, lead to minimal or absent response to the diuresis, thus resulting in an indeterminate study.

The degree of hydronephrosis may also affect the interpretation of the diuretic renogram. A markedly dilated, atonic urinary tract may diminish or negate the diuretic response by virtue of its large volume,

which slows down the rate of radionuclide washout, as well as because of the poor renal function, which often results from the existing parenchymal atrophy (ABRAMSON et al. 1983) (Fig. 5.15).

Factors which may further influence the outcome of the study include patient hydration (adequate hydration is recommended), patient posture (prone, sitting, or upright imaging may be indicated in certain cases), ectopic location of a kidney, the intravenous injection of radionuclide and diuretic (inadvertent subcutaneous extravasation may occur), bladder on drainage (it enhances ureteral emptying and prevents interference from reflux in patients who reflux), and selection of appropriate regions of interest for generation of the correct time versus activity curves.

The normal renogram curve shows prompt uptake and rapid biphasic washout of the tracer. Diuretic renography in patients with dilated urinary tracts yields in general three types of curve (THRALL et al. 1981; TALNER 1990). The first is the obstructed pattern, showing continued increase or plateau in the activity over time, with lack of diuretic response. The second type is the nonobstructed pattern, where the increase in activity responds promptly or soon after diuretic stimulus by displaying a significant decrease in the curve. The third type is the equivocal or indeterminate pattern, where the initial increase in activity shows some response to diuresis but, clearly, not a sufficient response to exclude obstruction.

Investigators further have tried to estimate the renal transit time of different tracers in an effort to establish presence or absence of urinary obstruction or parenchymal disease. The renal transit time calculates the time it takes a radionuclide to reach the collecting system from the point of its arrival in the kidney via the renal artery. Problems arise with these calculations depending on the radionuclide used (different renal handling results in different transit times) and the presence of glomerular and/or tubular disease, both of which may affect the transit times in the absence of obstruction. If renal parenchymal disease is unlikely, the transit time correlates reasonably well with the presence or absence of obstruction.

The obstructed and nonobstructed renogram curves obtained during investigation of a dilated upper urinary tract usually reflect accurately the presence or absence of obstruction respectively. The indeterminate curve, observed in 10%–15% of cases reported in the literature, provides no reliable information on the status of the hydronephrotic urinary tract and further evaluation is mandatory (THRALL et al. 1981; O'REILLY 1986; LANG 1984). Correlation

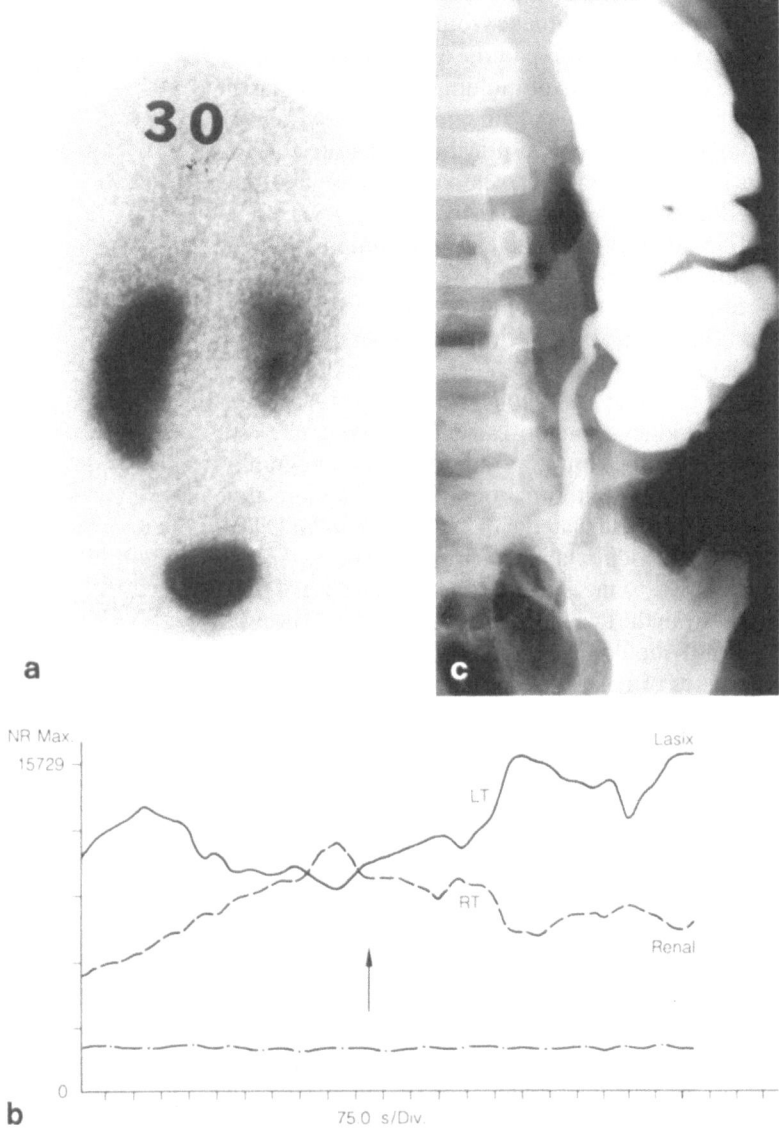

with clinical and additional radiographic data, such as a Whitaker test, or comparison with previous studies, when available, is helpful (KASS et al. 1985). Eliciting pain during the examination, similar to that experienced by symptomatic patients, often suggests the presence of obstruction. Asymptomatic patients with urinary tract dilatation and an equivocal renogram should be observed closely and restudied. A markedly dilated collecting system often complicated by coexisting poor renal function is a well-documented cause for false-positive results. The less frequently occurring false-negative diuretic renogram in compensated, high grade, and high intrapelvic pressure obstruction usually requires a Whitaker study. Since the patient often is symptomatic, a

Fig. 5.15 a–c. Marked hydronephrosis resulted in false-positive diuretic renogram in a 5-year-old boy post pyeloplasty for left ureteropelvic junction obstruction. **a** Thirty-minute posterior scan after Lasix diuresis (at 13 min) shows significant radionuclide retention in the left collecting system. **b** Computer generated time–activity washout curves show a left renogram more compatible with obstruction. **c** Pressure-flow study (Whitaker test) yielded normal differential pressures between the left collecting system and the bladder. The left ureter is patent. (PFISTER et al. 1986)

negative (nonobstructed) renogram should bot be the end of the investigation.

Quantification of individual kidney function is essential in the management of patients with long-standing obstruction in whom renal parenchymal atrophy has been documented by radiologic studies or suspected on clinical grounds. The decision to remove a kidney or repair the obstruction largely depends on the ability of radionuclides to estimate the existing, residual renal function. Similarly, quantifying the function of a previously obstructed postoperative kidney is a very good method of assessing the surgical outcome and detecting possible complications as early as possible. Another important issue resides in predicting the degree of functional renal recovery to be expected after relief of the obstruction, in an effort to decide wheter the patient will benefit from a corrective surgical procedure (CHIBBER et al. 1981; LANG 1984; PIEPZ et al. 1986). Individual kidney function can be approximately estimated during routine radionuclide renography. Noninvasive split functional indices and relative GFR can be calculated with technetium-99m DTPA or GH or iodine labeled hippuran, the latter also being used to measure relative effective renal plasma flow in the two kidneys (SCHLEGEL and HEMWAY 1976). It should be kept in mind that differences in estimates of renal function may exist between various tracers and should be expected since they may be handled in different mechanisms by the kidneys and measure separate parameters (glomerular vs tubular deficits) which are not equally depressed during obstruction (REHLING et al. 1988; LEAR et al. 1989; RUSSELL et al. 1988; WALLER et al. 1987).

Technetium-99m dimercaptosuccinic acids (DMSA) has been shown to be a reliable renal cortical imaging tracer has been extensively used as such in a variety of clinical conditions. Following its intravenous injection, DMSA concentrates mostly within the proximal renal tubules, while a fraction of it (up to 25%) is eliminated through the urine within the first several hours. Differential or relative renal uptake if DMSA can be estimated either as a split percentage between the two kidneys or as a percentage of the injected dose. It has been found that in patients with overall normal renal function, relative DMSA uptake correlates satisfactorily with differential GFR. Renal cortical DMSA uptake often is improved following repair of the obstruction, so that the preoperative uptake would be expected to be maintained or increased after surgical correction. A major technical error can occur when DMSA uptake is measured in obstructed kidneys, by including either the entire collecting system or part thereof in the region of interest. The tracer trapped in the obstructed urinary tract will then always overestimate renal parenchymal uptake; most centers now obtain a 24-h scintigram for measurements, at which time the collecting system may be relatively void of radio-

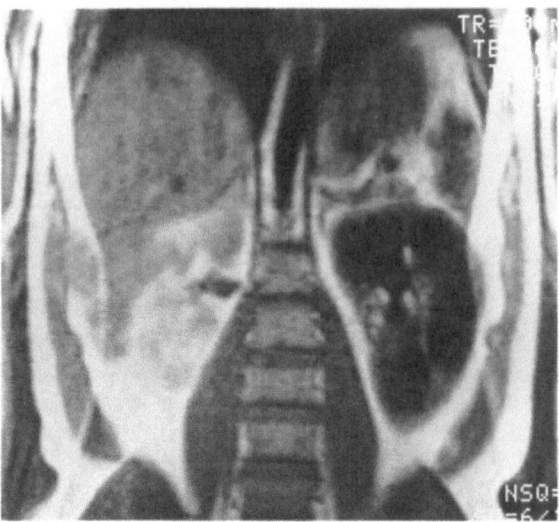

Fig. 5.16. Giant left hydronephrosis on T1-weighted spin-echo coronal MR imaging. There is marked dilatation of the low signal intensity left collecting system and enlargement of the overall renal size (same patient as in Fig. 5.6)

nuclide in the urine. Visual inspection of DMSA images early on or late in the presence of hydronephrosis may show a central photopenic area, corresponding to the dilated pyelocalyceal system. Renal parenchymal uptake may then be calculated more accurately.

5.3.8 Magnetic Resonance Imaging

Hydronephrosis may also be demonstrated by magnetic resonance (MR) imaging techniques. On T1-weighted spin-echo images the low signal intensity urine contrasts with the bright appearing renal sinus or retroperitoneal fat which surrounds the calyces, renal pelvis, or ureter (PAPANICOLAOU et al. 1986) (Fig. 5.16).

The differentiation of the corticomedullary junction is preserved in normal or briefly obstructed kidneys. Prolonged obstruction, as previously mentioned, produces parenchymal atrophy that can be demonstrated with MR imaging (KIKINIS et al. 1987). The corticomedullary junction is effaced in longstanding obstruction, but this is not a specific finding. Nonobstructive and obstructive dysfunction of transplant kidneys may be differentiated by MR imaging (VAN GANSBEKE et al. 1988). Perinephric urinomas also can be shown and differentiated from acute hemorrhage. P31 MR spectroscopy, similar to Tc-DMSA scintigraphy, may prove useful for the evaluation of renal effects of ureteral obstruction (VIGNERON et al. 1988).

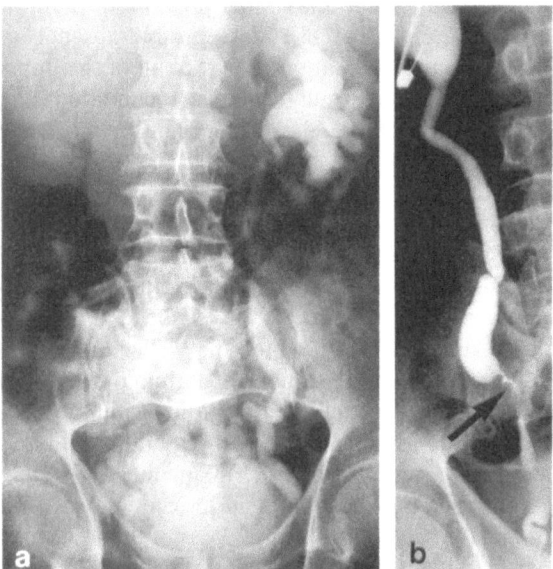

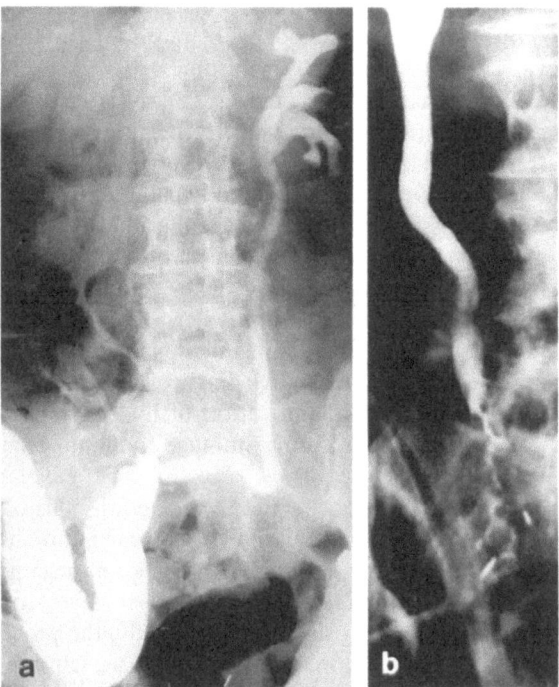

Fig. 5.17 a, b. Antegrade pyelography performed to define level and cause of right urinary obstruction. **a** Intravenous urogram shows an obstructed right kidney with delayed (absent) opacification of the calyceal system and ureter. **b** Antegrade pyelogram shows a tortuous, mildly dilated right ureter with a rather short stenotic segment overlying the sacroiliac joint *(arrow)*. Periureteral fibrosis was found at surgery from previous operation for colonic diverticulitis

Fig. 5.18 a, b. Antegrade pyelography in the investigation of urinary obstruction in a patient with ileal loop urinary diversion for bladder cancer. **a** Ileal loopogram shows prompt reflux into the left urinary system, but no retrograde opacification of the right urinary tract. **b** Antegrade pyelogram shows dilatation of the right urinary tract down to an abnormal ureteral segment near the ureteroileal anastomosis. Multiple filling mural defects and irregularity of the ureteral lumen indicated that recurrent transitional cell carcinoma was responsible for the obstruction

Coronal and sagittal images can be quite helpful in localizing the obstructing lesion along the ureteral course, especially in the presence of retroperitoneal disease. Calculi, however, are not visible on MR imaging unless they are large enough to appear as signal void foci.

5.3.9 Antegrade Pyelography and Pressure-Flow Study (Whitaker Test)

Percutaneous puncture of the intrarenal collecting system for antegrade pyelography remains the basic first step for assessment of upper urinary tract pathologic anatomy, pyeloureteral urodynamics, and many other interventional manipulations. Antegrade pyelography is a relatively simple, albeit an invasive, procedure with few complications; it usually can be performed rapidly under local anesthesia, yet the information gained is often crucial for patient management (PFISTER et al. 1986; RIEDY and LEBOWITZ 1986).

In most patients, the intravenous urogram will opacify the urinary tract adequately. In certain cases of hydronephrosis with possible obstruction or reduced renal function, the pathologic anatomy is inadequately defined, and antegrade or retrograde pyeloureterography is indicated (Fig. 5.17). Retrograde study through cystoscopic ureteric catheterization carries an increased risk of introduction of bacteria, may produce edema of the orifice, often utilizes general anesthesia, and may be very difficult to perform, such as in the male infant or those any age with urinary diversion.

Dilatation of part or all of the upper urinary tract may result from a diverse number of causes. However, in pediatric urology, the clinical entities encountered are usually distinctly different from those of the adult. Stones, urothelial tumors, and malignant (metastasis) or benign (retroperitoneal fibrosis) ureteral encasement are rare in children (Figs. 5.17, 5.18). Excluding vesicoureteral reflux, the majority of childhood disorders comprise congenital conditions of ureteropelvic junction obstruction, ureterocele, ectopic ureter, primary megaureter, and hydronephrosis associated with posterior urethral valves or the prune belly syndrome.

Occasionally, one or more renal cysts can pose difficult differential diagnostic imaging problems from or in association with hydronephrosis (CRONAN et al. 1982). Hydration, body habitus, and cutaneous dressing all may influence the ability of sonography to distinguish between peripelvic cysts and hydronephrosis in the adult or the multicystic kidney and hydronephrosis in the newborn. Antegrade needle puncture is a reliable investigative procedure in the event that a definitive diagnosis by imaging is not possible; the identification of hydronephrosis may warrant nephrostomy drainage and ultimate attempts at renal salvage.

Bleeding parameters are evaluated by history (anticoagulants, aspirin, known diathesis) and corrected, if abnormal. Antibiotics for gram-negative organisms should be administered if fever and possible pyonephrosis exist. Frequently, the procedure is performed on an outpatient basis. Children are sedated 30 min prior to the examination.

Patients are placed in the prone position on the fluoroscopy table, and the kidneys are localized by plain radiography, prior urography, concurrent urography, ultrasound, or CT, depending on the circumstances and individual preference.

Following antiseptic preparation and skin infiltration with a local anesthetic, usually 1–2 cm below the 12th rib to avoid pneumothorax, a 20- to 22-gauge needle is advanced toward the kidney. A direct posterior- or postero-oblique-directed tract into the lateral renal cortex is optimal for calyceal or infundibular entry. Puncture of the relatively bloodless Brödel's line region avoids the larger medially positioned blood vessels, avoids the free wall of the renal pelvis, and minimizes bleeding and urine leakage by providing a renal parenchymal seal about the needle and/or subsequent catheter if required.

Once a urine sample is obtained, the needle is attached to an extension tubing and manometer to determine the opening or resting pressure. If infection is suspected, opacification of the collecting system is indicated only after partial decompression by aspirating urine. This prevents overdistention, renal parenchymal or vascular backflow, and increased risk of bacteremia. In the absence of infected urine, full diagnostic evaluation of the pyeloureteral unit is performed after injection of contrast medium with fluoroscopy and spot and standard radiography.

Considerable information has been acquired in recent years toward an understanding of urine transport or urodynamics in the upper urinary tract and its relationship to bladder pressure in both the normal and diseased states. In the absence of ureteric reflux, dilatation of part or all of the upper urinary tract may result from several conditions that may or may not be related to current or active obstruction.

Hydronephrosis may be simulated by the calyceal dilatation of congenital megacalycosis or papillary necrosis of infection and analgesic abuse. The extrarenal pelvis is frequently a problem in determining wheter obstruction is associated. Generalized dilatation of the intrarenal collecting system and ureter may reflect only a high fluid output from the kidney, as in diabetes insipidus, which may or may not be associated with a structural renal alteration. The causes of a nonrefluxing megaureter are several and may result from intrinsic ureteral disease or may be related to abnormalities of the lower urinary tract, as in posterior urethral valves or the occult neurogenic bladder.

As a result of these and other factors, the evaluation of current or ongoing obstruction by glomerular filtered agents (urography and radionuclide renography with or without diuretic stimulation) or by contrast medium washout rates following retrograde or antegrade pyelography may be unreliable. Particularly difficult to evaluate by these techniques for the presence or absence of obstruction are cases in which renal function is poor, the ureter is markedly dilated with reduced elasticity, or dilatation of the upper urinary tract persists following surgical or percutaneous correction of an obstructing lesion and in those patients with concomitant high pressure bladders.

Opening or resting pressures of the kidney obtained at antegrade pyelography are helpful only when they are significantly elevated; in acute ureteral obstruction of a previously normal kidney, intrarenal pressures in excess of 50 cm H_2O are common. As obstruction continues toward a chronic state, intrarenal pressure falls toward lower levels owing to reduced renal function, altered compliance of the dilated ureter, and renal backflow with fluid absorption into venous and lymphatic channels.

The urodynamic antegrade pyelogram, ureteral perfusion test, or pressure-flow examination of Whitaker measures directly the ureters' resistance to a known flow rate with simultaneous pressure measurements of the kidney and bladder (WHITAKER 1979; PFISTER et al. 1982). The examination is performed with a small catheter in the bladder and a thin antegrade pyelogram needle in the kidney (Fig. 5.19). A simple water manometer is interfaced in each extension tubing to record pressure, while a variable rate pump continuously delivers diluted contrast media through the antegrade needle.

The Whitaker test is objective, reproducible, and unaffected by the kidney's glomerular filtrate rate. It provides excellent anatomic definition of the dilated ureter and permits direct measurement of the resistance to various known flow rates (10, 15, or 20 ml/min) along the course of the ureter, with controlled bladder volume and pressure. The lower urinary tract pressure reading is necessary to accurately interpret the upper tract pressures, particularly in the high pressure bladder of outlet obstruction or neurogenic disease, and after ureteral reimplantation or any other type of urinary diversion (loop) or undiversion.

The subtraction of absolute bladder pressure from absolute renal pressure provides the relative, differential, or step-off pressure (NEWHOUSE et al. 1981). At a flow rate of 10 ml/min, with the bladder empty, differential pressure below 13 cm H_2O is normal; arbitrary values of 14–20 cm H_2O indicate mild obstruction; 21–34 cm H_2O, moderate obstruction; and above 35 cm H_2O, severe obstruction.

When the normal bladder is filled, intravesical pressure rises, so that absolute renal pelvic pressure increases although the differential pressure drops. The kidney which is subjected to intermittent (reflux) or continuous (bladder obstruction) high absolute pressure above 20 cm H_2O is at risk even in the absence of ureteral obstruction defined as normal differential pressure between the kidney and bladder.

It is not clear at this time whether percutaneous ureteral perfusion answers all questions on the dilated upper urinary tract. Particularly bothersome is the compliant, atonic, and progressively distensible pyeloureteral unit which can accommodate large fluid volumes and thus dampen pressure response to induced flow rates. However, this type of upper tract abnormality may not be definitively evaluated by any single technique. Finally, the Whitaker examination must be carefully performed, without shortcuts or a slipshod approach if technical errors which alter pressure values are to be avoided.

5.4 Percutaneous Interventions

5.4.1 Introduction

After careful evaluation of the clinical, laboratory, and imaging data, the presence or absence of urinary obstruction can be ascertained in the vast majority of cases with confidence. In a small number of

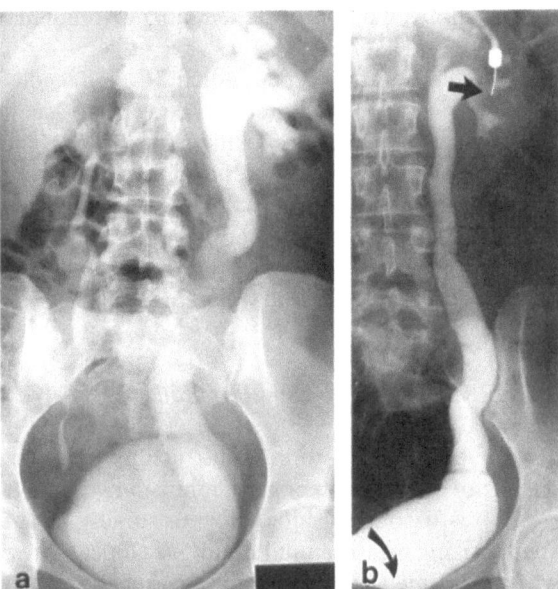

Fig. 5.19 a, b. Evaluation of left obstructing megaureter post reimplantation with the Whitaker test. **a** Preoperative intravenous urogram demonstrates a tortuous dilated left ureter and mild to moderate caliectasis. **b** The Whitaker test is performed with a bladder catheter in place *(curved arrow)* and a needle in the collecting system of the kidney *(arrow)*. The pressure-flow study yielded normal differential pressures between the kidney and the bladder

patients the exact nature and, possibly, level of the obstructing lesion may remain an enigma. Treatment planning commonly involves the efforts of a multidisciplinary team of physicians, with the radiologist being an integral member of it. Management choices are many and include among others, endoscopic (cystoscopic) stenting, percutaneous drainage, surgical exploration, or patient observation. The latter often is appropriate when the patient is afebrile, the obstructing lesion is a small (less than 5 mm) ureteral calculus very likely to pass spontaneously, or in a terminally ill patient in whom no intervention is indicated in the absence of infection. Surgical exploration is an option reserved for those likely to benefit from a single operative procedure that will relieve the obstruction and remove its cause as well. Most patients can be managed either temporarily or permanently with endoscopic or percutaneous drainage via stents or catheters. Both choices further allow the radiologist or the urologic access to the collecting system and ureter for further curative or palliative procedures. As a temporary treatment choice, retrograde or percutaneous stenting provides adequate drainage of the kidney(s), thus preserving renal function and relieving and/or preventing infection, while other therapeutic modalities are either applied (antibiotics, chemotherapy, radiation therapy) or pending (surgery).

The choice further depends on the overall medical condition of the patient (retrograde stenting usually requires general anesthesia), the nature and level of the obstructing process, the urinary tract anatomy (intestinal conduits, unusual ureteral reimplantations, bladder processes that render the ureteral orifice invisible, etc.), physician preference, and availability of certain skills and technology.

5.4.2 Patient Selection and Preparation

In the presence of urinary obstruction, the placement of a percutaneous nephrostomy catheter (PCN) is used as an alternative to surgery or as a temporizing measure until definitive clinical assessment and medical or operative correction can be carried out; it also acts as a means of gaining initial access to the urinary tract for secondary therapeutic percutaneous procedures (PFISTER et al. 1981; REZNEK and TALNER 1984) (Fig. 5.20). Critically ill patients can be managed by PCN at reduced morbidity and mortality; contributing factors to poor surgical risk of many patients include metabolic instability, limited cardiopulmonary reserve, and local tissue disruption due to recent surgery, radiation, local urine extravasation, or infection.

In preparation for nephrostomy, consultation with a urologist is advisable since most disorders requiring PCN are within their domain and certain severe untoward complications, while uncommon, may require urgent surgical exploration.

The procedure should be explained to the patient or his relatives so that informed consent can be obtained. The coagulation profile (prothrombin time, partial thromboplastin, platelet count, or others) is usually obtained. Careful inquiry is performed into any drugs which may affect bleeding parameters (SILVERMAN et al. 1990). Consulting with the hematologist may be required, especially in problem hemostasis cases where there is no overwhelming need for immediate action. Appropriate antibiotics and short acting analgesics or sedatives are obtained for administration as needed.

Placement of a peripheral intravenous line to simplify administration of medication or contrast media is desirable. While there is no absolute reason to give an antibiotic such as cefazolin routinely for simple PCN, its purpose is to decrease the development of septicemia (LANG 1983).

A commonly used antibiotic regiment in suspected bacterial pyonephrosis is ampicillin (1 g i.v.)

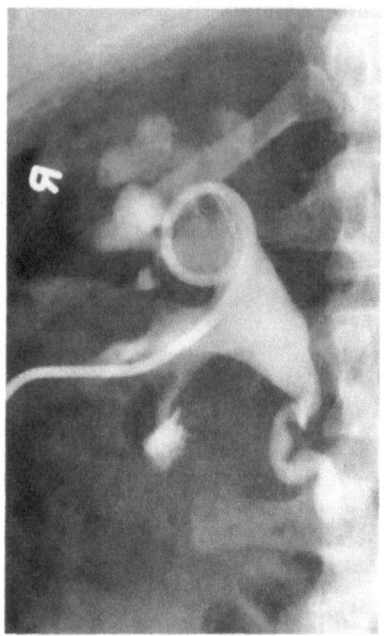

Fig. 5.20. Percutaneous nephrostomy tube placement for relief or urinary obstruction in patient with right ureteral compression by lymphoma (same patient as in Fig. 5.4). The 8-French pigtail catheter was placed using the Seldinger technique

combined with an aminoglycoside such as gentamicin or tobramycin (80 mg i.v. or i.m.) in a single dose 1 h prior to the procedure. The former is effective against enterococcus and most proteus bacteria while the latter is effective against all gram-negative organisms but not enterococcus. Fungal infection requires organism directed coverage; appropriate consultation is suggested.

Analgesic premedication such as diazepam and morphine or meperidine is desirable and those with severe azotemia often require less, being sedated by their disease. Intravenous midazolam in 0.5-mg increments and meperidine (25 mg) or fentanyl (in 25- to 50-μg increments) are administered intravenously as needed. Urinary diversion for simple obstruction and for pyonephrosis are the two most frequent indications for PCN.

In the sterile kidney, high grade obstruction may be tolerated up to 1 week before irreversible nephron damage begins; in most cases of ureteral calculi small stones will either pass within this time or the obstruction is incomplete. Conversely, obstruction with little likelihood of early reversal will require drainage. While drainage can be obtained by either the retrograde or the percutaneous route, the former method may be technically difficult or impossible in the case of obliterated ureteral orifice or ileal conduit. In other cases where other secondary manipulations are feasible, as in stricture dilatation or stone removal, the percutaneous approach may be the desirable choice.

Common causes of nonmalignant obstruction requiring temporary PCN, besides stones, are postsurgical ureteral anastomotic stenoses, vascular reconstruction with ureteral obstruction, gynecologic repairs with ureteral entrapment, and idiopathic retroperitoneal fibrosis. Percutaneous nephrostomy is also useful when the functional reserve capacity of an obstructed kidney is uncertain. Benign congenital lesions such as severe ureteropelvic junction and primary megaureter are common candidates for assessment of individual renal function and determination of subsequent management.

Frequently, malignancy from the bladder, prostate, uterus, colon, breast, and lung will result in renal obstruction. With the exception of lymphoma, many malignant obstructions have little expectation of response to further therapy. Sometimes, a PCN is necessary in kidneys obstructed by malignant disease, to ensure that all functional renal capacity is spared to help eliminate toxic chemotherapy agents that may benefit the patient. While palliative percutaneous drainage can be utilized, the technique should not be used merely to prolong life if the quality of living is intolerable (FALLON et al. 1980). In situations of malignant obstruction long-term nursing care is simplified by converting simple PCN to an external-type antegrade stent or, if this is not possible, to one of the extended nephrostomy catheter arrangements.

Regardless of the etiology, patients with urinary tract obstruction are at a high risk for pyohydronephrosis, which carries a high morbidity and mortality (YODER et al. 1983; LANG 1983, 1986). Percutaneous intervention in these febrile patients is safer than the operative approach; suspected bacterial and fungal pyonephrosis can be diagnosed by direct sampling of the urine from the kidney(s). If infected urine is present, PCN provides rapid decompression. However, even with antibiotic coverage, exacerbation of sepsis can occur even in the absence of performing diagnostic pyeloureterography; careful monitoring of the blood pressure and other vital signs is necessary during the first 12 h. Nephrostomy drainage affords a temporizing benefit while the septic episode subsides; additionally, many of these kidneys will demonstrate surprising ability for functional recovery. Subsequently, the obstruction lesion may then be treated surgically or percutaneously where feasible. In cases where malignant disease has caused obstruction, PCN frequently provides the definitive treatment.

5.4.3 Percutaneous Nephrostomy Placement

The first step towards establishing percutaneous access to the urinary tract is performing an antegrade pyelogram. The anatomic information gained from this study allows effective, safe, and appropriately positioned placement of the percutaneous catheter. Fluoroscopy or ultrasonography and, on occasion, CT can be used to guide the procedure. However, catheter placement and all guidewire–catheter–dilator manipulations and tube positioning in nondilated or mildly dilated collecting systems are best done with fluoroscopic control for safety purposes. Sonography allows accurate assessment of depth and is useful in pregnant women, those at risk from intravenous contrast media, and in nonopacifying kidneys or at the bedside. Considerable dilatation of the urinary tract usually makes sonographically guided PCN placement easier.

Antegrade pyelography and subsequent percutaneous nephrostomy are performed under fluoroscopic guidance with the patient in the prone or prone oblique (the side to be punctured elevated 30°) position. In either approach the tube tract is posterolateral through the renal parenchyma rather than directly into the free wall of the renal pelvis. The transparenchymal renal PCN tract ensures closer entry into the relative avascular zone (Brödel's line) of the kidney and provides a tight seal around the nephrostomy catheter. A transpelvic approach reduces intrarenal catheter length and increases the possibility of tearing the pelvis or lacerating a major vessel in the renal hilum. Most but not all urinomas and significant renal bleeding would appear to be related to entry attempts into the renal pelvis rather than the calyx or infundibulum.

Conversely in ectopic pelvic kidneys and renal transplants the approach is anterolateral (CURRY et al. 1984). In the latter situation it should be lateral to the surgical incision to avoid traversing the peritoneal cavity while in the former, CT guidance is helpful to document avoidance of bowel loops. In all other situations, however, the puncture site should be below the 12th rib to eliminate the potential for pneumothorax and damage to intercostal vessels, which are capable of significant bleeding.

For simple drainage, the point where the nephrostomy catheter enters the kidney is of limited concern; pressure is the same within all portions of the collecting system and the catheter will drain providing it is not wedged into the fornix of a calyx or a tapered obstructed segment of the ureter. If segmental obstruction is present, however, the obstructed calyx needs to be selectively drained or a percutaneous infundibuloplasty performed (LANG 1990).

The two main methods for placement of a PCN are the angiographic Seldinger and the trocar ones. Most other techniques are variations on these two types.

The Seldinger technique consists in placing a guidewire into the collecting system first, followed by dilatation of the fresh percutaneous track to the desired caliber and placement of the nephrostomy catheter (LEROY 1990). The usual working guidewire is a torque 0.038 in. and the size of the nephrostomy catheters vary from 8 to 12 French (Fig. 5.20). Larger catheters may be placed, if so indicated, usually for long-term or permanent nephrostomy drainage.

The trocar technique utilizes a pencil-point hollow metal trocar with a distal side hole that fits snuggly into a thin walled metallic or Teflon peelaway sheath cannula (PFISTER and NEWHOUSE 1979). The coned end of the trocar is noncutting and displaces the tissues rather than incising or lacerating them. Both parts together, the system is advanced on a straight trajectory through the retroperitoneal tissues and renal parenchyma until it reaches the collecting system. Upon puncturing a calyx, urine under pressure exits the lumen of the trocar through its distal side hole. The trocar is then removed and a fitting catheter is quickly fed into the collecting system and coiled in a calyx or the renal pelvis.

Once the PCN catheter is in the collecting system, adequate urine return and/or a nephrostogram confirm satisfactory tube position. The catheter then is attached to external drainage and is fixed to the skin with a variety of devices, from skin sutures to self-adhesive ostomy disks.

With some experience, PCN should be successful in 95%-98% of adult and pediatric cases. A lower initial success rate of 80%-90% will occur in nondilated collecting systems or when the target calyx or entire pyelocalyceal system is filled with calculus. In such situations the collecting system must be distended by a separate antegrade needle, a retrograde ureteral catheter, or intravenous contrast combined with a ureteral compression device.

Minor complications such as postnephrostomy transient bleeding or local transient extravasation are to be expected. Significant complications from PCN are relatively infrequent and substantially less than from surgical nephrostomy, where mortality ranges from 6% to 8%, and in septicemia, where it approaches 12% (PFISTER and NEWHOUSE 1979; HRUBY and MARBERGER 1984; KLEIST et al. 1984).

Complications requiring specific therapy or prolonged hospitalization occur in 3%-5% of PCNs compared to 25% of surgical nephrostomies. More serious complications of PCN such as pneumothorax, urinoma, and some catheter problems are avoidable while many of those involving bleeding are not.

The most frequent severe complication is hemorrhage; significant vascular trauma may occur in 1%-2% of patients (STABLES et al. 1978; PFISTER and NEWHOUSE 1979). Significant bleeding may be immediate, delayed with the formation of pseudoaneurysms and arteriovenous fistulae, or late when the nephrostomy catheter is removed or exchanged (COPE and ZEIT 1982).

Early arterial injury is manifest clinically by continued hematuria for 3-5 days and by the formation of new clots. Alternatively, if a drop in the hematocrit occurs, out of proportion to the observed hematuria, a perirenal hematoma should be suspected and investigated by CT or, if CT is unavailable, by ultrasound. If, after PCN, bleeding persists or spontaneously recurs, a renal arteriogram is indicated for diagnostic and therapeutic reasons since selective embolic occlusion of the involved segmental renal artery can be performed while preserving most of the remaining renal parenchyma.

About 15% of all patients undergoing PCN will have pyonephrosis; 1%-28% of these may have some exacerbation of their illness from tube placement; shaking chills, increased temperature, and transient hypotension are not infrequent while septic shock can occur in 7% of cases. Elevation of intrarenal pressure from contrast injection during PCN increases the risk of bacteremia and/or fungemia and should be avoided (LANG 1986).

The patient with a PCN in place requires regular monitoring of the function and tolerance of the catheter. The vast majority of patients tolerate the catheter very well and continue to live a relatively normal life-style. The patient or his/her family can be instructed to take care of the PCN and recognize a pending or existing malfunction or complication. Regular change of the catheter is advised every 2-3 months when long-term drainage is anticipated; exchange of the initial catheter for a self-retaining tube in this situation may be desirable.

5.4.4 Percutaneous Ureteral Stenting

Depending on the cause of the obstruction and the nature of the percutaneous or endoscopic intervention (curative or palliative), a PCN can be converted into a ureteral stent, either internal or with external access (FRITZSCHE and LANG 1990). The stent provides adequate internal drainage and, therefore, can be clamped at the skin level. However, it can be accessed easily for additional procedures or removal. The internal stent is indicated more often, mainly for patient comfort and elimination of the small risk of contaminating the urinary tract by keeping it exposed to the body surface.

5.4.5 Percutaneous Drainage of Fluid Collections

A urinoma or perinephric abscess may form concomitantly with urinary obstruction and should be drained simultaneously with the collecting system by placing a percutaneous retroperitoneal catheter in addition to the PCN. Sonography or CT are useful imaging adjuncts in evaluating the perinephric and retroperitoneal space in patients with urinary obstruction who may have developed a fluid collection concomitantly. Small urinomas can be left alone and expected to resolve completely provided the obstruction is relieved. Larger urinomas or infected retroperitoneal fluid collections require individual drainage in addition to treating the obstruction.

Seldinger or trocar introduced catheters under sonographic or fluoroscopic guidance provide satisfactory drainage (LANG 1990: YODER and PFISTER 1990). Repeat sonography or CT is advised prior to removing a catheter. Discovery of undrained collections may require catheter manipulation or insertion of additional drainage tubes. Longstanding retroperitoneal urinomas run the risk of becoming infected and inducing a fibrotic reaction, which may lead to ureteral strictures.

A ureteral stent can be placed for short- or long-term drainage. Percutaneous placement as opposed to retrograde insertion usually occurs in patients too sick to undergo a relatively short intraoperative procedure or when an attempt at retrograde stenting has failed either because of technical problems (anatomy of the urinary tract, lack of appropriate instrumentation) or because the tight obstruction has prevented such a stent placement. The percutaneous procedure may be performed as a primary study or, after urinary decompression with a PCN, at a later day, the latter often in patients with pyonephrosis, where a shorter procedure is initially preferable.

References

Abramson SJ, Papanicolaou N, Treves S, Colodny AH, Bauer SB, Retik AB (1983) Diuretic renography in the assessment of urinary tract dilatation in children. Pediatr Radiol 13:319

Amis ES Jr, Hartman DS (1984) Renal ultrasonography 1984: a practical overview. Radiol Clin North Am 22:315

Amis ES Jr, Cronan JJ, Pfister RC, Yoder IC (1982a) Ultrasonic inaccuracies in diagnosing renal obstruction. Urology 19:101

Amis ES Jr, Cronan JJ, Pfister RC (1982b) Pseudohydronephrosis on noncontrast computed tomography. J Comput Assist Tomogr 6:511

Berdon WE, Levitt SB, Baker DH, Becker JA, Uson AC (1970) Hydronephrosis in infants and children - value of high dosage excretory urography in predicting renal salvageability. AJR 109:380

Better OS, Arieff AJ, Massry SG, Kleeman CR, Maxwell MH (1973) Studies on renal function after relief of complete unilateral ureteral obstruction of three months' duration in man. Am J Med 54:234

Bigongiari LR, Davis RM, Novak WG, Wicks JD, Kass E, Thornbury JR (1977) Visualization of the medullary rays on excretory urography in experimental ureteric obstruction. AJR 129:89

Brock WA, Nachtscheim DA, Kaplan GW, Talner LB (1979) Congenital giant hydronephrosis. Urol Radiol 1:67

Cattell WR (1970) Excretory pathways for contrast media. Invest Radiol 5:473

Cattell WR, Fry IK, Spencer AG, Purkiss P (1967) Excretion urography-1. Factors determining the excretion of Hypaque. Br J Radiol 40:561

Chibber PJ, Chisholm GD, Hargreave TB, Merrick MV (1981) 99m Technetium DMSA and the prediction of recovery in obstructive uropathy. Br J Urol 53:492

Cooke GM, Bartucz JP (1974) Spontaneous extravasation of contrast medium during intravenous urography. Clin Radiol 25:87

Cope C, Zeit RM (1982) Pseudoaneurysms after nephrostomy. AJR 139:255

Cremin BJ, Stables DP (1971) Striation (longitudinal mucosal folds) in the upper urinary tract. II. A comparison of findings in children and adults. Br J Radiol 44:445

Cronan JJ, Amis ES Jr, Yoder IC, Kopans DB, Simeone JF, Pfister RC (1982) Peripelvic cysts: an imposter of sonographic hydronephrosis. J Ultrasound Med 1:229

Cronan JJ, Amis ES, Zeman RK, Dorfman GS (1986) Obstruction of the upper-pole moiety in renal duplication in adults: CT evaluation. Radiology 161:17

Curry NS, Cochran S, Barbaric ZL, Schabel SJ, Pagani JJ, Kangarloo H, Diament H, Gobian R, Vujic J (1984) Interventional radiologic procedures in the renal transplant. Radiology 152:647

Dalla-Palma L, Rocca-Rossetti S, Pozzi-Mucelli RS, Rizzato G (1981) Computed tomography in the diagnosis of retroperitoneal fibrosis. Urol Radiol 3:77

Davidson AJ (1985) The widened pelvocalyceal system. In: Davidson AJ (ed) Radiology of the kidney. W.B.Saunders, Philadelphia, p 537

De Maeyer P, Simons M, Oosterlinck W, De Sy WA (1982) A clinical study of 99m technetium dimercaptosuccinic acid uptake in obstructed kidneys: comparison with the creatinine clearance. J Urol 128:8

Dunbar JS, Nogrady MB (1970) The calyceal crescent - a roentgenographic sign of obstructive hydronephrosis. AJR 110:520

Earlam RJ (1967) Recovery of renal function after prolonged ureteric obstruction. Br J Urol 39: 58

Elkin M (1963) Radiological observations in acute ureteral obstruction. Radiology 81: 484

Elkin M, Boyarsky J, Martinez J, Kaplan N (1964) Physiology of ureteral obstruction as determined by roentgenologic studies. AJR 92: 291

Fallon B, Olney L, Culp DA (1980) Nephrostomy in cancer patients. To do or not to do? Br J Urol 52: 237

Friedland GW, Axman MM, Love T (1971) Neonatal "urinothorax" associated with posterior urethral valves. Br J Radiol 44: 471

Fritzsche P, Lang EK (1990) Stenting of the ureter – antegrade and retrograde techniques. In: Pollack HM (ed) Clinical urography. W. B. Saunders, Philadelphia, p 2767

Gillenwater JY (1986) The pathophysiology of urinary obstruction. In: Walsh PC, Gittes RF, Perlmutter AD, Stamey TA (eds) Campbell's urology, 5th edn. W. B. Saunders, Philadelphia, p 542

Griscom NT, Kroeker MA (1973) Visualization of individual papillary ducts (ducts of Bellini) by excretory urography in childhood hydronephrosis. Radiology 106: 385

Hann L, Pfister RC (1982) Renal subcapsular rim sign: new etiologies and pathogenesis. AJR 138: 51

Hinman F (1934) Pathogenesis of hydronephrosis. Surg Gynecol Obstet 58: 356

Hjortso E, Fugleberg S, Nielsen L (1988) Diuresis renography in patients with reduced renal function. Dan Med Bull 35: 294

Hodson CJ, Craven JD (1966) The radiology of obstructive atrophy of the kidney. Clin Radiol 17: 305

Hruby W, Marberger M (1984) Late sequelae of percutaneous nephrostomy. Radiology 152: 383

Hyde I, Wastie ML (1971) Striation (longitudinal mucosal folds) in the upper urinary tract. I. Striated renal pelvis and ureter. Br J Radiol 44: 445

Jaenicke JR (1970) The renal response to ureteral obstruction: a model for the study of factors which influence glomerular filtration pressure. J Lab Clin Med 76: 373

Kass EJ, Majd M, Belman AB (1985) Comparison of the diuretic renogram and the pressure perfusion study in children. J Urol 134: 92

Kerr WS Jr (1954) Effect of complete ureteral obstruction for one week on kidney function. J Appl Physiol 6: 672

Kikinis R, von Schulthess GK, Jager P, Durr R, Bino M, Kuoni W, Kubler O (1987) Normal and hydronephrotic kidney: evaluation of renal function with contrast enhanced MR imaging. Radiology 165: 837

Kleist H, Pettersson S, Wikholm G (1984) Percutaneous nephropyelostomy: a procedure not without complications. Scand J Urol Nephrol 18: 71

Koff SA, Thrall JH, Keyes JW Jr (1979) Diuretic radionuclide urography: a non-invasive method for evaluating nephroureteral dilatation. J Urol 122: 451

Lang EK (1984) The effect of percutaneous nephrostomy drainage upon renal plasma flow rate in the partially obstructed kidney. AJR 142: 236

Lang EK (1985) Antegrade ureteral stenting for dehiscence, strictures and fistulae. AJR 143: 795

Lang EK (1986) Percutaneous nephrostomy in treatment of renal infection. Estratto da Progressi in Radiologia. Uroradiologia 193

Lang EK (1990a) Renal, perirenal and pararenal abscesses: Percutaneous drainage. Radiology 174: 109

Lang EK (1990b) Percutaneous infundibuloplasty. AJR (in print)

Lang EK, Price EW (1983) Redefinition of indications for percutaneous nephrostomy. Radiology 147: 419

Lear JL, Feyerabend A, Gregay C (1989) Two compartment, two sample technique for accurate estimation of effective renal plasma flow, theoretical development and comparison with others methods. Radiology 172: 431

LeRoy AJ (1990) Percutaneous nephrostomy: techniques and instrumentation. In: Pollack HM (ed) Clinical urography. W. B. Saunders, Philadelphia, p 2725

Maillet PS, Pelle-Francoz DP, Laville M, Gay F, Pinet A (1986) Nondilated obstructive acute renal failure: diagnostic procedures and therapeutic management. Radiology 160: 659

Moncada R, Wang JJ, Love L, Bush I (1968) Neonatal ascites associated with urinary outlet obstruction (urine ascites). Radiology 90: 1165

Morin ME, Baker DA (1979) The influence of hydration and bladder distension on the sonographic diagnosis of hydronephrosis. J Clin Ultrasound 7: 192

Newhouse JH, Pfister RC (1979) The nephrogram. Radiol Clin North Am 17: 213

Newhouse JH, Pfister RC, Hendren WH, Yoder IC (1981) Whitaker test after pyeloplasty: establishment of normal ureteral perfusion pressures. AJR 137: 223

Nimmo MJ, Merrick MV, Allan PL (1987) Measurement of relative renal function. A comparison of methods and assessment of reproducibility. Br J Radiol 60: 861

O'Reilly PH (1986) Diuresis renography 8 years later: An update. J Urol 136: 993

O'Reilly PH, Testa HJ, Lawson RS, Farrer DJ, Edwards EC (1978) Diuresis renography in equivocal urinary tract obstruction. Br J Urol 50: 76

O'Reilly PH, Lawson RS, Shields RA, Testa HJ (1979) Idiopathic hydronephrosis – the diuresis renogram: a new non-invasive method for assessing equivocal pelvioureteral junction obstruction. J Urol 121: 153

Papanicolaou N, Hahn PF, Edelman RR et al. (1986) Magnetic resonance imaging of the kidney. Urol Radiol 8: 139

Pfister RC, Newhouse JH (1978) Radiology of ureter. Urology 12: 15

Pfister RC, Newhouse JH (1979) Interventional percutaneous pyeloureteral techniques. II. Percutaneous nephrostomy and other procedures. Radiol Clin North Am 17: 341

Pfister RC, Yoder IC, Newhouse JH (1981) Percutaneous uroradiologic procedures. Semin Roentgenol 16: 135

Pfister RC, Newhouse JH, Hendren WH (1982) Percutaneous pyeloureteral urodynamics. Urol Clin North Am 9: 41

Pfister RC, Papanicolaou N, Yoder IC (1986) Diagnostic morphologic and urodynamic antegrade pyelography. Radiol Clin North Am 24: 561

Piepz A, Ham HR, Roland JH (1986) Technetium-99m DMSA imaging and the obstructed kidney. Clin Nucl Med 11: 389

Platt JF, Rubin JM, Ellis JH (1989) Distinction between obstructive and nonobstructive pyelocaliectasis with duplex Doppler sonography. AJR 153: 997

Rabinowitz JG, Keller RJ, Wolf BS (1966) Benign peripelvic extravasation associated with renal colic. Radiology 86: 220

Rascoff JH, Golden RA, Spinowitz BS, Charytan C (1983) Nondilated obstructive nephropathy. Arch Intern Med 143: 696

Rehling M, Lund JO, Moller ML, Lange P, Gammelgaard J, Clausen E, Trap-Jensen J (1988) Acute unilateral obstruction of ureter. Disparity in divided renal function calculated from I-131 hippuran and 99mTc-DTPA renography. Urology 31: 51

Reznek RH, Talner LB (1984) Percutaneous nephrostomy. Radiol Clin North Am 22: 393

Riedy MJ, Lebowitz RL (1986) Percutaneous studies of the upper urinary tract in children, with special emphasis on infants. Radiology 160: 231

Russell CT, Thorstad BL, Yester MV, Stutzman M, Dubovsky EV (1988) Quantitation of renal function with technetium 99m MAG3. J Nucl Med 29: 1931

Salomon LL, Lanza FL (1962) Glomerular filtration in the rat after ureteral ligation. Am J Physiol 202: 559

Schlegel JU, Hemway SA (1976) Individual renal plasma flow determination in 2 minutes. J Urol 116: 282

Scola FH, Cronan JJ, Schepps B (1989) Grade I hydronephrosis: pulsed Doppler US evaluation. Radiology 171: 519

Shea TE, Pfister RC (1969) Opacification of the gallbladder by urographic contrast media: reflection of an alternate excretory pathway. AJR 107: 763

Siegelman SS, Bosniak MA (1965) Renal arteriography in hydronephrosis. Radiology 85: 609

Silverman SG, Mueller PR, Pfister RC (1990) Hemostatic evaluation before abdominal interventions: an overview and proposal. AJR 154: 233

Smellie JM, Ransley PG, Normand ICS, Prescol N, Edwards D (1985) Development of new scars: a collaborative study. Br J Urol 290: 1957

Sokoloff J, Talner LB (1973) The heterotopic excretion of sodium iothalmate. Br J Radiol 46: 571

Stables DP, Ginsberg NJ, Johnson ML (1978) Percutaneous nephrostomy: a series and review of the literature. AJR 130: 75

Talner LB (1990) Urinary obstruction. In: Pollack HM (ed) Clinical urography. W. B. Saunders, Philadelphia, p 1613

Thomsen HS, Hvid-Jacobsen K, Meyerhoff HH, Nielsen SL (1987) Combination of DMSA-scintigraphy and hippuran renography in unilateral obstructive nephropathy. Improved prediction of recovery after intervention. Acta Radiol 28: 653

Thrall JH, Koff SA, Keyes JW Jr (1981) Diuretic radionuclide renography and scintigraphy in the differential diagnosis of hydroureteronephrosis. Semin Nucl Med 11: 89

Upsdell SM, Leeson SM, Brooman JC, O'Reilly PH (1988) Diuretic-induced urinary flow rates at varying clearances and their relevance to the performance and interpretation of diuresis renography. Br J Urol 61: 14

Uson AC, Levitt SB, Lattimer JK (1969) Giant hydronephrosis in children. Pediatrics 44: 209

Van Gansbeke D, Segebarth C, Toussaint C, Matos C, Gevenois PA, Kinnaert P, Struyven J (1988) Nonobstructive kidney transplant dysfunction: Magnetic resonance evaluation. Br J Radiol 61: 473

Vaughan ED Jr, Sweet RE, Gillenwater JY (1973) Unilateral ureteral occlusion: pattern of nephron repair and compensatory response. J Urol 109: 979

Vigneron DB, Tzika AA, Hricak H, Price DC, Bretan P, Aboseit S, Mueller S, James TL (1988) Complete and partial ureteral obstruction: evaluation of renal effects with P31 MR spectroscopy and Tc-DMSA scintigraphy. Radiology 168: 645

Waller DG, Keast CM, Fleming JS, Ackery DM (1987) Measurement of glomerular filtration rate with technetium 99m DTPA: comparison of plasma clearance techniques. J Nucl Med 28: 372

Weiss RM (1976) Initiation and organization of ureteral peristalsis. Urol Survey 26: 2

Weiss RM, Wagner ML, Hoffman BF (1967) Localization of the pacemaker for peristalsis in the intact canine ureter. Invest Urol 5: 42

Weller MH, Miller K (1973) Unusual aspects of urine ascites. Radiology 109: 665

Whitaker RH (1975) Some observations and theories on the wide ureter and hydronephrosis. Br J Urol 47: 377

Whitaker RH (1979) An evaluation of 170 diagnostic pressure flow studies of the upper urinary tract. J Urol 121: 602

Wilson DR (1975) Mechanisms of post-obstructive diuresis in the solitary hydronephrotic kidney of the rat. Clin Sci Mol Med 48: 167

Wilson DR (1977) Renal function during and following obstruction. Ann Rev Med 28: 329

Wilson DR, Honrath U (1976) Cross-circulation study of natriuretic factors in postobstructive diuresis. J Clin Invest 57: 380

Wilson DR, Know W, Hall E, Sen AK (1974) Renal sodium- and postassium-activated adenosine triphosphate deficiency during post-obstructive diuresis in the rat. Can J Physiol Pharmacol 52: 105

Yoder IC, Pfister RC, Lindfors KK, Newhouse JH (1983) Pyonephrosis: imaging and intervention. AJR 141: 735

Yoder IC, Pfister RC (1990) Drainage of abscess and fluid collections. In: Pollack HM (ed) Clinical urography. W. B. Saunders, Philadelphia, p 2818

6 Therapy for Caculus Disease of the Kidney and Ureter

Andrew J. LeRoy

CONTENTS

6.1 Introduction 177
6.2 Radiologic Evaluation of the Calculus Patient . 177
6.3 Historical Overview
    of Surgical Calculus Therapy 179
6.4 Modality Review 180
6.4.1 Extracorporeal Lithotripsy 180
6.4.1.1 Technique 180
6.4.1.2 Applications 181
6.4.1.3 Advantages 182
6.4.1.4 Disadvantages 182
6.4.2 Transurethral Ureteroscopy 182
6.4.2.1 Technique 183
6.4.2.2 Advantages 184
6.4.2.3 Disadvantages 184
6.4.3 Percutaneous Stone Removal 184
6.4.3.1 Technique 184
6.4.3.2 Applications 185
6.4.3.3 Advantages 185
6.4.3.4 Disadvantages 185
6.4.4 Open Surgery 186
6.4.4.1 Technique 186
6.4.4.2 Advantages 186
6.4.4.3 Disadvantages 186
6.5 Clinical Applications: Summary 187
6.6 Future Trends 187
    References 187

6.1 Introduction

Symptomatic calculi in the collecting systems of the kidney and ureter are a frequent cause of patient morbidity in modern medical practice. The disability and discomfort associated with this disease are well documented and have influenced the progressive development of successful treatment modalities. Improved diagnostic modalities have also been developed, using increasingly more sophisticated laboratory and imaging procedures. Research has continued into the underlying etiologies of calculus formation and the appropriate therapy directed at inhibiting initial calculus development.

Andrew J. LeRoy, M.D., Associate Professor of Diagnostic Radiology; Mayo Medical School and Consultant in Diagnostic Radiology, Mayo Clinic, 200 1st Street, SW, Rochester, MN 55905, USA

The overall beneficiaries of this continuing medical progress are the many patients who are annually afflicted with renal calculus disease.

The role of diagnostic radiology in the care of stone patients has also expanded. While the initial diagnostic evaluation of patients with renal and ureteral calculi begins with a standard medical history and physical examination, imaging procedures are frequently required for absolute verification of the suspected clinical diagnoses. The rapid technological developments which have been introduced into diagnostic radiology practice in the past decade have all had an impact on the imaging evaluation and therapy of such patients. Standard radiologic examinations are essential in the initial diagnosis of calculus disease, in therapy planning, in assessing the results of therapy, and in subsequent evaluations of renal calculus status (Van Arsdalen et al. 1990).

6.2 Radiologic Evaluation of the Calculus Patient

The radiologic evaluation of patients with renal calculus disease has traditionally consisted of the plain abdominal radiograph (KUB film), coupled with localized body section radiography of the kidneys. This examination defines the number, size, intrarenal location, and interval change of the renal or ureteral calculi present. Small calyceal stones may be easily overlooked on plain film examination of the abdomen and are much better defined on renal body section radiographs. Although small uric acid calculi may not be identified with this technique, nearly all other calculi larger than 1–2 mm can be readily identified because of their inherent radiopacity. Because this examination is relatively inexpensive, easily reproducible, and widely available, it serves as the baseline evaluation for renal calculi in most clinical practices.

Although it has become much less important in the diagnosis of many urologic diseases, excretory urography continues to be a primary component of calculus patient evaluations. This examination readily identifies the location of calculi within the col-

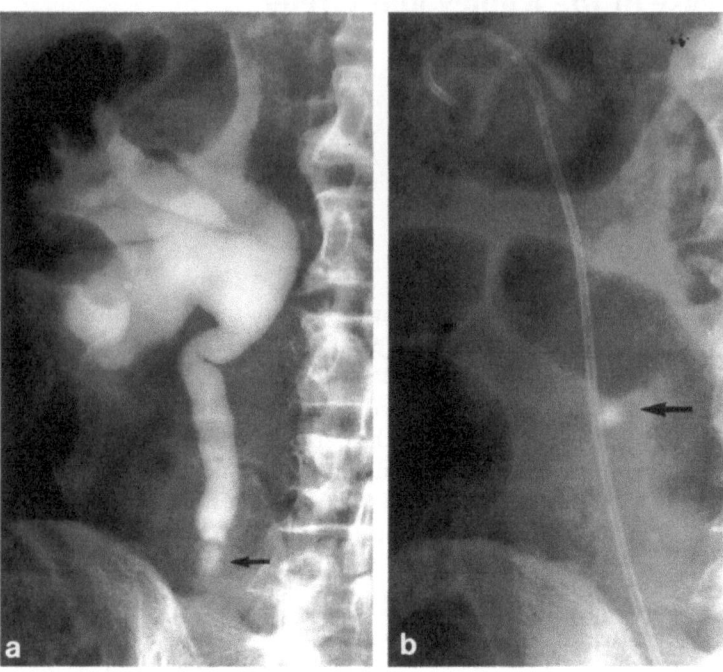

Fig. 6.1. a Urogram film of the right kidney and ureter shows a moderately obstructing 6 mm upper ureteral stone *(arrow)*. **b** Prior to EL therapy, a ureteral stent has been inserted to assist in stone *(arrow)* localization and allow subsequent fragment passage down the ureter along the stent

lecting systems, provides a baseline level of function in the stone-bearing kidney, and outlines anatomic features essential to therapy decisions (Fig. 6.1). Urography also helps exclude the coexistence of other renal diseases, such as renal mass lesions, which would alter the planned therapeutic approach. Because urograms are widely available, relatively noninvasive, reproducible, and reasonably priced, they may be repeatedly obtained on individual calculus patients of follow changing stone status and the results of therapy.

The introduction of high quality diagnostic ultrasonography into medical practice within the last 15 years has greatly enhanced the noninvasive imaging of the renal calculus patient. Most authors feel that real-time ultrasound examination of the kidneys, specifically to identify renal calculi, is a valuable clinical procedure, although very operator dependent. The reliability of ultrasound detection of renal calculi varies with the size and location of the stone as well as the degree of collecting system dilatation (Fig. 6.2). Most calyceal and renal pelvic calculi can be identified by dedicated ultrasonographers. The detection of most ureteral calculi, however, is very difficult, primarily due to the inability to identify accurately small stone reflections within the retroperitoneal adipose tissues surrounding the ureter. Perhaps the more important aspect of the renal ultrasound examination in the calculus patient is the detection of stone-induced alterations in the kidney or collecting systems. Ultrasonography

has become the standard for noninvasive diagnosis of collecting system dilatation. The status of the renal parenchyma is evaluated well with ultrasound, detecting potential renal atrophy, focal parenchymal loss due to calculus disease, or concurrent renal mass. Ultrasonography may identify perinephric processes as well as the surrounding retroperitoneal structures, although some experts prefer computed tomography (CT) in this setting, especially in obese patients. The preoperative delineation of urographically identified collecting system filling defects is an important clinical problem which can often be resolved with a simple ultrasound examination. In this setting, small stones can usually be readily differentiated from nonshadowing soft tissue urothelial neoplasms.

The development of CT of the kidneys has also changed the evaluation of the stone-afflicted patient in the past decade. Because of its great inherent sensitivity to differences in contrast of adjacent tissues, CT is the most sensitive modality available to detect the presence of renal or ureteral calculi. Some attempts have been made to distinguish between physiochemically different types of renal calculi based upon their CT densities using standard CT

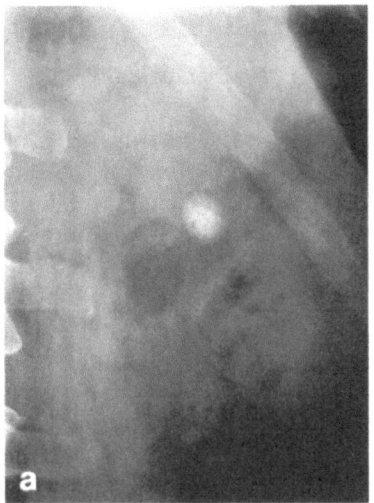 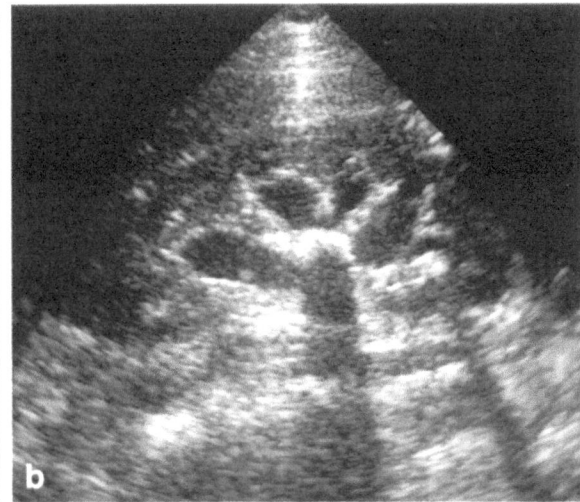

Fig. 6.2. **a** Plain film of the left kidney displays a 1 cm central renal pelvic calculus in an ideal EL patient. **b** Ultrasound examination readily demonstrates the shadowing pelvic calculus and the calyceal dilatation present due to the ureteropelvic junction stone. A tiny shadowing lower pole calculus is also present

techniques. Although all renal calculi are equally white on CT scans of the kidneys displayed at the usual CT window and level settings, the actual CT densities do vary considerably. Because there is considerable overlap in the range of CT densities between various stone types, this utilization of CT has not developed into a clinically practical examination. The application of CT scanning to calculus patients instead has evolved in a manner similar to that of diagnostic ultrasound. CT scans excel at defining the status of the renal parenchyma, the perinephric space, and the entire retroperitoneum. Urographic filling defects in the collecting systems are well seen with CT, which has a marked advantage over ultrasound in ureteral evaluation and in obese patients.

Magnetic resonance imaging (MRI) of the kidneys has primarily been clinically applied to distinguish medullary-cortical differences and renal masses in a multiplanar display format. No definitive work has been published in the area of renal calculus disease. Because of the inherently poor MRI signal of renal calculi on proton imaging sequences, it is not anticipated that MRI will have any rapid application to the calculi themselves. The potential of MRI to evaluate renal functional impairment due to previous or existing calculus disease awaits further investigation.

6.3 Historical Overview of Surgical Calculus Therapy

The therapeutic modalities available for the treatment of symptomatic renal and ureteral calculi have changed tremendously in the past decade. A variety of effective treatment modalities have evolved which must be individually applied to each patient and clinical situation to best effect the dual goals of stone treatment: first, complete removal of the symptomatic renal calculi, and second, minimization of patient disability.

Despite the proliferation of treatment modalities, the underlying indications for the treatment of renal and ureteral calculi have not changed over the past several decades. Most clinicians still believe that small asymptomatic calyceal stones need not be treated except in special circumstances. The classical indications for surgical intervention in the therapy for renal and ureteral calculi are (a) obstruction, (b) infection, (c) hematuria, and (d) symptomatic pain. An equally important part of all treatment modalities is the physiochemical evaluation of the symptomatic calculus and subsequent proper patient counseling to prevent future stone recurrence.

Historically, open flank surgery under general anesthesia has been the accepted treatment of urolithiasis since the development of these methods in the 1880s at the start of the modern era of surgery. In the 2000 years prior to that, sporadic historical reports described the manual expression of stone material through spontaneous flank wounds. These were invariably cases of pyohydronephrosis with severe renal impairment and advanced calculus disease. In the past century of standard flank surgery, a wide variety of innovative surgical techniques were developed to deal with the myriad variations in stone disease presentations. Simple stone disease was treated with surgical pelviolithotomy, ureterolithotomy, or nephrolithotomy, while complex stone disease led to development of extended or anatrophic nephrolithotomy. These surgical procedures were widely practiced and successful, and were essential components in the development of modern urologic surgery.

Percutaneous removal of renal and ureteral calculi was developed in the late 1970s and early 1980s as an alternative to standard surgical flank procedures. This method offered greatly reduced patient disability and ease of repeated access into the collecting systems to effect complete stone removal, and generated a wide variety of complex endourologic procedures. The close cooperation of interventional radiologists and urologists was essential for the evolution of most of these procedures.

Concurrent to the introduction of percutaneous techniques, retrograde transurethral ureteroscopy was developed by the urologic community. As ureteroscopic equipment has evolved and improved, diagnostic and therapeutic indications have extended to position ureteroscopy as a prime component of the urologic armamentarium. Modification of percutaneous stone fragmentation devices and ureteral access techniques have extended the utilization of the relatively inexpensive ureteroscopic equipment into all components of the urologic community. Retrograde ureteroscopy is now widely considered the prime modality for the treatment of calculi in the mid and lower ureter.

Extracorporeal lithotripsy is the most recently clinically introduced technology for treatment of symptomatic calculi. Readily accepted by the general population because of limited postprocedural patient disability, as well as by the urologic community because of its relatively simple operational requirements and utility, extracorporeal lithotripsy has become the dominant form of therapy of renal calculi in those populations in which this technology is available. Continuing evolution of lithotripsy technology has allowed the development of minimal anesthesia outpatient therapy and a continued reduction in patient disability associated with extracorporeal lithotripsy treatment.

6.4 Modality Review

6.4.1 Extracorporeal Lithotripsy

Extracorporeal lithotripsy (EL) of renal and ureteral calculi was developed by CHAUSSY and associates in Munich in conjunction with the Dornier Company, with research beginning in the mid 1970s and the first patient applications in 1980 (CHAUSSEY 1982). Following initial success, the Dornier term "extracorporeal shock wave lithotripsy" (ESWL) spread rapidly throughout Europe and North America. The vast majority of clinical studies have been performed using the Dornier HM-3 lithotriptor (DRACH et al. 1986).

Because of the success of the initial Dornier model, numerous other manufacturers have developed alternative lithotriptors. Variations in stone localization equipment, shock wave initiation devices, wave transmission systems, and other technical components have produced multiple lithotriptors with varying potentials (RASSWEILER et al. 1988). Clinical applications of all of these models are underway and the results of these trials, as well as market forces, will determine future trends in this equipment.

6.4.1.1 Technique

All extracorporeal lithotriptors function by generation of a shock wave outside the patient's body. This wave is focused onto the symptomatic calculus, which has previously been identified with either x-ray or ultrasound localization. Sequential shock waves are delivered to the stone until adequate fragmentation is achieved. Depending upon the power source and application, patient anesthesia requirements vary from the initial use of general anesthesia with the HM-3 model to only intravenous sedation or no anesthesia on newer machines. After the targeted stone is completely fragmented, the small pieces pass spontaneously down the ureter and through the bladder. Up to 50% of patients require no pain medication during the 2 days to 2 months during which the stone fragments pass.

The currently available lithotriptors can be divided into groups based upon their shock wave generation device (Table 6.1). The original Dornier HM-3 system used an underwater spark-gap electrode, a reliable and powerful shock wave source. This technology has been modified by other manufacturers but it continues to be popular and prominent technology. The second type of shock wave

Table 6.1. Lithotriptor manufacturers listed by shock wave generation device

Spark gap	Piezoelectric	Electromagnetic
Direx (Israel)	Diasonics (USA)	Siemens (FRG)
Dornier (FRG)	EDAP (France)	Stortz (FRG)
Medstone (USA)	Wolf (FRG)	
Northgate (USA)		
Technomed (France)		

generation system employs an electromagnetic source, commercially available in lithotriptors from Siemens and Storz. The third form of shock wave generation is the use of piezoceramic technology in which a field of crystals are simultaneously stimulated, producing a focused shock wave at a defined distant point. The power output of all these technologies is variable, dependent upon the input energy provided to the source.

The focal point volume of the focused shock wave is determined by the underlying shock wave generation system and the focusing apparatus. The piezoelectric systems produce the smallest focal point volume and considerable power gain at the focal point. Conversely, the spark-gap systems produce a considerably larger focal zone, but this power diffusion is compensated for by the underlying superior input power of this technology. While the end result of calculus fragmentation may not significantly differ between these technologies, the focal volume size inversely corresponds to the precision of stone localization which is required to most effectively use each generated shock wave.

Accurate renal calculus localization is achieved on these lithotriptors by either ultrasonographic or x-ray applications. The original Dornier system used a biplane fluoroscopic localization system which was precise, reliable, and easily learned. In an effort to reduce cost and overall equipment size and complexity, this system has been abandoned by most current manufacturers. One alternative is the use of a single movable x-ray source (C-arm type fluoroscope). Many manufacturers have alternatively chosen ultrasound localization for their guidance systems. The use of an inline, real-time ultrasound probe for constant fragmentation monitoring and focal point alignment permits extremely accurate localization and optimizes the utilization of each shock wave. Unfortunately, many investigators have noted that ultrasound localization of small stones within the kidney can be very difficult and extremely time consuming. Localization of stones in the ureter and even at the ureteropelvic junction is often impossible with ultrasonography, even in experienced hands. The determination of degree of stone frag-

mentation using ultrasound guidance also requires considerable experience and may be impossible in larger stones which generate considerable shadowing debris, obscuring the operating field. Significant-sized fragments generated during EL may spontaneously move to other portions of the collecting systems not immediately in the viewing plane of the ultrasound guidance system and subsequently may be obscured by small fragments, requiring retreatment at a later session.

6.4.1.2 Applications

Extracorporeal lithotripsy is the most widely used method of stone therapy for renal and upper ureteral stones. Nearly all stones can be fragmented into sufficiently small pieces that they will spontaneously pass. Following accurate stone localization, serial shock waves (2000–4000, depending on shock wave generator type) are used in a dedicated fragmentation session. Treatment of larger stones or more resistant stones such as those made of calcium oxalate monohydrate may require several sessions to achieve adequate fragmentation.

The use of ureteral stents to assist the effectiveness of lithotripsy is widely practiced. The accurate localization of small ureteral stones is improved by prelithotripsy retrograde placement of a ureteral stent. The subsequent stone fragment passage along the indwelling ureteral stent while maintaining renal function and minimizing patient disability permits outpatient lithotripsy therapy in many institutions. The retrograde passage of a ureteral stent often will dislodge a small ureteral stone back into the renal pelvis, where experience has shown these stones will fragment more readily. If a ureteral stone is not displaced by the stent, most urologists attempt to pass the stent around the stone and up the ureter. This was originally thought to be necessary to enhance stone fragmentation by providing a fluid layer around the stone, but recent experience has questioned this nearly universal need for stenting (PREMINGER et al. 1989). In those lithotriptors which use fluoroscopic localization, radiolucent urinary calculi are best visualized with contrast media injected through retrograde stents placed prior to lithotripsy.

In addition to stent placement, other accessory procedures are occasionally required to complete EL therapy. Retrograde ureteroscopy is performed to remove large obstructing fragments or the accumulation of a column of stone fragments in the lower ureter *("Steinstrasse")* (WEINERTH et al. 1989). Rare patients will require percutaneous nephrostomy placement for urinary diversion because of ureteral obstruction by stone material. While transient ureteral obstruction does not require collecting system decompression, the development of clinical signs of sepsis mandates intervention for fragment-caused obstruction.

6.4.1.3 Advantages

Extracorporeal lithotripsy is highly effective at fragmentation of nearly all calculi. Because of the rapidly decreasing anesthesia requirements for these treatments and the associated minimal patient post-procedural disability, patient acceptance of this technology is enthusiastic (LINGEMAN et al. 1986a). Long-term studies of lithotripsy results show that about 70% of all treated patients will be stone free at 3-6 months. In ideal patients with renal pelvic stones of 1 cm or less in size, the eventual stone-free rate will be over 90%. The lithotriptors themselves have been shown to be mechanically reliable with relatively simple operational requirements.

6.4.1.4 Disadvantages

Despite its minimal invasiveness and rapid clinical acceptance, the limitations of this technique must be constantly reevaluated. The major clinical disadvantage of EL relative to other stone treatment modalities is that the stone fragments are still within the renal collecting system at the conclusion of the procedure. This requires natural passage of these fragments out of the collecting systems, whereas with all other treatment modalities the stone is actively removed by the operator during the procedure. This results in a 30% residual stone fragment rate in treated patients, even with adequate fragmentation and retreatments. Factors associated with decreased rates of complete stone discharge include (a) increasing stone size, (b) initial lower pole position of the treated stone, (c) collecting system anomalies, (d) incomplete initial stone fragmentation, and (e) particularly fragmentation-resistant stone composition such as cystine.

Lithotripsy of large stones produces a large fragment burden, leading to multiple episodes of ureteral obstruction *(Steinstrasse)* requiring repeated interventions (Fig. 6.3). Because many patients seek extracorporeal therapy but fail to return for post-procedural clinical follow-up, ureteral obstruction and renal atrophy resulting from unrecognized and asymptomatic incomplete stone passage can occur.

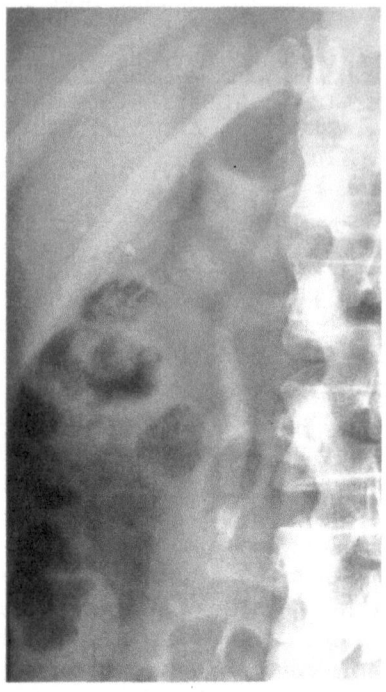

Fig. 6.3. After EL of a 2.5 cm right pelvic calculus, a large collection of stone fragments has accumulated in the upper ureter. Because of repeated episodes of ureteral obstruction, the fragments were eventually removed from the lower ureter with ureteroscopy

Acute perinephric bleeding or subcapsular hematomas develop in about 1% of treated patients (Fig. 6.4). Although initial studies have shown acute interrenal hemorrhage and segmental renal dysfunction in a large percentage of treated kidneys, long-term renal complications appear to be minimal, with only a very small incidence of new systemic hypertension or renal function deterioration. Rare patient mortality from lithotripsy has been reported, due to either cardiopulmonary collapse or acute hemorrhage. Extracorporeal lithotriptors continue to be expensive medical technology. The initial cost of 1-2 million dollars (U.S.) must be balanced against the relatively limited number of patients on whom this technology can be clinically applied.

6.4.2 Transurethral Ureteroscopy

Transurethral ureteroscopy was developed as a natural extension of cystoscopy by urologists. With the improvement of lens systems and accessories, rigid and flexible ureteroscopes ranging from 8 to 14 French were developed which can be passed in a retrograde manner through nearly all ureteral orifices and subsequently up the ureter (LYON et al.

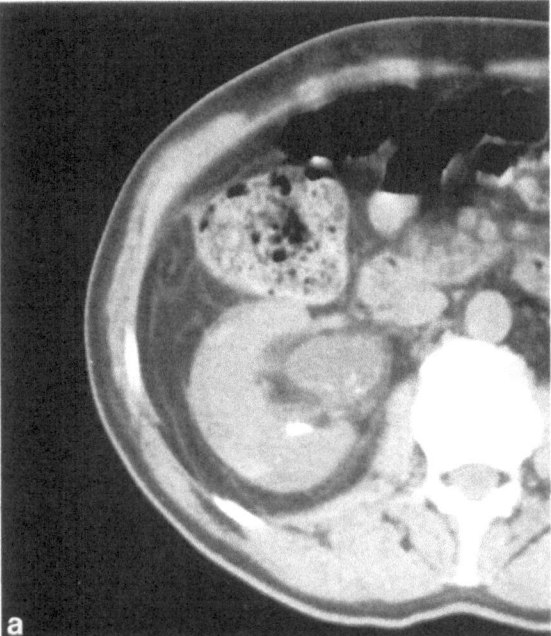

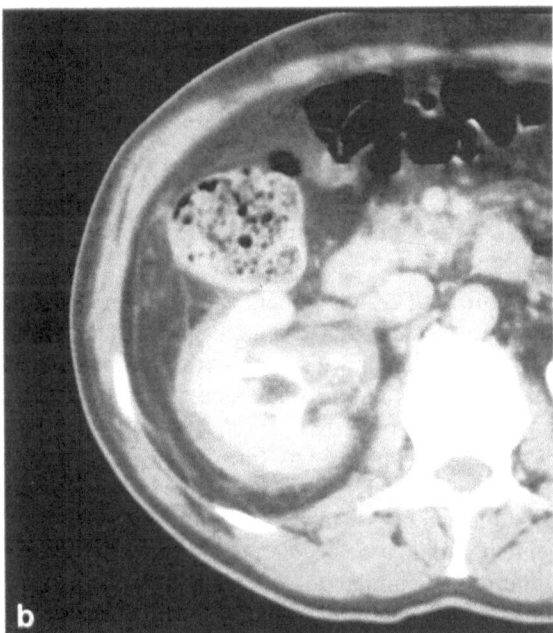

Fig. 6.4. a CT scan of the right kidney immediately after EL shows a small acute subcapsular hematoma and multiple stone fragments in the renal pelvis and calyx. **b** Contrast-enhanced CT at the same level also demonstrates an intrapelvic blood clot containing stone debris. A repeat examination at 1 month was normal

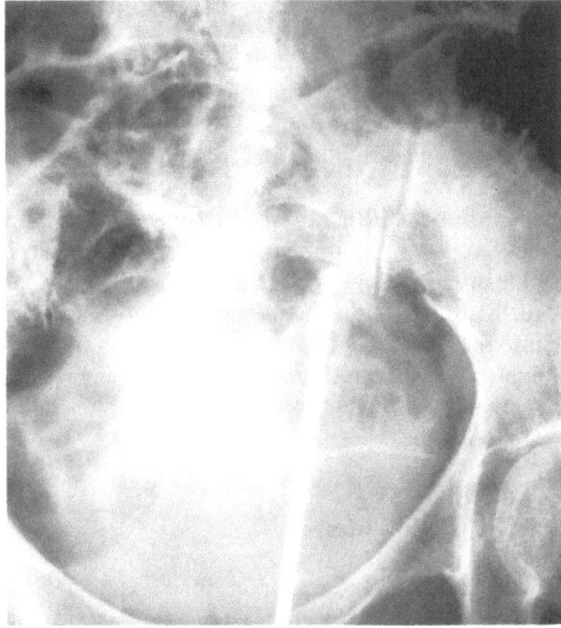

Fig. 6.5. Ultrasonic lithotripsy of a left lower ureteral stone under direct ureteroscopic visualization facilitates subsequent extraction of the resultant stone debris

1984). Fragmentation and extraction of ureteral stones with this technology is highly successful and has become widely available.

6.4.2.1 Technique

Following routine cystoscopy and location of the appropriate ureteral orifice, small ureteroscopes may be passed directly into the ureteral orifice and then up the ureter. Larger endoscopes (10–14 French) require dilatation of the ureteral orifice with either balloon catheters or progressive dilators prior to ureteroscopic insertion. While small ureteral calculi can be directly extracted, larger stones require initial fragmentation using either ultrasonic, electrohydraulic, or laser lithotripsy (Fig. 6.5). Because of instrumentation limitations, lithotripsy through the commercially available small flexible ureteroscopes is limited to laser or electrohydraulic lithotripsy. In addition to stone therapy, ureteroscopy facilitates urothelial biopsy or diagnostic endoscopy throughout the ureter. Access to the upper ureter and renal pelvis with the rigid scopes is often limited by the natural anatomy of the ureter, but the diagnostic flexible ureteroscopes frequently can be advanced into the pelvis for complete renal endoscopy. The progressive development of smaller endoscopes has permitted the treatment of pediatric calculus patients ureteroscopically as well.

6.4.2.2 Advantages

Ureteral calculus removal with ureteroscopy is highly successful. The available fragmentation techniques facilitate the removal of stones of nearly any
size or composition from the ureter (HUFFMAN
1988). Postprocedural patient disability is minimal
with outpatient therapy possible in selected cases.
Ureteroscopic equipment has become widely available and is relatively inexpensive ($ 30000 U.S.). Its
further applications as the extension of endoscopy
into the remainder of the urinary tract for diagnostic
evaluation in non-calculus-bearing patients greatly
increases the potential utilization of ureteroscopic
technology.

6.4.2.3 Disadvantages

Transurethral ureteroscopic stone extraction is a
safe procedure in experienced hands, with the major
complications of ureteral tears occurring infrequently once experience has been achieved (STACKL and
MARBERGER 1986). Large dense calcium oxalate
monohydrate ureteral stones can still present somewhat of a problem in fragmentation and removal.
Ureteral anatomic abnormalities or previous surgical or radiation therapy may preclude adequate endoscopic manipulations. General anesthesia is required for these therapeutic endoscopic procedures,
but this may slowly change as smaller and more
manipulable endoscopes and fragmentation devices
become available.

6.4.3 Percutaneous Stone Removal

Percutaneous stone removal developed in the late
1970s in Europe and quickly spread to the United
States and then worldwide. Because of greatly decreased postoperative patient disability when compared to standard flank incision surgical procedures, this therapeutic method proliferated until EL
was developed. A wide variety of instrumentation
for percutaneous procedures was developed, facilitating complex endourologic stone therapy procedures. Because of EL limitations, primarily with
treatment of large calculi, percutaneous stone removal methods are still actively used.

6.4.3.1 Technique

Percutaneous stone removal procedures are technically demanding on the operating physicians. Suc-

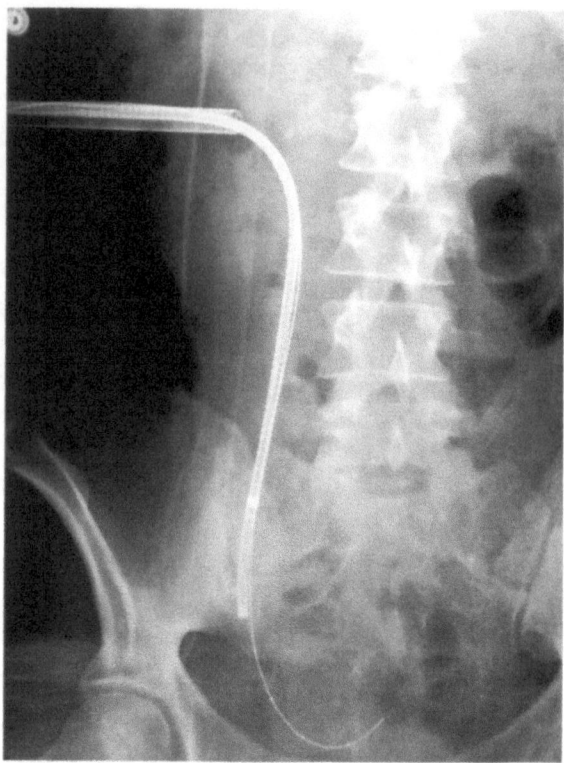

Fig. 6.6. Following percutaneous removal of a large right renal
pelvic calculus, a flexible endoscope was advanced through
the working sheath and then down the ureter to remove a
coexisting ureteral calculus

cessful final results depend upon the initiation of
safe and accurate access into the renal collecting systems. In most clinical situations this is performed via
percutaneous nephrostomy access, although a few
authors have preferred the retrograde ("inside-out")
creation of nephrostomy tracts. Antegrade percutaneous of the collecting systems and subsequent tract
establishment is widely successful, primarily using
angiographic-type needle-guidewire-catheter access
equipment, similar to other radiologic procedures
such as angiography and related interventional procedures. The access to particular stone configura-
tions requires a thorough knowledge of renal anatomy and access techniques. Once percutaneous
access to the renal collecting systems and ureter has
been established, the tract may be acutely dilated to
the appropriate size for subsequent stone removal.
In most cases, this requires dilatation to up to
30 French, using a variety of commercially available
equipment. This includes balloon dilatation catheters, progressive angiographic-type fascial dilators,
concentric polyurethane dilators, or metal telescop-
ing dilators. All these systems are safe, effective, and
can be used under local anesthesia in the appropri-

ate medical setting. Once the tract is adequately dilated, stone removal can proceed. Fluoroscopic removal of renal or upper ureteral stones using baskets through a sheath is very effective but limited to stones less than 1 cm in size. Most percutaneous stone removal is performed endoscopically, facilitating fragmentation of large stones prior to removal, using either ultrasonic, electrohydraulic, or laser lithotripsy (Fig.6.6). Ultrasonic lithotripsy has been shown to be particularly effective since it not only fragments the stone but also simultaneously extracts the stone debris produced. Following complete stone removal, the tract is tamponaded and the collecting system drained with a large caliber nephrostomy tube. This also maintains the tract for future access in case of unexpected retained stone fragments at the conclusion of the initial procedure.

6.4.3.2 Applications

Percutaneous stone removal techniques can be applied to nearly any clinical calculus presentation. Because EL is ideally suited to the majority of clinical presentations, percutaneous lithotripsy in the current stone therapy setting is used as the initial mode of therapy in only about 10% of patients. These are patients whose body habitus precludes EL or those who have large stone volumes in whom EL fragmentation would subsequently require multiple additional interventional procedures to help clear the stone debris. Percutaneous stone removal is also the ideal backup procedure for failed primary ureteroscopic or EL procedures (LeRoy et al. 1987).

6.4.3.3 Advantages

Since complete stone removal is frequently possible with percutaneous procedures, it is clinically advantageous to use these techniques when complete stone removal is required, such as with infected stones. Percutaneous stone removal also facilitates the correction of underlying anatomic abnormalities such as in those patients with isolated calyceal stones behind an infundibular stricture, ureteropelvic junction obstruction requiring endopyelotomy, or distal ureteral obstruction limiting lithotripsy fragment passage (Fig.6.7). The wide variety of equipment available for percutaneous procedures permits the treatment of nearly all clinical stone presentations (Segura et al. 1985).

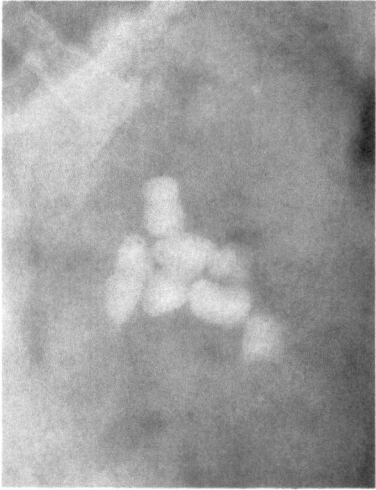

Fig.6.7. Multiple faceted renal pelvic calculi are present in a patient who has a recurrent ureteropelvic junction obstruction. At the time of the percutaneous calculus removal procedure, an endopyelotomy was also performed on the postoperative stricture

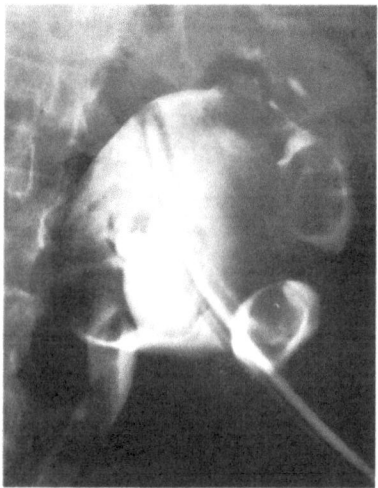

Fig.6.8. Considerable blood clot fills the left renal pelvis on this nephrostogram 3 days after a percutaneous stone removal procedure. In this patient, bleeding spontaneously ceased and intervention was no required

6.4.3.4 Disadvantages

The technical requirements of percutaneous access and subsequent stone removal procedures now may be somewhat limited to larger stone referral centers because of the limited number and complexity of these residual patient presentations. Major complications of percutaneous stone removal procedures include (a) sepsis (usually with struvite stone manipulation), (b) collecting system perforation, and

(c) hemorrhage (LANG 1987). In less than 0.5% of patients, massive life-threatening bleeding may occur from iatrogenic arteriovenous fistulas or renal pseudoaneurysms, requiring angiographic evaluation and embolization (Fig. 6.8; see also Fig. 7.35). Injury to adjacent organ systems can occur with inadvertent access tract creation or endoscopic manipulation. Long-term studies have shown no major impact on renal parenchymal anatomy or function from percutaneous procedures in the majority of patients (MARBERGER et al. 1985). The physician time commitment required for percutaneous procedures is considerably greater than for EL. Postoperative patient disability is also usually greater with percutaneous stone removal than with extracorporeal procedures.

6.4.4 Open Surgery

Flank incision open surgical procedures have been a standard component of urologic therapy for stone disease since the 1880s. The wide availability of other less debilitating procedures has reduced open surgical cases to less than 2% of all stone therapy (BOYLE et al., to be published). Nevertheless, to effect complete stone removal, open surgical intervention continues to be a necessary part of the available options for stone therapy.

6.4.4.1 Technique

Standard flank incisional surgery has changed little in the last 30 years. The classic techniques of nephrolithotomy, pelviolithotomy, and ureterolithotomy are all well described and standard operations. The most widely practiced stone surgical procedure now is that of extended or anatrophic nephrolithotomy for removal of large staghorn calculi. The open surgical results and residual stone fragment rate compare favorably with extensive repeated endourologic and extracorporeal combination procedures. In those patients who require complete stone removal, such as those with infected stones, this procedure continues to be a necessary part of the surgical armamentarium. However, patients with marked unilateral renal deterioration coupled with extensive stone disease are often best treated with nephrectomy.

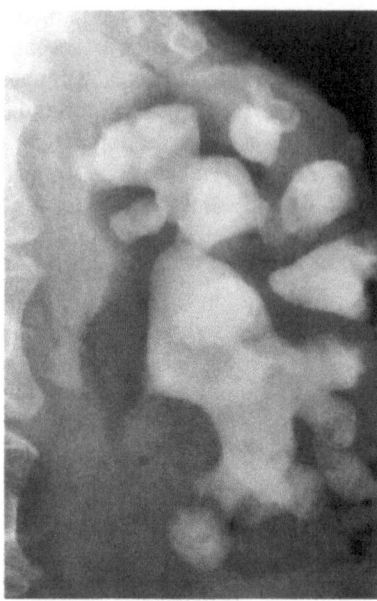

Fig. 6.9. The complexity of this large renal calculus precludes complete removal with EL or percutaneous techniques. Open flank surgical therapy permits complete stone removal in a single procedure

6.4.4.2 Advantages

Open surgical intervention provides intraoperative access to all the renal calyces. This permits complete stone removal combined with plastic procedures for those stone-containing calyces with highly stenotic infundibula (Fig. 6.9). Other rare surgical procedures such as ureterolithotomy or pelviolithotomy are still occasionally performed in conjunction with other plastic surgical procedures of the urinary tracts.

6.4.4.3 Disadvantages

The major disadvantage of open flank surgery compared to other available stone therapy modalities is that of greater postoperative patient disability. Total hospital days are higher than with other treatment options and patient disability prior to resumption of normal daily activities extends over a longer period of time. Because of the perinephric scar tissue created by these extensive renal surgical procedures, repeat surgical intervention at a later date is more complicated. Open surgical procedures, especially those like anatrophic nephrolithotomy, require considerable time commitment by the operating physician when compared to other treatment modalities.

6.5 Clinical Applications: Summary

The vast majority of small symptomatic renal pelvic, calyceal, or upper ureteral stones are best treated with EL. This results in 70%–80% of all stone patients undergoing extracorporeal therapy. As stone volume increases, the use of EL becomes controversial (LINGEMAN 1987). Certainly very large stones can be adequately fragmented using EL, but the resulting fragment burden will produce repeated bouts of ureteral obstruction and associated complications requiring repeated interventions. In addition, the final rate of complete stone clearance decreases as initial stone volume increases. Some practitioners respond to this situation by utilizing EL "monotherapy," which consists of repeated lithotripsy sessions coupled with ureteral stenting and intervening as necessary. Other authors favor precutaneous stone removal of large renal calculi to better achieve complete stone removal in a single session with a limited amount of postprocedural intervention. The combination procedure of initial percutaneous stone debulking followed by selective EL of residual calyceal calculi, followed by final complete endoscopic percutaneous stone removal, may be the best alternative therapy for large calculi.

For those stones in the mid and lower ureter, most clinicians advocate transurethral ureteroscopy as the therapeutic modality of choice. The recent clinical introduction of relatively pain-free extracorporeal lithotriptors has led some investigators to extend the application of EL to all ureteral stones. This use of EL is compromised by patient positioning difficulties in fixed geometry machines, by the complexity of accurate stone localization over the pelvic bones and near the bladder, and by the more intensive patient follow-up needed to assure success compared to ureteroscopy (LINGERMANN et al. 1986b).

Percutaneous stone removal methods are the primary modality applied to large renal stones or other non-EL candidates, or as the backup method of therapy when EL or ureteroscopy fails. Currently, about 10% of all stone patients undergo primary percutaneous procedures. Open flank surgery is extremely limited in its current clinical application, as detailed above. Because of the wide variations in referrals and practice, as well as the underlying stone populations, these statements can only be considered as guidelines.

6.6 Future Trends

Extracorporeal lithotripsy has become the major mode of renal stone therapy because of its excellent clinical results as well as the high degree of patient acceptability. Newer generation lithotriptors have been developed which now require little or no anesthesia, creating truly outpatient procedures. Patient acceptance of multiple repeated pain-free noninvasive lithotripsy procedures will continue to change the clinical utility of lithotripsy. The application of similar technology to biliary tract calculi (SACKMANN et al. 1988) has produced multipotential machines, further enhancing the treatment of those patients with symptomatic renal and ureteral calculi. The development of smaller and better endoscopes will continue to facilitate the widespread acceptance and utility of ureteroscopy. Finally, continued research on initial stone formation etiologies may produce appropriate chemotherapeutics to preclude the requirement for any of these interventional therapeutic modalities.

References

Boyle ET Jr, Segura JW, LeRoy AJ (in press) Open stone surgery in current urologic practice. J Urol

Chaussy C (1982) Extracorporeal shock wave lithotripsy. New aspects in the treatment of kidney stone disease. S Karger, Publishers, Inc, Basel

Drach GW, Dretler S, Fair W, et al. (1986) Report of the United States cooperative study of extracorporeal shock wave lithotripsy. J Urol 135: 1127–1133

Huffman JL, Bagley DH (1988) Ureteropyeloscopic removal of upper urinary tract calculi. In: Huffman JL, Bagley DH, Lyon ES (ed) Ureteroscopy, W. B. Saunders, Philadelphia, pp 85–105

Lang EK (1987) Percutaneous nephrostolithotomy and lithotripsy: A multiinstitutional survey of complications. Radiology 162: 25–30

LeRoy AJ, Segura JW, Williams H Jr, Patterson DE (1987) Percutaneous renal calculus removal in an extracorporeal shock wave lithotripsy practice. J Urol 138: 703–706

Lingeman JE (1987) Current concepts in the relative efficacy of percutaneous nephrostolithotomy and extracorporeal shock wave lithotripsy. World J Urol 5: 229–236

Lingeman JE, Newman D, Mertz JHO, et al. (1986)a Extracorporeal shock wave lithotripsy: The Methodist Hospital of Indiana experience. J Urol 135: 1134–1137

Lingeman JE, Sonda LP, Kahnoski RJ, et al. (1986)b Ureteral stone management: Emerging concepts. J Urol 135: 1172–1174

Lyon ES, Huffman JL, Bagley DH. (1984) Ureteroscopy and ureteropyeloscopy. Urology 23: 29–36

Marberger M, Stackl W, Hruby W, Kroiss A (1985) Late sequelae of ultrasonic lithotripsy of renal calculi. J Urol 133: 170–173

Preminger GM, Kettelhut MC, Elkins SL, Seger J, Fetner CD (1989) Ureteral stenting during extracorporeal shock wave lithotripsy: Help or hindrance? J Urol 142: 32–36

Rassweiler J, Westhauser A, Bub P, Eisenberger F (1988) Second-generation lithotripters: A comparative study. J Endourol 2: 193–204

Sackmann M, Delius M, Sauerbruch T, et al. (1988) Shockwave lithotripsy of gallbladder stones. The first 175 patients. N Engl J Med 318: 393–396

Segura JW, Patterson DE, LeRoy AJ, et al. (1985) Percutaneous removal of kidney stones: Review of 1000 cases. J Urol 134: 1077–1081

Stackl W, Marberger M (1986) Late sequelae of the management of ureteral calculi with the ureterorenoscope. J Urol 136: 386–389

Van Arsdalen KN, Banner MP, Pollack HM (1990) Radiographic imaging and urologic decision making in the management of renal and ureteral calculi. Urologic Clinics of North America 17: 171–190

Weinerth JL, Flatt JA, Carlson CC III (1989) Lessons learned in patients with large Steinstrasse. J Urol 142: 1425–1427

7 Renal Trauma

ERICH K. LANG

CONTENTS

7.1 Introduction 189
7.2 Concepts of Management 189
7.3 Diagnostic Assessment 190
7.3.1 Excretory Urography 190
7.3.2 Computed Tomography 191
7.3.2.1 Technique 191
7.3.2.2 CT Categorization of Renal Injuries 194
7.3.3 Arteriography 203
7.3.4 Radionuclide Imaging 205
7.3.5 Retrograde Pyelography 206
7.3.6 Ultrasonography 206
7.3.7 Magnetic Resonance Imaging 207
7.4 Coexistent Renal and Intraabdominal Injury . . 209
7.5 Approach to Radiologic Assessment
 of Renal Trauma 209
 References 210

7.1 Introduction

The past decade has seen the emergence of a new management strategy for renal injuries. Increased acceptance of conservative management for some types of renal injury combined with improved confidence in the information provided by a new generation of imaging modalities has made feasible the clinical implementation of new management concepts, which also address the quest for curtailment of medical cost.

Renal contusion and corticomedullary lacerations with an intact renal capsule account for approximately 75% of all renal injuries. Lacerations with disruption of the renal capsule but without communication to the collecting system account for about 10%–12% of renal injuries, while lacerations extending into the collecting system account for about 7%. Injuries resulting in fragmentation of the kidney account for 3%–5%, as do pedicle injuries. Avulsion of the ureteropelvic junction and laceration of the renal pelvis are relatively rare.

ERICH K. LANG, Professor and Chairman; Department of Radiology, School of Medicine in New Orleans, Louisiana State University, Medical Center, 1542 Tulane Avenue, New Orleans, LA 70112-2822, USA

Subcapsular, perinephric, and intrarenal hematomas may be present in any of the categories. To some degree, their presence and size parallel the magnitude of the underlying injury and in patients with blunt injury reflect the magnitude of the acceleration or deceleration force.

7.2 Concepts of Management

Renal contusions and minor lacerations not extending into the collecting system and not associated with a substantial volume of devascularized renal parenchyma are prone to heal spontaneously. In the absence of associated abdominal injury, such injuries may therefore be managed conservatively (CASS 1983; EVINS et al. 1980). Conversely, surgical intervention is mandatory in patients with pedicle injuries, renal rupture, fragmentation of the kidney, subintimal tears, or occlusion of the renal artery, renal vein, or its major branches (CASS et al. 1979; GOLDBERGER et al. 1982; SAGALOWSKY et al. 1983).

Disagreement exists on the management of parenchymal injuries extending into the collecting system and to some degree on parenchymal injuries attendant upon penetrating trauma (CASS 1983; HEYNES et al. 1983). In recent years, conservative management has been advocated for subsets of such injuries (DEMETRIADES and RABINOWITZ 1984). Parenchymal tears or penetrating injuries extending into the collecting system but without formation of massive urinomas (small urinoma collections are easily drainable by percutaneous methods) are no longer considered definitive indications for surgical intervention (CASS et al. 1985). Likewise, penetrating trauma per se is no longer considered a mandatory indication for surgical management (HEYNES et al. 1985). Particularly if the route of penetrating trauma is exclusively retroperitoneal, conservative management is favored by most, provided there is no evidence of concomitant injury to other organs and there is but a small volum of devascularized renal parenchyma attendant upon the injury (BERNATH et al. 1983; DEMETRIADES and RABINOWITZ 1984;

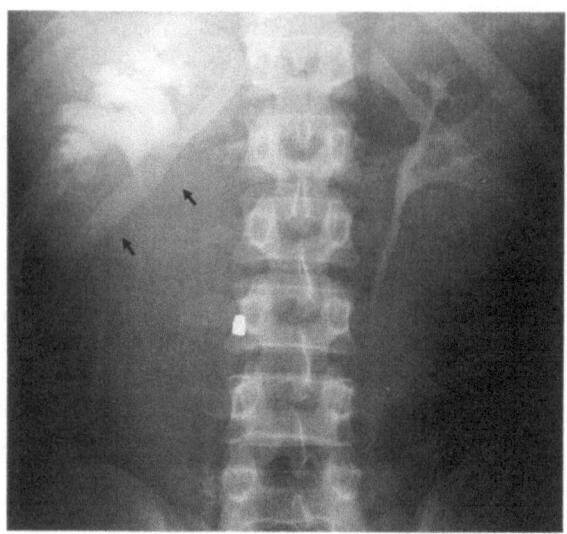

Fig. 7.1. Intravenous urogram demonstrating superior and lateral displacement of the right kidney, and a moderate degree of hydronephrosis attributable to a mass compressing the ureteropelvic junction *(arrows)*. On exploration, this mass proved to be a massive hematoma

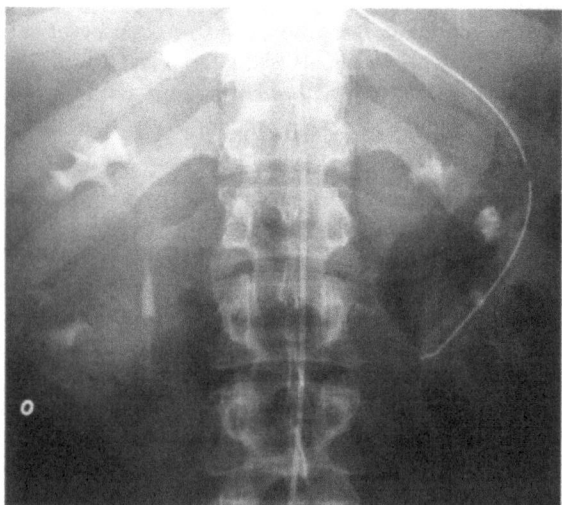

Fig. 7.2. Intravenous urogram demonstrating excellent opacification of the superior and inferior calyceal group of the right kidney. The midcalyceal group has failed to opacify. There is a suggestion of a space-occupying nonenhancing mass in the midpole of the right kidney, implying only minor injury, perhaps an intrarenal hematoma. Other examinations (17) proved a through and through fracture of the kidney. (LANG 1983 a)

EVINS et al. 1980). Conversely, support for early surgical intervention is based upon the supposition that it reduces the likelihood of later complications such as abscess and hemorrhage, which often complicate secondary nephrectomy, and perhaps fosters an ear-

lier and better restoration of physiologic function of the kidney (COLAPINTO 1977; GASKE et al. 1984; GOLDBERGER et al. 1982; JASKE et al. 1984).

Gunshot wounds, because of the prevalence of associated intraabdominal injuries, contamination by foreign material, and, particularly, creation of massive amounts of devitalized tissues as a result of the blast effect, mandate surgical exploration, debridement, and definitive management by surgery (CARROLL and McANINCH 1985). Conservative management of penetrating injury is therefore largely reserved for stab wounds via a retroperitoneal pathway (BERNATH et al. 1983; DEMETRIADES and RABINOWITZ 1984; I. M. THOMPSON et al. 1977; J. S. THOMPSON et al. 1980; WEIN et al. 1977).

7.3 Diagnostic Assessment

7.3.1 Excretory Urography

Excretory urography offers the advantage of ready availability and in general is capable of establishing the presence or absence and function of the kidneys. Staging of renal injury by urography is generally considered unreliable, though some laudatory reports have indicated an accuracy of 87% in patients who sustained blunt trauma (CARROLL and McANINCH 1985; NICOLAISEN et al. 1985). In 30% of his patients, ERTURK could neither stage renal injury nor differentiate minor from major renal injury (ERTURK et al. 1985). Above all, the excretory urogram offers no information on concomitant injury to other parenchymal organs or viscera. While there are findings on plain radiographs such as visceral displacement, obscuring of the psoas outline, lumbar scoliosis, and displacement of the kidney by perinephric fluid collection, correlation of these findings with the degree of renal damage was present in less than one-third of the renal injuries reviewed by HESSEL and SMITH (1974) (Fig. 7.1). Even the presence of a urographically normally functioning kidney does not exclude serious renal injury (CASS and VIEIRA 1987). WILSON and ZIEGLER (1987) found massive renal injury in patients with a urographically normal appearing kidney (Fig. 7.2).

Diminished excretion of contrast medium, once again, is non-specific. It may occur with simple contusion but has also been observed in severely shattered kidneys. The patchy nephrogram may be seen with a mere contusion, segmental infarction, or injuries causing massive parenchymal separation by clots (RUBIN and SCHLIFTMAN 1979). A frank disruption of the nephrogram would of course indicate a renal laceration or at least an interposed hematoma, at times associated with underlying renal pathology (GON-ZALES and GUERRIERO 1985; BERGREN et al. 1987).

Unilateral absence of excretion on urograms may herald severe renal injury (CASS and LUXENBERG 1984; STABLES 1976). However, unfortunately non-function has been observed with relatively minor parenchymal injuries and contusion. It may also occur attendant upon obstruction by blood clots, though this is usually heralded by an intensifying ne-phrogram (CASS and LUXENBERG 1984; CARROLL and McANINCH 1985; KISA and SCHENK 1986).

Extravasation of opacified urine indicates lacera-tion of the collecting system (CASS et al. 1985). This may be a ureteropelvic junction avulsion, pelvic tear, or merely a laceration into the intrarenal collecting system. However, minor extravasation may be missed on the intravenous urogram. Extravasation from a functioning kidney tends to be more pro-nounced and hence is readily discovered on in-travenous urograms (Fig. 7.3).

Intravenous drip nephrotomography has been ad-vocated in the past to evaluate dehiscence of paren-chymal tears (MAHONEY and PERSKY 1968). This technique has today been superseded by computed tomography (CT).

Nonetheless, the intravenous urogram is useful in select circumstances in patients in whom significant abdominal or renal injury is held unlikely on the basis of historical information and injury mechan-ism, and when confirmation of bilateral normal renal function suffices to expedite disposition and discharge from the hospital (CASS et al. 1986). Con-versely, patients with an abnormal urogram must then be investigated further, usually by CT (FEDERLE et al. 1981; NICOLAISEN et al. 1985).

The single intraoperative urogram also provides useful information to the surgeon faced with ex-panding retroperitoneal hematomas and the need to verify the presence of a second functioning kidney prior to emergency exploration and management of a presumably severely injured kidney (NICOLAISEN et al. 1985).

7.3.2 Computed Tomography

Computed tomography is the examination of choice for categorization and classification of renal injury as well as for like assessment of injury to other intra-peritoneal, retroperitoneal, and pelvic organs (CASS and VIEIRA 1987; FEDERLE 1990; FEDERLE and BRANT-ZAWADZKI 1986; FEDERLE et al. 1981, 1987; McANINCH and FEDERLE 1982; PEITZMAN et al.

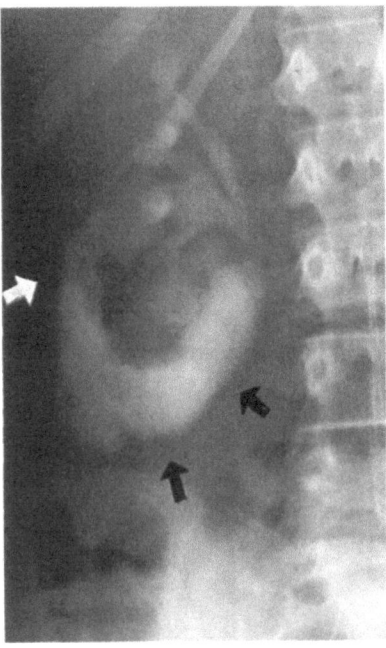

Fig. 7.3. Late phase intravenous urogram demonstrating an opacified urinoma in the dependent portion of Gerota's space *(arrows)*. This proves communication to the collecting system. (LANG 1987a)

1986). To extract maximal information, computed tomograms are performed preenhancement, during the phase of contrast medium transit (dynamic phase), and in the postenhancement phase (BRETAN et al. 1986; BRETAN and McANINCH 1988; LANG 1983a, 1989; LANG et al. 1985).

The preenhancement study is utilized to identify potential problem areas which are then studied in greater detail during the phase of dynamic transit and in the postenhancement phase.

7.3.2.1 Technique

Preenhancement computed tomograms are usually obtained at 10 mm slice thickness through all areas of potential interest. Their greatest value is to dem-onstrate fresh hematomas, which are characterized by a relatively high CT number, in the range of 50-70 Hounsfield units (Fig. 7.4). Subcapsular hemato-mas of the liver, spleen, and kidney, as well as peri-renal, intrarenal, and intrahepatic hematomas, are well shown by this technique (DRUY and RUBIN 1979; FEDERLE and BRANT-ZAWADZKI 1986; LANG 1990). Periduodenal hematomas and hematomas ex-tending into the base of the mesentery or the mesen-tery of the colon are likewise readily demonstrated. The technique is also uniquely sensitive for identifi-

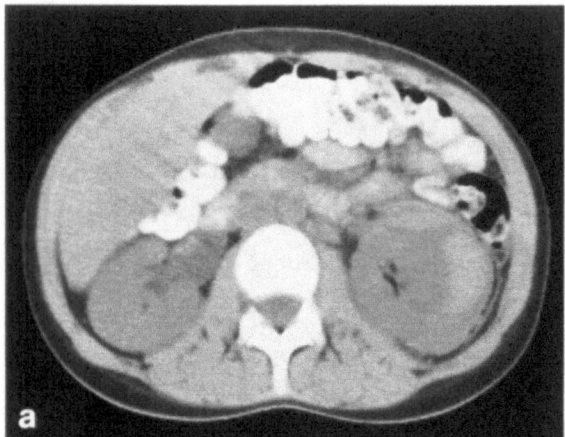

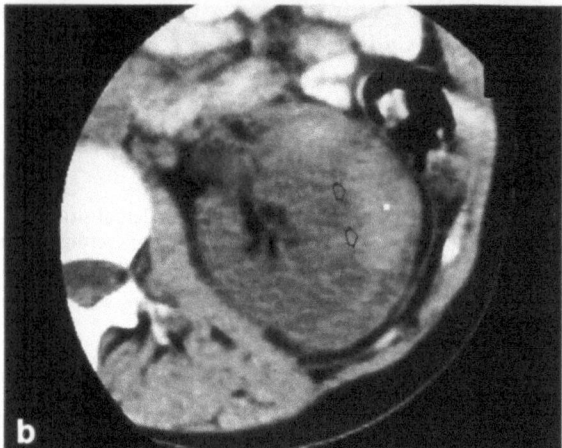

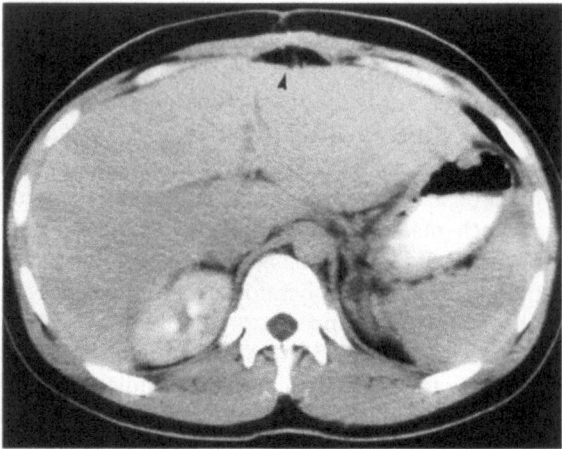

Fig. 7.5. Computed tomogram demonstrating free air in the intraperitoneal space. In the absence of penetrating injury, this is indicative of dehiscence of viscera

Fig. 7.4 a, b. Computed tomograms demonstrating high density material (70 Hounsfield units) in the anterior perirenal space indicative of a fresh hematoma. The narrow window setting shows the hematoma to better advantage *(arrows).* (LANG 1989)

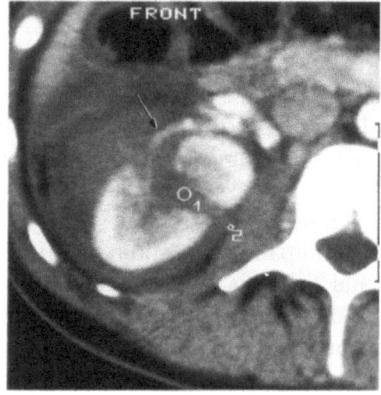

Fig. 7.6. A computed tomogram during the arterial capillary phase of contrast transit, demonstrating the classical differential enhancement pattern of cortex and medulla as well as opacified vessels *(arrow).* A fracture through the kidney is clearly seen. Nonenhancing yet high density material indicates the presence of a fresh hematoma separating the fragments *(1)* as well as a similar hematoma in the perinephric space *(2).* (LANG 1989)

cation of minimal amounts of free air in the intraperitoneal cavity, which tends to puddle just below the xiphoid or in the retroperitoneal space (FEDERLE and BRANT-ZAWADZKI 1986). In the absence of penetrating or open injury, this is indicative of visceral injury and/or laceration (Fig. 7.5). Dynamic computed tomograms depict tissues during the early phases of contrast medium transit and to some degree simulate the information provided by the capillary phase arteriograms (LANG 1983a) (Fig. 7.6). However, because of the time interval between slices, somewhat different phases of contrast medium transit are shown on each successive slice. Only the very first slices depict the truly capillary phase of transit; later slices reflect a composite of capillary enhancement and early parenchymal phase, i.e., beginning excretion of contrast medium into tubules and intracellular accumulation (LANG 1983a, 1987a, 1989).

The sequence is determined by the clinical findings and the regions implicated by history, physical findings, and findings on the preceding nonenhanced computed tomograms. Protocols have been developed relegating two or three slices to the upper liver and spleen region, four of five slices to the mid and lower liver and kidney regions, and the remaining four to six slices to the lower region of the aorta, the pelvis, or even the region of the descending thoracic aorta. This type of dynamic study tends to deploy slices in 20- to 30-mm increments. By one such series, the lower thoracic aorta, liver, spleen, kidneys, and lower abdominal aorta and pelvis can be

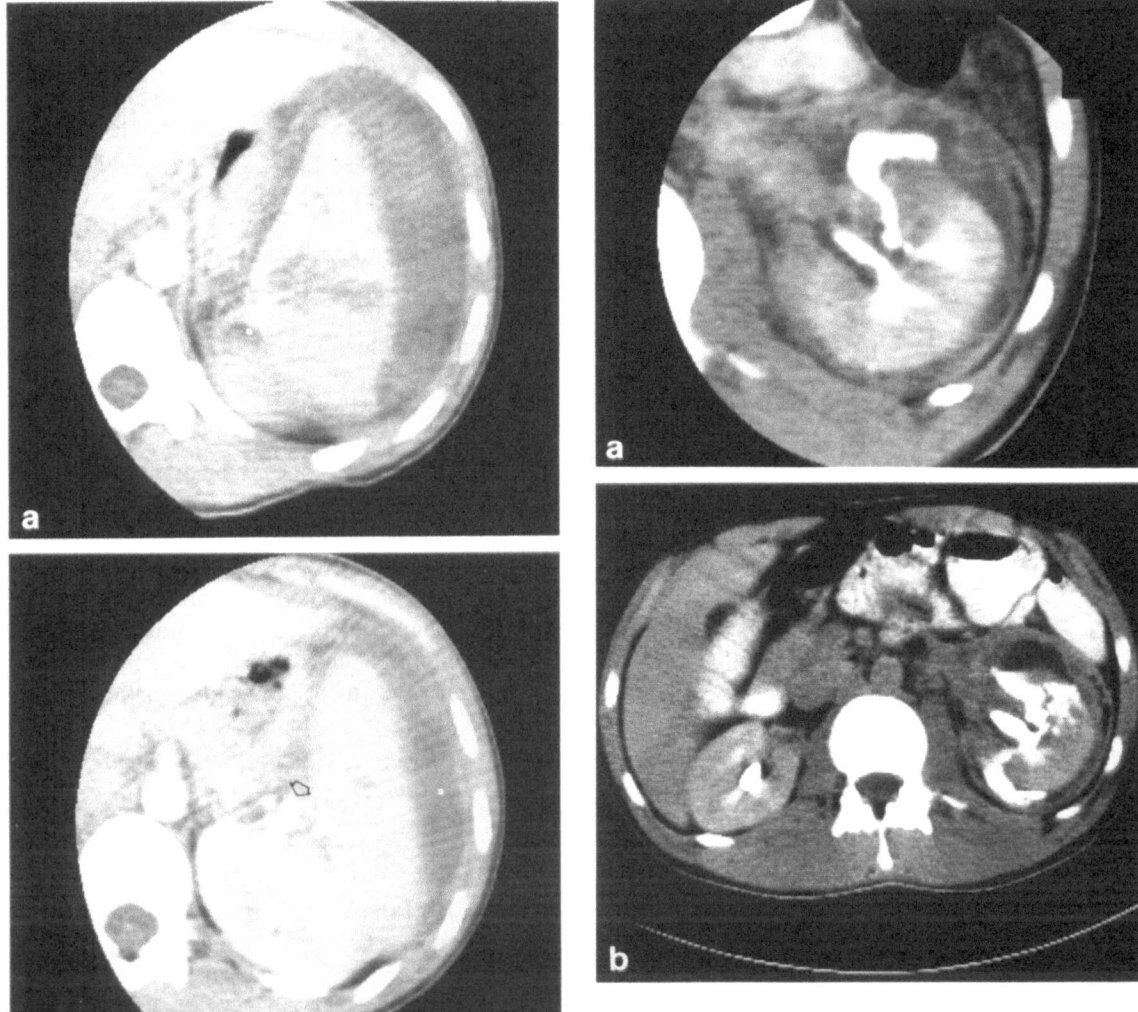

Fig. 7.7. a Dynamic computed tomogram demonstrating a dumbbell-shaped and other irregularly contoured areas, lacking enhancement, in the spleen. These were felt to represent fractures and pulp hematomas. A crescentic subcapsular hematoma compresses the lateral margin of the spleen. There is evidence of a hematoma dissecting into the splenorenal ligament. **b** A slightly lower cut demonstrating puddling of contrast material in the region of the splenic hilus and splenorenal ligament. This reflects active bleeding from branches of the splenic artery as well as from torn branches of the superior capsular artery of the kidney *(arrow)*

Fig. 7.8. a Postenhancement computed tomogram demonstrating a tract from the anterior midcalyceal group, into the perirenal space. Urinoma appears to be well incapsulated. **b** At a slightly lower cut level, tracts communicating to the intrarenal pelvis are demonstrated. These end in a perinephric urinoma. In addition, there is extravasation into the renal parenchyma

surveyed for the presence of compromised perfusion of parenchymal organs, vascular occlusion, and dissecting aneurysm (BRETAN and MCANINCH 1988; LANG 1987a, 1990; PHILLIPS et al. 1986) (Fig. 7.7).

Some 15–20 min after administration of a bolus of 50–100 ml of contrast medium for the dynamic series and often also after administration of dilute oral contrast medium, postenhancement computed

tomograms are obtained. The slices are concentrated in the region implicated on the preceding dynamic computed tomograms (LANG 1983a; LANG et al. 1985). An unlimited number of slices can be obtained to document all areas of interest since there is no longer a time constraint such as governs the sequence on the dynamic series. Not infrequently, computed tomographic cuts of the head are ob-

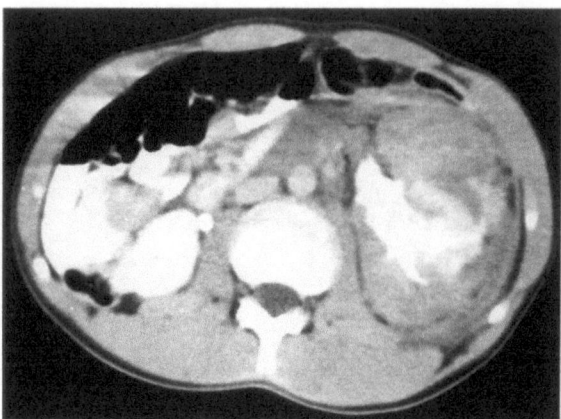

Fig. 7.9. Extravasation of contrast medium laden urine is seen in the peripelvic space. A fracture extends from the lateral circumference into the renal pelvis

tained at this time in patients with suspicion of coexistent head injury. Postenhancement computed tomogram are particularly useful for identification of extravasation of contrast medium laden urine indicating the presence of parenchymal tears extending into the collecting system and/or injury to the pelvis, ureter, or ureteropelvic junction (Figs. 7.8, 7.9). The high sensitivity for detecting minimal differences in attenuation coefficients facilitates recognition of minute extravasation of contrast medium laden urine. Moreover, spotty or absent enhancement of parenchyma along fracture margins on the dynamic computed tomograms raises suspicion of inadequate vascular supply because of either thrombosis of vessels or spasm (Fig. 7.10).

Extravasation of contrast medium administered per os or rectal klysis can indicate dehiscence of bowel and usually reveals the location of such injury (PHILLIPS et al. 1986).

The combined criteria generated by the pre-enhancement, dynamic, and postenhancement computed tomograms make possible accurate categorization and assessment of most traumatic injuries to kidneys, liver, spleen, pancreas, bowel, bladder, and to a lesser degree blood vessels, particularly aorta.

7.3.2.2 CT Categorization of Renal Injuries

Contusion of the kidney is characterized by minute extravasation of contrast medium laden urine into the interstitial spaces, best seen on delayed (1 h +) postenhancement CT (BRETAN et al. 1986; RUBIN and SCHLIFTMAN 1979; LANG 1983a) (Fig. 7.11). Somewhat decreased enhancement of the afflicted segment may be shown on dynamic computed tomograms, reflecting the spasm of vessels and reduced perfusion. Overall staining quality on both dynamic and postenhancement computed tomograms, apart from the speckled appearance caused by extravasated contrast medium laden urine, tends to be within normal limits (BRETAN et al. 1986; BRETAN and MCANINCH 1988) (Fig. 7.12). The initially prevailing spasm dissipates after use of hypertonic contrast medium which moderates akin to intra-

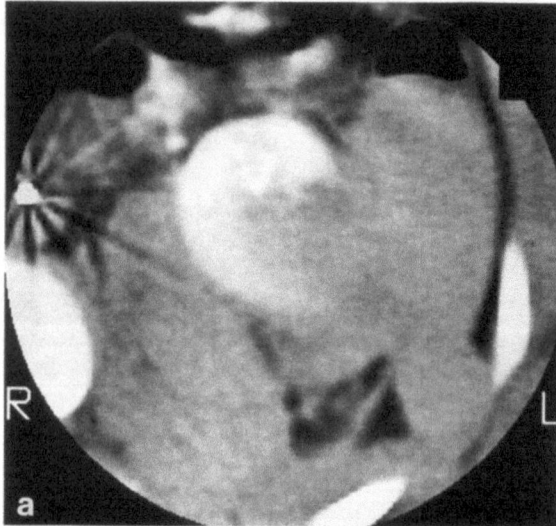

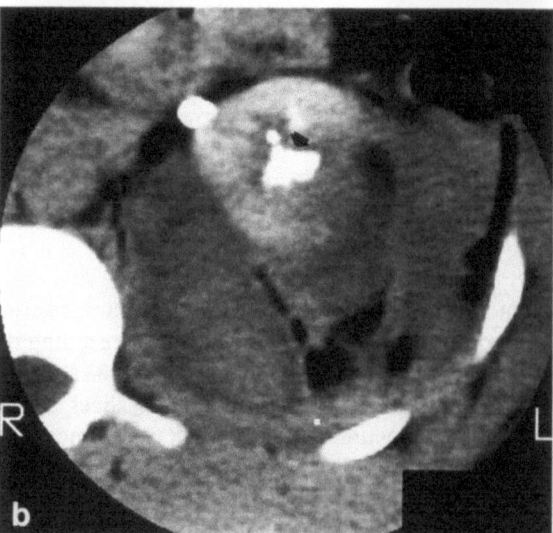

◁

Fig. 7.10. a Enhancement of the fracture margins is inhomogeneous and spotty, suggesting a compromised vascular supply. Note the high density fresh hematoma in the perirenal space tamponading the fracture as well as the large fresh hematoma extending into the pararenal space *(arrows)*. **b** Eight days later, after lysis of the clot, there is extravasation of contrast medium laden urine from the lower polar calyx *(arrow)*. The vascular supply to the fracture margin was inadequate to support the healing process. (LANG 1985)

arterial vasodilators, e.g., Priscoline (LANG et al. 1985; LANG 1987a).

Parenchymal tears are categorized and assessed on both axial sections as well as reconstructions along an oblique, sagittal, or coronal plane (FEDERLE 1990; ERTURK et al. 1985; LANG 1983a, 1989; HAYNES et al. 1984; SCLAFANI and BECKER 1985; YALE-LOEHR et al. 1989). The enhancement of the parenchyma seen during the phase of capillary transit of contrast medium reflects accurately parenchymal perfusion and therefore viability (Figs. 7.13, 7.14). A mottled enhancement on both dynamic and postenhancement computed tomograms indicates compromised perfusion (LANG 1983a; LANG et al. 1985) (Figs. 7.10, 7.15). Depending on the magnitude of parenchymal involvement, this predisposes to later slough of affected tissues and may be considered an indication for preemptive debridement (BRETAN and MCANINCH 1988; CASS and VIEIRA 1987; SAGALOWSKY et al. 1983; THOMPSON et al. 1980).

The staining quality of the parenchymal margins on postenhancement computed tomograms reflects accumulation of contrast medium in tubules, and therefore an intact vascular supply to the region as well as adequate pressure to attain perfusion and excrete contrast medium. However, excretion is moderated by the pressure existing in the collecting system. During the early nephrographic phase, obstruction of the collecting system by blood clots may result in decreased parenchymal stain attendant upon reduced perfusion caused by high pressure in the collecting system. On later nephrographic phase computed tomograms, there is an increasing stain.

Extension of a tear into the collecting system, severance of the ureteropelvic junction, and dehiscence of the pelvis are heralded by extravasation of urine (CASS et al. 1979: STEINBERG et al. 1984; KENNEY et al. 1987) (Fig. 7.9). The high sensitivity for detection of minimal differences in attenuation coefficients makes possible identification of minute extravasation of contrast medium laden urine. Lack of demonstrable extravasation of contrast medium laden urine in patients with parenchymal dehiscence known to extend into the collecting system implies a temporary or permanent seal of the tear by blood clot or fibrocytic healing (Fig. 7.16). The location of extravasated contrast medium laden urine is

▷

Fig. 7.12. Dynamic phase computed tomogram, in another patient with renal contusion, demonstrating satisfactory enhancement of all parenchyma. From prior administration of contrast medium, there is still some extravasated contrast medium laden urine causing a speckled appearance of the anterior pole. A very small perirenal hematoma is also present *(arrow)*. (LANG 1983a)

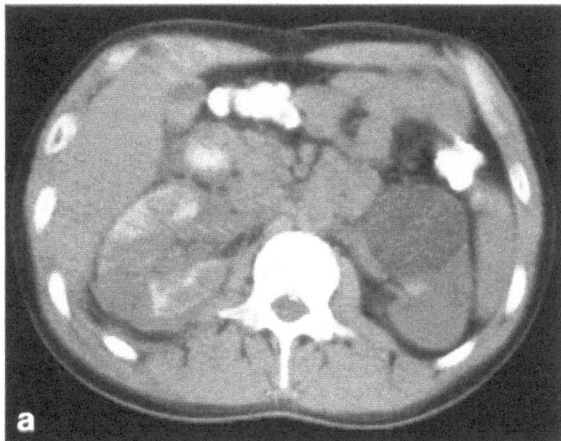
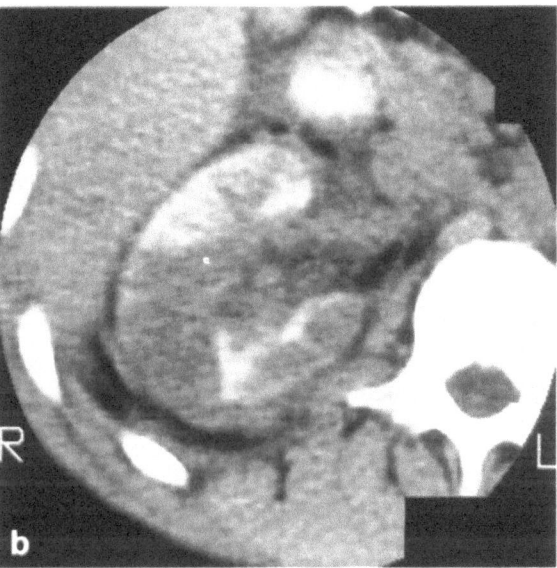

Fig. 7.11a, b. Computed tomograms obtained some 4 h after administration of intravenous contrast medium, demonstrating the classical interstitial extravasation of contrast medium laden urine characteristic for renal contusion. (LANG 1989)

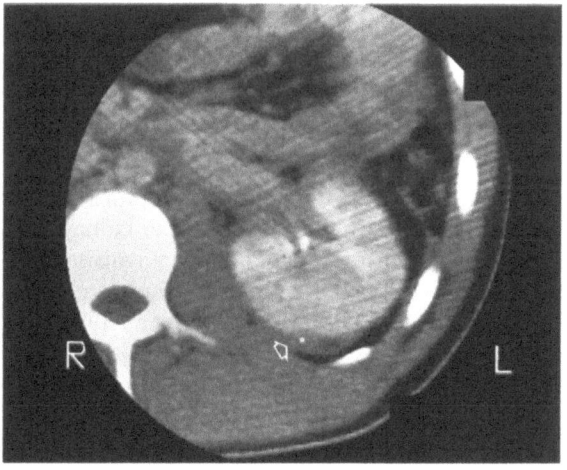

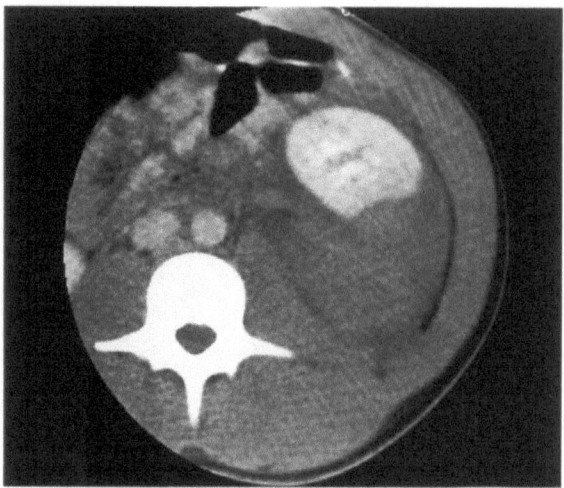

Fig. 7.13. Dynamic phase computed tomogram demonstrating homogeneous staining of the lower pole of the left kidney with the exception of a crescentic defect indicating severance of a small fragment by a stileto injury. There is a large hematoma in the perirenal space. Unlike the patient shown in Fig. 7.10a, the staining quality of the margins are excellent, indicating a favorable prognosis for primary healing

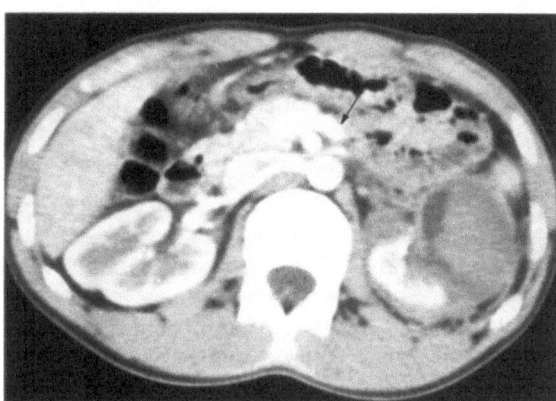

Fig. 7.14. Dynamic phase computed tomogram demonstrating a small posterior fragment of normally staining left kidney. Anteriorly, a large high density hematoma and a low density urinoma are present in the perinephric space. The excellent staining quality of the fragment indicates viability, salvageable by autotransplantation. A fracture through the body of the pancreas with active bleeding is noted *(arrow)*. (LANG 1989)

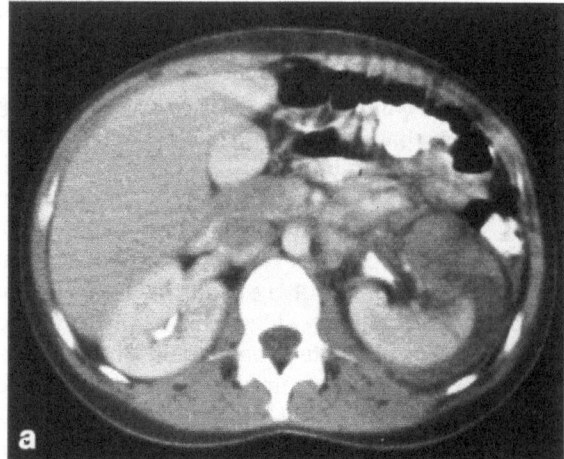

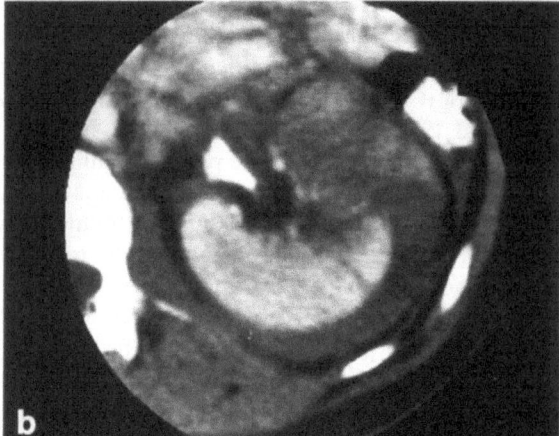

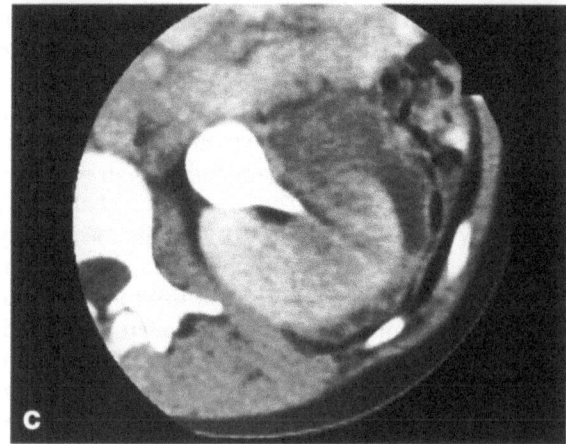

an important indicator of the site of injury. Thus exclusive or initial extravasation of contrast medium laden urine at a point medial to the kidney pelvis and ureteropelvic junction indicates avulsion of the ureteropelvic junction or injury to the kidney pelvis (SCLAFANI et al. 1985; STEINBERG et al. 1984; KENNEY et al. 1987).

Containment of extravasated contrast medium laden urine in a defined space, i.e., localized urinoma, suggests a seal against abutting tissues or curtail-

Fig. 7.15. a, b Dynamic computed tomogram demonstrating mottled staining quality of the anterior segment of the mid pole of the left kidney and a large enveloping perirenal hematoma. Conservative therapy was pursued, since only a small segment of renal parenchyma showed evidence of vascular compromise. **c** The follow-up computed tomogram 9 days later shows evidence of healing. The perirenal hematoma is gradually reabsorbing (same patient as Fig. 7.4). (LANG 1989)

Fig. 7.16. Despite what appears to be a shattered kidney, there is only minimal extravasation of contrast medium laden urine along the tract *(arrows)*. A huge blood clot curtails extravasation into the perirenal space

Fig. 7.17. a A computed tomogram depicting the arterial capillary phase demonstrates excellent opacification of a fragment of the posterior half of the right kidney as well as of vessels leading to that fragment. **b** A cut some 3 cm lower demonstrates the anterior fragment likewise featuring excellent staining quality. Extravasation of contrast medium during the capillary phase *(arrows)* indicates active bleeding. **c** A sagittal reconstruction demonstrates to advantage the oblique through and through fracture *(arrowheads)* as well as the large enveloping hematoma. The excellent viability of the fragments should make possible salvage of this kidney by appropriate surgical intervention. (LANG et al. 1985)

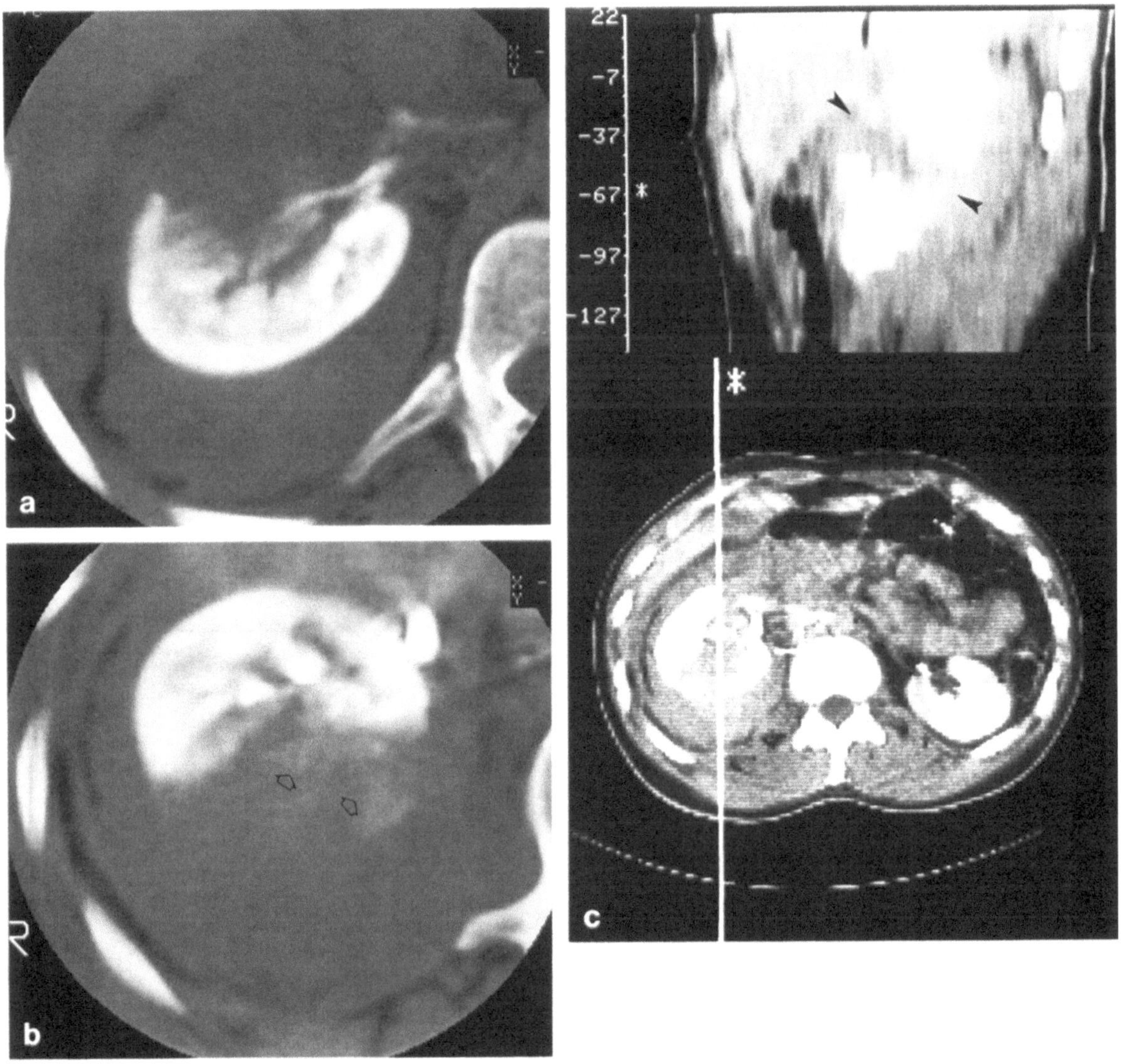

▽

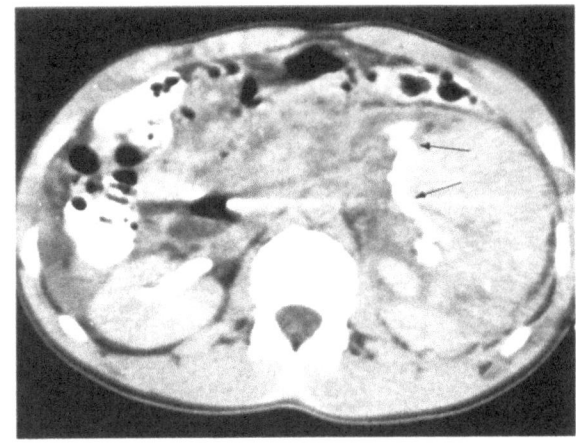

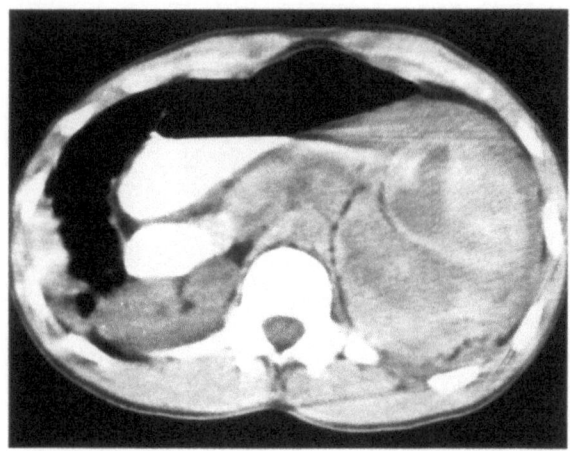

Fig. 7.18. There is evidence of liquefaction of a huge blood clot in the posterior perirenal space. Layering occurs, the corpuscular elements of the lysing clot seeking the dependent position, the supernatant the upper layers

Fig. 7.19. a Angio computed tomogram demonstrating anterolateral displacement of the left kidney. Note minimal extravasation of contrast medium laden urine *(arrows)*. The overall staining quality of the fracture margin is satisfactory, indicating a favorable prognosis (LANG et al. 1985). **b** A percutaneous drainage tube has been introduced into the large hematoma and urinoma in the posteromedial perirenal space (LANG et al. 1985). **c** Injection into the drainage catheter demonstrates the extent of the urinoma. The filling defects reflect residual blood clots. **d** Following drainage for 1 week, the urinoma and hematoma have all but disappeared. Staining of the renal parenchyma margins is excellent. Note some enhancement of a membrane that has formed around the residual urinoma and hematoma

▽

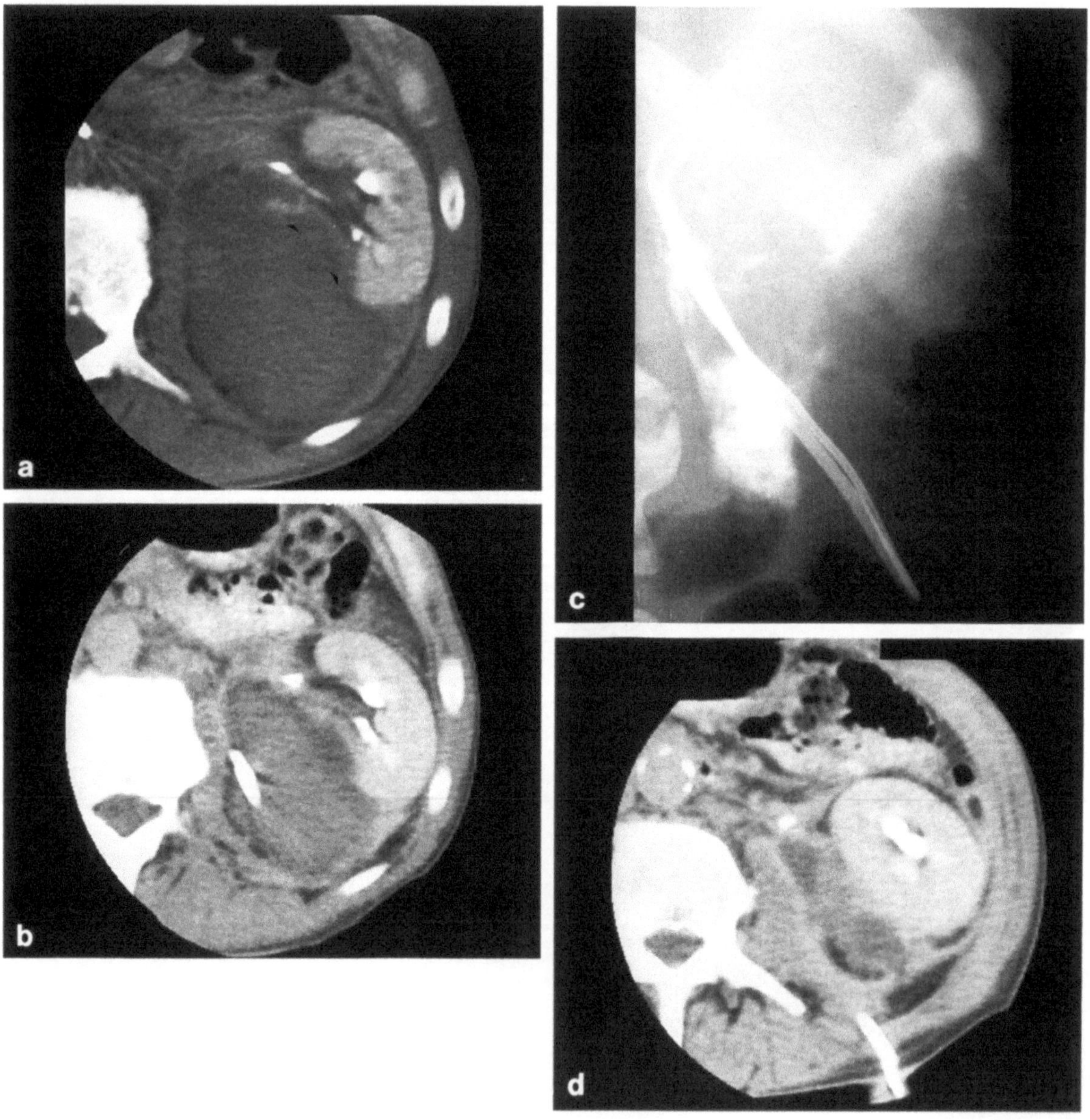

ment by intact fascial planes and is an important criterion supporting continued conservative management of such patients provided they are otherwise stable (Fig. 7.15).

Urinomas and hematomas frequently coexist. Often, the hematoma may be a temporary barrier to extravasation of urine or curtail extravasation by formation of a wall containing the urinoma. The propensity of such hematomas to lyse between the 7th and 10th day may occasion expansion of urinomas at that point in time (PETERS and SAGALOWSKY 1986; SAGALOWSKY et al. 1983; WILSON and ZIEGLER 1987) (Figs. 7.8, 7.10). By then, however, the hematoma is usually replaced by fibrocytes and healing by cicatricial tissue and, hence, formation of a wall is on the way.

The diagnosis of a shattered kidney is suggested on dynamic and postenhancement computed tomograms. The location of the fracture fragments and fracture lines can be defined further by appropriate oblique, sagittal, and coronal reconstructions (Fig. 7.17). Most importantly, the staining quality of fragments and fracture margins on a dynamic series is an important criterion indicating viability and hence salvageable parenchyma (CASS 1983; 1988; LANG et al. 1985; LANG 1987a). Surgical repair of appropriately located and well perfused fragments may be possible. Even if this is not the case, autotransplantation of large fragments into the pelvis and closure of the collecting system by a watertight suture may salvage functioning parenchyma (MARBURGER 1988; WEIN et al. 1977; YALE-LOEHR et al. 1989).

Location and size of subcapsular intra-, peri-, and pararenal hematomas are readily definable on computed tomograms (McCORT 1983). Urinomas, chylomas, and hematomas can be differentiated on the basis of characteristic attenuation coefficients (DRUY and RUBIN 1979; FEDERLE et al. 1981; McANINCH and FEDERLE 1982). Fresh hematomas tend to be hyperdense provided the hematocrit of the patient was within the normal range (Fig. 7.4). Older hematomas or seromas are usually hypodense. Liquefaction of hematomas results in a characteristic layering effect (Fig. 7.18).

The hematoma, urinoma, or hygroma itself lacks enhancement; however, a vascularized capsule or membrane enveloping such lesions may enhance, reflecting the presence of inflammatory neovascularity in its fibrous wall (Fig. 7.19d). Once a membrane has formed, evacuation by percutaneous, CT – or ultrasound – guided drainage is usually feasible (Fig. 7.19).

Subcapsular hematomas have a lenticular or crescentic configuration and eccentric location. They

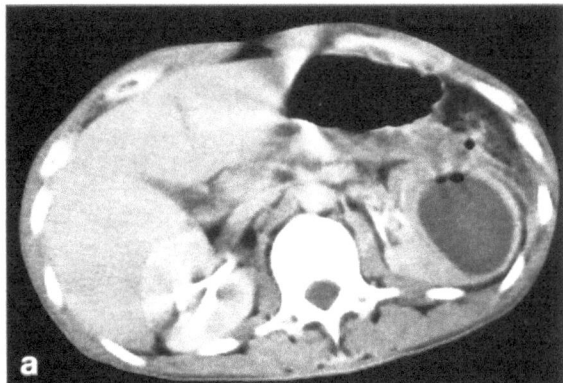
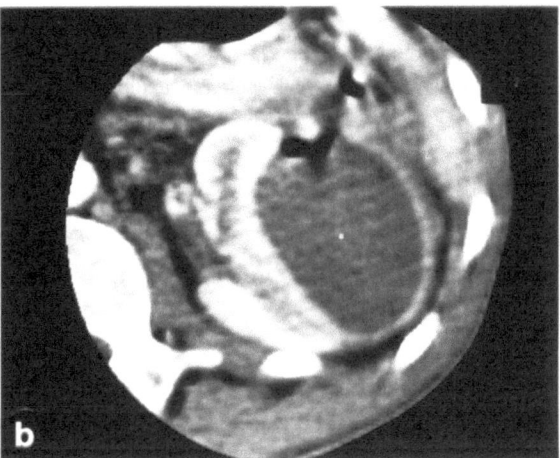

Fig. 7.20. a Postenhancement computed tomogram demonstrating a large subcapsular hematoma with two ominous air bubbles. **b** The dynamic computed tomogram shows crescentic deformity of the left kidney but unimpeded staining quality of cortical parenchyma. Prominent enhancement of the capsule indicates age and presence of inflammatory neovascularity. (LANG et al. 1985)

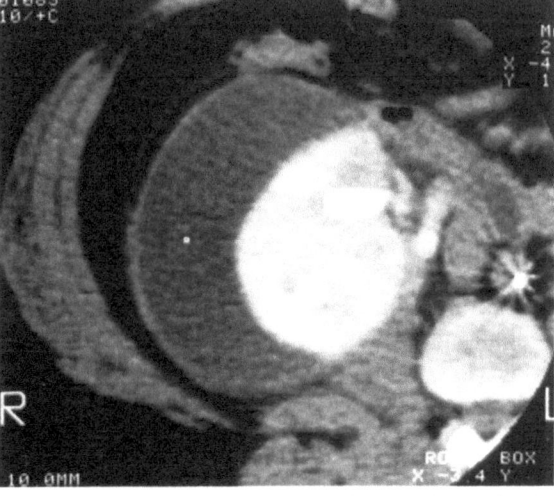

Fig. 7.21. The unusually low attenuation coefficient in the perirenal fluid collection suggests fat content and therefore a traumatic chyloma

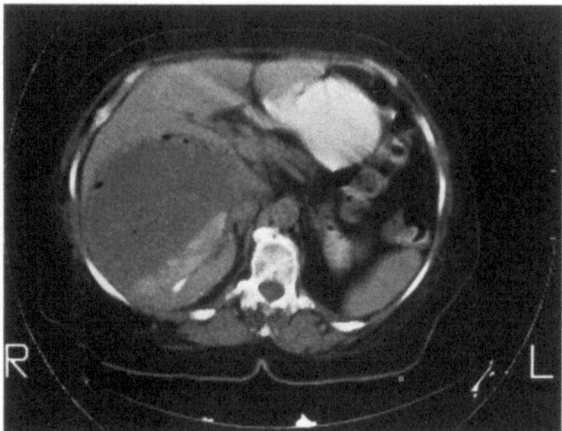

Fig. 7.22. Postenhancement computed tomogram demonstrating a crescentic deformity of the anterior circumference of the right kidney. The mottled staining quality indicates compromised perfusion, possibly spasm or small infarcts. Dispersed gas bubbles in the subcapsular fluid collection suggest an abscess. (LANG 1987a)

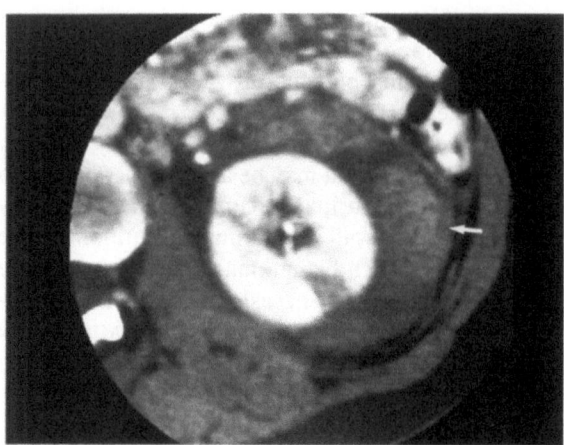

Fig. 7.24. Dynamic computed tomogram demonstrating a small wedge-shaped area of decreased enhancement with the apex toward the hilus and the base toward the periphery. The appearance indicates a traumatic infarct. Note the perirenal hematoma *(white arrow)*

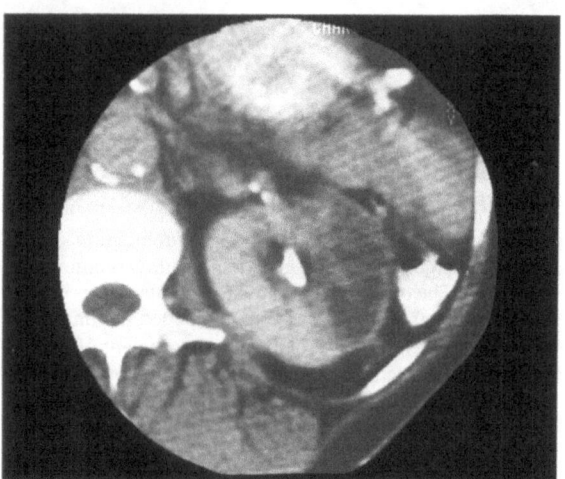

Fig. 7.23. Postenhancement computed tomogram demonstrating a wedge-shaped area of decreased staining with the apex toward the hilus and the base toward the periphery. There is enhancement of a very thin rim of cortex. This appearance is characteristic of an infarct. (LANG 1987a)

tend to compromise perfusion of abutting renal parenchyma. This is heralded by a decreased enhancement on the dynamic phase computed tomograms and sometimes also on the subsequent postenhancement computed tomograms (TAKAHASHI et al. 1977) (Fig. 7.20). Large intrarenal and even perirenal hematomas may likewise compromise perfusion of abutting parenchyma subjected to compression.

Substantial subcapsular hematomas compromising perfusion of the renal cortex may initiate renin and angiotensin production and hence hyperten-sion. As a late complication, they predispose to formation of a "Page kidney." Compromised perfusion of renal parenchyma is, therefore, an indication for evacuation of the responsible hematoma by surgical or interventional radiologic techniques (TAKAHASHI et al. 1977; LANG 1985, 1987b).

Attenuation coefficients provide criteria for differentiation of chylomas (range −40 to −80) (Fig. 7.21), urinomas (unenhanced urine range 0 to +15), seromas (+20 to +40), fresh hematomas (+45 to +70), and sometimes abscesses (−10 to +30) (FEDERLE 1990; FEDERLE et al. 1981; LANG et al. 1985; LANG 1987a) (Fig. 7.22). Moreover, attenuation coefficients provide most sensitive criteria for ascertaining residual communication between the collecting system and urinomas. Lack of step up of attenuation coefficients in a urinoma some 40 min after administration of intravenous contrast medium and in the presence of an otherwise well functioning renal unit is considered conclusive for a seal of any preexisting rent (LANG et al. 1985; LANG 1987a).

Traumatic infarct may be the consequence of thrombosis or embolism of the renal artery or its branches and rarely of the renal vein. Focal traumatic infarcts present classically as a wedge-shaped area (the base of the wedge oriented toward the periphery, the apex toward the hilum) lacking enhancement in both the dynamic and the postenhancement phase (GLAZER et al. 1983; WONG et al. 1984) (Figs. 7.23, 7.24). A thin rim of cortex over the infarcted area frequently enhances. This is the result of collateral flow from capsular vessels to perforating cortical branches (GLAZER et al. 1983). The

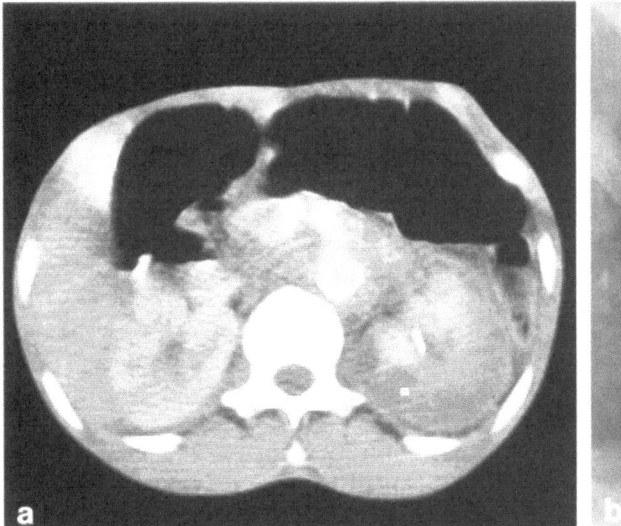
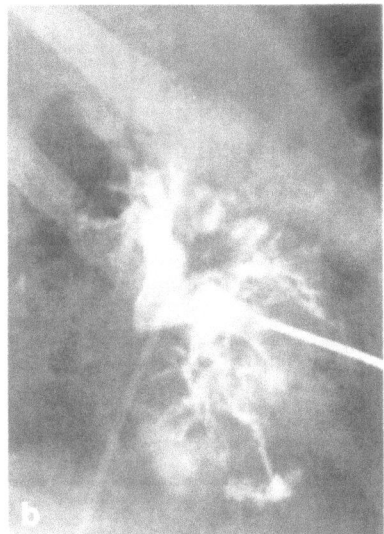

Fig. 7.25. a The left kidney shows a progressively intensifying but inhomogeneous stain. There is evidence of both subcapsular seroma and fluid collection in the anterior perirenal space. **b** A selective percutaneous renal venogram demonstrating huge thrombi in the main renal veins, confirming the diagnosis of renal vein thrombosis

size of focal infarcts and the magnitude of collateral supply determine the capability for self-healing. The CT appearance of infarcts, however, is mimicked by focal pyelonephritis.

Demonstration of a thrombus in the renal vein on CT is confirmatory for the diagnosis of renal vein thrombosis (GLAZER et al. 1984). Often the diagnosis of renal vein thrombosis is suggested on CT by an increasing, commonly inhomogeneous stain and perirenal hematomas (Fig. 7.25).

Vascular injuries present with a spectrum ranging from prominent findings to relative silence as well as a plethora of secondary manifestations indicative of such injury.

Initially, intimal flaps in the main or segmental renal arteries may not produce any findings on dynamic or postenhancement computed tomograms. However, once such injuries progress to thrombosis of the vessels, lack of enhancement and loss of function of the afflicted parenchyma on dynamic and postenhancement computed tomogras result (LANG 1983b, 1985) (Fig. 7.26). Retrograde filling of the renal vein indicates disruption of arterial flow, usually attendant upon avulsion of the renal artery (CATES et al. 1986) (Fig. 7.26). Traumatic severance and/or thrombosis of the main renal artery of any of its major branches result in lack of parenchymal enhancement during the phase of capillary transit and

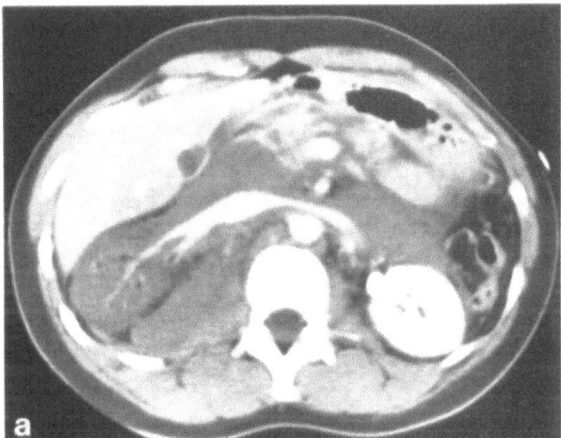
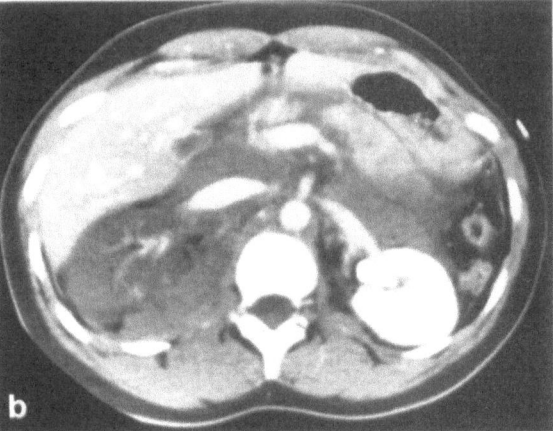

Fig. 7.26. a Renal artery thrombus. Dynamic computed tomogram demonstrating lack of parenchymal contrast enhancement of the right kidney and retrograde opacification of the renal veins. **b** A section more cephalad in the same patient indicates, in addition, transection of the body of the pancreas. (CATES et al. 1986)

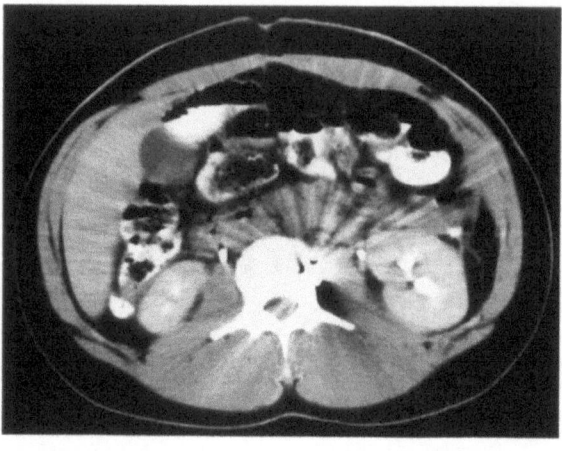

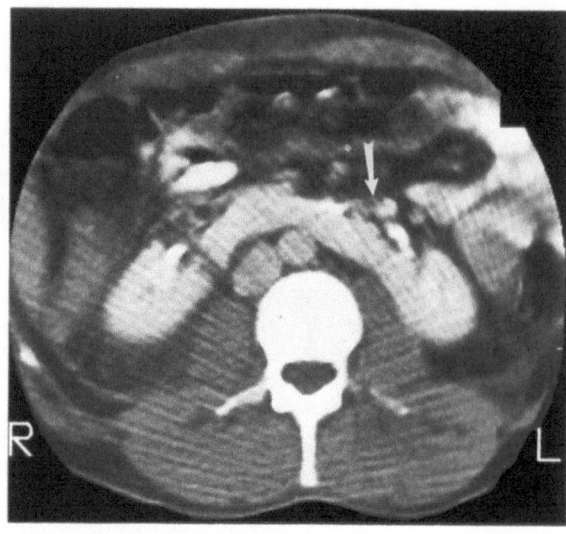

Fig. 7.27. Computed tomogram demonstrating displacement of the left kidney by a high density mass interposed between aorta and kidney. The interposed mass represents a hematoma resultant from partial avulsion of the renal artery

Fig. 7.29. Dynamic computed tomogram demonstrating a parenchymal tear extending into the medially displaced medial inferior calyceal group of a horseshoe kidney *(arrow)*. History indicated only minimal trauma

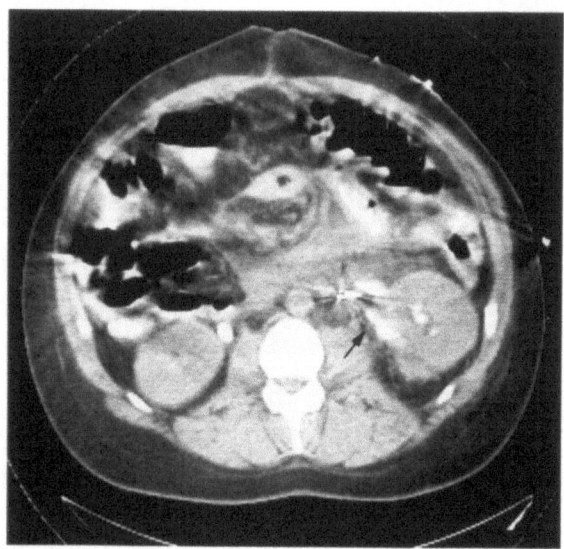

Fig. 7.28. Angio computed tomogram demonstrating extravasation of contrast medium in the left paraaortic space *(arrow)*. The left kidney is displaced anteriorly and laterally. There is some contrast medium in the calyces of the lower pole. Extravasation and displacement of the kidney were due to avulsion of the main renal artery, into which a small injection of 6 ml of dilute dye had been carried out for the purpose of angio CT. The lower polar artery was intact, explaining function of the lower pole of the kidney. Displacement of the kidney was due to a hematoma interposed between aorta and kidney

the subsequent parenchymal phase. Lateral displacement of the kidney by a medially located perihilar mass often with an attenuation coefficient suggesting a fresh hematoma is a helpful observation indicating laceration or severance of the main renal artery or vein (SCLAFANI et al. 1985) (Figs. 7.27, 7.28).

Importantly, CT often reveals the presence of small renal cell carcinomas, angiomyolipomas, benign cysts, polycystic disease, or hydronephrosis as the cause for disproportionate subcapsular, perirenal, or intrarenal hematoma formation in patients who have sustained trivial trauma (BROWER et al. 1978; KARP et al. 1986; MILLER et al. 1966; NEWMAN and SMITH 1987; RHYNER et al. 1983) (Fig. 7.29).

Criteria advocated for assessment of renal parenchymal injury are equally applicable to the diagnosis of injury to liver, pancreas, and spleen. Likewise, criteria for diagnosis of renal hematomas are transferable to hematomas in the liver, spleen, wall of the bowel, periduodenal space, base of the mesentery, pelvis, and other retroperitoneal locations (LANG 1990) (Fig. 7.30). The location of the hematoma indicates the probable site of injury to vessels, e.g., aorta, celiac axis, or superior, inferior mesenteric, or pelvic arteries. Attenuation coefficients are once again pivotal for establishing the age of such hematomas, as is layering in aged hematomas.

Arteriovenous fistulae such as aortocaval fistulae can be diagnosed on dynamic CT on the basis of premature opacification of the communicating vein or inferior vena cava (LANG 1987a; POLLACK and

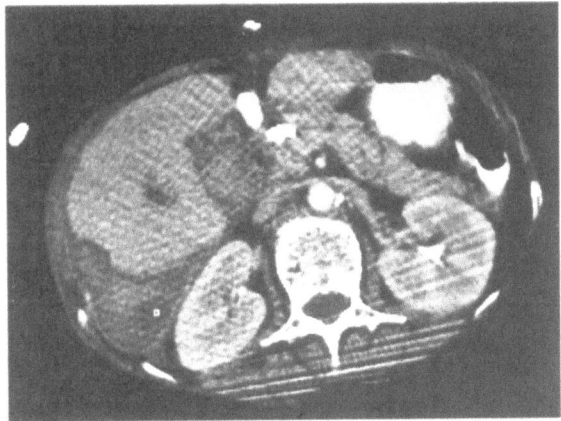

Fig. 7.30. Dynamic computed tomogram demonstrating a substantial subcapsular hematoma below Glisson's capsule. An area of decreased enhancement in the center of the liver is felt to reflect a hematoma. The kidneys appear unremarkable. (LANG 1987a)

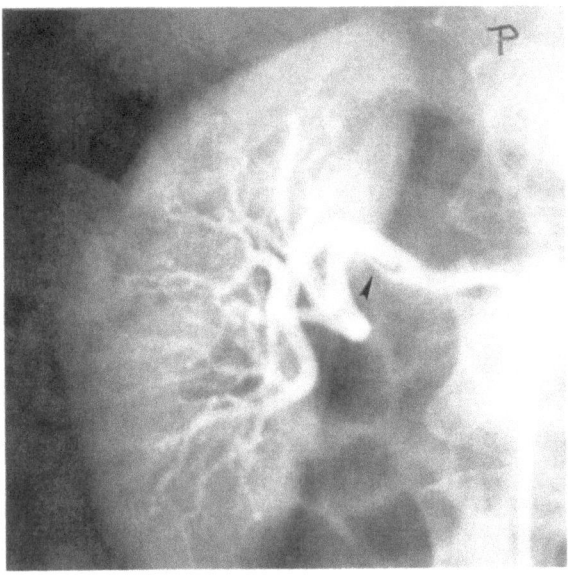

Fig. 7.32. Selective arteriogram demonstrating a typical intimal flap in the main renal artery *(arrowhead)*. (LANG 1989)

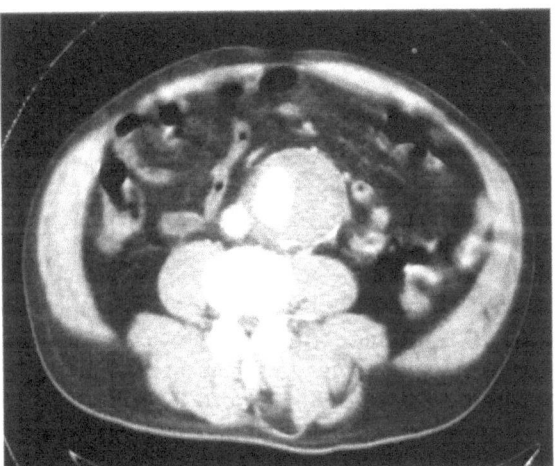

Fig. 7.31. Dynamic computed tomogram demonstrating simultaneous opacification of aorta and inferior vena cava. The traumatic aortocaval fistula is responsible

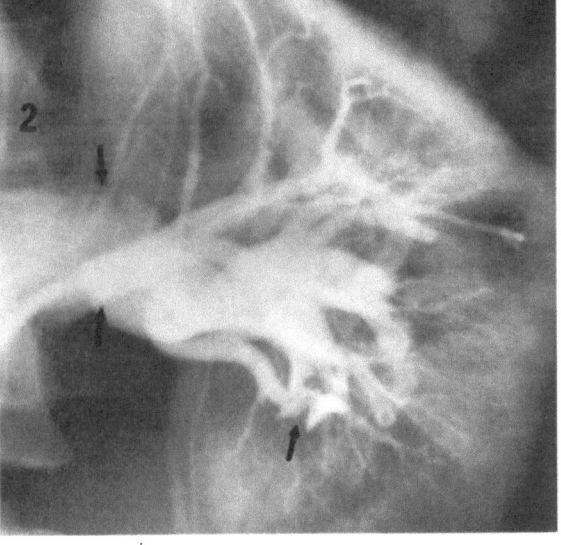

Fig. 7.33. Selective arteriogram demonstrating premature opacification of a massively dilatd renal vein *(arrows)*. Multiple arteriovenous fistulae are demonstrated in the lower pole of the left kidney. These are the consequence of a stiletto injury. (LANG 1971)

WEIN 1989) (Fig. 7.31). Assessment of injuries to the CNS and particularly subdural hematomas or intracerebral hemorrhage is carried out in a like fashion.

Because of the frequent coexistent injury to muscle tissues and attendant myoglobinuria, the amount of contrast medium administered should be kept to a minimum. Fifty milliliters will generally suffice to carry out the proposed protocol and this amount is tolerated even by critically injured patients.

7.3.3 Arteriography

While arteriography has been superseded by CT as the preferred method for evaluating most renal injuries, there remains a well-defined subset of traumatic injuries for which angiography is recommended for categorization (COSGROVE et al. 1973;

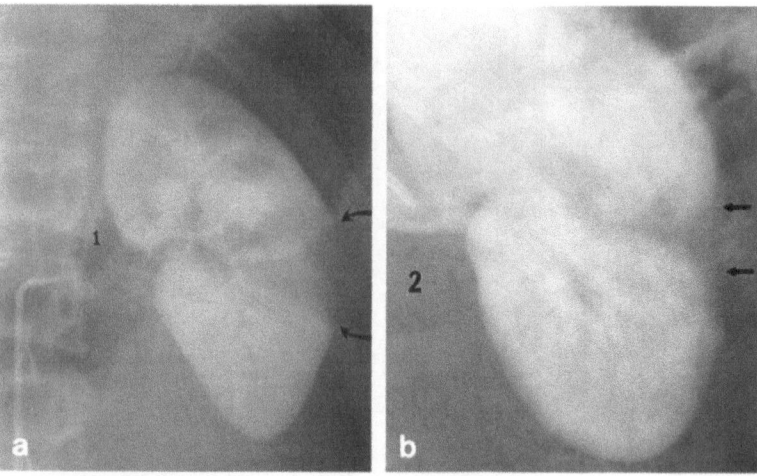

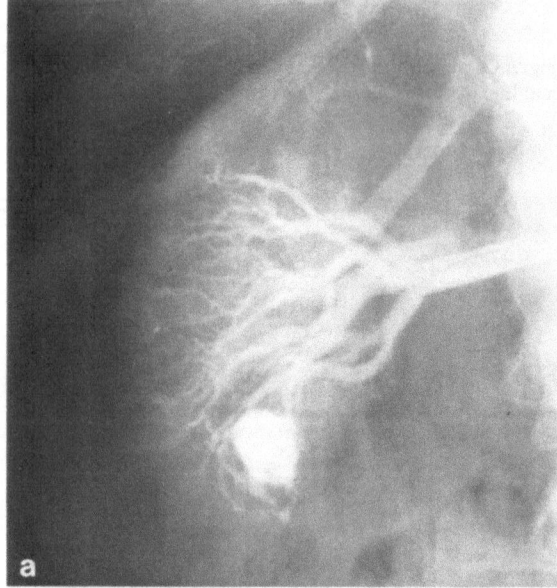

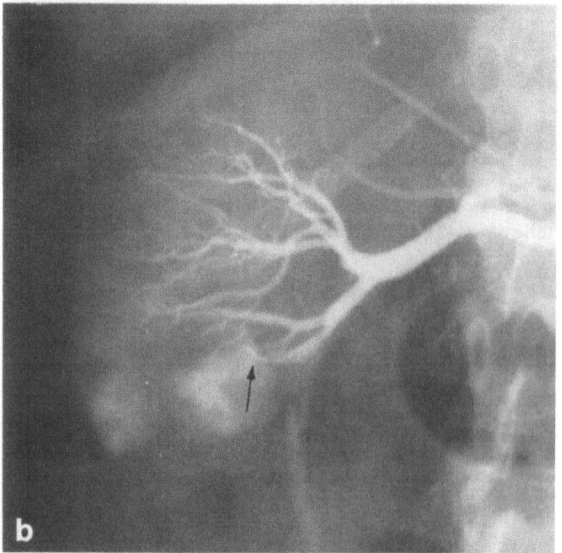

△

Fig. 7.34. a The capillary phase of an arteriogram demonstrating dehiscence of the cortex of the left kidney with an interposed hematoma splaying the margins *(arrows)*. Staining quality of the fracture margins is excellent, suggesting a favorable prognosis. **b** An arteriogram performed almost 1 year later demonstrates a recessed scar *(arrows)* but otherwise satisfactory healing

Fig. 7.35. a Selective arteriogram demonstrating a traumatic pseudoaneurysm resulting from a stab wound to the lower pole of the right kidney (LANG 1989). **b** A 2-French Tracker catheter has been advanced superselectively in the branch supplying the traumatic pseudoaneurysm *(arrow)*. The lesion is occluded with Avacryl (6-cyanoacrylate). Only a very small amount of parenchyma is lost employing this superselective intervention

LANG 1975, 1976; LOHSE et al. 1982). These include patients with clinical findings consistent with vascular injury and an injury mechanism predisposing to such. Rapid acceleration and deceleration subject the renal artery attached to the aorta and immobilized by spine and multiple lumbar branch vessels to potential shearing force causing tear of the intima and formation of an intimal flap (LOHSE et al. 1982) (Fig. 7.32). Penetrating injury prone to produce arteriovenous fistulae or aneurysms is one other indication for arteriography (FISHER et al. 1989) (Fig. 7.33).

Optimal evaluation includes midstream aortography followed by selective renal arteriography. Digital subtraction techniques, though lauded for reducing the amount of contrast medium, lack detail for assessment of small vessel injuries, intimal flaps, and arteriovenous fistulae (COSGROVE et al. 1973; FISHER et al. 1989). Digital subtraction venography is marred by inadequate detail and does not reduce contrast medium use. Arteriographic findings range from small perfusion defects to large devitalized segments of renal parenchyma and demonstration of

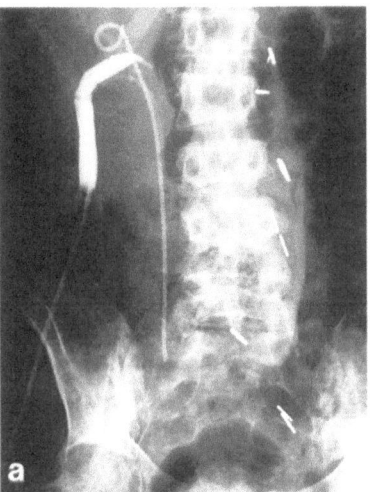 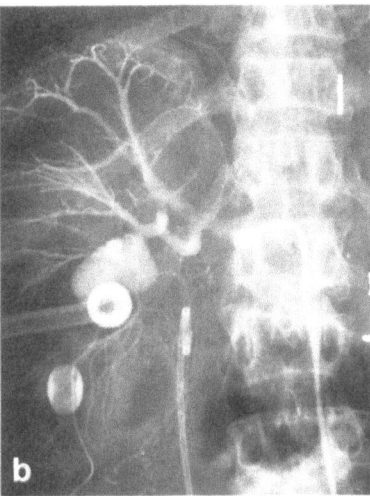 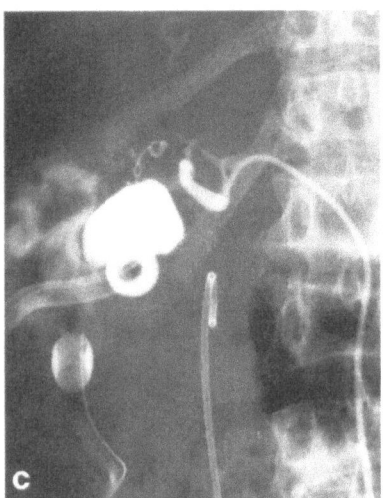

Fig. 7.36. a Following percutaneous extraction of a renal calculus, a J-stent is seen in position from the superior calyceal
group into the distal right ureter; a 10-ml 12-cm Olbert balloon
is inflated in position, attempting to tamponade massive
bleeding from the entry site. b A selective arteriogram demonstrates a pseudoaneurysm fed from an interlobar artery as the
cause for the bleeding. c Superselective catheterization of the
offending interlobar artery has been carried out. Several 3-mm
Gianturco coils have been used to occlude the interlobar
branch. The pseudoaneurysm, itself, has been "casted" with a
combination of two parts Avacryl, one part contrast medium.
Bleeding was satisfactorily and immediately controlled. There
were no sequelae

displacement and occlusion of arteries, arteriven-
ous fistulae, and intimal flaps. Arteriography offers
important criteria for establishing viability and salvageability of tissues (LANG 1975, 1976) (Fig. 7.34).

Active bleeding sites or arteriovenous fistulae are
not only diagnosed but can be therapeutically occluded (COSGROVE et al. 1973; FISHER et al. 1989)
(Figs. 8.35, 8.36). The impact of such occlusion on
parenchymal perfusion can be predicted with great
accuracy. Moreover, detailed information about vascular supply is provided that can serve as a road map
for subsequent surgical intervention, and particularly for bench surgery attempting to salvage parts of
the kidney. Following arterial surgery, arteriography
is the procedure of choice to demonstrate the nature
and site of complications, should they develop.

7.3.4 Radionuclide Imaging

The computed radionuclide urogram offers physiologic information on renal function. Technetium
99 m glucoheptonate is the radiopharmaceutical of
choice to produce perfusion, static, and drainage

images (ROSENTHAL 1986; LANG 1985; CHOPP et al.
1980). The radiopharmaceutical is injected intravenously as a bolus in a dose of approximately 15 mCi.
Images are obtained in a rapid sequence (2 s). Static
images are begun 1 min later and repeated at 3-min
intervals. Radionuclide imaging is useful to ascertain the state of global and regional perfusion as well
as parenchymal function and also to demonstrate
urinary extravasation (CHOPP et al. 1980).

The Schlegel technique is favored for extrapolat-
ing renal plasma flow rate (SCHLEGEL and LANG
1980). Renal plasma flow rate is a particularly sensitive indicator for deterioration of renal perfusion
attendant upon a variety of underlying conditions
(Fig. 7.37). Imaging studies indicate the presence of
fractures with interposed blood clots or regions of
reduced perfusion as a photopenic area (Fig. 7.38).
If the latter area is well defined and corresponds to
an anatomic unit, it usually indicates compromise of
the respective segmental artery.

Extrarenal collections of the radiotracer during
the perfusion phase reflect active bleeding whereas
later accumulations are most likely attributable to
urine extravasation (ROSENTHAL 1986).

Renal radionuclide imaging can be combined
with technetium 99 m sulfur colloid hepatosplenic
imaging. This combination offers anatomic, morphologic information of injury to kidney, spleen,
and liver as well as physiologic data. It is a useful
triage examination in patients with low suspicion of
renal, hepatic, or splenic injury.

Renal radionuclide imaging can be used also for
assessing long-term results of treatment of renal
fragments of questionable viability and for investigating delayed complications such as resultant
hypertension. Its noninvasive nature and lack of de-

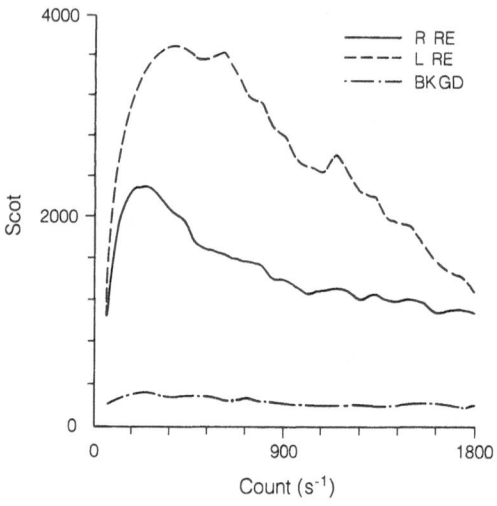

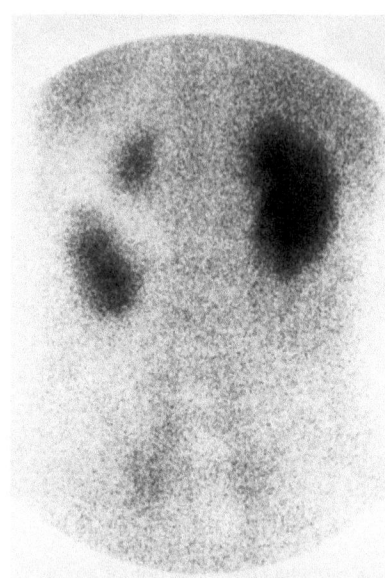

Fig. 7.37. Radionuclide renogram demonstrating significantly reduced perfusion of the right kidney, proved to be due to temporary spasm attendant upon minor trauma

Fig. 7.38. Delayed scintiscanogram after administration of technetium DTPA demonstrating a fracture through the mid portion of the left kidney with two perfused fragments. (LANG 1989)

pendence on contrast media make it attractive in patients with known sensitivity to contrast media.

7.3.5 Retrograde Pyelography

Retrograde ureterography and pyelography are of value to confirm lacerations of the renal pelvis or ureteropelvic junction (Fig. 7.39). Precise characterization and localization of the nature of disruption aids in deciding whether surgery or percutaneous stenting is of benefit (MENDEZ 1977). However, with the exception of categorization of this type of injury, retrograde pyelography is contraindicated in renal trauma since it carries the risk of introducing an infection.

7.3.6 Ultrasonography

Until the advent of Doppler ultrasonography, sonograms lacked physiolgic information. In the past, they were primarily used for monitoring extrarenal fluid collections (KAY et al. 1980). Differentiation of urinomas from fresh hematomas and older hematomas is possible on the basis of characteristic echogenicity. Urinomas tend to be anechoic with good through transmission, while fresh hematomas tend to be hypoechoic and older hematomas may be quite echogenic (Fig. 7.40). Obviously, ultrasonography is

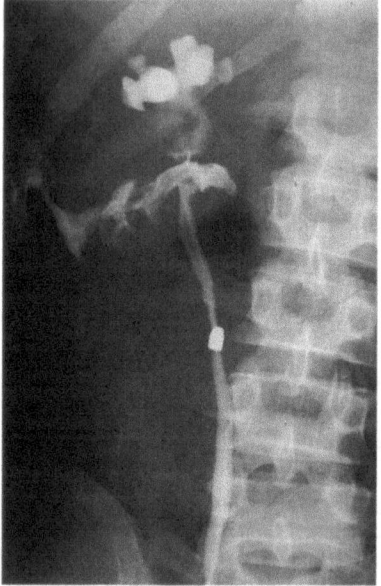

Fig. 7.39. Retrograde pyelogram demonstrating extravasation of contrast material from a partial dehiscence at the ureteropelvis junction, localizing the precise site of injury

useful for monitoring spontaneous reabsorption or drainage of such fluid collections. Since lacerations can be visualized as a linear defect, the technique is also useful for monitoring progressive separation of renal fragments by enlarging interposed hematomas or urinomas (FURTSCHEGGER et al. 1988).

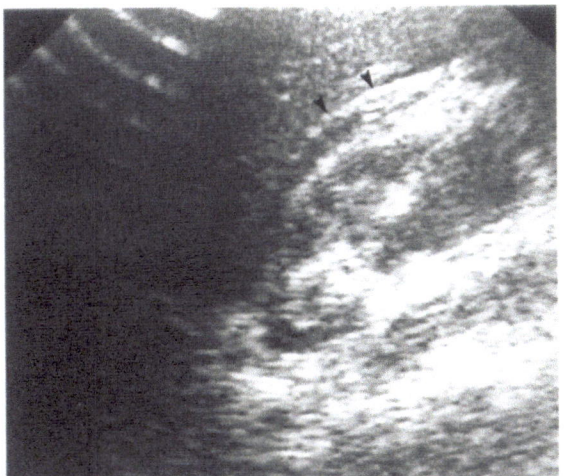

Fig. 7.40. Ultrasonogram in sagittal direction suggesting a relatively echoic collection in the anterior perirenal space. This proved to be an ancient hematoma

Doppler ultrasonography may offer important information as to the patency of main renal vessels (WONG 1989; MARTIN et al. 1988) (Fig. 7.41). If the original enthusiasm regarding the diagnostic yield of Doppler ultrasonography is borne out in larger series, this modality may assume a major role in triage of major vessel injury which, hitherto, has often been subjected to immediate exploration.

7.3.7 Magnetic Resonance Imaging

Magnetic resonance (MR) imaging offers the advantage of multiplanar imaging and sensitivity for differentiation of different types of fluid collections as well as ischemic changes (TERRIER et al. 1987). Focal areas of high signal intensity may be related to hemorrhage with a short T1, while extravasated urine or edema with a long T1 tends to cause focal areas of decreased signal intensity. The earliest findings of minimal renal contusion may be a loss of the corticomedullary junction, which should be distinct on T1-weighted images (BAUMGARTNER et al. 1987). Small collections of blood are readily demonstrated by MR imaging. This has proven particularly useful for the demonstration of small hematomas associated with renal contusion attendant upon extracorporeal shock wave lithotripsy (ESWL) (BAUMGARTNER et al. 1987; RUBIN et al. 1987) (Figs. 7.42, 7.43–7.45). Even minor changes such as resultant edema in the perinephric space or adjacent organs are manifested by prominent strands and fascial thickening (RUBIN et al. 1987). Obviously, small collections of blood in the subcapsular, peri- or pararenal space attendant upon blunt or penetrating

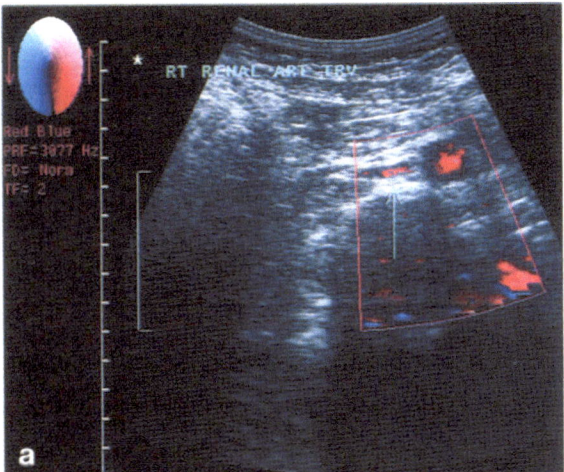

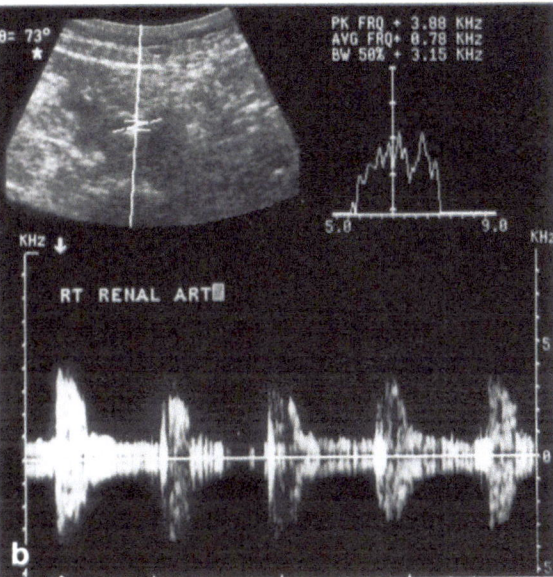

Fig. 7.41. Color Doppler ultrasonogram of the renal artery suggesting reduced flow. Exploration proved the presence of a traumatic flap with fresh thrombus formation

trauma could be demonstrated similarly by this modality. Moreover, thrombosis of renal artery or vein is diagnosable by this technique (YUASA and KUNDEL 1985). Even ischemic changes attendant upon lack of perfusion can be demonstrated and differentiated against edema, which is difficult, if not impossible, for imaging examinations diagnosing on the basis of an absorption differential of x-ray beam energies (TERRIER et al. 1987). There are logistic factors that make difficult general use of MR imaging in acute trauma patients, who are often on life support systems. However, once the patient is stable, MR imaging is an excellent method for evaluating progression or regression of retroperitoneal effusions and for differentiating between urine and blood content.

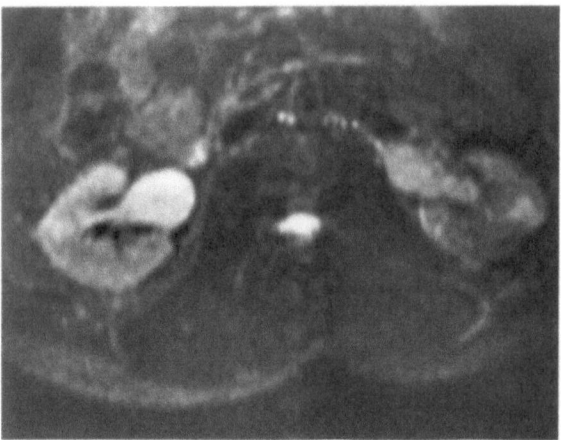

Fig. 7.42. A T2-weighted image (TR 2500, TE 80, spin echo) demonstrating an area of increased signal intensity within the kidney, indicating the presence of a fresh hematoma attendant upon an ESWL procedure. T1-weighted images showed some loss of definition of the corticomedullary junction, a relatively nonspecific finding indicative of edema. (Courtesy of Dr. HOWARD M. POLLACK)

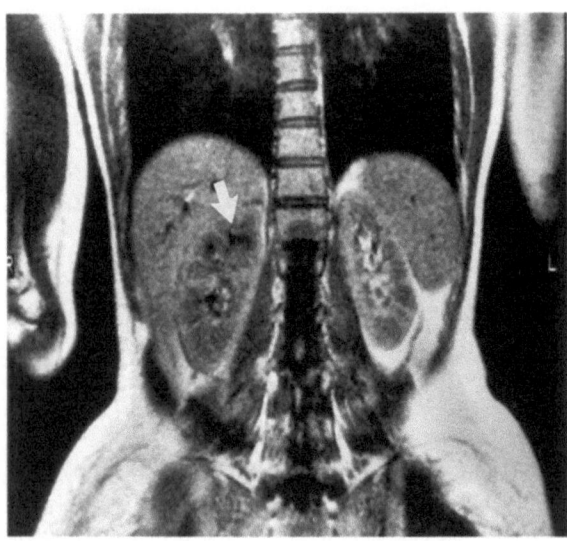

Fig. 7.44. Coronal MR image (SE 500/30) obtained after ESWL with 2250 shockwaves showing an area of decreased signal intensity *(arrow)* in the upper pole of the right kidney. (BAUMGARTNER et al. 1987).

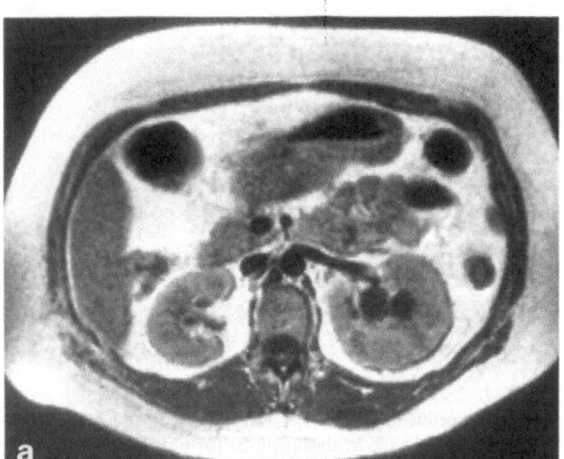

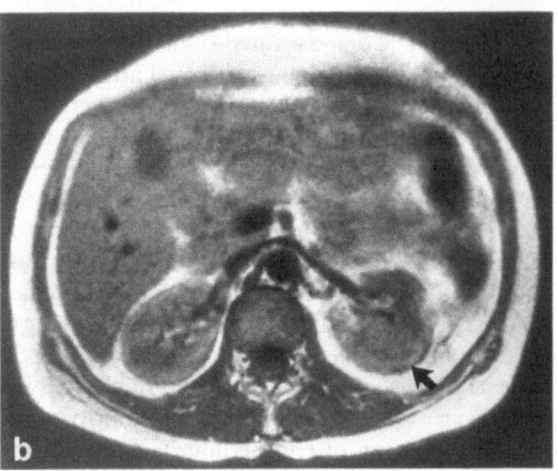

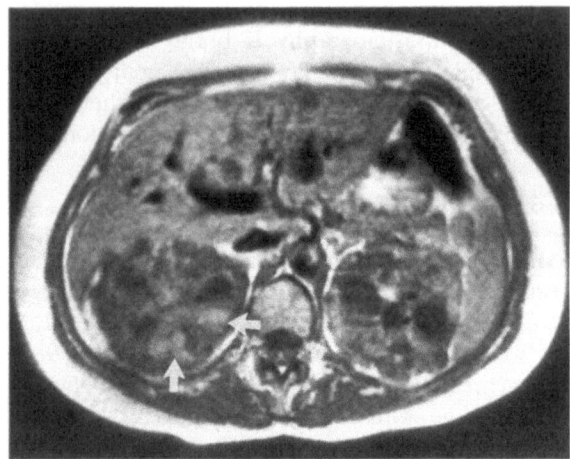

Fig. 7.45. Axial MR image (SE 900/30) revealing high intensity signals *(arrows)* in the upper pole of the right kidney after ESWL with 3000 shockwaves. The areas of varying signal intensity in the remainder of both kidneys indicate the presence of adult polycystic disease. (BAUMGARTNER et al. 1987)

◁

Fig. 7.43. a Axial MR images (SE 900-30) obtained after ESWL with 1500 shockwaves shows a swollen left kidney with loss of the corticomedullary junction. **b** After ESWL with 1700 shockwaves, there are focal areas of increased signal intensity *(arrow)* posterior in the left kidney, again with poor definition of the corticomedullary junction. (BAUMGARTNER et al. 1987)

7.4 Coexistent Renal and Intraabdominal Injury

Penetrating, but also blunt renal injuries resulting from motor vehicle accidents have a high incidence of associated abdominal injuries, many of which require laparotomy (CASS 1983; LANG 1990; MON-STREY et al. 1988). In a series of some 1176 renal injuries due to blunt trauma, CASS (1983) found 874 associated injuries of which 384 (33% of all patients) required immediate laparotomy.

Computed tomography, particularly if combined with dynamic mode recording, has proven highly effective in diagnosing such coexistent injuries. In our group of 337 patients with confirmed renal injury due to either blunt or penetrating trauma, 525 coexistent abdominal or retroperitoneal injuries were diagnosed (LANG 1990). In general, the severity of abdominal organ injury bore a linear relationship to the severity of renal injury (Table 7.1). Moreover, intraabdominal and retroperitoneal organ injuries tended to be more severe in patients who had sustained penetrating injury. Major intraabdominal or retroperitoneal organ injuries occurred in 79 of 83 such patients. There is, however, a major difference in the predominant target organ of such injury. Among our 361 patients who sustained blunt abdominal trauma, we noted 29 injuries to bowel; among 83 patients who sustained penetrating trauma, there were 73 injuries to bowel and stomach (Fig. 7.46). Major injuries to liver and spleen occurred with equal frequency in blunt and penetrating trauma patients. However, minor injuries to liver and spleen were more common with blunt trauma (42% incidence rate) than with penetrating trauma (15%). Injuries to the skeletal system, CNS, and pelvic organs were likewise more common among patients who sustained blunt trauma (54%) than those with penetrating trauma (28%). The accuracy of clinical vs radiologic diagnosis varied for different organs and different injury mechanisms. In general, CT diagnosis was vastly superior in blunt trauma. The diagnosis of associated abdominal or retroperitoneal organ injury was correctly established by CT

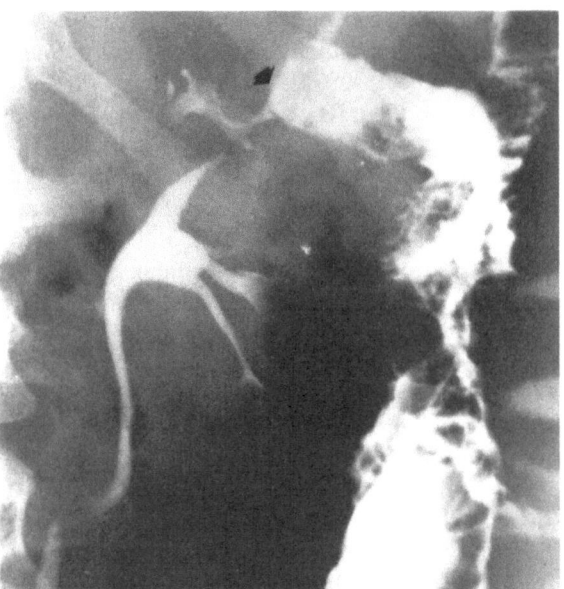

Fig. 7.46. Intravenous urogram demonstrating a jejunal-calyceal fistula and a jejunal-colic fistula. Both the jejunum and finally the left colon are opacified by contrast laden urine

in 277 (85%) of 324 patients who sustained blunt trauma, whereas clinical examinations established the correct diagnosis in only 86 (26%) (LANG 1990). CT was particularly useful for diagnosing fractures involving the pancreas, hematomas in the wall of the bowel or mesentery, rupture of the bowel due to blunt trauma, and major injuries to liver and spleen (JEFFREY et al. 1982; KARNAZE et al. 1981; LANG 1990) (Figs. 7.14, 7.17).

7.5 Approach to Radiologic Assessment of Renal Trauma

Although many variables influence the choice of imaging examinations of the acutely traumatized kidney, a preferential approach has emerged capable of answering the questions which determine our treatment protocols at today's standards (KARP et al. 1986; MONSTREY et al. 1988; POLLACK and WEIN 1989; SCLAFANI and BECKER 1985).

Though hematuria is one of the criteria indicating renal injury, many patients, particularly those with microscopic hematuria, may have sustained only very minor injury (NICOLAISEN et al. 1985; HARDE-MAN et al. 1987).

In patients with a history of injury mechanism and clinical findings indicating probability of only minimal renal injury without associated abdominal or retroperitoneal organ injury, intravenous uro-

Table 7.1. Coexistent major abdominal or other organ injuries in patients who sustained no or minor vs major renal injury due to blunt or penetrating trauma[a]. (LANG 1990)

Other site	Minimal renal injury	Major renal injury
Total no.	349 (77)	12 (6)
Liver	24 (6)	1 (1)
Spleen	25 (4)	2 (1)
Pancreas	7 (2)	1 (0)
Bowel	17 (23)	1 (4)

[a] Figures within parentheses relate to penetrating trauma.

graphy or computed radionuclide urography suffices for triage examination (Cass and Luxenberg 1984; Cass et al. 1986; Hardeman et al. 1987; Kisa and Schenk 1986; Kuzmarov et al. 1981; Liev et al. 1988; Monstrey et al. 1988; Oakland et al. 1987; Rubin and Schliftman 1979; Stables 1976; Wilson and Ziegler 1987). These techniques are generally readily available, inexpensive, and noninvasive. Demonstration of normally functioning kidneys suffices for determining the clinical management of such patients (Cass et al. 1986; Lieu et al. 1988).

In the presence of clinical findings indicating renal injury and of persistent hematuria, and with an injury mechanism prone to produce substantial renal parenchymal injury, CT with both dynamic and postenhancement recordings is recommended. It must be emphasized that absence of hematuria does not exclude major renal injury; in fact, one-third of patients with pedicle injury failed to exhibit hematuria (Cass 1983, 1988). An injury mechanism prone to produce other intraabdominal and/or retroperitoneal organ injuries intensifies the need for examination by CT. In this setting, intravenous urography can be withheld since it is not likely to contribute substantial additional information; in fact it may actually delay treatment and sometimes increases the amount of contrast medium deployed (Nicolaisen et al. 1985; Cass and Vieira 1987; Oakland et al. 1987). In this scenario, the dynamic and postenhancement computed tomograms are capable of identifying and categorizing not only renal injuries but also coexistent intraabdominal and retroperitoneal organ injuries (Moore et al. 1989). In the latter categories, the diagnostic sensitivity is 300% greater than with clinical examination and competitive studies (Lang 1990). Although there are a substantial number of false-positive diagnoses of some such injuries, specifically of the liver, the ability to follow such injuries and intervene only if follow-up imaging examination indicates incipient clinical complications, or in the presence of clinical deterioration, tends to minimize this problem (Lang 1990). Failure to diagnose minor hepatic and splenic injuries by CT and even more so by clinical examinations does not appear to influence the ultimate outcome adversely since such lesions heal without further treatment.

A properly staged sequence of computed tomograms assessing the abdomen and sometimes chest by dynamic mode, and regions incriminated by clinical findings or by prior examinations by postenhancement computed tomograms, offers an unequalled criteria constellation for diagnosis and categorization of multiple injuries. If necessary, im-

plicated regions of the chest, pelvis, and head can be evaluated further by postenhancement computed tomograms without the need for additional i.v. contrast medium.

For diagnosis and categorization of the magnitude of renal parenchymal injuries, the combination of dynamic and postenhancement computed tomograms offers extraordinarily sensitive criteria. Contusion, parenchymal tears, viability of parenchymal margins, abutting hematomas, resultant traumatic infarcts, and extravasation of contrast medium laden urine are diagnosed with high accuracy and specificity. While the presence and location of arterial injuries may well be suggested by findings on computed tomograms, detailed categorization of this injury requires selective angiography.

Follow-up of identified parenchymal injuries treated conservatively can be performed by CT, ultrasonography, and sometimes radionuclide studies or intravenous urography (Furtschegger et al. 1988). A change in management, and perhaps surgical intervention, is indicated if progressive loss of parenchymal viability, increasing size of hematomas or urinomas, and failure to seal parenchymal communications to the collecting system with resultant continued extravasation into urinomas or fistulas are observed (Fig. 7.41). Obviously, deterioration of clinical condition and certain laboratory indicators, such as a rapid rise in amylase, might militate toward a change in therapy, i.e., surgical intervention to debride and/or close the defect, create a watertight suture to prevent further extravasation of urine, or correct injuries to liver, spleen, or pancreas that show progressive devascularization (Guerriero 1988; Peters and Bright 1977; Taylor et al. 1988).

While protocols furnish useful algorithms for our approach, flexibility must be maintained for each patient and the ultimate diagnostic assessment as well as the treatment approach individualized to meet specific circumstances.

References

Baumgartner BR, Dickey KW, Ambrose SS, Walton KN, Nelson RC, Bernerdino ME (1987) Kidney changes after extracorporeal shock wave lithotripsy (appearance on MR imaging). Radiology 163: 531–534

Bergren CT, Chan FN, Bodzin JH (1987) Intravenous pyelogram results in association with renal pathology in therapy and trauma patients. J Trauma 27: 515–518

Bernath AS, Schutte H, Fernandes RRD, et al. (1983) Stab wounds of the kidney: conservative management in flank penetration. J Urol 129: 468–470

Bretan PN, McAninch JW (1988) Evaluation of renal trauma: indications for computed tomography and other diagnostic techniques. In: Lypton D, Catalona WJ, Lipshultz LI, McQuire EJ (eds) Advances in urology, vol 1. Yearbook Medical, Chicago, p 65

Bretan PN, McAninch JW, Federle MP, Jeffrey RB Jr (1986) Computerized tomography staging of renal trauma: 85 consecutive cases. J Urol 136: 561

Brower P, Paul J, Brosman SA (1978) Urinary tract abnormalities presenting as result of blunt abdominal trauma. J Trauma 18: 719–722

Carroll PR, McAninch JW (1985) Operative indications in penetrating renal trauma. J Trauma 25: 587–593

Cass AS (1983) Blunt renal trauma in children. J Trauma 23: 123–127

Cass AS (1988) Discussion. In: Guerriero WG (ed) Problems in Urology, vol 2. Lippincott, Philadelphia, p 184

Cass AS, Luxenberg M (1983) Conservative or immediate surgical management of blunt renal injuries. J Urol 130: 1116

Cass AS, Luxenberg M (1984) Unilateral nonvisualization in excretory urography after external trauma. J Urol 132: 220–227

Cass AS, Vieira J (1987) Comparison of IVP and CT findings in patients with suspected severe renal injury. Urology 29: 484–487

Cass AS, Susset J, Khan A, Godec CJ (1979) Renal pedicle injury in multiple injured patients. J Urol 122: 728

Cass AS, Luxenberg M, Gleich P, et al. (1985) Type of blunt renal injury rather than associated extravasation should determine treatment. Urology 26: 249–251

Cass AS, Luxenberg M, Gleich P, Smith CS (1986) Clinical indications for radiographic evaluation of blunt renal trauma. J Urol 136: 370–371

Cass EJ (1988) Renal injury in children. In: Cass AS (ed) Genitourinary trauma. Blackwell Scientific, Boston, p 58

Cates JW, Foley WD, Lawson TL (1986) Retrograde opacification of renal vein: a CT sign of renal artery avulsion. Urol Radiol 8: 92–94

Chopp RT, Hekmant-Ravan H, Mendez R (1980) Technetium 99 m glucoheptonate renal scan in diagnosis of acute renal injury. Urology 15: 201

Colapinto ND (1977) Early exploration or laparotomy for stab wounds of the abdomen. Can Med Assoc J 117: 157

Cosgrove MD, Mendez R, Morrow JW (1973) Traumatic renal arteriovenous fistula: a report of 12 cases. J Urol 110: 627–631

Demetriades D, Rabinowitz B (1984) Selective conservative management of penetrating abdominal wounds: a prospective study. Br J Surg 71: 92

Druy EM, Rubin BE (1979) Computed tomography in the evaluation of abdominal trauma. J Comput Assist Tomogr 3: 40–44

Erturk E, Sheinfeld J, DeMarco PL, et al. (1985) Renal trauma: evaluations by computerized tomography. J Urol 133: 946–949

Evins SC, Thomason WB, Rosenblaum R (1980) Nonoperative management of severe renal laceration. J Urol 123: 247–249

Federle MP (1990) Evaluation of renal trauma. In: Pollack H (ed) Urologic radiology, Sect 5, Trauma, EK Lang (ed) Chapter 51. Lippincott, Philadelphia, pp 1472–1493

Federle MP, Brant-Zawadzki M (1986) Computed tomography in evaluation of trauma. 2nd edn. William & Wilkins, Baltimore, pp 265–270

Federle MP, Kaiser JA, McAninch JW, et al. (1981) The role of computer tomography in renal trauma. Radiology 141: 455–460

Federle MP, Brown TR, McAninch JW (1987) Penetrating renal trauma: CT evaluation. J Comput Assist Tomogr 11: 1026–1030

Fisher RG, Ben-Menachen Y, Whigham C (1989) Stab wounds of the renal artery branches: angiographic diagnosis and treatment by embolization. AJR 152: 1231–1235

Furtschegger A, Egender G, Jakse G (1988) The value of sonography in the diagnosis and follow-up of patients with blunt renal trauma. Br J Urol 62: 110–116

Glazer GM, Francis IR, Brady TM, Teng SS (1983) Computed tomography of renal infarction: clinical and experimental observation. AJR 140: 721–727

Glazer GM, Francis IR, Gross BH, Amendola MA (1984) Computed tomography of renal vein thrombosis. J Comput Assist Tomogr 8: 288–293

Goldberger JH, Bernstein DM, Rodman GH Jr, Suarez CA (1982) Selection of patients with abdominal stab wounds for laparotomy. J Trauma 22: 476

Gonzalez EP Jr, Guerriero WG (1985) Genitourinary tract trauma in children. In: Kelalis PK, King LR, Belman AB (eds) Clinical pediatric urology, vol 2. W. B. Saunders, Philadelphia, pp 1125–1126

Guerriero WG (1988) Genitourinary trauma. In: Guerriero WG (ed) Problems in urology, vol 2. Lippincott, Philadelphia, pp 186–187

Hardeman SW, Husmann BA, Chinn HKW, Peters PC (1987) Blunt urinary tract trauma: identifying those patients who require radiologic diagnostic studies. J Urol 138: 99

Haynes JW, Walsh JW, Brewer WH, Vick CW, Allen HA (1984) Traumatic renal artery occlusion: CT diagnosis with angiographic correlation. J Comput Assist Tomogr 8: 731–733

Hessel SJ, Smith EH (1974) Renal trauma: a comprehensive review in radiologic assessment. CRC Crit Rev Clin Radiol Nucl Med 5: 251–293

Heynes CF, DeClerk BP, DeKock MLS (1983) Stab wounds associated with hematuria – a review of 67 cases. J Urol 130: 228

Heynes CF, DeClerk BP, DeKock MLS (1985) Nonoperative management of renal stab wounds. J Urol 134: 239–242

Jaske G, Furtschegger A, Egender G (1987) Ultrasound in patients with blunt renal trauma managed by surgery. J Urol 138: 21

Jeffrey PB, Federle MP, Stein SM, et al. (1982) Intramural hematoma of the cecum following blunt trauma. J Comput Assist Tomogr 6: 404–407

Karnaze GC, Sheedy PF, Stephens DH, et al. (1981) Computed tomography in duodenal rupture due to blunt abdominal trauma. J Comput Assist Tomogr 5: 267–271

Karp MP, Jewett TC Jr, Kuhn JP, et al. (1986) The impact of computed tomography, scanning in a child with renal trauma. J Pediatr Surg 21: 617–623

Kay CJ, Rosenfield AB, Armm M (1980) Grayscale ultrasonography in the evaluation of renal trauma. Radiology 134: 461–466

Kenney PJ, Panicek DN, Witanowski LS (1987) Computed tomography of ureteral disruption. J Comput Assist Tomogr 11: 480–484

Kisa E, Schenk WG III (1986) Indications for emergency intravenous pyelography (IVP) in blunt abdominal trauma: a reappraisal. J Trauma 26: 1086–1089

Kuzmarov IW, Morehouse DD, Gibson S (1981) Blunt renal trauma in the pediatric population: a retrospective study. J Urol 126: 448

Lang EK et al. (1971) Renal arteriography in the assessment of renal trauma radiology. 98: 103

Lang EK (1975) Arteriography in the assessment of renal trauma: The impact of arteriographic diagnosis on preservation of renal function and parenchyma. J Trauma 15: 553-560

Lang EK (1976) The role of arteriography in trauma. Radiol Clin North Am 14: 353-359

Lang EK (1983a) Assessment of renal trauma by dynamic computer tomography. Radiographics 3: 566-584

Lang EK (1983b) Current concepts in diagnosis of renal trauma. Contemp Diagn Radiol 6 (15): 1-5

Lang EK (1985) Imaging examinations in management of renal trauma. Sem US CT MR 6 (2): 11-108

Lang EK (1987a) Trauma of the urinary tract. In: Taveras JM, Ferrucci JT (eds) Radiology. Lippincott, Philadelphia, pp 1-24

Lang EK (1987b) Percutaneous nephrostomy, lithotomy and lithotripsy: multi-institutional survey of complications. Radiology 162: 25-30

Lang EK (1989) Assessment of traumatic injury to the kidney by imaging examinations. Probl Urol 3 (4): 704-730

Lang EK (1990) Intraabdominal and retroperitoneal organ injuries diagnosed on dynamic computed tomograms obtained for assessment of renal trauma. J Trauma 30 (9): 1161-1168

Lang EK, Sullivan J, Frentz G (1985) Renal trauma: radiologic studies comparison of urography, computed tomography, angiography and radionuclide studies. Radiology 154: 1-6

Lieu TA, Fleischer GR, Mahboubi S, et al. (1988) Hematuria and clinical findings as indications for intravenous pyelography in pediatric blunt renal trauma. Pediatrics 82: 216-222

Lohse JR, Pothan RJ, Waters RF (1982) Traumatic bilateral renal artery thrombosis: case report and review of the literature. J Urol 127: 522-527

Mahoney SA, Persky L (1968) Intravenous drip nephrotomography as adjunct in evaluation of renal injury. J Urol 99: 513-516

Marburger H (1988) Blunt injuries of the kidneys. In: Cass AS (ed) Genitourinary trauma. Blackwell Scientific, Boston, pp 21-24

Martin KW, McAlister WH, Shackelford GD (1988) Acute renal infarction: diagnosis by Doppler ultrasound. Pediatr Radiol 18: 373-376

McAninch JW (1985) Urogenital trauma. Thieme-Stratton, New York

McAninch JW, Federle MP (1982) Evaluation of renal injuries with computerized tomography. J Urol 128: 456-460

McCort JJ (1983) Perirenal fat infiltration by hemorrhage: radiographic recognition and CT confirmation. Radiology 149: 665-667

Mee SL, McAninch JW, Robinson AS, et al. (1989) Radiographic assessment of renal trauma: a 10 year prospective study of patient selection. J Urol 141: 1095-1098

Mendez R (1977) Renal trauma. J Urol 118: 698-703

Miller RC, Sterioff F Jr, Drucker WR, Persky L, Wright HK, Davis IH (1966) The incidental discovery of occult abdominal tumors in children following blunt abdominal trauma. J Trauma 6: 99-106

Monstrey SJM, Vander Werken C, Debruyne FMJ, Goris RJA (1988) Rational guidelines in renal trauma assessment. Urology 31: 469-473

Montie JE, Ross G Jr (1977) Results of nonoperative management. J Urol 117: 122-126

Moore EE, Shacford SR, Pachter HL, et al. (1989) Organ injury scaling: spleen, liver, kidney. J Trauma 12: 1664-1666

Newman B, Smith S (1987) Unusual renal mass in a newborn infant. Radiology 163: 193-194

Nicolaisen GS, McAninch JW, Marshall GA, Bluth RF Jr, Carroll PR (1985) Renal trauma re-evaluation of the indications for radiography assessment. J Urol 133: 183-187. Proc R Soc Med 80: 21

Oakland CDH, Britton JM, Charlton CAC (1987) Renal trauma in the intravenous urogram. Proc R Soc Med 80:21

Peck JJ, Berne TV (1981) Posterior abdominal stab wounds. J Trauma 21: 298

Pietzman AB, Makaroun MS, Slasky S, et al. (1986) Prospective study of computed tomography in initial management of blunt abdominal trauma. J Trauma 26: 585-592

Peters PC, Bright TC (1977) Blunt renal injuries. Urol Clin North Am 4: 17-28

Peters PC, Sagalowsky AI (1986) Genitourinary trauma. In: Walsh PC, Gittes RF, Perlmutter AB, Stamey TA (eds) Campbell's urology, vol 1. 5th edn. W. B. Saunders, Philadelphia, PA, Chap 26

Phlillips T, Sclafani SJA, Goldstein A, et al. (1986) Use of contrast enhanced CT enema in management of penetrating trauma to flank and back. J Trauma 26: 593-601

Pollack HM, Wein AJ (1989) Imaging of renal trauma. Radiology 172: 297-308

Ralls PW, Barakos JA, Kaptein EM, et al. (1987) Renal biopsy related hemorrhage: frequency in comparison of CT and sonography. J Comput Assist Tomogr 11: 1031

Rhyner B, Federle MP, Jeffrey RB (1984) CT of trauma to the abnormal kidney. AJR 142: 747-750

Rosenthal L (1986) Renal and urinary tract trauma. In: O'Reilly PH, Shields RA, Testa HJ (eds) Nuclear medicine in urology and nephrology, 2nd edn., Butterworths, London, p 16

Rubin BE, Schliftman R (1979) The striated nephrogram in renal contusion. Urol Radiol 1: 119-121

Rubin JI, Arger PH, Pollack HM, et al. (1987) Kidney changes after extracorporeal shock wave lithotripsy: CT evaluation. Radiology 162: 21-25

Sagalowsky AL, McConnell JB, Peter PD (1983) Renal trauma requiring surgery: an analysis of 185 cases. J Trauma 23: 128-131

Schlegel JU, Lang EK (1980) Computed radionuclide urogram for assessing acute renal failure. AJR 124: 1029-1034

Sclafani SJA, Becker JA (1985) Radiological diagnosis of renal trauma. Urologic Radiol 7: 192

Sclafani SJA, Goldstein AS, Panetta T, et al. (1985) CT diagnosis of renal pedicle injury. Urol Radiol 7: 63

Stables EP (1976) Unilateral absence of excretion at urography after abdominal trauma. Radiology 121: 609

Steinberg DL, Jeffrey RB, Federle MP, McAninch JW (1984) A computerized tomographic appearance of renal pedicle injury. J Urol 132: 1163-1164

Takahashi M, Tamakawa Y, Shibata A, Fukushima Y (1977) Computed tomography of "page" kidney. J Comput Assist Tomogr 1: 344

Taylor GA, Eichelberger MR, Polter BM (1988) Hematuria, a marker of abdominal injury in children after blunt trauma. Ann Surg 208: 688-693

Terrier F, Hricak H, Berry I, et al. (1987) Edema and lack of blood perfusion produce opposite effects on the magnetic resonance characteristics of acutely ischemic rate kidneys. Invest Radiol 22: 118-125

Thompson IM, Latournett H (1977) Results of nonoperative management of blunt trauma. J Urol 118: 522-524

Thompson JS, Moore EE, Van Duzer-Moore S, Moore JB, Galloway AC (1980) The evolution of abdominal stab wound management. J Trauma 20: 478

Wein AJ, Murphy JJ, Mulholland SG, et al. (1977) A conservative approach to the management of blunt renal trauma. J Urol 117: 425–427

Wilson RF, Ziegler BW (1987) Diagnostic and treatment problems in renal injuries. Am Surg 53: 399–402

Wong SN, Lorns, Yu ECL (1989) Renal blood flow pattern by noninvasive doppler ultasound in normal children and acute renal failure patients. J US Med 8: 135–139

Wong SW, Moss AA, Federle MP, et al. (1984) Renal infarction: CT diagnosis and correlation between CT findings and etiology. Radiology 150: 201–205

Yale-Loehr AJ, Kramer SS, Quinlan DM, et al. (1989) CT of severe renal trauma in children, evaluation and course of healing with conservative therapy. AJR 152: 109

Yuasa Y, Kundel H (1985) Magnetic resonance imaging following unilateral occlusion of renal circulation in rabbits. Radiology 154: 151

8 Benign Renal Tumors

Jeffrey H. Newhouse

CONTENTS

8.1   Introduction 215
8.2   Oncocytoma 215
8.3   Renal Adenoma 217
8.4   Juxtaglomerular Cell Tumor (Reninoma) 218
8.5   Angiomyolipomas 218
8.6   Multiocular Cystic Nephroma 222
8.7   Congenital Mesoblastic Nephroma
        (Fetal Renal Hamartoma) 223
8.8   Medullary Fibroma
        (Renal Medullary Interstitial Cell Tumor) 223
        References 224

8.1 Introduction

Benign renal neoplasms are surprisingly common (SOMEREN et al. 1989), but since many of them are very small and have virtually no potential to produce clinically significant disease, the important benign renal tumors encountered in an imaging practice appear relatively infrequently. Often, benign renal tumors can be distinguished from malignant ones by their imaging features (WILLIAMSON 1990), which permits appropriate therapeutic decisions to be made, and certain clinical events may raise the strong likelihood of particular benign tumors; for both reasons, a familiarity with these lesions is important for practicing radiologists (AMIS and NEWHOUSE 1991). This chapter will discuss first those tumors which are of epithelial origin, and then those which are felt to be mesenchymal or hamartomatous.

8.2 Oncocytoma

An oncocytoma is a relatively rare tumor (JOHNSON et al. 1979; MORALES et al. 1980; PEARSE and HOUGHTON 1979; ROTHENBERGER et al. 1978). It has been described by a number of names, including granular cell adenoma, oncocytic tubular adenoma,

JEFFREY H. NEWHOUSE, M.D., Professor of Radiology; Columbia Presbyterian Medical Center, 177 Ft. Washington Avenue, New York, NY 10032, USA

and oxyphilic tubular adenoma. It arises in the cortex of the kidney and is usually supposed to contitute a tumor of the proximal convoluted tubular cells; some investigators, however, feel it may arise from distal tubular cells as well. Oncocytomas may appear in other organs, including the salivary glands, nasal mucosa, thyroid and parathyroid glands, lacrimal glands, lung, and adrenal cortex. Rarely, patients with tuberous sclerosis may have oncocytomas and a few oncocytomas have been found in conjunction with renal cell carcinomas (MAATMAN et al. 1984). Rarely, the tumors may be multicentric or bilateral (MOURA and NASCIMENTO 1982).

Oncocytomas have been found in patients from the teenage years through late old age; there is a peak incidence in the fifties, sixties, and seventies. There is a male predominance.

Their natural history is not very well known. Certainly, most oncocytomas are entirely benign, but a few have demonstrated evidence of local fat invasion or metastasis to local nodes (LIEBER et al. 1981; MAATMAN et al. 1984; PSIHRAMIS et al. 1988). Patients who have had oncocytomas resected usually develop no evidence of recurrence. However, since some renal cell carcinomas have portions of the tumor which look histologically like oncocytomas, and since some oncocytomas, as mentioned above, may reveal evidence of metastatic behavior, some investigators believe that the oncocytoma may be a low grade variant of renal cell carcinoma rather than a distinct tumor.

Most oncocytomas are treated by radical nephrectomy (MAATMAN et al. 1984), both because they frequently cannot be distinguished from renal cell carcinomas with absolute certainty, and because of their admittedly infrequent tendency to display local invasion. At least one patient has been reported in whom a biopsy-proven oncocytoma has not been resected; over a period of several years, the tumor has appeared to progress very little.

Oncocytomas may be asymptomatic and come to attention only because the affected kidney has been imaged for other reasons. Symptomatic oncocyto-

mas have been documented as producing pain, hematuria, and palpable masses.

The pathology of oncocytomas (AKHTAR and
KOTT 1979; CHOI et al. 1983; YU et al. 1980) varies
relatively little from tumor to tumor. Grossly, they
are seen to be round tan or brown tumors which
range in size from less than 1 cm to over 26 cm in
diameter; the most common tumors are approximately 5 cm in diameter. A bisected tumor may reveal a central cleft or stellate scar. The tumors
usually do not have a true capsule, but are clearly
demarcated from adjacent kidney and other tissues
in most cases. They rarely contain regions of hemorrhage, necrosis, or calcifications; a very few of these
tumors have been reported as having multiple small
cystic regions within them (OGDEN et al. 1987). Very
rarely, the tumors may extend into the renal vein.

Microscopic examinations of these lesions
(LIEBER et al. 1981) reveal relatively large eosinophilic cells (oncocytes) with many mitochondria.
These cells are arranged in sheets, nests, or clusters.
The central cleft or stellate scar usually consists of a
cellular hyalinized or edematous stroma. Nuclear
pleomorphism, if present, is usually only focal; mi-
toses are very rarely seen.

Histologic diagnosis of an oncocytoma requires
the examination of many parts of the tumor, since
some renal cell carcinomas contain regions which
have tissue which looks identical with that found
within oncocytomas. For this reason, needle biopsies or small open biopsies of the tumors are not
usually felt to be sufficient for absolute diagnosis.

If the tumors are large, they may appear on plain
films as upper abdominal masses. Calcification,
visible either on radiographs (WASSERMAN and
EWING 1983) or computed tomographic (CT) examinations, is very rare.

A urogram reveals evidence of a round renal mass
which is usually indistinguishable from a renal cell
carcinoma. It may distort the collecting system, but
since the tumor very rarely occludes the vasculature
or invades the entire kidney, the tumor-bearing kidney almost always functions. The lesion is usually
well demarcated.

On ultrasound, the tumor is seen to be a solid
mass with relatively homogeneous echogenicity
which is usually little different from that of normal
renal parenchyma (Fig. 8.1). But there may be a central echo-poor or echo-dense cleft or stellate region.

On CT, the tumors are usually found to be round
and of relatively homogeneous density except for
the central cleft or scar (COHAN et al. 1984; LEVINE
and HUNTRAKOON 1983; QUINN et al. 1984). They
usually enhance relatively homogeneously, but do

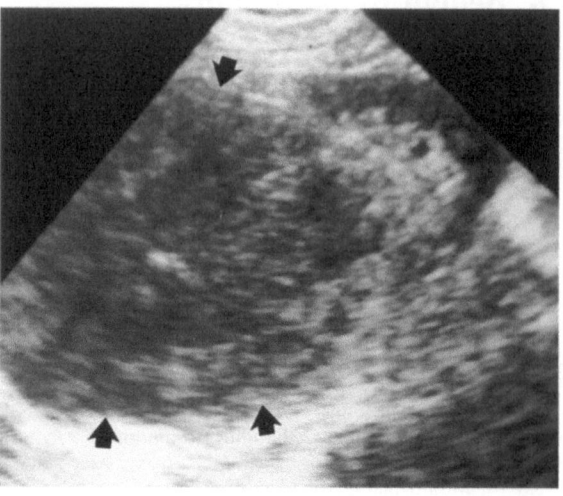

Fig. 8.1. Renal oncocytoma. Ultrasound reveals large renal
mass *(arrows)* with moderate slightly heterogeneous echogenicity

not become as dense as normal renal parenchyma
(Fig. 8.2). The very rare tumor which extends into the
renal vein may have the venous thrombus demonstrable by CT. The tumor has a distinct margin more
often than does renal carcinoma.

Angiography usually reveals a relatively vascular
tumor (Fig. 8.3), although occasionally the tumors
may be hypovascular (AMBOS et al. 1978; CLARK and
PALUBINSKAS 1972; COMPTON et al. 1976; SCHMIDT
and TAENZER 1980; SOS et al. 1976). The characteristic appearance of the lesion is that of a spoke-
wheel arrangement of radial vessels (QUINN et al.
1984) which rarely show marked puddling or arteriovenous shunting. The nephrogram phase is
usually relatively homogeneous, with the exception
of the lucency in the central scar.

Magnetic resonance imaging (MRI) reveals a
well-defined tumor (SOHN et al. 1987) which may approximate the intensity of normal renal parenchyma
on both T1-weighted and T2-weighted images;
some of the tumors are less intense than kidney on
T2-weighted images.

One case of an oncocytoma which displayed persistent uptake of Tc-DTPA has been reported
(CHOUDHRI et al. 1987).

Investigators differ with regard to the degree that
they feel that a definite diagnosis of oncocytoma can
be made preoperatively (JANDER 1979; OLDER et al.
1978). Some feel that if a homogeneous lesion with a
central scar is seen at CT and ultrasound, and if angiography reveals a spoke-wheel vascular pattern,
one can be certain enough about the diagnosis to
recommend treating it as a benign tumor and therefore recommending conservative tumor excision or

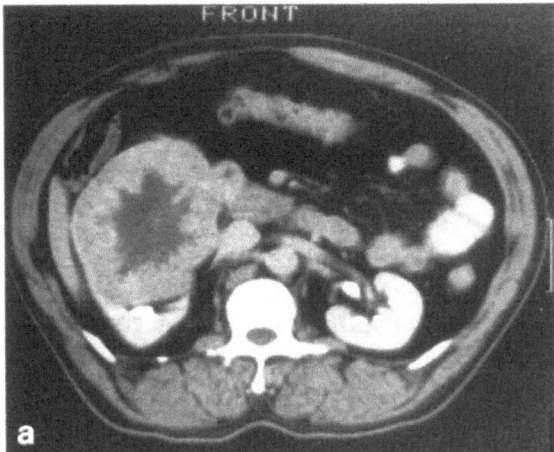

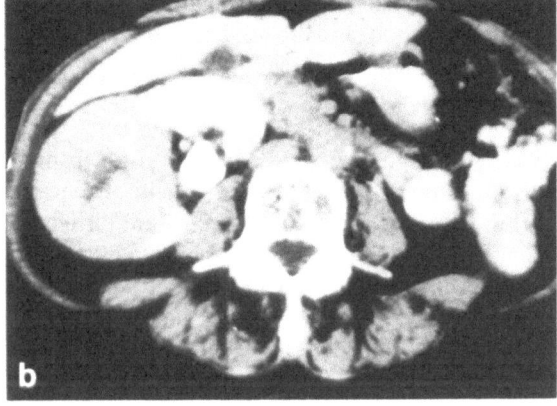

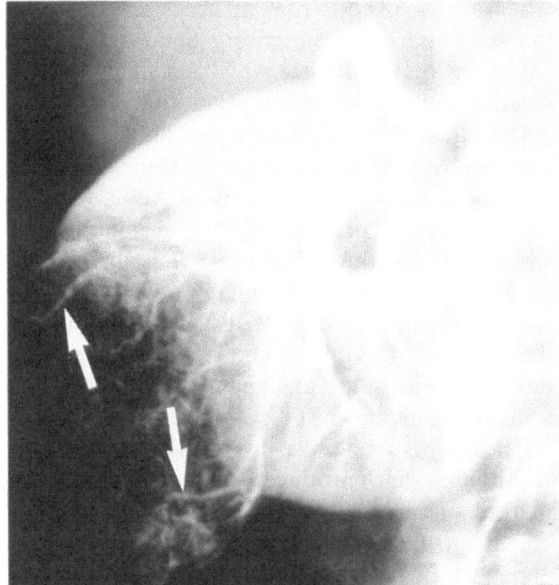

Fig. 8.3. Oncocytoma. Angiogram reveals moderate vascularity with peripheral curved vessels and a few radial penetrating arteries *(arrows)*

◁

Fig. 8.2 a, b. CT of renal oncocytomas. **a** Right renal mass with large central stellate scar. **b** Another case, showing small stellate scar and homogeneous opacification of the tumor

partial nephrectomy. Other investigators feel that although it is relatively unusual for a renal cell carcinoma to exhibit all of these characteristics of an oncocytoma, renal cell carcinomas are so much more numerous than oncocytomas that demonstration of oncocytoma-like imaging features still does not permit a definitive diagnosis to be made, so that the patient needs to be treated as if he has a renal cell carcinoma until the entire tumor has been resected and can be examined.

8.3 Renal Adenoma

There has been a long-standing controversy with regard to whether such a lesion as a renal adenoma even exists, at least if the term *adenoma* is meant to designate a tumor which, without some sort of degeneration into another lesion, does not metastasize or exhibit other signs of malignant behavior. Currently, few investigators believe that a clear distinction can be made between renal adenomas and renal cell carcinomas; instead, most feel that there exist renal epithelial tumors with a wide range of malig-

nant potential (BENNINGTON 1987). Nevertheless, renal adenomas deserve at least a short discussion since the term *adenoma* persists and is used by some pathologists and other physicians to refer to a particular kind of lesion.

Small cortical epithelial tumors in the kidney are quite common, appearing in 7%–23% of all autopsies. They may often be multiple and bilateral. They are more common in males and in patients who use tobacco, increase in frequency with increasing age, and are more common in patients with renal small vessel disease (BUDIN and MCDONNELL 1984) (an association which is independent of age), clearcut renal cell carcinoma (AMBOS et al. 1981), or von Hippel-Lindau disease. Most are quite small and discovered only at autopsy; they may be encountered serendipitously in CT examinations of the kidney; due to their small size, however, they are probably usually missed by intravenous urography, ultrasound, nuclear medicine, and MRI.

Their potential to metastasize is, of course, of critical importance, since it determines the necessity for therapy. It seems to be true that renal adenomas and carcinomas together form a spectrum of tumors which are less likely to have metastasized the smaller they are at the time of discovery. Some authors have suggested that a diameter of 3 cm might be considered a cut-off point, all renal epithelial tumors smaller than this being adenomas, but even smaller tumors have been found to produce metastases (TALAMO and SHONNARD 1980). In addition, there are no histologic, biochemical, or imaging features which permit differentiation of renal epithelial tumors into malignant and benign forms, so that when renal epithelial tumors are discovered premortem the most practical thing to do is to treat them all as having at least some malignant potential, with the potential increasing as the size increases.

The tumors are almost always asymptomatic. The rare tumors which produce symptoms may cause hematuria or mild pain; very rarely does a tumor which anyone would call an adenoma become large enough to be palpated.

Therapy consists of excision. The exact surgical technique to be used has not been universally agreed upon. Some practitioners feel that a small tumor has sufficiently small potential for recurrence that a local excision with a margin of renal parenchyma may suffice. This practice is not universally accepted, however, since a few small renal tumors have been found in which local invasion beyond the resection margin was encountered after partial nephrectomy. Surgical plans should therefore be individualized, with the patient's age, general medical condition, and tumor size and stage being considered.

The pathology of renal adenomas is that of cortical tumors, which may be extremely small (small enough to be missed by all imaging techniques) or may range up to several centimeters in size. The cellular morphology may be papillary, alveolar, or tubular, and the cells themselves may be eosinophilic, basophilic, or clear cell.

The imaging of renal adenomas differs relatively little from the imaging of renal cell carcinomas except with regard to the average size of the tumors. As we have noted, a very large majority of tumors are too small to be seen by any imaging modality. Very rarely, an adenoma may become large enough to be recognizable as a space-occupying renal cortical lesion on urography. Ultrasound and CT features of the tumors differ in no discernible way from those of small renal cell carcinomas. If they are discovered in the setting of chronic dialysis (LEVINE et al. 1984), the imaging features of some sort of end-stage renal disease and the acquired renal cystic disease of dialysis will usually be seen simultaneously. The angiographic patterns of renal adenomas are like those of renal cell carcinomas: the papillary forms are usually hypovascular or avascular with a faint or absent tumor blush, whereas tubular forms are more likely to be hypervascular and to have a distinct tumor blush.

8.4 Juxtaglomerular Cell Tumor (Reninoma)

Juxtaglomerular cell tumor is a rare benign neoplasm which arises from the juxtaglomerular cells in the renal cortex (SQUIRES et al. 1984). The cells in the tumor produce renin, so that the patients usually present with hyperreninemic hypertension; they also usually have hyperaldosteronemia, with its subsequent hypokalemia. The patients often present in young adulthood, and the tumor has not infrequently been encountered in children. There is a female predominance.

The tumors are usually small (DUNNICK et al. 1983). Although they occasionally protrude from the surface of the kidney, they may be entirely encased within the renal cortex, so that they are difficult to identify on plain films or urography. On ultrasound, they usually appear echogenic. CT examinations without contrast may reveal the tumors if they are exophytic but may miss them entirely if they are intraparenchymal; when contrast is administered, the tumors enhance less than the normal cortex and thus become visible. Arteriography usually reveals the tumors to be hypovascular; renal vein sampling may provide evidence of hypersecretion of renin.

8.5 Angiomyolipomas

Angiomyolipomas are benign renal tumors which may present either as a solitary abnormality or as part of the tuberous sclerosis syndrome (CHONKO et al. 1974; McCULLOUGH et al. 1971; PEROU and GRAY 1960; SCULLY et al. 1980). Of all patients with tuberous sclerosis, 40%–80% have been estimated to have angiomyolipomas. Of all patients with angiomyolipomas, 50% have been said to have tuberous sclerosis. The latter figure may require revision, however; careful autopsy studies have shown small angiomyolipomas to be present in kidneys more frequently than had been previously supposed, and high quality CT and ultrasound examinations have revealed small asymptomatic tumors in a sufficiently high percentage of all patients that it is probably true that the large majority of patients in whom angiomyolipomas can be found do not have tuberous sclerosis.

Tuberous sclerosis (GLASSBERG et al. 1987), or Bourneville's disease, is a rare disease affecting approximately 1 in every 150000 live births. It is an autosomal dominant inherited condition with variable penetrance; it appears clinically more frequently in females than in males. The manifestations of the disease are usually multiple. Symptoms of epilepsy or mental retardation may be present. In the brain (INGLIS 1954), hamartomatous or phakomatous lesions consisting of clusters of neuroglial cells may be found, especially in the basal ganglia and around the ventricles. Plain films or CT may reveal intracerebral calcifications (VIAMONTE et al. 1960). There may be phakomatous lesions in the retina or optic nerve. A variety of integumentary lesions may appear. These consist of adenoma sebaceum, which may appear in a butterfly distribution on the face, along with subungual or periungual fibromas, café au lait spots, or shagreen patches (these are regions of rough skin found in the lumbar area). The lungs may be involved and display small cystic regions with a disorganized interstitial pattern on chest films. Rhabdomyomas may be encountered in the heart. Occasionally, the adrenals may contain hamartomas. The kidneys frequently display multiple angiomyolipomas (INGLIS 1954; STILLWELL et al. 1987; THELMO et al. 1978; WRIGHT et al. 1974) and may contain multiple cysts as well (FELDMAN et al. 1975; MITNICK et al. 1983). There are reports of association of adult-type polycystic renal disease and of renal cell carcinoma (GUTIERREZ et al. 1979; TAYLOR et al. 1989; WEINBLATT et al. 1987) with tuberous sclerosis (LYNNE et al. 1979; PEREZ-ATAYDE et al. 1981; SNOWDON 1974), but it is not clear whether this is a meaningful association or merely represents a chance occurrence, nor is it certain that the multiple renal cysts which may be part of the tuberous sclerosis syndrome have not been mistaken for adult-type polycystic renal disease. Adenomas have appeared in small bowel and in liver. Small cystic lesions and sclerotic lesions have been described in the bones (SMULEWICZ and TAFRESHI 1977), especially in the phalanges.

Both the number and severity of findings in tuberous sclerosis may vary considerably from patient to patient. Some investigators have suggested that patients who only have angiomyolipomas may in fact have a forme fruste of tuberous sclerosis; lymphangiomatosis is also considered by some to be a possible mild form of the disease.

Angiomyolipomas in the absence of tuberous sclerosis also appear more often in females than in males. They may be multiple (BECHTOLD 1976). The classic age at presentation is in the third to fifth de-

cades of life, but, on rare occasions, these tumors have been encountered in teenagers (BERNIE 1973) and even in younger children (HAGOOD et al. 1976).

Angiomyolipomas, especially when small, may be completely asymptomatic, and are then diagnosed only serendipitously when the kidneys are imaged for other clinical reasons. The tumors may be symptomatic as well (CAMPBELL et al. 1974; KHILNANI and WOLF 1961; KLAPPROTH et al. 1959; MOUDED et al. 1978; PRICE and MOSTOFI 1965); rarely, they may grow large enough to present as palpable masses. More often, they make themselves known by undergoing spontaneous hemorrhage (HOEL and TOLLEFSEN 1976). The bleeding may occur into the retroperitoneum (BEH et al. 1976) and be sufficiently severe to cause serious shock. Rarely, the bleeding may be into the intraperitoneal cavity (MACDOUGALL 1960). Gross hematuria may also appear, and the bleeding may be associated with abdominal, flank, or back pain. The likelihood of hemorrhage is thought to be roughly proportional to the size of the tumor. Little is known about the growth rate of the tumors, since few have been followed for any length of time. No tumor has ever been demonstrated to grow (BLUTE et al. 1988), but, since tuberous sclerosis is an inherited condition and since the tumors are extremely rarely diagnosed in early childhood, it is reasonable to assume that they grow very slowly, ultimately to produce clinical symptoms in adulthood. The tumors have never been shown to exhibit malignant behavior although very rare malignant mesenchymal tumors with similar cell types appear (MAAR et al. 1976). Rarely, angiomyolipomas in the absence of tuberous sclerosis have been shown to be associated with adult-type polycystic disease and with renal cell carcinoma (BARBOUR and CASALI 1978; MALONE et al. 1986; UEDA et al. 1987); these associations, like those found in patients with tuberous sclerosis, have not conclusively been shown to represent anything other than chance occurrence.

Several courses of therapy are possible for patients with renal angiomyolipomas. Relatively small ones probably require no treatment at all (BRET et al. 1985), since they do not become malignant and are probably relatively unlikely to bleed. Larger ones are often surgically resected, either because they have presented with acute bleeding or because their size raises concern that serious hemorrhage might occur later. Resection is usually conservative, since sparing of renal parenchyma is desirable; occasionally, renal angiomyolipomas have been subjected to nephrectomy either because the tumors could not be technically removed from the remainder of the kidney or because preoperative diagnosis did not permit the exclusion of renal cell carcinoma from the differential diagnosis. Angiomyolipomas which have bled, or which are felt to be at risk of bleeding, may also be treated by angiographic means (MOOR-HEAD et al. 1977): both Gelfoam emboli and ablation by absolute ethanol have been shown to be effective if the branches of the renal artery supplying the tumor can be selectively catheterized.

Gross pathology examination of angiomyolipomas reveals them to be gray or yellow tumors ranging in size from about 1 cm in diameter to as much as 40 cm in width (SHERMAN et al. 1981). Histologic examination reveals varying proportions of mature fat cells, smooth muscle cells which may be grouped in disorganized fascicles, and tortuous thick-walled blood vessels with a paucity of elastic tissue (SHERMAN et al. 1981). Evidence of interstitial hemorrhage may be seen, and occasionally the tumors contain calcification.

The tumors may appear in the renal cortex or medulla, and may extend into the perinephric space, the renal sinus, or even the renal vein (KUTCHER et al. 1982); there are rare reported cases which have extended from the renal vein through the inferior vena cava (WEIGERT et al. 1983) into the right atrium (ROTHENBERG et al. 1986). The tumors may be single or multiple, and may be associated with angiomyolipomatous tissue in juxtarenal lymph nodes (BUSCH et al. 1976; TAYLOR et al. 1989); lymph node involvement represents the tendency of the tumors to be multicentric in origin, rather than to metastasize. Occasionally, only two of the tissues may be present (RUMANCIK et al. 1984), so that the tumor may be termed an angiolipoma, angiomyoma, or myolipoma.

Imaging studies reveal findings which reflect gross pathology (BAGLEY et al. 1980; KHILNANI and WOLF 1961; KLAPPROTH et al. 1959).

Plain films are abnormal only when the tumors are very large, in which case upper abdominal masses may be seen; these may appear lucent (BARON et al. 1977).

Intravenous urography and nephrotomography may reveal no abnormalities whatsoever if the tumors are single and small. A single large tumor may look like any other space-occupying lesion in the kidney. If the tumor contains a large proportion of fat, the lesion may appear relatively lucent. The tumors usually arise from the renal parenchyma, but may appear in the renal sinus (DIAMOND et al. 1977). Multiple tumors may present urographically as multiple space-occupying lesions throughout the kidney which stretch and distort the collecting system in a way which mimics adult-type polycystic

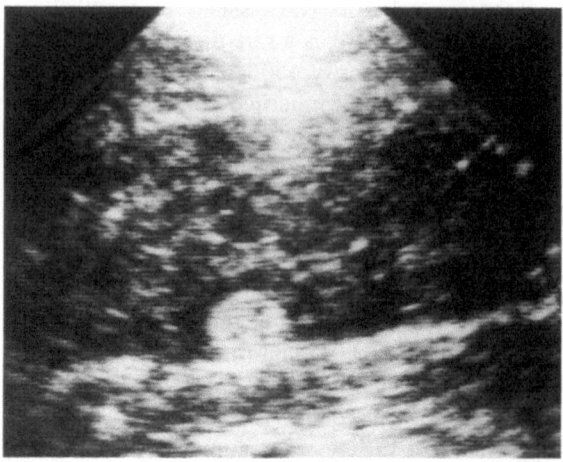

Fig. 8.4. Angiomyolipoma. Renal ultrasound reveals a small, circular, very echogenic, cortical mass

renal disease. On rare occasion, a portion of the tumor may project into the collecting system and form a filling defect. If there has been massive retroperitoneal hemorrhage, the renal and psoas muscle outlines may be obscured. The tumors rarely calcify (DEETHS and MELSON 1975).

The commonest ultrasound appearance of an angiomyolipoma ist that of a very echogenic mass (Fig. 8.4) (BUSH et al. 1979; HARTMAN et al. 1981; KUIJPERS and JASPERS 1989; LEE et al. 1978; SCHEIBLE et al. 1978; SHAWKER et al. 1979). The dense echogenicity is presumed to be due to fatty tissue, so that tumors which have small amounts of fat may appear less echogenic. The echogenicity may be homogeneous or heterogeneous. Although the average angiomyolipoma is considerably more echogenic than the average renal cell carcinoma, the echogenicity of relatively echodense carcinomas and the least dense angiomyolipomas overlap, so that an exact diagnosis by ultrasound is not always possible. Certainly, for any large tumor, confirmation that a tumor is definitely an angiomyolipoma should be provided by CT. There is some controversy over whether a small very echogenic tumor seen by ultrasound needs to be confirmed as an angiomyolipoma by CT; this appearance is much less likely to be caused by a renal carcinoma.

Since CT is able to demonstrate fat, it probably is the modality which is most reliable in the specific diagnosis of angiomyolipoma (HANSEN et al. 1978; KRATZ and HAMPER 1982; SCHWEDEN et al. 1983; SHAWKER et al. 1979; SHERMAN et al. 1981). At CT, angiomyolipomas may appear of virtually any size (Fig. 8.5) and are diagnosed by virtue of finding portions of the tumor which have CT numbers which are unquestionably in the negative range (BUSH et al. 1979). Demonstration of fat within a renal tumor almost certainly means that the tumor is an angiomyolipoma; the only entities which might be in the differential diagnosis include the rare Wilms' tumor, which contains small amounts of fatty material, and lipomas and liposarcomas. If the tumor has undergone hemorrhage, the hemorrhagic portion may not have negative CT numbers, and evidence of perirenal or peritumoral hematoma may be visible. The tumors which extend into the renal vein or vena cava will be visible as lucent defects in the vessels. Tumors with small amounts of fat may not have fatty regions demonstrable by CT; using thin slices may demonstrate small fatty regions in an angiomyolipoma in circumstances where relatively thick slices fail to do so (BOSNIAK et al. 1988). Tumors which have no fat at all will have no lucent regions, and angiomyomas may therefore be undistinguishable from renal cell carcinomas by CT. If intravenous contrast is used, inhomogeneous enhancement may be demonstrated within the tumors.

Relatively few angiomyolipomas have had their MRI experience described (EARTHMAN et al. 1986; ZERRIB et al. 1988). In general, the MRI features mirror those seen at CT: the fatty regions of the tumor appear like fat elsewhere in the body; that is, they are relatively bright on T1-weighted and T2-weighted images. A differential diagnostic problem arises when comparing angiomyolipomas to renal cell carcinomas with focal areas of hemorrhage, since intratumoral hematomas may appear bright on both T1-weighted and T2-weighted images. In some cases, distinction may be made in the T2-weighted images, where some hematomas will appear brighter than normal fat.

Currently, angiography is rarely used in the diagnosis of angiomyolipomas, but occasionally an angiogram may be necessary for preoperative surgical planning (WALKER et al. 1976) or as part of an embolization (BUCHELER et al. 1975) or ablation procedure (EARTHMAN et al. 1986). The visualized pattern of blood vessels is usually that of a hypervascular tumor (Fig. 8.6), but hypovascular tumors may occasionally be encountered (BARRILERO 1977; BECKER et al. 1973; KHALIL and LOY 1978; KRATZ and HAMPER 1982; LEE 1977; LOVE and FRANK 1965; PALMISANO 1967; SOOD et al. 1975; VIAMONTE et al. 1960). Small multiple aneurysms may be seen arising from the branches of the arteries; contrast may pool within these aneurysms. Arteriovenous shunting is rare but occasionally occurs (BARZILAIet al. 1987). Sometimes vessels parasitized from vascular beds other than that supplied by the renal artery may be seen

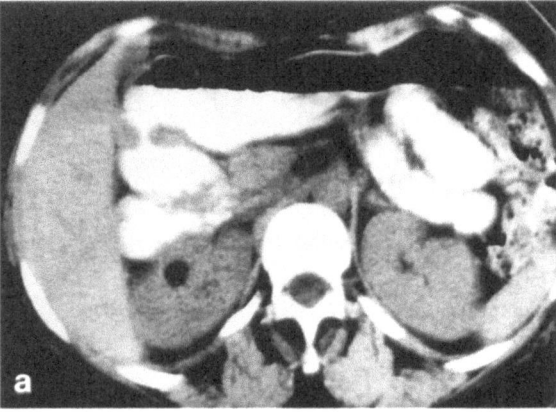

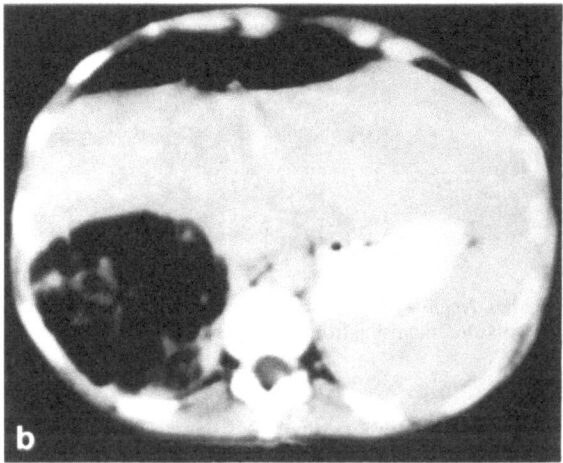

Fig. 8.5 a, b. Renal angiomyolipomas. **a** CT reveals small fat density mass in right renal parenchyma. **b** Another case. CT shows large heterogeneous fatty tumor which has extended superior to the right kidney

(DAVIS 1978); this finding does not indicate malignancy, however. The nephrogram phase of an arteriogram may reveal inhomogeneous opacification of the tumor, occasionally with a whorled or onion-peel appearance. Although the classic angiographic appearance of angiomyolipomas differs from that of renal cell carcinomas in that the former is more likely to show small aneurysms and a whorled nephrogram, and less likely to have arteriovenous shunting, vascular patterns of the two tumors are sufficiently variable that distinction cannot always be made on the basis of the angiographic pattern alone. In those unusual tumors which have extended into the renal vein or inferior vena cava (BRANTLEY et al. 1985), venography will reveal the tumor thrombus as a lucent filling defect.

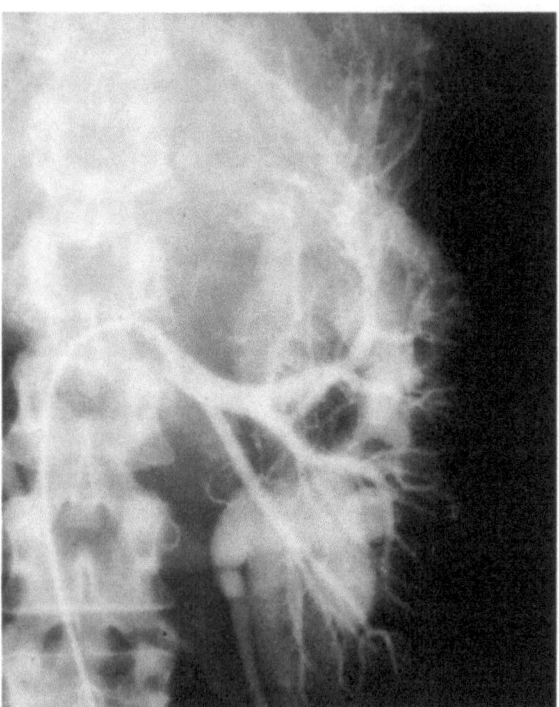

Fig. 8.6. Angiomyolipoma. Selective renal arteriogram reveals vascular lesion arising from the upper renal pole

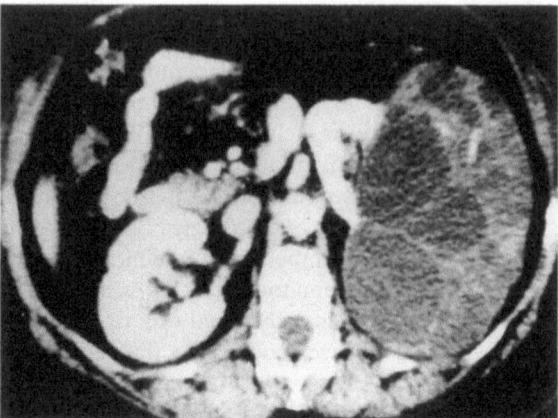

Fig. 8.7. Multilocular cystic nephroma. CT reveals large ovoid lesion arising from left kidney. Septae divide the lesion into many fluid-filled locules

8.6 Multilocular Cystic Nephroma

Multilocular cystic nephroma is an uncommon benign renal tumor which has engendered a great deal of confusion in the literature. Investigators have different with regard to whether it represents a true neoplasm or is an example of a kind of congenital dysplasia, about whether it has the potential to develop focal areas of malignant renal cell carcinoma, about the exact histologic findings in the lesion, and about what it should be called. For the moment, we will assume that it represents a benign neoplasm with insignificant potential for malignant degeneration. This is a tumor with a peculiar bimodal age and sex distribution. It may appear within the first few years of life. Boys up to 2 years of age may be afflicted and a few older girls have been found with the disease; the tumor has also been found to be prevalent in women between 40 and 60 years of age. It may present with a mass, hematuria, or infection.

Pathologic examination usually reveals the tumor to be solitary (MADEWELL et al. 1983). It consists of a roughly spherical mass with a fibrous capsule. The tumor has been found to range from 3 to 33 cm in diameter. There is a tendency for the tumor to contain multiple noncommunicating cysts; the septae between the cysts contain fibrous tissue and the cysts

do not communicate with the collecting system. The lining of the cysts consists of cuboidal or flattened epithelium. Some authors claim that the septae should not contain any tubules, glomeruli, or identifiable precursors of these structures; others permit lesions with small amounts of these structures to be called multiocular cystic nephromas. The ratio between the volume of cystic lesions and solid portions of the tumor varies tremendously from lesion to lesion.

Plain films may reveal evidence of a soft tissue mass if the tumor is sufficiently large (MADEWELL et al. 1983); some of the tumors have grossly visible calcification within the septae or capsule. Urography usually reveals a mass; occasionally, nephrotomography may reveal that it has septae. The mass may distort or protrude into the collecting system and has occasionally been known to obstruct the affected kidney.

Ultrasound patterns vary, depending upon the ratio of cystic regions to solid tissue (CARLSON et al. 1979; MADEWELL et al. 1983). The tumor may be almost entirely cystic, with just a few septae, or relatively echogenic throughout without clear-cut cysts. In the latter case it may resemble a Wilms' tumor or a renal cell carcinoma. At CT, the pattern may also vary between that of a primarily solid tumor and a lesion with multiple cysts and only a few septae (SLASKY and WOLFE 1982); if sufficiently thick, the septae and solid portions may be seen to enhance slightly with contrast (Fig. 8.7). Calcification may be noted on either ultrasound or CT examinations. A few cases examined by MRI have been reported; in them the multiple cystic regions have been visualized as regions with different intensity on T1-

weighted and T2-weighted images, presumably having to do with the protein content or degree of hemorrhage within each locule.

Angiography has shown a very variable pattern of vascularity in these tumors, ranging from those with a large degree of neovascularity to those which are nearly completely without vessels (CARLSON et al. 1979; MADEWELL et al. 1983).

Treatment of the tumors is surgical. They could presumably be cured by local resection, but since the preoperative imaging studies often do not permit malignancy to be excluded, a total nephrectomy is usually performed.

8.7 Congenital Mesoblastic Nephroma (Fetal Renal Hamartoma)

Congenital mesoblastic nephroma ist the most common renal tumor to appear within the first few months of life; it is very rare in late childhood or adulthood. It is occasionally diagnosed in utero. There is a very slight male predominance. The tumor is benign (BECKWITH 1986; BERDON et al. 1973; BO-LANDE 1974; NEZELOF et al. 1975; SNYDER et al. 1981); technically successful resection is usually curative, but the patient may need chemotherapy.

The clinical presentation is often that of a palpable abdominal mass. The patients may also present with hematuria, hypertension, jaundice, vomiting, and even hypercalcemia.

Gross pathologic examination reveals a tumor which is usually solid (HARTMAN et al. 1981); necrosis is rare although cystic internal regions occasionally appear (JOSHI and BECKWITH 1989). The tumor may be white, yellow, or tan. Histologic examination reveals spindle-like fusiform cells which may arise from muscle or fibrous tissue; the tumor can be distinguished from Wilms' tumor by the absence of neoplastic epithelial cells.

The tumors range from 8 to 30 cm in diameter and are almost always large enough to produce a detectable soft tissue mass on plain films (HARTMAN et al. 1981). Calcification is rarely seen. Urography reveals a renal mass which often distorts the affected kidney and its collecting system. Ultrasonic examination reveals that the tumor is solid and has relatively low level echoes (Fig. 8.8). Cystic regions may appear relatively anechoic if the are present. On CT, the tumor is heterogeneous and demonstrates irregular enhancement with contrast (Fig. 8.9). Angiography reveals some neovascularity with an inhomogeneous capillary phase.

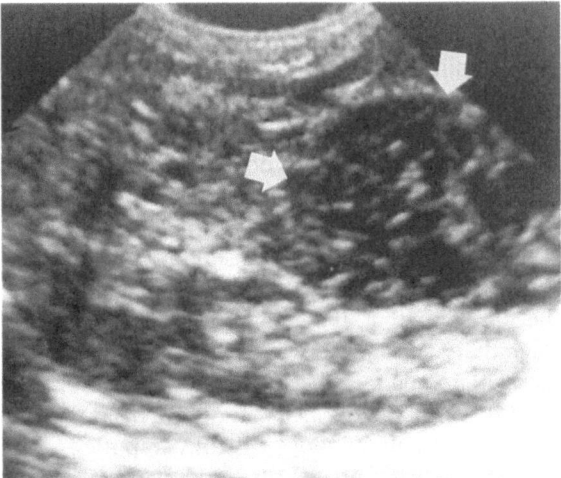

Fig. 8.8. Mesoblastic nephroma. Ultrasound reveals heterogeneous, primarily hypoechoic lesion *(arrows)* arising from the anterior renal surface and compressing the kidney. (Case courtesy of SUSAN KLEIN, M.D., Dept. of Radiology, Westchester County Medical Center, Valhalla, N.Y.)

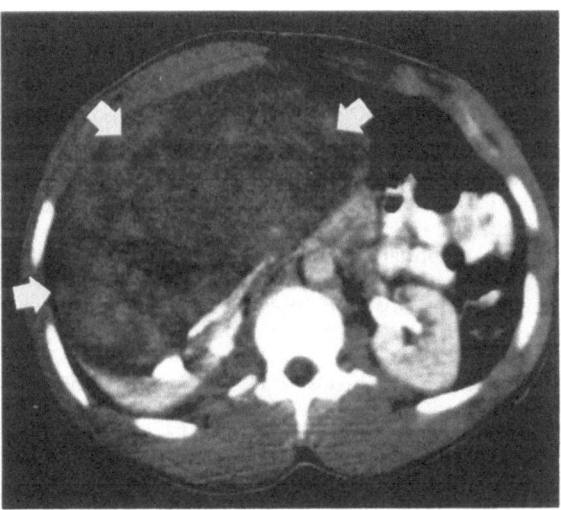

Fig. 8.9. Mesoblastic nephroma. CT reveals large ovoid lesion *(arrows)* arising from and distorting the right kidney. Faint heterogeneous opacification is seen within the tumor. (Case courtesy of DZORAH BALSAM, M.D., Nassau County Medical Center, Plainview, N.Y.)

8.8 Medullary Fibroma (Renal Medullary Interstitial Cell Tumor)

Medullary fibroma is an extremely common neoplasm. Although it very rarely appears in any clinical imaging studies, some familiarity with it is worthwhile given its extremely high prevalence.

Pathologically, these are small tumors, ranging from a few millimeters to a centimeter or so in diameter. They appear in the renal medulla, and may be seen in up to 40% of autopsies. There is no sex predilection, but they become more common with advancing age. They are round gray nodules which, upon histologic examination, are seen to be composed primarily of spindle-shaped cells. Calcification is occasionally noted.

Almost always, these tumors are clinically silent. When they produce symptoms, flank pain or hematuria may appear. When they are sufficiently large to become apparent, they may present as small renal medullary space-occupying lesions which may encroach upon the collecting system (LENNOX and CLARK 1975), rarely calcify, and have been noted to have neovascularity (POLGA 1976). A report of a case studied by MRI showed the tumor to have low signal intensity on both T1-weighted and T2 spin-echo sequences (CORMIER et al. 1989).

References

Akhtar M, Kott E (1979) Oncocytoma of kidney. Urology 14: 397-400

Ambos MA, Bosniak MA, Valensi QJ, Madayag MA, Lefleur RS (1978) Angiographic patterns in renal oncocytomas. Radiology 129: 615-622

Amos MA, Bosniak MA, Lefleur RS, Mitty HA (1981) Adrenal adenoma associated with renal cell carcinoma. AJR 136: 81

Amis ES JR, Newhouse JH (1991) Essentials of Uroradiology. Little, Brown & Co., Boston

Bagley D, Appell R, Pingoud E. McGuire EJ (1980) Renal angiomyolipoma. Urology 15: 1-5

Barbour GL, Casali RE (1978) Bilateral angiomyolipomas and renal cell carcinoma in polycystic kidney. Urology 12: 694-698

Baron M, Leiter E, Brendler H (1977) Preoperative diagnosis of renal angiomyolipoma. J Urol 117: 701-707

Barrilero AE (1977) Renal angiomyolipoma: a study of 13 cases. J Urol 117: 547-552

Barzilai IM, Braden GL, Ford LD, Goodman LH, Delima RJ, Germain MJ, Fitzgibbons JP (1987) Renal angiomyolipoma with arteriovenous shunting. J Urol 137: 483-484

Bechtold IR (1976) Multiple bilateral renal angiomyolipoma. Scand J Urol Nephrol 10: 160-164

Becker JA, Kinkhabwala M, Pollack H, Bosniak M (1973) Angiomyolipoma (hamartoma) of the kidney. Acta Radiol [Diagn] (Stockh) 14: 561-568

Beckwith JB (1986) Wilms tumor and other renal tumors of childhood: an update. J Urol 136: 320-324

Beh WP, Barnhouse DH, Johnson III SH, Marshall M Jr, Price SE Jr (1976) A renal cause for massive hemorrhage-renal angiomyolipoma. J Urol 116: 372-374

Bennington JL (1987) Renal adenoma. World J Urol 5: 66-70

Berdon WE, Wigger HJ, Baker DH (1973) Fetal renal hamartoma – a benign tumor to be distinguished from Wilms' tumor. AJR 118: 18-27

Bernie J (1973) Renal angiomyolipoma in an adolescent: a case report. J Urol 109: 492-494

Blute ML, Reza SM, Segura JW (1988) Angiomyolipoma: clinical metamorphosis and concepts for management. J Urol 139: 20-24

Bolande RP (1974) Congenital and infantile neoplasia of the kidney. Lancet II: 1497-1504

Bosniak MA, Megibow AJ, Hulnick DH, Horii S, Raghavendra BN (1988) CT diagnosis of renal angiomyolipoma: the importance of detecting small amounts of fat. AJR 151: 497

Bosniak MA, Subramanyam BR (1990) Renal parenchymal and capsular tumors in adults. In: Taveras JM, Ferrucci JT (eds) Radiology/Diagnosis-Imaging-Intervention. Lippincott, Philadelphia

Brantley RE, Mashni JW, Bethards RE, Chernys AE, Chung WM (1985) Computerized tomographic demonstration of inferior vena caval tumor thrombus from renal angiomyolipoma. J Urol 133: 836-837

Bret PM, Bretagnolle M, Gaillard D et al. (1985) Small, asymptomatic angiomyolipomas of the kidney. Radiology 154: 7-10

Bucheler VE, Weibbach L, Muller R, Thelen M (1975) Katheterembolisation eines blutenden Nierenhamartoms. Zugleich ein Beitrag zur angiographischen Diagnostik. Fortschr Röntgenstr 122: 107-112

Budin RE, McDonnell PJ (1984) Renal cell neoplasms – their relationship to arteriolonephrosclerosis. Arch Pathol Lab Med 108: 138-140

Busch FM, Bark CJ, Clyde HR (1976) Benign renal angiomyolipoma with regional lymph node involvement. J Urol 116: 715-724

Bush WH Jr, Freeny PC, Orme BM (1979) Angiomyolipoma. Urology 14: 531-540

Campbell EW, Brantley R, Harrold M, Simson LR (1974) Angiomyolipoma presenting as fever of unknown origin. Am J Med 57: 843-846

Carlson DH, Carlson D, Simon H (1979) Benign multilocal cystic nephroma. AJR 131: 621-625

Cass AS (1980) Large renal adenoma. J Urol 124: 281-282

Choi H, Almagro UA, McManus JT, Norback DH, Jacobs SC (1983) Renal oncocytoma. Cancer 51: 1887-1896

Chonko AM, Weiss SM, Stein JH, Ferris TF (1974) Renal involvement in tuberous sclerosis. Am J Med 56: 124-132

Choudhri AH, Patel PR, Cunnigham DA (1987) Uptake of 99m Tc-DTPA by a renal oncocytoma. Eur J Nucl Med 13: 311-312

Clark RE, Palubinskas AJ (1972) The angiographic spectrum of renal hamartoma. AJR 114: 715-721

Cohan RH, Dunnick NR, Degesys GE, Korobkin M (1984) Computed tomography of renal oncocytoma. J Comput Assist Tomogr 8: 284-287

Compton WR, Lester PD, Kyaw MM, Madsen JA (1976) The abdominal angiographic spectrum of tuberous sclerosis. AJR 126: 807-813

Cormier P, Patel SK, Turner DA, Hoeksema J (1989) MR imaging findings in renal medullary fibroma. AJR 153: 83-84

Davis TJ (1978) Parasitic arterial supply to renal angiomyolipoma. J Urol 119: 271-274

Deeths TM, Melson GL (1975) Calcification in an angiomyolipoma: a case report. J Urol 114: 613-614

Diamond A, Kodroff M, Ravitz G (1977) Renal sinus angiomyolipoma. Urology 9: 221-223

Dooms GC, Hricak H, Sollitto RA, Higgins CB (1985) Lipomatous tumors and tumors with fatty component: MR imaging potential and comparison of MR and CT results. Radiology 157: 479-483

Dunnick NR, Hartman DS, Ford KK, Davis CJ Jr, Amis ES Jr (1983) The radiology of juxtaglomerular tumors. Radiology 147: 321

Earthman WJ, Mazer MJ, Winfield AC (1986) Angiomyolipomas in tuberous sclerosis: subselective embolotherapy with alcohol, with long-term follow-up study. Radiology 160: 437-441

Feldman S, Libertino JA, Dowd JB (1975) Hamartoma and renal transplant implications. J Urol 114: 460-462

Glassberg KI, Stephens FD, Lebowitz RL et al. (1987) Renal dysgenesis and cystic disease of the kidney: a report of the Committee on Terminology, Nomenclature and Classification, Section on Urology. American Academy of Pediatrics. J Urol 138: 1085-1092

Gutierrez OH, Burgener FA, Schwartz S (1979) Coincident renal cell carcinoma and renal angiomyolipoma in tuberous sclerosis. AJR 132: 848-850

Hagood CO Jr, Garvin DD, Lachina FM, Polsky WS, Ball TP, Bobroff LM (1976) Abdominal aortic aneurysm and renal hamartoma in an infant with tuberous sclerosis. Surgery 79: 713-715

Hansen GC, Hoffman RB, Sample WF, Becker R (1978) Computed tomography diagnosis of renal angiomyolipoma. Radiology 128: 789-791

Hartman DS, Goldman SM, Friedman AC, Davis CJ Jr, Madewell JE, Sherman JL (1981 a) Angiomyolipoma: ultrasonic-pathologic correlation. Radiology 139: 451-458

Hartman DS, Lesar MSL, Madewell JE, Lichtenstein JE, Davis CJ Jr (1981 b) Mesoblastic nephroma: radiologic-pathologic correlation of 20 cases. AJR 136: 69-74

Hoel R, Tollefsen I (1976) Renal angiomyolipoma (hamartoma). Scand J Urol Nephrol 10: 165-169

Inglis K (1954) The relation of the renal lesions to the cerebral lesions in the tuberous sclerosis complex. Am J Pathol 30: 739-755

Jander HP (1979) Renal oncocytoma: a nonentity. Radiology 130: 815-817

Johnson JR, Thurman AE, Metter JB, Bannayan GA (1979) Oncocytoma of kidney. Urology 14: 181-189

Joshi VV, Beckwith JB (1989) Multilocular cyst of the kidney (cystic nephroma) and cystic, partially differentiated nephroblastoma. Cancer 64: 466-479

Khalil VM, Loy V (1978) Das Angiomyolipom der Niere aus angiographischer und morphologischer Sicht. Fortschr Röntgenstr 129: 323-327

Khilnani MT, Wolf BS (1961) Hamartolipoma of the kidney: clinical and roentgen features. AJR 86: 830-841

Klapproth HJ, Poutasse EF, Hakard JB (1959) Renal angiomyolipomas. AMA Arch Pathol 67: 56/400-67/411

Kratz HW, Hamper P (1982) Präoperative radiologische Diagnostik des renalen Angiomyolipoms. Fortschr Röntgenstr 137: 183-189

Kuijpers D, Jaspers R (1989) Renal masses: differential diagnosis with pulsed Doppler US. Radiology 170: 59-60

Kutcher R, Rosenblatt R, Mitsudo SM, Goldman M, Kogan S (1982) Renal angiomyolipoma with sonographic demonstration of extension into the inferior vena cava. Radiology 143: 755-756

Lee TG, Henderson SC, Freeny PC, Raskin MM, Benson EP, Pearse HD (1978) Ultrasound findings of renal angiomyolipoma. J Clin Ultrasound 6: 150-155

Lee WJ (1977) Angiographic manifestations of renal hamartoma. Angiology 28: 416-420

Lennox KW, Clark RE (1975) Renal medullary fibroma: report of a case presenting as a submucosal pelvic tumor. J Urol 113: 288-290

Levine E, Huntrakoon M (1983) Computed tomography of renal oncocytoma. AJR 141: 741-746

Levine E, Grantham JJ, Slusher SL, Greathouse JL, Krohn BP (1984) CT of acquired cystic kidney disease and renal tumors in long-term dialysis patients. AJR 142: 125-131

Lieber MM, Tomera KM, Farrow GM (1981) Renal oncocytoma. J Urol 125: 481-485

Love L, Frank SJ (1965) Angiographic features of angiomyolipoma of the kidney. AJR 95: 406-408

Lynne CM, Carrion HM, Bakshandeh K, Nadji M, Russel E, Politano VA (1979) Renal angiomyolipoma, polycystic kidney, and renal cell carcinoma in patient with tuberous sclerosis. Urology 14: 174-176

Maar K, Bocker KMR, Stolze T (1976) Maligne entartetes Angiolipoleiomyom der Niere - Renovasographie und Pathohistologie bei Nierenhämartomen. Urologe [A] 15: 297-299

Maatman TJ, Novick AC, Tancinco BF, Zissis V, Levin HS, Montie JE, Montague DK (1984) Renal oncocytoma: a diagnostic and therapeutic dilemma. J Urol 132: 878-885

MacDougall JA (1960) Renal hamartoma causing intraperitoneal haemorrhage. Br J Urol 32: 280-281

Madewell JE, Goldman SM, Davis CJ Jr, Hartman DS, Feigin DS, Lichtenstein JE (1983) Multilocular cystic nephroma: a radiographic-pathologic correlation of 58 patients. Radiology 146: 309-321

Malone MJ, Johnson PR, Jumper BM, Howard PH, Hopkins TB, Libertino JA (1986) Renal angiomyolipoma: 6 case reports and literature review. J Urol 135: 349-353

McCullough DL, Scott R Jr, Seybold HM (1971) Renal angiomyolipoma (hamartoma): review of the literature and report of 7 cases. J Urol 105: 32-44

Mitnick JS, Bosniak MA, Hilton S, Raghavendra BN, Subramanyam BR, Genieser NB (1983) Cystic renal disease in tuberous sclerosis. Radiology 147: 85-87

Moorhead JD, Fritzsche P, Hadley HL (1977) Management of hemorrhage secondary to renal angiomyolipoma with selective arterial embolization. J Urol 117: 122-123

Morales A, Wasan S, Bryniak S (1980) Renal oncocytomas: clinical, radiological and histological features. J Urol 123: 261-264

Mouded IM, Tolia BM, Bernie JE, Newman HR (1978) Symptomatic renal angiomyolipoma: report of 8 cases, 2 with spontaneous rupture. J Urol 119: 684-688

Moura ACF, Nascimento AG (1982) Renal oncocytoma: report of a case with unusual presentation. J Urol 127: 311-313

Nezelof C, Laurent M, Imbert MC, Jaubert F (1975) Le cystadenome renal de l'enfant. Arch Fr Pediatr 32: 815-834

Ogden BW, Beckman EN, Rodriguez FH Jr (1987) Multicystic renal oncocytoma. Arch Pathol Lab Med 111: 485-486

Older RA, Cleeve DM, Fetter BF, Jackson DA (1978) "Spoke-wheel" angiographic pattern in renal masses: nonspecificity. Radiology 128: 836

Palmisano PJ (1967) Renal hamartoma (angiomyolipoma). Radiology 88: 249-252

Pearse HD, Houghton DC (1979) Renal oncocytoma. Urology 8: 74-77

Perez-Atayde AR, Iwaya S, Lack EE (1981) Angiomyolipomas and polycystic renal disease in tuberous sclerosis. Urology 17: 607-610

Perou ML, Gray PT (1960) Mesenchymal hamartomas of the kidney. J Urol 83: 240-261

Polga JP (1976) Renal medullary fibroma presenting as a calcified mass with neovascularity. J Urol 116: 105-106

Price EB Jr Mostofi FK (1965) Symptomatic angiomyolipoma of the kidney. Cancer 18: 761-774

Psihramis KE, Cin PD, Dretler SP, Prout GR Jr, Sandberg AA (1988) Further evidence that renal oncocytoma has malignant potential. J Urol 139: 585-587

Quinn MJ, Hartman DS, Friedman AC et al. (1984) Renal oncocytoma: new observations. Radiology 153: 49-53

Rothenberg DM, Brandt TD, D'Cruz I (1986) Computed tomography of renal angiomyolipoma presenting as right atrial mass. J Comput Assist Tomogr 10: 1054-1056

Rothenberger K, Kramann B, Steuer G (1978) Onkozytom der Niere. Urologe [A] 17: 91-93

Rumancik WM, Bosniak MA, Rosen RJ, Hulnick D (1984) Atypical renal and pararenal hamartomas associated with lymphangiomyomatosis. AJR 142: 971-972

Scheible W, Ellenbogen PH, Leopold GR, Slao NT (1978) Lipomatous tumors of the kidney and adrenal: apparent echographic specificity. Radiology 129: 153-156

Schmidt VM, Taenzer V (1980) Angiographisches Erscheinungsbild seltener Nierentumoren. Onkozytom und benignes Hypernephrom. Fortschr Röntgenstr. 132: 417-421

Schweden VF, Klose KJ, Schild H, Engelmann U, Riedmiller H, Weber M (1983) Computertomographie des renalen angiomyolipoms. Fortschr Röntgenstr 139: 269-273

Scully RE, Galdabini JJ, Neely BU (1980) Case records of the Massachusetts General Hospital: case 12-1980. N Engl J Med 302: 736-741

Shawker TH, Horvath KL, Dunnick NR, Javadpour N (1979) Renal angiomyolipoma: diagnosis by combined ultrasound and computerized tomography. J Urol 121: 675-676

Sherman JL, Hartman DS, Friedman AC, Madewell JE, Davis CJ, Goldman SM (1981) Angiomyolipoma: computed tomographic-pathologic correlation of 17 cases. AJR 137: 1221-1226

Slasky BS, Wolfe PW (1982) Cross-sectional imaging of multiocular cystic nephroma. J Urol 128: 128-131

Smulewicz JJ, Tafreshi M (1977) Angiographic changes in tuberous sclerosis. Angiology 28: 300-322

Snowdon JA (1974) Cerebral aneurysm, renal cysts and hamartomas in a case of tuberous sclerosis. Br J Urol 46: 583

Snyder HM III, Lack EE, Chetty-Baktavizian A, Bauer SB, Colodny AH, Retick AB (1981) Congenital mesoblastic nephroma: relationship to other renal tumors of infancy. J Urol 126: 513-516

Sohn HK, Kim SY, Seo HS (1987) MR imaging of a renal oncocytoma. J Comput Assist Tomogr 11: 1085-1087

Someren A, Zaatari GS, Campbell WG Jr et al. (1989) The kidneys. In: Someren A (ed) Urologic Radiology with Clinical and Radiologic Correlations. Macmillan, New York

Sood S, Mancini A, Kropp K (1975) Tuberous sclerosis: emphasis on the angiographic findings. J Urol 114: 185-197

Sos TA, Gray GF Jr, Baltaxe HA (1976) The angiographic appearance of benign renal oxyphilic adenoma. AJR 127: 717-722

Squires JP, Ulbright TM, DeSchryver-Kecskemeti K, Engleman W (1984) Juxtaglomerular cell tumor of the kidney. Cancer 53: 516-523

Stillwell TJ, Gomer MR, Kelalis PP (1987) Renal lesions in tuberous sclerosis. J Urol 138: 477

Talamo TS, Shonnard JW (1980) Small renal adenocarcinoma with metastases. J Urol 124: 132-134

Taylor RS, Joseph DB, Kohaut EC, Wilson ER, Bueschen AJ (1989) Renal angiomyolipoma associated with lymph node involvement and renal cell carcinoma in patients with tuberous sclerosis. J Urol 141: 930-932

Thelmo WL, Lefkowitz M, Seemayer TA (1978) Renal failure secondary to angiomyolipoma. Urology 11: 389-392

Ueda J, Kobayashi Y, Itoh H, Itatani H (1987) Angiomyolipoma and renal cell carcinoma occurring in same kidney: CT evaluation. J Comput Assist Tomogr 11: 340-341

Viamonte M Jr, Ravel R, Politano V et al. (1960) Angiographic findings in patient with tuberous sclerosis. AJR 98: 723

Walker DE, Barry JM, Hodges CV (1976) Angiomyolipoma: diagnosis and treatment. J Urol 116: 712-714

Wasserman NF, Ewing SL (1983) Calcified renal oncocytoma. AJR 141: 747-749

Weigert F, Ringelmann W, Voeth C (1983) Diagnostisches Vorgehen beim solitären Angiomyolipom der Niere. Fortschr Röntgenstr 139: 525-530

Weinblatt ME, Kahn E, Kochem J (1987) Renal cell carcinoma in patients with tuberous sclerosis. Pediatrics 80: 898-903

Williamson B (1990) Benign neoplasms of the renal parenchyma. In: Pollack HM (ed) Clinical Urography. W.B. Saunders, Philadelphia

Wright FW, Ledingham JGG, Dunnill MS, Grieve NWT (1974) Polycystic kidneys, renal hamartomas, their variants and complications. Clin Radiol 25: 27-43

Yu GSM, Rendler S, Herskowitz A, Molnar JJ (1980) Renal oncocytoma. Cancer 45: 1010-1018

Zerbib M, Marichez M, Taieb A, Boccon-Gibod L, Debre B, Steg A (1988) L'angiomyolipome renal. Presse Med 17: 463-466

9 Renal Cystic Disease

ERICH K. LANG

CONTENTS

9.1   Overview 227
9.2   Simple Renal Cysts 229
9.2.1 Radiologic Findings 229
9.2.2 Cyst Puncture and Aspiration Test Complex .. 231
9.3   Inflammatory (Infected) Cysts 232
9.4   Hemorrhagic Cysts 234
9.5   Calcified Cysts 235
9.6   Multilocular Cysts 237
9.7   Autosomal Dominant Polycystic Disease 238
9.8   Autosomal Recessive Polycystic Disease 240
9.9   Acquired Renal Cystic Disease 241
9.10   Multicystic Dysplastic Kidney 242
9.11   Medullary Cystic Disease of the Kidney 244
9.12   Cysts of the Renal Sinus 244
9.13   Medullary Sponge Kidney 246
9.14   Cystic Disease Associated with Malignant
       and Benign Neoplasms 246
       References 248

9.1 Overview

Cystic lesions are one of the most common abnormalities of the kidneys and are the most common asymptomatic space-occupying lesions (LANG 1973, 1980, 1986). While the vast majority of renal cysts are of the uncomplicated simple cyst variety, renal cystic disease comprises a heterogeneous group of developmental, acquired, and hereditary entities. A number of classifications based on appearance, location, associated disease, and hereditary factors have been proposed. Those that take into consideration radiographic findings have been found most useful for categorizing renal cystic disease for the radiologist's use (ELKIN and BERNSTEIN 1969; GLEASON et al. 1967; GROSSMAN et al. 1968) (Table 9.1). Other classifications that have contributed greatly to our understanding of the disease have been based upon microdissection studies clarifying the morphology of different renal cystic disease entities (OSATHANONDH and POTTER 1964).

ERICH K. LANG, M.D., Professor, Department of Radiology, School of Medicine in New Orleans, Louisiana State University, Medical Center, 1542 Tulane Avenue, New Orleans, LA 70122-2822, USA

Table 9.1. Classification of cystic disease of the kidney. (Modified from ELKIN, BERNSTEIN, GLEASON, et al.)

I.   Renal dysplasia
     a) Multicystic
        1. Pelvioinfundibular atresia
        2. Hydronephrotic multicystic kidney
     b) Focal and segmental dysplasia

II. Polycystic disease
     a) Autosomal recessive polycystic disease
        1. Newborn
        2. Childhood
     b) Autosomal dominant polycystic disease

III. Simple renal cyst
     a) Uncomplicated simple renal cyst
     b) Hemorrhagic cyst
     c) Hyperdense cyst
     d) Cyst with calcifications
     e) Inflammatory cyst

IV. Cyst of the renal sinus
     a) Peripelvic cyst
     b) Perinephric cyst

V.   Medullary cystic disease
     a) Medullary sponge kidney
     b) Uremic medullary cystic disease

VI. Multiloculated renal cyst
     a) Associated with neoplastic disease
        1. Multilocular cystic nephroma
        2. Wilms' tumor
        3. Miscellaneous tumors
     b) Associated with inflammatory disease
     c) Associated paracytic disease (echinococcosis)
     d) Associated with trauma
     e) Associated with cystic diseases
        1. Subseptation
        2. Segmental multicystic kidney

VII. Miscellaneous cystic diseases
     a) Pluricystic kidney disease
     b) Glomerulocystic kidney disease
     c) Microcystic disease
     d) Associated with or caused by neoplasms
     e) Associated with syndromes (various types of cyst)

The ubiquity of the benign simple renal cyst, particularly in older patients, has made it necessary to develop criteria to differentiate such innocuous lesions from others which may require therapy. Increased utilization of abdominal ultrasonography and computed tomography (CT) has brought to the attention of the clinician an unprecedented number of renal cystic lesions. In general, differentiation from other masses is straightforward.

However, some renal cysts may be complicated by hemorrhage or infection or may present in an atypical fashion with calcifications, hyperdensity, or subseptation. In such circumstances, differentiation from cystic neoplasms or other renal cystic masses may be difficult. Moreover, some renal neoplasms may be associated with or cause cysts. von Hippel-Lindau disease is often associated with renal cystic disease but, unfortunately, also with renal adenomas and carcinomas. Up to 40% of patients treated for end-stage renal disease by hemodialysis develop renal cysts but such patients are also prone to develop adenomas and renal cell carcinoma.

Renal dysplasia may occasion multicystic disease or present with segmental dysplasia and focal multicystic disease. Depending on the point at which nephrogenesis was disturbed, either pyeloinfundibular atresia (early form) or hydronephrotic multicystic kidney (interference later during gestation) results.

Two forms of polycystic disease are readily differentiated. Autosomal dominant polycystic disease (adult type) is the common form of polycystic disease; it is characterized by cysts arising in the collecting ducts or nephron and also presents with hepatic and pancreatic cysts and cerebral aneurysms. Neonatal or juvenile polycystic disease is an autosomal recessive type which, depending on the time of presentation, may show predominantly periportal fibrosis and hepatic disease with liver failure or severe renal cystic disease with renal failure. The latter form, which is encountered in neonates, appears incompatible with prolonged survival.

Medullary cystic disease can be divided into (a) medullary sponge kidney with characteristic dilatation of collecting tubules in the renal pyramids and (b) medullary cystic disease with cyst formation in the medulla, tubular atrophy, and salt-loosing nephropathy.

The term "multiloculated renal cyst" reflects the anatomic pathological appearance of such cysts, which have a variety of causes.

Multilocular cystic nephroma is a benign neoplasm that presents in this fashion. However, a number of malignant neoplasms, and specifically Wilms' tumor, may present in an identical fashion. Inflammatory disease can occasion loculation in a preexisting renal cyst, causing presentation as a multiloculated renal mass. Parasitic disease, and specifically echinococcosis, is also prone to develop cysts with loculation (in fact with invaginated daughter cysts).

Table 9.2. Syndromes presenting with renal cyst among other malformations

Apert syndrome
Beckwith-Wiedemann syndrome
Brachmann-de Lange syndrome
Brachymesomelia-renal syndrome
Caroli's disease
Congenital rubella
Cutis laxa
DiGeorge syndrome
Duplication, long or short arm chromosome 10
Down syndrome (trisomy 21)
Ehlers-Danlos syndrome
Elajalde syndrome
Goldenhar's syndrome
Gorlin's syndrome
Hajdu-Cheney syndrome
Ivemark's syndrome
Kaufman McKusick syndrome
Laurence-Moon-Biedl syndrome
Marden Walker syndrome
Meckel-Gruber syndrome
Miranda syndrome
Myotonic dystrophy
Noonan's syndrome
Oculorenal syndrome
Patau's syndrome (trisomy 13-15)
Pseudothalidomide syndrome
Short-rib polydactyly syndrome
Spherocytosis
Triploidy
Trisomy 16-18
Tuberous sclerosis
Turner's syndrome
von Hippel-Lindau disease
Zellweger syndrome (cerebrohepatorenal syndrome)

Cysts of the renal sinus are frequently the result of lymphangiectasia and represent peripelvic lymphatic cysts. Other inflammatory diseases, however, can likewise cause cyst formation in this location.

A large group of miscellaneous cysts defy assignment to a specific category in such classifications. Glomerulocystic disease is characterized by dilatation of Bowman's space and adjacent tubules (McAlister 1979). Microcystic disease results from cystic dilatation of proximal convoluted tubules and is associated with nephrotic syndrome (Glassberg and Filmer 1985).

The term "pyelogenic cyst" simply denotes any cyst with an inflammatory round cell infiltrate in its base.

A large number of syndromes have renal cysts as one of their features (Table 9.2). These may be of the simple, hemorrhagic, calcified, multilocular, or multicystic variety.

A number of cystic entities, such as cystic renal cell carcinoma, cystic Wilms' tumor, renal abscess, renal hydatid disease, multilocular cystic nephroma, medullary sponge kidney, perinephric pseudocyst, perinephric urinoma, calyceal diverticulum, pyelogenic cyst, and traumatic cyst, are discussed in detail in the appropriate chapters of this book.

9.2 Simple Renal Cysts

Simple renal cysts occur in the renal cortex or at the corticomedullary junction. The lining of the cyst wall is smooth. Microscopically, it consists of a flattened epithelium. Collagenized fibrous tissue may form a pseudocapsule; mononuclear infiltrates in the base reflect past or present inflammatory manifestations.

It has been suggested that simple cysts form as a consequence of tubular obstruction. This is often initiated by medullary interstitial fibrosis, which increases with age. Experimentally cysts have been produced by simultaneously infarcting the vascular supply of a region and obstructing the draining tubule (HEPLER 1946).

Increased use of intravenous urography in the 1960s resulted in a sharp increase in the diagnosis of benign renal cysts in older males (LANG 1973). Increased use of abdominal ultrasonography and CT has shown simple renal cysts to be present in about 30% of patients over 50 years of age (LANG 1980, 1984, 1986; TADA et al. 1983). The incidence of benign renal cysts appears to be somewhat higher in males than in females, particularly in the older age group.

Benign renal cysts tend to be asymptomatic. Only large cysts may present with discomfort, pain, and a palpable mass. Rarely, hypertension ensues. Activation of the renin-angiotensin mechanism attendant upon compression and vascular compromise of abutting cortical parenchyma is thought to be the cause.

9.2.1 Radiologic Findings

On intravenous urograms and nephrotomograms, renal cysts are characterized as a sharply defined spherical mass lacking enhancement and, if extending to the cortical margins, causing "cortical spurs." An infinitely thin wall delineates extrarenal components of such cysts (LANG 1973). Depending on their location, they may displace calyces and infundibula or may even cause relative obstruction and blunting of calyces (Figs. 9.1, 9.2 a). Large cysts may distort the renal contour. Tomograms obtained during the nephrographic phase best depict some of the pivotal

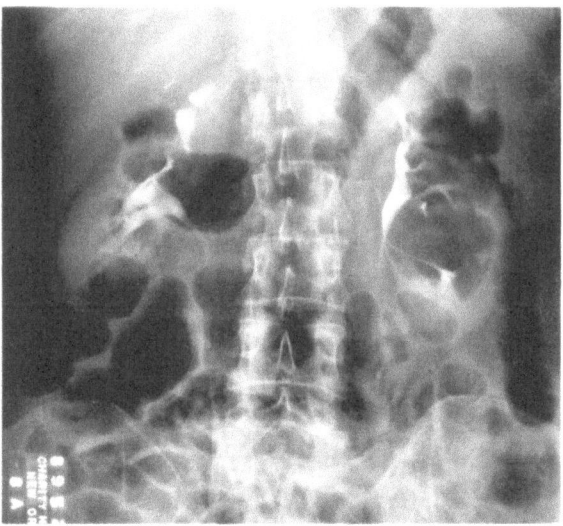

Fig. 9.1. Intravenous urogram showing splaying of infundibula and calyces, indicating the presence of a mass. The smooth displacement favors a cyst or solid lesion remote from displaced calyces

criteria. If such criteria as water density, no enhancement after intravenous contrast administration, a wall thickness no greater than a pencil line, and sharp definition against abutting parenchyma are met, the accuracy of nephrotomographic diagnosis is close to 95% (BOSNIAK 1986).

Ultrasound provides highly diagnostic criteria for simple renal cysts. Absence of internal echoes, excellent through-transmission, distinct and smooth margins of the distal wall, acoustic enhancement, and documentation of a spherical or ovoid shape are the pertinent sonographic criteria for the diagnosis of a benign simple cyst (Fig. 9.3). If these criteria are met, diagnostic accuracy approaches 98% (POLLACK et al. 1982; LINGARD and LAWSON 1979).

Some deep-seated cysts may cause diagnostic difficulty because of beam diversions. If the width of the beam exceeds the diameter of the mass, echoes from adjacent structures may appear to originate from within the mass (POLLACK et al. 1979).

Since criteria are based on fluid content of the intrarenal mass, arteriovenous fistulae must be differentiated from benign renal cyst by pulsed Doppler ultrasound to assess flow within the lesion (PLATT et al. 1989; KJER et al. 1990) (Fig. 9.4). Likewise, differentiation of neoplasms, hydronephrosis, and cysts at the corticomedullary junction can be improved by the use of pulsed Doppler ultrasound (SCOLA et al. 1989; KJER et al. 1990).

On computed tomograms, benign renal cysts present a sharply delineated round or elliptical mass

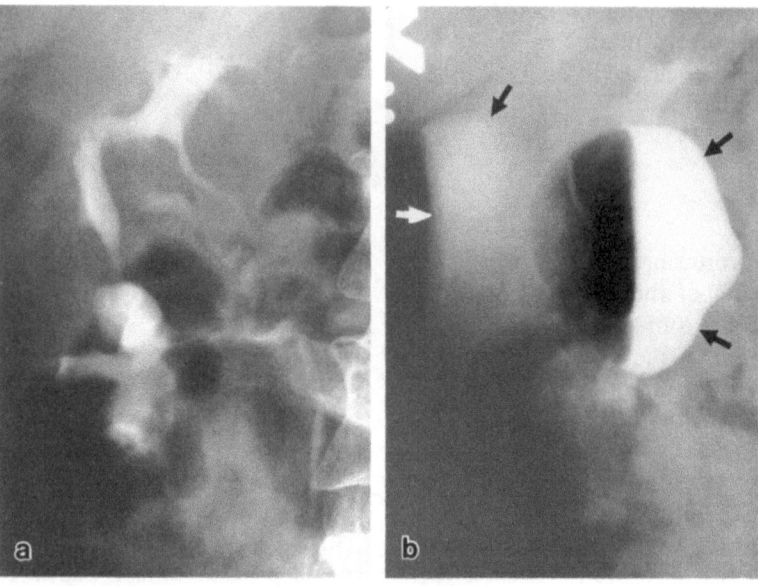

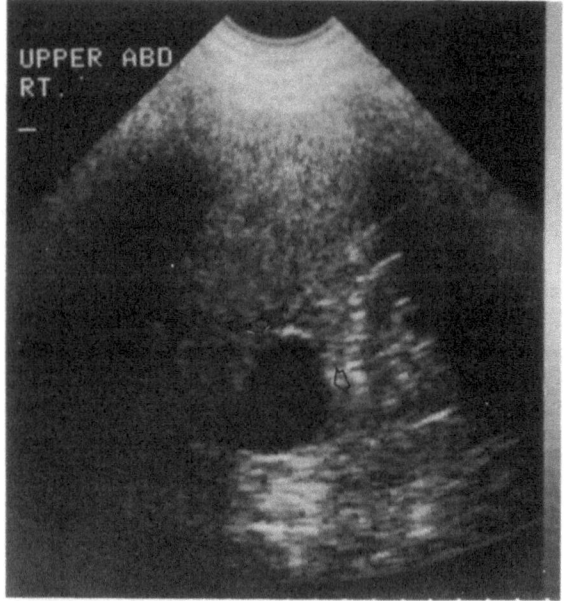

Fig. 9.3. Coronal scan through the right kidney demonstrating a spherical and sharply demarcated cystic mass (*broken arrows*). Note excellent through-transmission and lack of internal echoes characteristics of a benign renal cyst

△

Fig. 9.2. a Intravenous urogram suggesting displacement of the infundibulum of the superior calyceal group and of the posterior mid calyx by a space occupying lesion. **b** Following cyst puncture, and introduction of both air and contrast medium, a dumbbell shaped intercommunicating cyst is demonstrated (*arrows*) explaining the displacement pattern seen on the intravenous urogram

injections performed several days earlier. In general, such an elevation does not persist more than a few days (SHANSER 1978; MAYER et al. 1982).

False-positive elevation of attenuation coefficients has been reported in small intrarenal cysts less than 1 cm in diameter. This fictitious enhancement is caused by a partial volume effect (MCCLENNAN et al. 1979). Another false-positive observation, that of a thick wall, may result from imaging the parenchymal peak in cross-section (SEGAL and SPARTARO 1982).

Documentation of CT criteria consisting of a sharply defined elliptical or round mass, attenuation coefficients in the range from −10 to +10 HU, and lack of enhancement following administration of intravenous contrast medium establish the diagnosis of benign renal cyst with an accuracy of about 99%.

Correlation to sonographic studies is often capable of affirming the diagnosis in dubious cases. Guided cyst puncture and aspiration are advocated if a diagnosis cannot be established with acceptable confidence by ultrasound and CT.

with smooth border. Attenuation coefficients tend to range from −10 to +10 Hounsfield units (HU) (Fig. 9.5). Following administration of intravenous contrast medium, neither during the phase of capillary transit nor on postenhancement CT scans should there be a step-up of the attenuation coefficient. However, occasionally the attenuation coefficient may be slightly elevated as a result of contrast

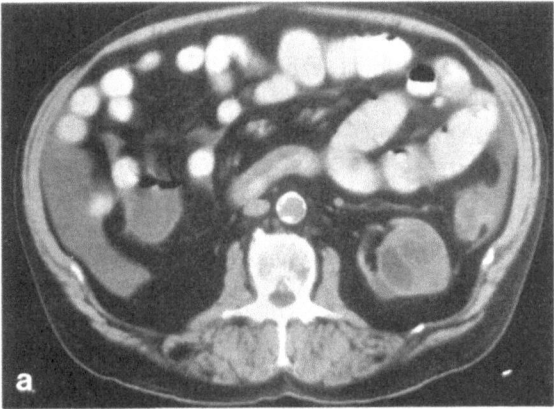

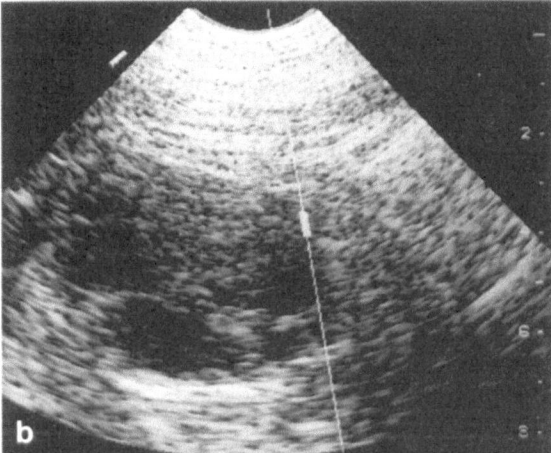

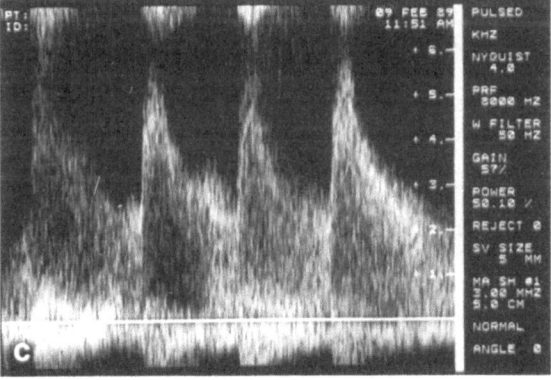

Fig. 9.4a-c. Patient with chronic renal failure undergoing peritoneal dialysis. **a** CT demonstrates a complex cystic mass in the left kidney. Adjacent images demonstrated a simple cyst in the atrophic native kidney. **b** Sonogram of the left kidney demonstrates a complex cystic mass. **c** The Doppler spectrum of the left renal mass demonstrates peak systolic frequencies of almost 6 kHz, consistent with malignancy. (KIER et al. 1990)

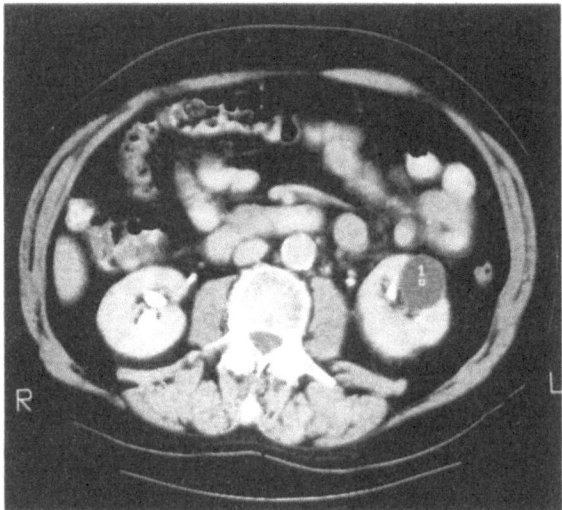

Fig. 9.5. Dynamic CT showing a classical sharply defined nonenhancing mass with a thin wall, diagnostic of a benign cyst

9.2.2 Cyst Puncture and Aspiration Test Complex

Guided cyst puncture can be performed under fluoroscopic, ultrasound, or CT guidance. This procedure is usually reserved for cysts that pose a diagnostic dilemma (LANG 1966, 1973, 1980; AMIS et al. 1987).

The aspirate is evaluated for color and turbidity, and biochemically for fat, lactic acid dehydrogenase (LDH), protein content, and sometimes amylase levels. Cytopathologic studies can be carried out on the cyst fluid or on the micropore filtrate. Culture of the aspirate is advocated if infection is suspected.

A simple or double contrast cystogram is then performed, introducing iodinated contrast medium and air (LANG 1966, 1973, 1980; GROSS 1979). The cystogram should be documented in multiple projections utilizing horizontal and vertical beam direction to demonstrate the different wall segments in double or single contrast (FIg. 9.2b).

Aspiration of clear and straw colored fluid with low fat and protein content and an LDH content commensurate with that of plasma transudate, a negative cytology, and smooth walls on double contrast cystograms establish the diagnosis of a benign renal cyst with a very high accuracy, approaching 100%. At times, technical errors such as inadequate replacement of cyst fluid with iodinated contrast medium and air or delay of the radiologic examination after instillation of the contrast medium cause artifacts due to incomplete expansion and, therefore, preclude definitive interpretation. Complica-

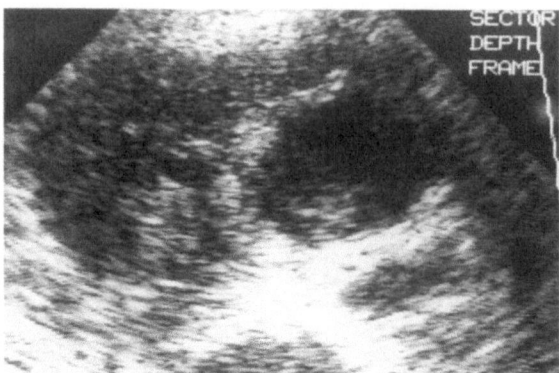

Fig. 9.6. Ultrasonogram showing scattered internal echoes and suggesting the present of a debris-fluid level. The cystic lesion appears to be thick walled. The findings are characteristic for an inflammatory cyst

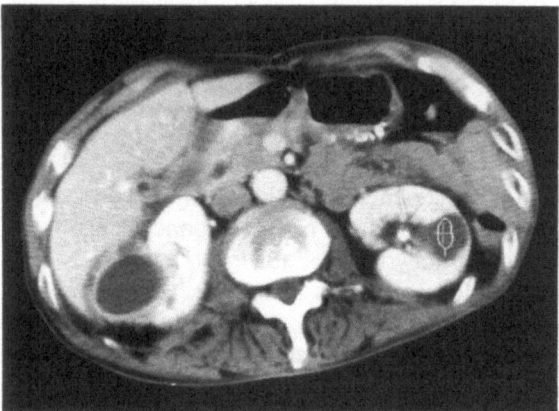

Fig. 9.7. A typical benign cyst is shown in the left kidney. On the right side, a low density subcortical cystic mass with a thickened enhancing wall as well as enhancement in the abutting perirenal tissues is noted; these are characteristics of an inflammatory cyst

tions of cyst puncture and aspiration studies are rare and basically attributable to faulty technique (LANG 1977).

9.3 Inflammatory (Infected) Cysts

Inflammatory cysts result when benign renal cysts become infected. The walls of such cysts are thickened; a round cell infiltrate beneath the cuboidal lining of the cyst is the classical histologic criterion. The normally thin wall of a benign cyst is converted to a thick inflammatory rind with inflammatory neovascularity (LANG 1973, 1980).

Plain radiographs or intravenous urograms produce no specific criteria. However, the thick wall of the infected and inflammatory cyst is sometimes appreciated on nephrotomograms (BOSNIAK 1986). Rarely, a gas-fluid level heralds the presence of a gas forming organism (FELDBERG and MALI 1980).

Ultrasonograms characteristically show a thick walled cystic mass with scattered internal echoes. Often, a debris-fluid level is shown (Fig. 9.6). The presence of gas bubbles results in intense echoes and "dirty shadowing." Occasionally, echogenic mural masses may be shown that simulate a necrotic tumor but are caused by exudate adherent to the cyst wall.

Computed tomograms, particularly the dynamic phase recordings, provide criteria suggesting an inflammatory cyst. During the phase of capillary transit, the wall appears to be thickened and shows enhancement consistent with inflammatory hyperemia (Figs. 9.7, 9.8a). In contradistinction to tumors projection into a cyst or cystic and necrotic tumors, an enhancing mass is not demonstrable (LANG 1984). The perirenal fat, however, assumes a ground glass density and a synechial pattern, which reflect edema but may be difficult to differentiate against lymphatic spread of a neoplasm.

The attenuation coefficients of the unenhanced cyst are often relatively high, in a range of 20–40 HU. A high protein content, necrotic debris, and perhaps some hemorrhage may be the cause (BALFE et al. 1982; COLEMAN 1984; FISHMAN et al. 1983; SUSSMAN et al. 1984). Alteration of the permeability of the cyst wall attendant upon inflammatory disease encourages transmission of protein molecules but also of contrast medium. This may explain the step-up of attenuation coefficients recorded over inflammatory cysts hours after urography or arteriography (SHANSER et al. 1978). However, in the vast majority of inflammatory cysts, such a step-up of attenuation coefficients after intravenous administration of contrast medium is not observed. Heterogeneity of attenuation coefficients recorded over different areas of a cyst may be attributable to layering of debris and hence higher or lower protein concentration in a given sample.

On rare occasions, a debris-fluid or air-fluid level may be demonstrated.

Nuclear medicine studies indicate the presence of an inflammatory rind by increased accumulation of indium 111 labeled white cells and gallium 67.

On angiograms, infected cysts tend to demonstrate inflammatory neovascularity in the cyst wall (LANG 1971; CHO et al. 1976).

On T1 weighted Magnetic resonance (MR) images, the infected cyst is characterized by an intensified signal intensity as compared to the benign uncomplicated cyst. Based on signal intensity, an

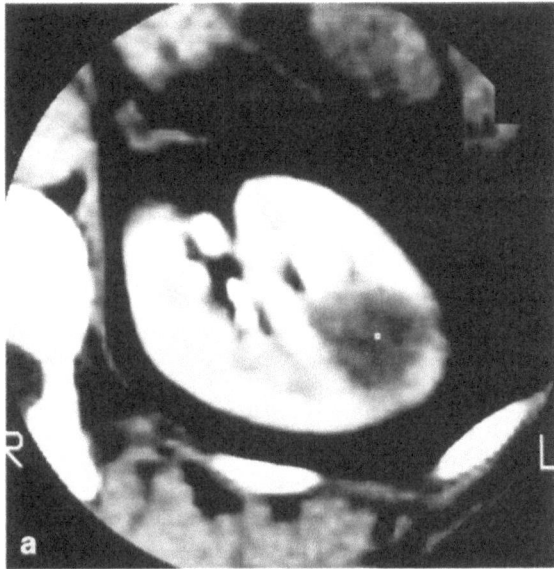

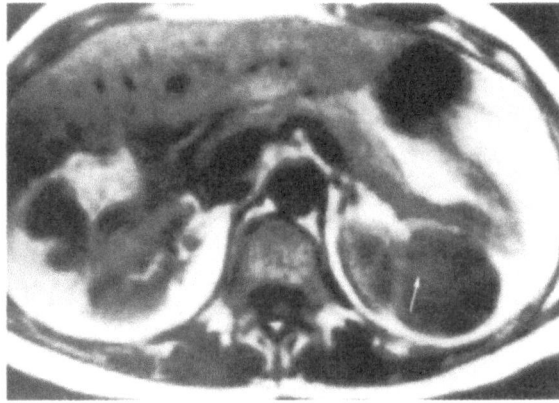

Fig. 9.9. MR image (SE 500-30) showing a fluid containing lesion of low signal intensity in the left kidney. Septa within the cyst (*arrow*) are of higher signal intensity compared to the low intensity fluid. (MAROTTI et al. 1987)

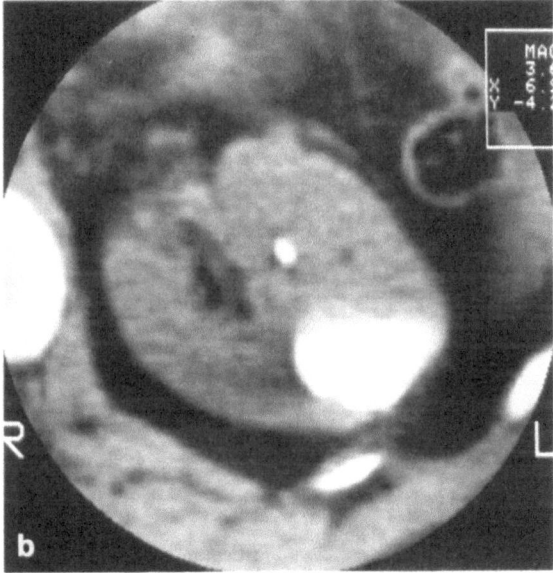

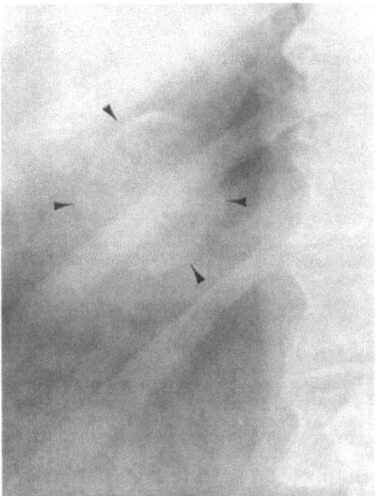

Fig. 9.8. a Dynamic CT showing a thick walled lesion with some fronds projecting into the lumen. The attenuation coefficient of 27 HU is higher than customarily seen in a benign renal cyst. **b** CT guided cyst puncture yielded fluid with elevated LDH and protein but only minimally elevated fat and normal cytology and thereby indicated an inflammatory cyst. Irregularities of the wall reflect fibrinous deposits on the cyst wall

Fig. 9.10. A KUB of the abdomen demonstrates shell-like calcifications in the region of the upper pole of the right kidney (*arrowheads*). These could represent calcifications in a benign or hemorrhagic renal cyst

infected cyst may be indistinguishable from a chronic hemorrhagic cyst, though signal intensity on T1 weighted images should be greater with a subacute or acute hemorrhagic cyst. The thick wall is, once again, readily identified on MR studies (Fig. 9.9a). Inflammatory cysts may also demonstrate septa (Fig. 9.9b).

Guided cyst puncture and aspiration and histochemical and cytologic assessment of the aspirate are the final arbiters in equivocal cases (LANG 1971, 1973, 1980). The fat content of the aspirate of an inflammatory cyst tends to be low. The LDH is usually less than 250 imu/ml. These biochemical criteria offer differentiation of an inflammatory exudate against the debris resulting from necrotic neoplasms. The protein content, however, may be high both in an inflammatory infected cyst and in a necrotic cystic neoplasm. Absence of neoplastic cells

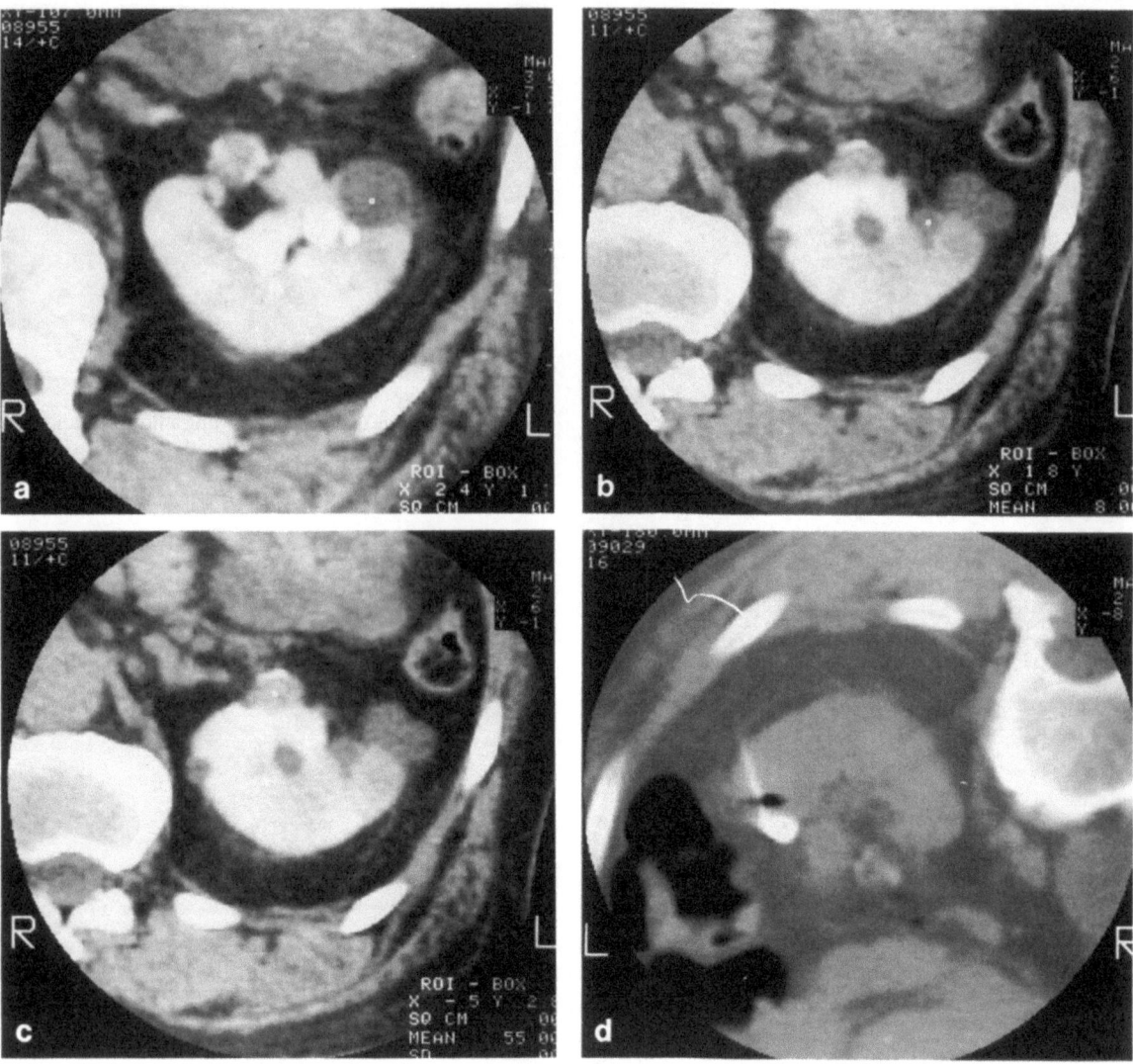

graded higher than 4 on cytologic examination should eliminate necrotic and cystic neoplasms from differential consideration. The double contrast cystogram may, at times, show filling defects attributable to necrotic exudate adherent to the cyst wall (Fig.9.8b). Gram stain and cultures may reveal the offensive organism.

9.4 Hemorrhagic Cysts

The term "hemorrhagic cyst" refers to a cyst into which bleeding has occurred. This may be attendant upon trauma, bleeding diathesis, or factors of unknown etiology. Up to 6% of all renal cysts present as hemorrhagic cysts (BERNSTEIN and WOODSIDE 1977; JACKMAN and STEVENS 1974).

Fig.9.11a–d. Multiple cysts are demonstrated in the upper pole of the left kidney. Attenuation coefficients vary from − 12 to + 55 HU. Shell-like calcifications are demonstrated in the rim of the hyperdense cyst. Cyst puncture and aspiration were carried out, confirming the benign nature. The hyperdense cyst with calcifications in its wall proved to be a hemorrhagic cyst

Pathologic examination of such cysts often discloses thick fibrous walls with rust colored material and sometimes plates of calcification. Many of these lesions are multiloculated. Histologically, an organized hemorrhage is enveloped by a thick walled cystic mass.

On intravenous urograms, there are no specific findings other than shell-like calcifications that may occur relatively frequently in chronic hemorrhagic cysts (Fig9.10). On ultrasound, chronic hemorrhagic

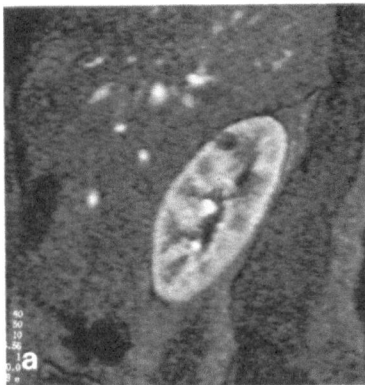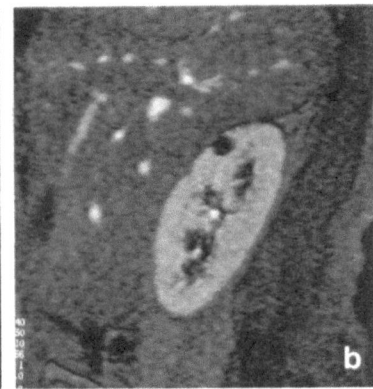

cysts may appear multiloculated, feature a thick wall, and frequently show shadowing calcifications in the wall. Particularly in chronic hemorrhagic cysts, echoes are elicited from the liquefying blood clots. Since clots are immersed in a liquid medium which offers an acoustic interface, a complex pattern results; fragmentation of clots increases the number of echoes. However, fresh bleeding or serosanguinous fluid without formation of blood clots is indistinguishable from a benign uncomplicated renal cyst on ultrasonograms.

On computed tomograms, hemorrhagic cysts are characterized by a high attenuation coefficient, reflecting hemoglobin or iron content (COLEMAN 1984; SUSSMAN et al. 1984). Characteristically, attenuation coefficients of such cysts are in a range of 50–90 HU on the unenhanced scan. Thus, the lesions appear hyperdense on the unenhanced scan but hypodense on the postenhancement scan (Fig. 9.11 a, c).

Enhancement of the wall of hemorrhagic cysts is commonly seen on dynamic CTs during the late capillary phase of contrast medium transit, reflecting the presence of inflammatory neovascularity (LANG 1984). The pathophysiologic mechanism is the same as described for inflammatory cysts. Calcifications in the wall of such cysts occur relatively frequently and are readily shown on CT.

Magnetic resonance imaging can differentiate between hemorrhagic cyst and uncomplicated simple cyst. The signal intensity varies with the age of the hemorrhagic cyst (HRICAK et al. 1983). The signal intensity is highest in hemorrhagic cysts during the phase of subacute hemorrhage (LIPUMA 1984). However, MR imaging cannot differentiate between a hemorrhagic cyst and a hemorrhage in a cystic and necrotic neoplasm with any degree of confidence (NEWHOUSE et al. 1986). Gadolinium-DPTA enhanced dynamic MR imaging offers a diagnostic criterion, i.e., enhancement of the carcinoma, which

Fig. 9.12. a Sagittal images of a dynamic contrast enhanced MR study demonstrating a small simple renal cyst, which is hypointense relative to the cortex. Ninety seconds after administration of Gd-DTPA conspicuity of the cyst increases attendant upon peak cortical signal intensity occurring at that time in parenchyma, yet there is lack of enhancement of the cyst itself. **b** Later, cortex and medulla are nearly isointense. The nonenhancing cyst remains well defined

may prove useful in differentiation of such lesions (EILENBERG et al. 1990) (Figs. 9.12, 9.13).

Cyst puncture and aspiration offer additional criteria to differentiate between a benign hemorrhagic cyst and a hemorrhage into a cyst containing a neoplasm. A relatively low fat and LDH content (below 250 imu/ml), the presence of cholesterol clefts, and a cytologic grade of less than 3 suggest a benign hemorrhagic cyst (Fig. 9.11 d). However, in many instances, cytology may reveal a grade 4 and an LDH content considered borderline for neoplasms. Double contrast study may demonstrate filling defects attributable to blood clots or neoplasm (Fig. 9.14). In this scenario, a definitive differentiation is not possible and surgical exploration must be resorted to as the final arbiter.

In the case of hemorrhage provoked by a traumatic puncture, a changing blood content typically will be seen while aspirating fluid from the cystic lesion, whereas a true hemorrhagic cyst produces a constant murky aspirate.

9.5 Calcified Cysts

Mural calcifications occur in about 1% of simple serous cysts but in a much higher percentage of inflammatory and hemorrhagic cysts. They present as thin eggshell layers of calcifications in a cyst wall (Fig. 9.10). Calcifications in tumors are of the dystrophic variety, presenting throughout the necrotic

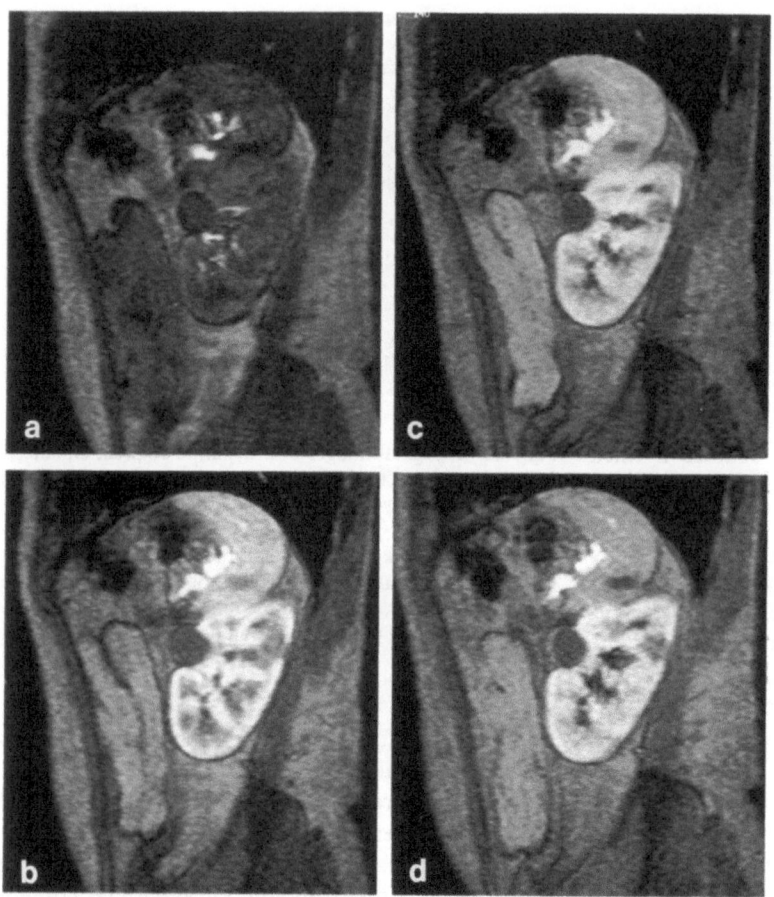

△
Fig. 9.13. a Precontrast study demonstrating a hypointense cyst. The carcinoma is not appreciated. **b** At 100 s after instillation of Gd-DTPA, an irregularly contoured carcinoma is demonstrated as an enhancing cortical mass. The cyst increased in conspicuity, failing to enhance and contrasting clearly against the peak cortical signal intensity. **c** At 200 s, the carcinoma continues to enhance, though considerably less than cortex and medulla. **d** At 15 min, the carcinoma remains conspicuous while the cyst fails to enhance. (EILENBERG et al. 1990)

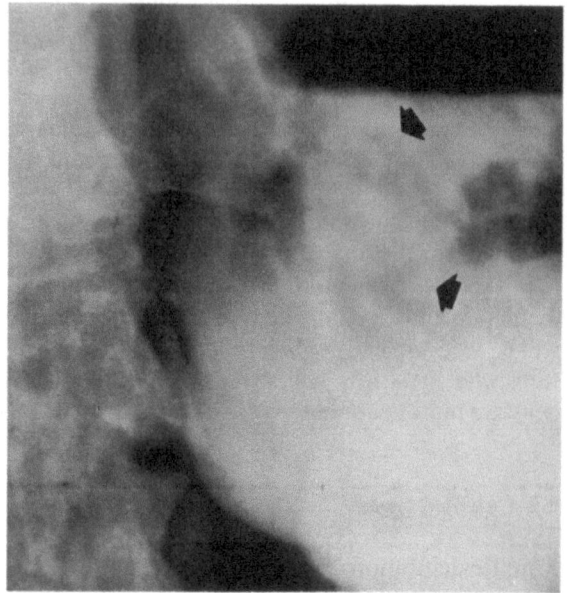

Fig. 9.14. A double contrast cyst study showing innumerable nodular filling defects in the cyst (*arrowheads*). The murky aspirate revealed a grade 5 cytology and high protein, fat, and LDH contents consistent with a neoplasm, which was subsequently proven

tumor elements and causing clusters of mortar-like calcifications.

Ultrasonograms offer no information because of shadowing and reverberation artifacts produced by the calcifications. At times, because of the reduced through-transmission a solid mass is mimicked.

Computed tomography is the most sensitive technique for detecting and properly localizing calcifications. It has been suggested that calcifications localized to the perimeter of the lesion and not associated with a soft tissue mass projecting beyond its perimeter are dependable criteria indicating a benign cyst (WEYMAN et al. 1982) (Fig. 9.15). Unfortu-

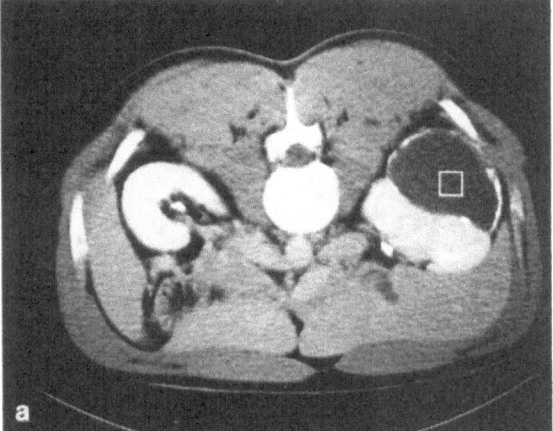

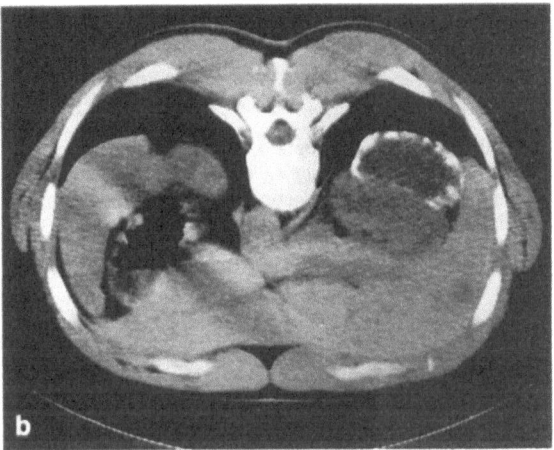

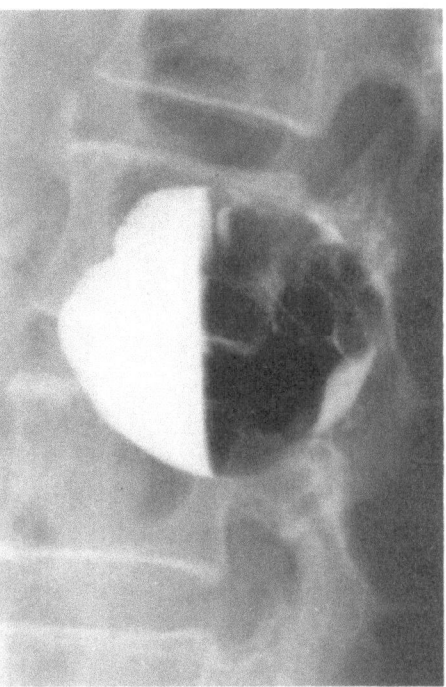

Fig. 9.16. A double contrast cyst study shows to advantage multiple septa existing within this cyst. These represent a subseptated multilocular benign cyst. Biochemical and cytologic examinations of the aspirate confirmed the diagnosis. Irregularities of the cyst wall reflect fibrinous deposits

Fig. 9.15. a Dynamic CT demonstrating a nonenhancing low density oval shaped subcortical mass in the right kidney. Shell-like calcifications are noted. There is no soft tissue mass extending beyond the confines of the calcifications. **b** At a slightly lower cut level (supine position), the calcifications appear thicker. This is due to the tangential cut through the circumference of the cyst wall. Lack of calcifications in the central region and lack of a soft tissue mass lateral to the calcifications are criteria supporting the diagnosis of a benign calcified cyst

9.6 Multilocular Cysts

The designation "multilocular cyst" is based on morphologic observations. A wide variety of entities can produce multilocular cysts. Septa in benign renal cysts produce a multilocular cyst. Frequently, this is a consequence of infection and inflammatory disease or hemorrhage into a benign cyst. The septa are formed by fibrous tissue lined with cuboidal epithelium.

Other common multiloculated renal masses are of neoplastic etiology. The multilocular cystic nephroma, a benign lesion, presents in this fashion, as does multiloculated renal cell carcinoma.

In rare instances, the septa can be appreciated on nephrotomograms. High resolution ultrasonograms and computed tomograms show the presence of septa with ease. Cyst puncture and aspiration studies demonstrate multiple compartments, which may communicate with one another or present as segregated and loculated compartments (Fig. 9.16). Usually, aspiration yields clear, yellowish fluid, although at times (particularly in cysts with a hemorrhagic background) a murky aspirate is retrieved. On MR images, the septa may be suggested by com-

nately, these criteria have not stood up to the test of time.

Guided cyst puncture and aspiration is the best means of establishing benign versus malignant etiology of a calcified cyst. Histochemical and cytopathologic criteria can establish the diagnosis with higher confidence than those generated by imaging examinations (Fig. 9.11 d). Nonetheless, there remain a substantial number of indeterminate lesions, particularly those yielding a grade 4 cytology on examination of the aspirate. For such lesions, exploration is strongly advocated (KIM et al. 1981; LANG 1980).

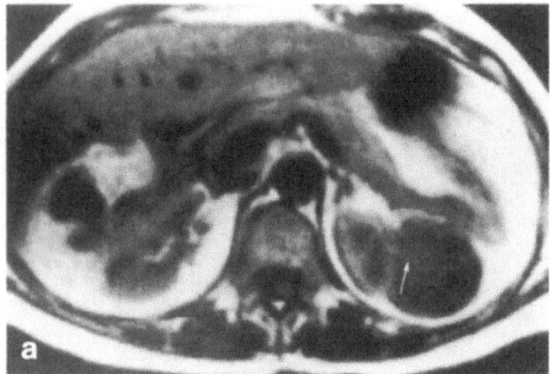

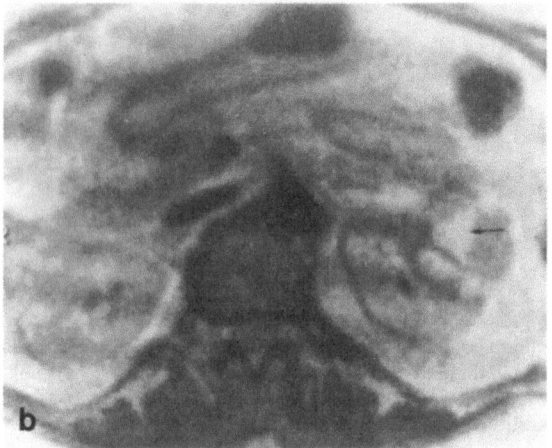

Fig. 9.17. a MR image (SE 500-30) showing a multilocular lesion of low signal intensity with one central focus of higher signal intensity in the left kidney (*arrow*). The signal intensity of the central area is similar to that of renal cortex. **b** MR image (SE 2000-30) showing a significant increase in the signal intensity of the central focus (*arrow*) while that of the surrounding lesion shows only a moderate increase. The lesion with the high signal intensity corresponds to a hemorrhagic cyst found at surgery. (MAROTTI et al. 1987)

partmentalized components with vastly different signal intensity, such as is caused by hemorrhagic contents (Fig. 9.17).

9.7 Autosomal Dominant Polycystic Disease

Autosomal dominant polycystic disease of kidney, liver, and pancreas is a genetically transmitted disorder. A large number of cysts of varying size, located predominantly in the cortex but also in the medulla of the kidneys, liver, and pancreas, are hallmarks of this entity.

The kidneys are enlarged, commensurate with the size and number of cysts. There is resultant distortion of the renal contour. Pelvis and calyces are intrinsically normal but are subject to compression and displacement by larger cysts.

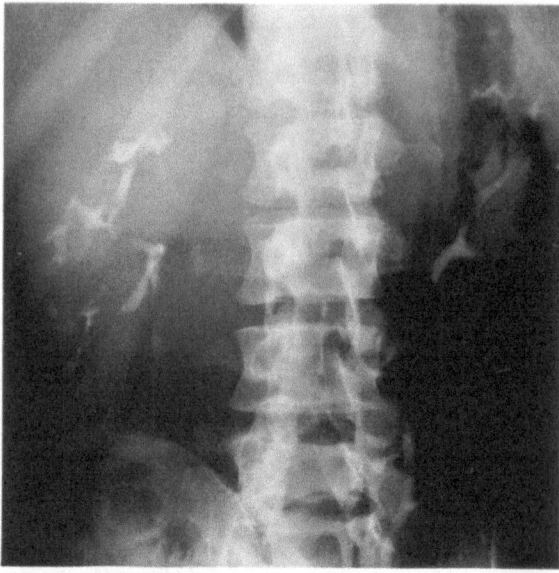

Fig. 9.18. Intravenous urogram demonstrating innumerable areas of effacement and displacement of calyces. The kidneys are large and of an irregular contour. These findings are characteristic of adult polycystic disease

The cysts vary in size and can attain diameters of many centimeters. They contain clear straw-colored fluid. Often, however, there is hemorrhage into one or more of the cysts, resulting in a hemorrhagic cyst. Microdissections show the cyst to arise from the nephron and draining tubules and therefore continuity exists with the nephron (OSATHANONDH and POTTER 1964).

Associated cystic disease of the liver is found in 30%–60% of the patients (LEVINE et al. 1985). Approximately 10% of the patients have cysts in the pancreas, and on rare occasions also in the ovary, endometrium, lungs, pituitary gland, breast, parathyroid, and epididymis (HARTNETT and BENNETT 1976).

The most common presenting signs and symptoms are palpable mass, abdominal pain, hematuria, and hypertension. Polycythemia may develop attendant upon erythropoietin production from the afflicted kidney. Progressive uremia heralds the end-stage of the disease. The abnormal kidneys are susceptible to trauma and hence intracystic or retroperitoneal hemorrhage.

The excretory urogram demonstrates enlarged kidneys with irregular contours. The nephrogram shows numerous sharply marginated radiolucencies of different size throughout the cortex and medulla (Swiss cheese appearance). Effacement and displacement of calyces is common and attributable to larger cysts (Fig. 9.18). In children, diffuse puddling

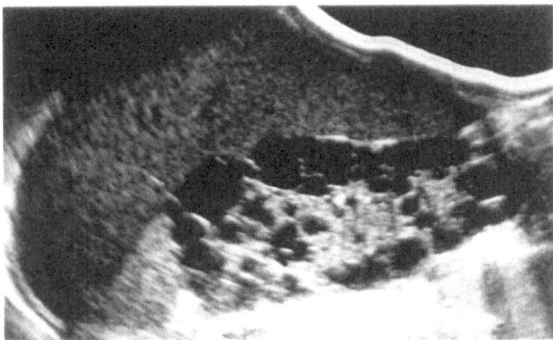

Fig.9.19. Adult autosomal dominant polycystic kidney disease. An ultrasonogram in a sagittal scan direction demonstrates innumerable cysts of different size, primarily in a cortical location. The central sinus echoes are normal. This is a differentiating feature against hydronephrosis and dilated calyces

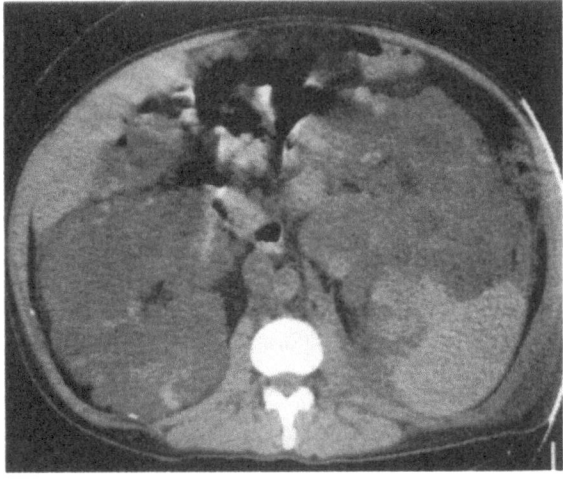

Fig.9.21. Computed tomogram demonstrating slight anterior displacement of the left kidney studded with innumerable cysts. High density material is identified in the posterior perinephric space attendant upon rupture of one of the cysts and bleeding into the posterior perinephric space. This is not an uncommon complication of adult polycystic disease. (Courtesy of Dr. ERROL LEVINE)

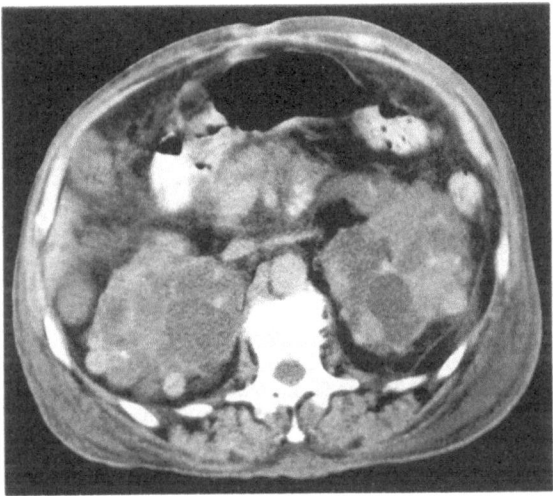

Fig.9.20. Computed tomogram in the postenhancement phase demonstrating innumerable cysts of variable size throughout both kidneys. Some cysts feature a substantially higher attenuation coefficient. The appearance is characteristic of autosomal dominant adult polycystic disease. The higher attenuation coefficient reflects recent hemorrhage into the cyst

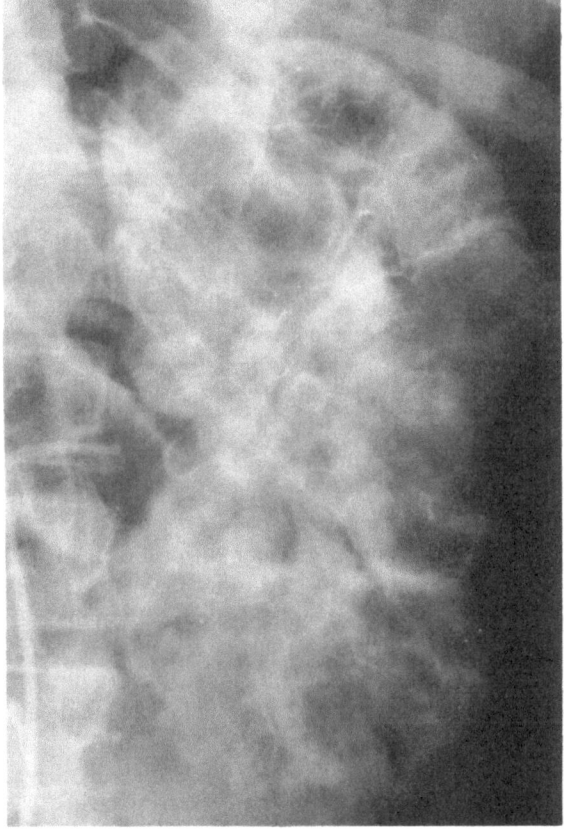

of contrast medium throughout the parenchyma of both kidneys is the characteristic finding distinguishing this entity from autosomal recessive polycystic disease, which shows contrast collections in a radiating striate pattern.

On ultrasonograms, enlarged kidneys with irregular contours are demonstrated. Innumerable sonolucent cysts are visualized (Fig.9.19). The central echo complex may be distorted by larger cysts (LARSON et al. 1978); there is, however, no continuity between pelvis and cystic lesions. Cysts with secondary hemorrhage or infection may show some internal

Fig.9.22. A late phase arteriogram demonstrating innumerable cysts of variable size throughout the cortex and medulla of the kidney (Swiss cheese appearance). This is characteristic for adult autosomal dominant polycystic disease

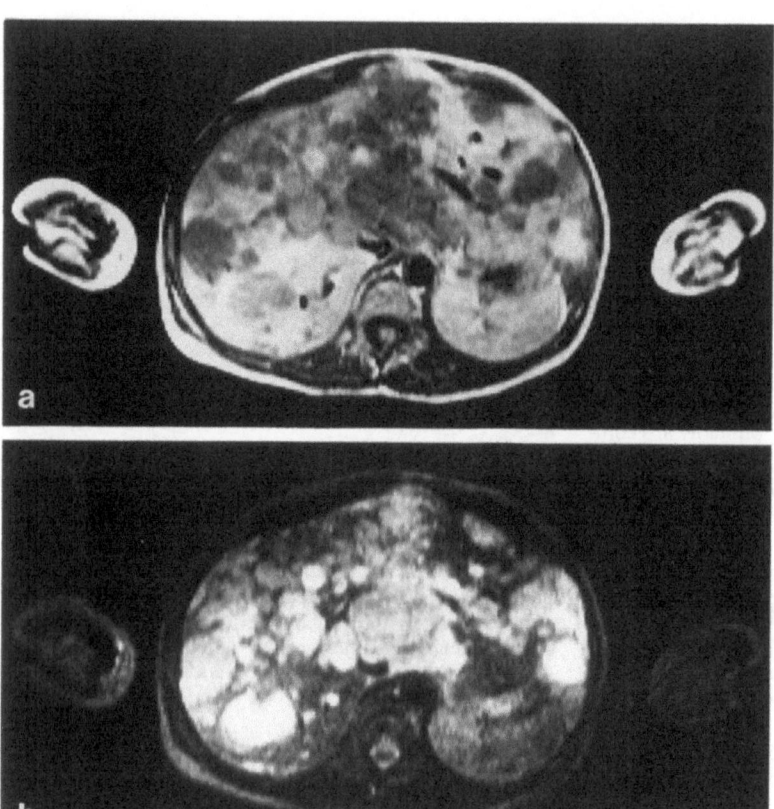

echoes. Cysts of the liver and pancreas likewise present as a sonolucent mass.

Computed tomograms demonstrate innumerable round to oval shaped cysts of various sizes throughout the cortex and medulla. In general, the attenuation coefficient is near to that of water. Occasionally, a high attenuation coefficient indicates hemorrhage into some of the cysts (Fig. 9.20). With progressive disease, the size and number of cysts and the renal volume increase (LARSON et al. 1978). Also in advanced disease, calcification within cyst walls or parenchyma may be identified.

High density cysts are common, occurring in up to 75% of all patients (LEVINE and GRANTHAM 1985, 1987). CT can also suggest infected cysts on the basis of thick and enhancing walls, occasionally with calcifications. Coexistence of neoplasms and polycystic disease is sometimes suggested on dynamic and postenhancement computed tomograms. Rupture of cysts into the perinephric space is readily identified on computed tomograms (SOFFER et al. 1987) (Fig. 9.21). Angiography indicates the presence of numerous cysts on the basis of splaying of intrarenal arterial branches and a Swiss cheese appearance on the nephrogram (Fig. 9.22).

Fig. 9.23a, b. T1 and T2 weighted magnetic resonance images demonstrating innumerable cystic lesions with signal intensity characteristic of fluid and some others characteristic of blood. Recent hemorrhage into cyst of this adult polycystic kidney is incriminated as being responsible for this appearance. (Courtesy of Dr. R. FRIEDENBERG)

On MR images, uncomplicated polycystic disease resembles multiple simple cysts, featuring a low signal intensity on T1 weighted images and a homogeneous and high intensity on T2 weighted images. The appearance of cysts complicated by hemorrhage varies, depending on the age of the hemorrhage (LEVINE and GRANTHAM 1987; LUENG et al. 1984) (Fig. 9.23).

On radionuclide scans, adult polycystic disease presents with multiple photopenic mass lesions.

9.8 Autosomal Recessive Polycystic Disease

Autosomal recessive polycystic disease is characterized by dilatation of renal collecting tubules, hepatic cysts, and periportal fibrosis. Depending upon the individual's age and onset of manifestations, the disease is categorized into perinatal, neonatal, infantile, and juvenile forms. The spectrum varies from predominantly renal and minimal hepatic involvement in the infant to predominantly hepatic and minimal renal involvement in the juvenile.

The perinatal form features massive enlargement of the kidney, which often weights as much as several hundred grams. The surface of the kidney demonstrates hugely dilated collecting ducts in the subcapsular region. The cut surface shows a spongy appearance owing to the dilated collecting tubules radiating from the cortex to the calyces. There is usually some form of associated hepatic disorder, often ectatic and tortuous bile ducts.

In the childhood form there is predominant hepatic disease. Marked periportal fibrosis causes focal dilatation of biliary radicals, portal hypertension, hepatofugal blood flow, splenomegaly, and gastric and esophageal varices. Changes in the kidneys, however, are less prominent. Caroli's disease may be a variant of the same underlying pathological process (NAKANUMA et al. 1982).

Pulmonary hypoplasia is often associated with the perinatal form and is a major contributory factor to the cause of death in the neonates (MADEWELL et al. 1979). In patients with long-term survival portal hypertension is to be expected.

The excretory urogram of neonates with manifestation of the perinatal form of autosomal recessive polycystic kidney disease demonstrates diminished renal function and massively enlarged kidneys with striations arranged radially and extending from cortex to medulla (Fig. 9.24). Contrast medium may be retained in tubules for days, attesting to the poor function. Ultrasonograms demonstrate enlarged reniform, highly echogenic kidneys with poor definition of cortical boundaries (BOAL and TEELE 1980). High resolution real-time scans often show a sonolucent rim around the echogenic kidney (HAYDEN et al. 1986). This sonolucent rim probably reflects compressed cortex. The central echoes may be difficult to differentiate from the echogenic medullary component of the kidney. A presumptive diagnosis of autosomal recessive polycystic kidney disease can be made in the fetus when bilateral large echogenic kidneys and oligohydramnios are demonstrated (see Chap. 14).

Computed tomograms demonstrate nephromegaly. Postenhancement scans show prolonged corticomedullary differentiation and a striated nephrogram extending prominently into the medulla (HOWIE and NICHOLSON 1980). Computed tomograms of the liver may demonstrate bands reflecting hepatic fibrosis.

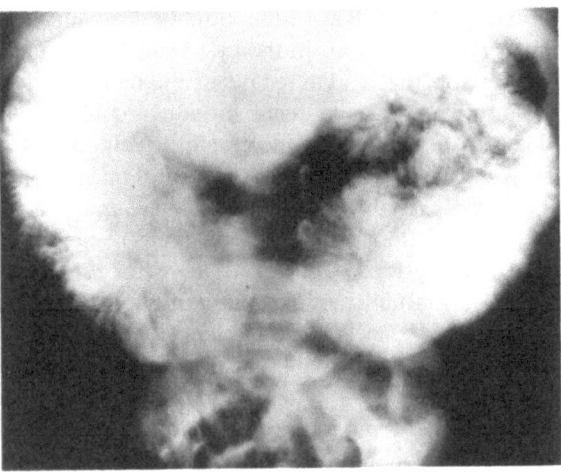

Fig. 9.24. In this neonate, a delayed intravenous urogram demonstrates massively enlarged kidneys with striations radiating from cortex to medulla. The apperance is characteristic for autosomal recessive polycystic kidney disease

The childhood form demonstrates a striate appearance in the apices of the pyramids similar to medullary sponge kidney on intravenous urograms. Otherwise, however, function appears unimpeded. Esophageal varices may be shown on gastrointestinal examination. On ultrasound increased parenchymal echogenicity and a few discrete medullary cysts may be identifiable. Heptomegaly, splenomegaly, and increased hepatic echogenicity are hallmarks of this disease.

Computed tomograms of the liver may demonstrate discrete cysts corresponding to focal bile duct dilatation. Hepatofugal flow may be suggested by prominent portal and splenic veins.

Technetium 99m sulfur colloid scans tend show numerous photopenic areas in the liver. These same lesions can be demonstrated accumulating radiotracer on hida or pipida scans (MORENO et al. 1984).

9.9 Acquired Renal Cystic Disease
(see also Chap. 13)

Acquired cystic disease of the kidney occurs with an overall incidence of 43.4% in patients with chronic renal failure, and particularly patients whose lives are prolonged by dialysis (BOMNER et al. 1980; FEINER 1981; LEVINE et al. 1984; VAZIRI et al. 1984). This disease is sometimes associated with renal cell carcinoma and retroperitoneal hemorrhage (LEVINE et al. 1987).

Pathologically, acquired cystic kidney disease is characterized by multiple small cysts permeating the cortex and medulla of both kidneys. Calcium oxalate crystals are seen in the cyst walls and lumina. The factors that lead to renal cyst and neoplasm formation in end-stage renal disease are unknown. There appears to be an increase in size and number of cysts once dialysis begins in these uremic patients. Following renal transplantation, there may be regression of the acquired cystic disease, suggesting that some cystogenic chemicals are being removed.

The important complications of acquired cystic disease are renal hemorrhage and renal neoplasia. Interestingly, most renal tumors in uremic patients are asymptomatic.

Computed tomograms demonstrate innumerable cysts throughout both kidneys (Chap. 7) (Fig. 9.4a). Calcification of cyst walls is common. High density hemorrhagic cysts occur commonly and are difficult to differentiate against solid tumors (LEVINE et al. 1984). Perinephric hemorrhage is a not uncommon complication of renal cystic disease. CT is invaluable to identify small carcinomas as a possible source of the hemorrhage.

On ultrasonograms, multiple cysts and increased echogenicity of small kidneys are the hallmarks of this entity. Doppler ultrasound may be capable of identifying renal neoplasms abutting complex cysts on the basis of characteristic high (2.5 kHz or greater) peak systolic Doppler shift (KIER et al. 1990) (Fig. 9.4b, c). MRI may prove useful in identifying coexistent tumor and hemorrhagic cyst.

Selective renal angiography and digital renal arteriography can identify the source of active hemorrhage and can be expanded to selective transcatheter embolization of the bleeding vessels or supply vessels to a small neoplasm.

9.10 Multicystic Dysplastic Kidney

Multicystic dysplastic kidney is the result of failed or improper interaction between the ureteric bud (ampulla) and the metanephric blastema. Obstruction early in fetal life, such as atresia at the ureteropelvic junction, causes severe malformations; incomplete obstruction in later pregnancy results in lesser malformations.

Two types are recognized: pelvioinfundibular atresia and the hydronephrotic multicystic dysplastic kidney.

Pelvioinfundibular atresia is associated with complete atresia of the pelvis and ureter, occurring early in fetal life. The resultant malformation does not have a reniform contour, but consists of grape-like clusters of thick walled cysts. These are held together by connective tissue, collagen fibers, and sometimes hyaline cartilage. Some primitive ducts are lined by cuboidal or low columnar epithelium. Collagenous walls envelop these structures. Pelvis and calyceal system cannot be identified. The vascular pedicle tends to be atretic; ureter is absent or obliterated.

Hydronephrotic multicystic dysplastic kidney shows similar changes except that the pelvis is dilated and communicates with cysts. Multicystic dysplastic kidney presents as a large mass in an otherwise asymptomatic neonate. It is one of the most common abdominal masses in neonates (65%). Usually, the contralateral kidney has other serious congenital anomalies. Therefore, careful evaluation of the contralateral kidney is important to exclude an associated life threatening anomaly that might require immediate surgery.

The radiologic findings of multicystic dysplastic kidney vary depending on whether pelvioinfundibular atresia or severe hydronephrosis is associated, whether the involvement is segmental or total, and whether the disease is uni- or bilateral.

Plain films demonstrate a large noncalcified abdominal mass that displaces bowel gas and frequently extends across the midline. Total body opacification shows multiple lucencies reflecting cysts (MADEWELL et al. 1979).

The hydronephrotic multicystic kidney may demonstrate excretion on delayed films and particularly contrast accumulation within the cystic spaces (COOPERMAN 1976). Patients with segmental multicystic dysplastic kidney show multiloculated masses displacing normal components of the kidney. The malformed segment is most often in the upper pole of the duplicated moiety.

Ring calcifications in the renal fossa may herald the presence of multicystic dysplastic kidney in adults (Fig. 9.25).

In patients with pelvioinfundibular atresia, high quality real-time sonograms demonstrate cysts of varying size and shape lacking communication with each other, absence of renal parenchyma, and absence of a sonolucent structure corresponding to a pelvis as well as echogenic areas in an eccentric location indicating tiny cysts. Hydronephrotic multicystic kidney, conversely, demonstrates multiple peripheral cysts communicating to a large medial cystic space, which represents the renal pelvis (Fig. 9.26). Very small cysts present as a highly echogenic mass. Multicystic dysplastic kidney can be detected prenatally on the maternal ultrasonograms (see Chap. 13).

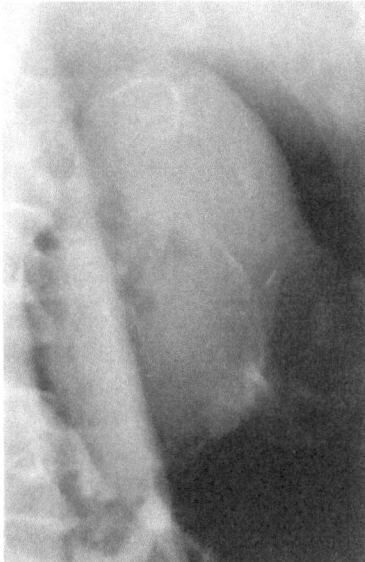

Fig. 9.25. Shell-like calcifications arranged in a grape-like fashion in the left renal fossa, reflecting a cystic dysplastic kidney in an adult

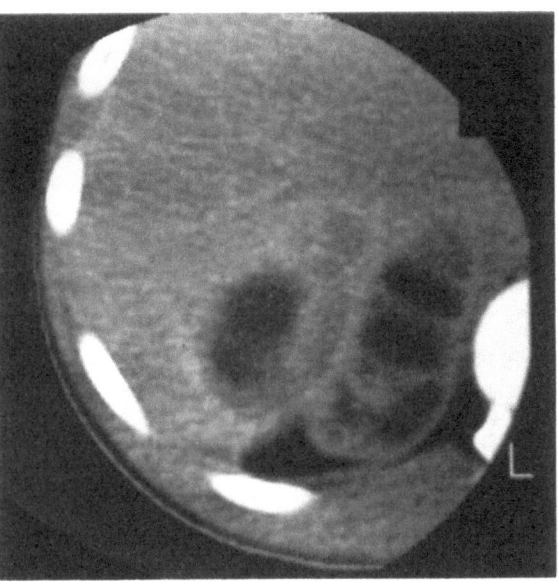

Fig. 9.27. Computed tomogram demonstrating innumerable cysts replacing the upper pole of the kidney; this appearance is indicative of a cystic dysplastic upper moiety. Benign simple cysts are seen in the remainder of both kidneys

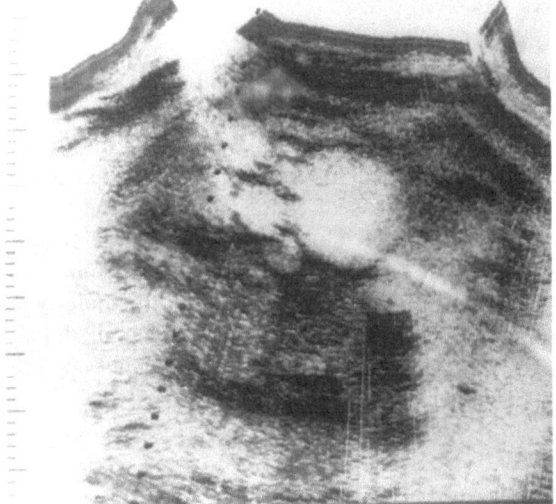

Fig. 9.26. Sonogram showing large cysts communicating with a hydronephrotic pelvis – a hallmark of a hydronephrotic multicystic dysplastic kidney

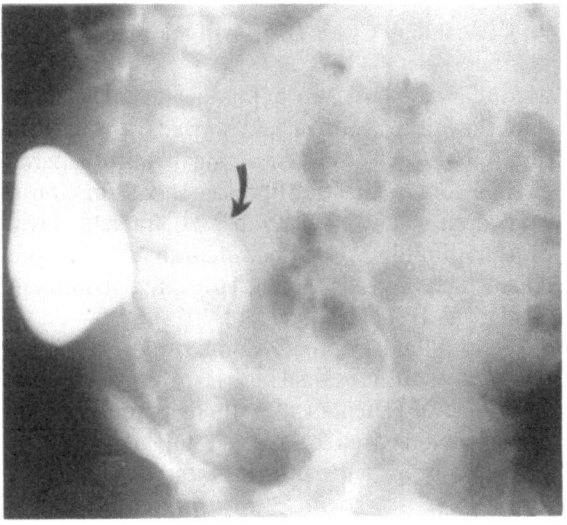

Fig. 9.28. Percutaneous cyst contrast study demonstrating contiguous opacification of cysts and pelvis (*arrow*) in this infant with hydronephrotic multicystic dysplastic kidney

On computed tomograms multicystic dysplastic kidney appears as a grape-like mass lacking reniform configuration. Innumerable small cystic lesions of water density are identified. The septa may be visible particularly after contrast enhancement. Segmental multicystic dysplastic malformations often involve only the upper moiety, the lower moiety of the kidney being normal (Fig. 9.27). Hy-dronephrotic multicystic kidney may demonstrate crescentic puddling of contrast medium. In adults, cyst wall calcifications are the classic manifestation (Fig. 9.25).

Technetium 99m glucoheptonate scintiscano-grams can provide both morphologic and functional information about the multicystic dysplastic kidney.

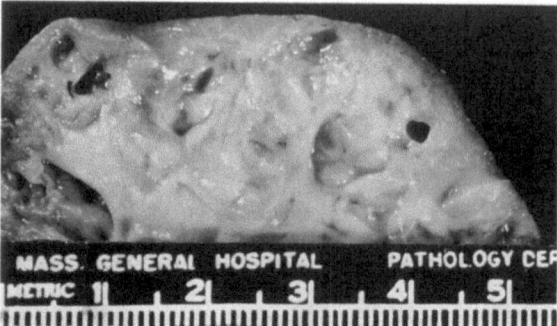

Fig. 9.29. Cut gross specimen showing classical cortical thinning and cysts of variable size throughout the medulla, establishing the diagnosis of medullary cystic disease. (Courtesy of R. PFISTER, Maryland)

In cases of pelvioinfundibular atresia, cyst puncture and aspiration demonstrates noncommunicating cysts. Conversely, in patients with hydronephrotic multicystic kidney, communications from cysts to the pelvis are documented (Fig. 9.28). The aspirate is usually of crank oil consistency.

9.11 Medullary Cystic Disease of the Kidney

Medullary cystic disease or familial juvenile nephronophthisis is a disorder characterized by progressive tubulointerstitial disease resulting in uniform parenchymal loss, interstitial fibrosis, and formation of small cysts in the medulla (Fig. 9.29). Interstitial lymphocytic infiltrates surround deposits of mucoproteins which represent Tamm-Horsfall glycoproteins (GARDNER 1976; RESNICK et al. 1978).

The childhood form of medullary cystic disease is inherited as an autosomal recessive disorder. It is encountered in patients with retinitis pigmentosa, the entity being referred to as renal retinal dysplasia.

Clinically, patients present with polyuria, polydipsia, enuresis, anemia, growth retardation, progressive renal failure, lethargy, weakness reflecting salt wasting, and symptoms due to hypokalemia attendant upon tubular damage. Laboratory findings tend to show elevated BUN, creatinine, phosphorus, acidosis, and hypokalemia.

Plain radiographs demonstrate small kidneys. Intravenous urograms show poor visualization of small kidneys with a smooth contour. These cysts do not communicate to the collecting system, as can be shown when selectively opacifying such cysts by percutaneous cyst puncture (Fig. 9.30). Occasionally, lucencies may be demonstrated at the cortical junction on nephrotomograms (LINK et al. 1979). A

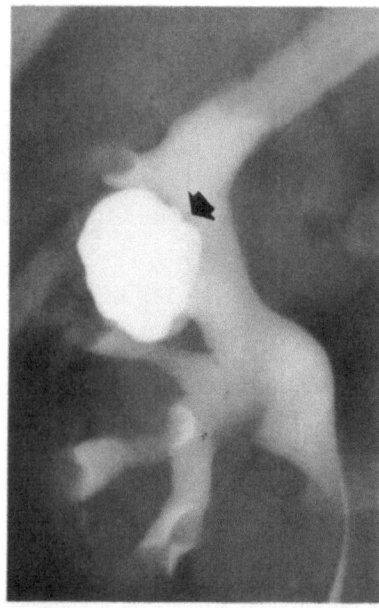

Fig. 9.30. Under ultrasound guidance, one medullary cyst was aspirated and opacified with contrast medium (*arrow*). Note a small kidney. Contrast excretion from prior intravenous injection results in an unusually dense opacification for a forme fruste of medullary cystic disease. The diagnosis was confirmed by the clinical observation of salt loosing

striated appearance in the medulla may be noted on late urograms.

High resolution ultrasonograms can demonstrate cysts at the cortical medullary junction in small kidneys with increased echogenicity (GAREL et al. 1984). On computed tomograms, cysts at the cortical medullary junction are demonstrated in otherwise small but smooth kidneys. Angiography similarly reveals avascular masses at the cortical medullary junction. To date, the role of MRI has not been established.

9.12 Cysts of the Renal Sinus

"Cyst of the renal sinus" has been coined as an inclusive term for both cysts arising in tissues of the sinus and those that arise from renal parenchyma but present in the renal sinus. "Peripelvic cysts", "parapelvic cysts", "parapelvic lymphatic cysts", and "parapelvic lymphangiectasia" are other terms that have been used for this entity. Etiologically, these cysts are most often attributable to lymphatic ectasia, probably secondary to pelvic lymphatic obstruction. This theory is supported by the low pressure and lymphatic type of fluid existing in such cysts, the lining that resembles lymphatic channels,

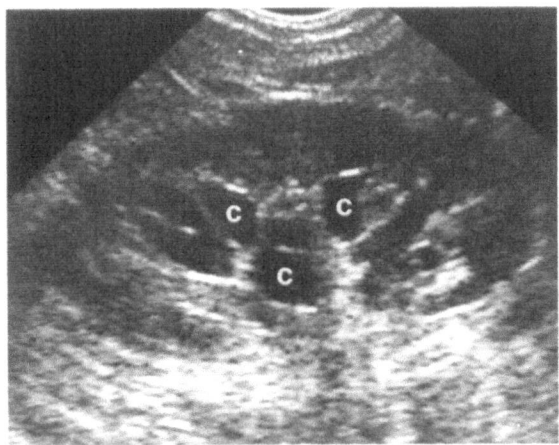

Fig. 9.31. Ultrasonogram in a sagittal scan direction demonstrating multiple renal cysts (*c*) within the renal sinus; these represent peripelvic cysts. (POLLACK and BANNER 1982)

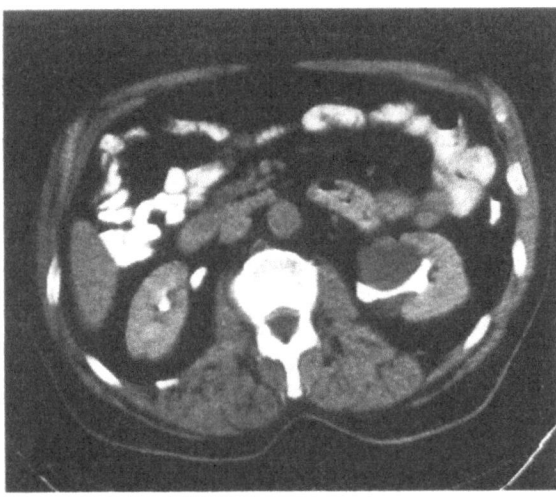

Fig. 9.32. Postenhancement computed tomogram demonstrating a low density cystic mass compressing the opacified pelvis of the left kidney, a characteristic location for a peripelvic cyst

and the observation that contrast medium extravasation into lymphatics attendant upon either obstruction or excessive injection pressure during retrograde pyelography will result in later opacification of such sinus cysts (MAYER et al. 1982). Remnants of the wolffian body, mesonephric remnants, and posttraumatic extravasation of urine with rents of the pyocalyceal system extending into renal sinus as well as familial renal lymphangiomatosis have been advocated as other causes (AMIS et al. 1983).

Renal sinus cysts occur most often in the fifth and sixth decades and are found in 1%–1.5% of autopsy cases. Parapelvic cysts are only rarely symptomatic since the cyst pressure only rarely exceeds intrapelvic urine pressure.

On excretory urograms, renal sinus cysts may present as a mass in the region of the renal hilus. Large cysts may displace the kidney laterally. A cyst of hilar origin tends to displace renal sinus fat and present with a radiolucent ring (peripheral fat sign). However, under certain circumstances, cysts originating from renal parenchyma may likewise displace infundibular or hilar fat and present with a peripheral lucent ring composed of fatty tissues.

On ultrasonograms, renal sinus cysts present as multiple sonolucent mass lesions in the region of the renal sinus (Fig. 9.31). Real-time sonograms demonstrating communications of dilated calyces with the dilated renal pelvis may be used to establish the diagnosis of hydronephrosis, which is a differential diagnostic consideration. On postenhancement computed tomograms, nondilated infundibula may be splayed around renal sinus cysts. Solitary renal sinus

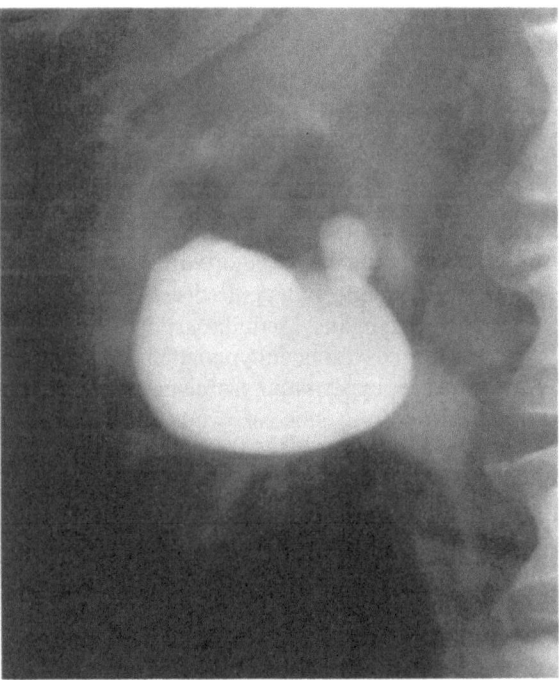

Fig. 9.33. A peripelvic cyst has been punctured under fluoroscopic control, aspirated, and contrast medium infused. The peripelvic cyst is outlined with contrast medium of greater density than the pelvis and calyces opacified from excreted and intravenously administered contrast medium. This proves that the peripelvic cyst does not communicate with the pelvis

cysts may show focal displacement of the pelvis (HI-DALGO et al. 1982) (Fig. 9.32). To allow opacification of the pelvis, computed tomographic cuts should be obtained a considerable time after administration of intravenous contrast medium so as not to confuse a nonopacified portion of a dilated renal pelvis with a parapelvic cyst.

Fluoroscopic, CT, or ultrasound guided cyst puncture and aspiration can be used to confirm the nature of such cysts on the basis of the visual apearance and biochemical characteristics of the aspirate. Injection of contrast medium will define the cystic cavity in its relation to pelvis and infundibula (LANG 1984) (Fig. 9.33). Symtomatic sinus cysts can be ablated by meticulous evacuation of the contents, by displacement with air, and by subsequent instillation of 95% alcohol. Instillation of 1–2 g Acromycin likewise tends to obliterate the renal sinus cyst. On T1 weighted MR images, cysts should present with low intensity signals.

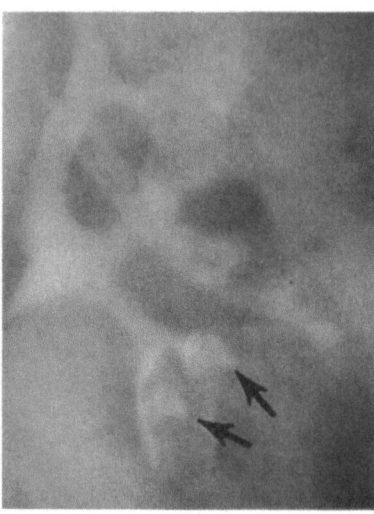

Fig. 9.34. Innumerable opacified small cysts in the pyramids (*arrows*) of the kidneys establish the diagnosis of medullary sponge kidney

9.13 Medullary Sponge Kidney

Medullary sponge kidney is characterized by small tubular or cystic cavities ranging from 1 to 5 mm in diameter and located in the pyramids. The cysts represent a dilatation of the terminal collecting tubules and ducts of Bellini. Interstitial fibrosis and inflammation may occur. Calculi may develop within these cysts. In contradistinction to polycystic disease, no cysts are found in other organs. Medullary sponge kidney has been associated with hemihypertrophy, Ehlers-Danlos syndrome, hyperparathyroidism, congenital hypertrophic pyloric stenosis, and Caroli's disease (PARKKER and SKALKO 1969; STELLA et al. 1976). A male predilection has been reported; the reported urographic incidence is 0.5% (PALUBINSKAS 1961).

On plain films, nephrocalcinosis or nephrolithiasis may be demonstrated. Medullary calculi clustering in the tips of renal pyramids are the characteristic finding. On intravenous urograms, the findings vary from discrete linear densities (benign tubular ectasia) to radiodense linear striae or cystic dilatation of the collecting ducts in the tips of the papillae (Fig. 9.34). In advanced cases, beaded cavities may be present in the papillae, with contrast medium surrounding calcifications in the cavities.

The natural history of medullary sponge kidney is unknown. Follow-up examinations only rarely show progression of disease such as an increased size and number of beaded cavities or calcifications.

The condition must be differentiated against a papillary blush resulting from concentration of contrast medium in nondilated terminal ducts. The papillary blush is homogeneous in nature and individual tubules cannot be identified. Moreover, the blush is best seen on early roentgenograms and tends to fade on delayed films, unlike manifestations of medullary sponge kidney, which intensify on delayed films.

Papillary necrosis described in detail in another chapter results in destruction of the apex and tip of the pyramid, causing an irregular cavitation rather than multiple cystic cavities in an otherwise intact papilla.

Computed tomography may demonstrate extracalyceal accumulation of contrast medium within a cyst of the papilla, which is considered diagnostic for this entity (BOAG and NOLAN 1988). On ultrasonograms, medullary nephrocalcinosis presents as discrete hyperechoic foci with acoustic shadowing within the pyramids and particularly the tips. Increased echogenicity is the telltale characteristic (GLAZER et al. 1982).

9.14 Cystic Disease Associated with Malignant and Benign Neoplasms

Entities such as multilocular cystic nephroma, cystic renal cell carcinoma, and cystic Wilms' tumor are discussed in detail in appropriate chapters in this volume.

Renal cysts occurring in von Hippel-Lindau disease are benign renal cysts filled with clear yellowish fluid and lined by cuboidal epithelium. About 15%

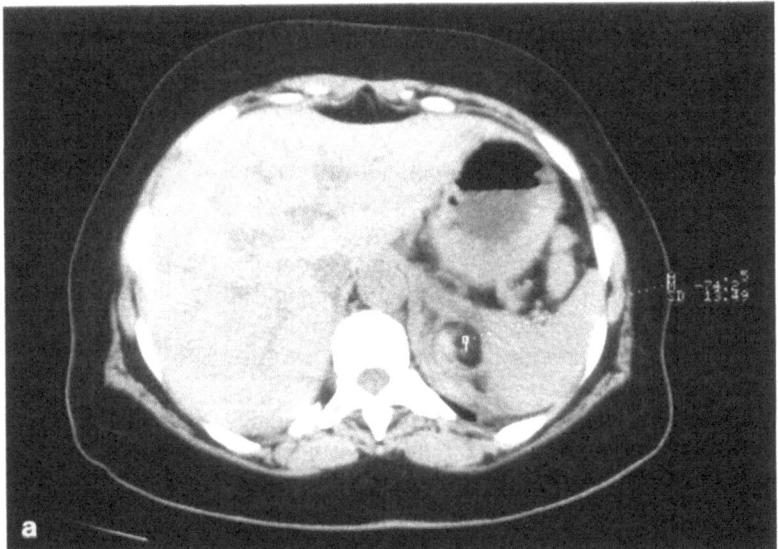

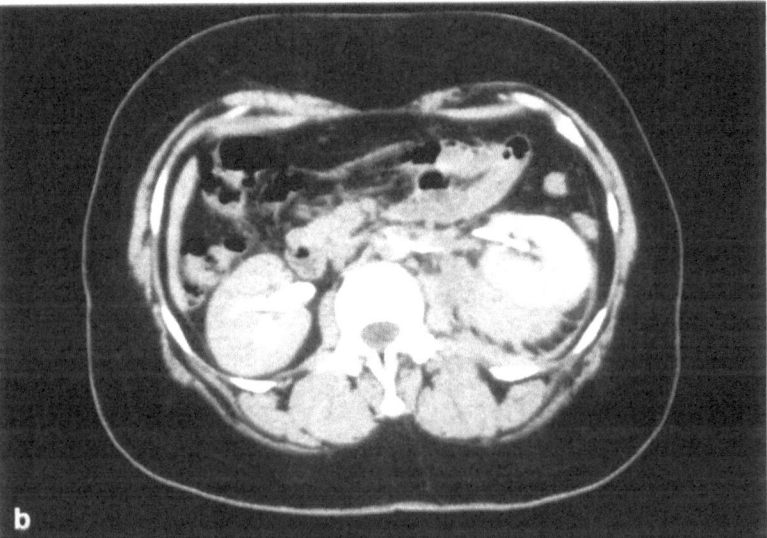

Fig. 9.35 a, b. Computed tomograms demonstrating a low density mass (-74 HU) in the upper pole of the kidney. Note some high density material representing hemorrhage into the tumor as well as a mantle of high density material in the posterior perirenal space attendant upon hemorrhage from this angiomyolipoma. Cysts are present in other segments of the kidney. Facial angiofibromas confirmed the diagnosis of tuberous sclerosis

of patients with von Hippel-Lindau disease also harbor pheochromocytomas (LEVINE et al. 1982). The pancreas may likewise be involved. Most commonly, multiple small cysts are the presenting feature; however, microcystic adenoma, nonfunctioning islet cell tumors, and pancreatic carcinoma may be associated with von Hippel-Lindau disease.

Renal cell carcinomas occur in more than one-third of patients with von Hippel-Lindau disease. In 75% of these, the neoplasms are bilateral and in 87%, multifocal (FILL et al. 1979).

Computed tomography is the method of choice for depicting small cortical renal cysts as well as cysts in the pancreas. CT is also most sensitive for the detection of asymptomatic renal tumors and pheochromocytomas (particularly bilaterally occur-

ring pheochromocytomas). Associated cerebellar angioblastomas and retinal angiomatosis are, likewise, identifiable on computed tomograms.

Renal cysts also occur in patients with tuberous sclerosis (Bourneville's disease). The cysts vary in size from microscopic to several centimeters in diameter. They tend to be lined by a columnar epithelium with hypochromatic nuclei. Often there is stratification of cells. Intraluminal papillary excrescences are commonly found projecting into these cysts (KUNTZ 1988). In the space between the cysts, one often encounters angiomyolipomas (PEREZ-ATAYDE et al. 1981).

The hallmark of the syndrome is cortical cerebral hamartomas. Subependymal masses, particularly giant cell astrocytomas, may protrude into the lateral ventricles. Facial angiofibromas (adenoma sebaceum) are characteristic cutaneous manifestations. Cardiac rhabdomyomas and subpleural cysts occasioning spontaneous pneumothorax are other common manifestations.

Computed tomography is an excellent modality to demonstrate both the cysts and renal hamartomas. The latter contain fat and are characterized by low attenuation coefficients in the range of −100 HU (SHERMAN et al. 1981; MITNICK et al. 1983) (Fig. 9.35). High resolution sonograms can establish the diagnosis on the basis of demonstrating anechoic cysts and hyperechoic angiomyolipomas. However, nonfatty tumors or tumors into which hemorrhage has occurred may be difficult to differentiate from other solid or composite mass lesions. On angiograms, angiomyolipomas are characterized by low density fatty tissue and innumerable aneurysms arranged in a pearl-string array. Hemorrhaging angiomyolipomas can be managed by superselective transcatheter embolization.

Erosions of the distal ungual tufts attendant upon subungual angiofibromas are characteristic skeletal manifestations.

References

Amis ES Jr, Cronan JJ (1988) The renal sinus: an imaging review and proposed nomenclature for sinus cyst. J Urol 139: 1151

Amis ES Jr, Cronan JJ, Pfister RC (1983) The spectrum of peripelvic cysts. Br J Urol 55: 150–153

Amis ES Jr, Cronan JJ, Pfister RC (1987) Needle puncture of cystic renal masses: a survey of the Society of Uroradiology. AJR 148: 297–304

Balfe DM, McClennan BL, Stanley RJ et al. (1982) Evaluation of renal masses considered indeterminate on computed tomography. Radiology 142: 421–428

Bernstein J, Woodside JR (1977) Malignant hemorrhagic renal cyst with occult neoplasm. Radiology 123: 599–605

Boag GS, Nolan R (1988) CT visualization of medullary sponge kidney. Urol Radiol 9: 220

Boal D, Teele R (1980) Sonography of infantile polycystic disease. AJR 135: 575–580

Bomner J, Waldherr R, Van Kaick G et al. (1980) Acquired renal cyst in uremic patients - in vivo demonstration by computed tomography. Clin Nephrol 14: 299–303

Bosniak MA (1986) The current radiological approach to renal cysts. Radiology 158: 1–10

Cho KJ, Maklad N, Curran J, Ting YM (1976) Angiographic and ultrasonic findings in infected simple cysts of the kidney. AJR 127: 1015–1019

Choyke PL, Filling-Catz MR, Shawker TH et al. (1990) von Hippel-Lindau disease: radiologic screening for visceral manifestations. Radiology 174: 815–820

Coleman BG, Arger PH, Mintz MC et al. (1984) Hyperdense renal masses: a computed tomographic dilemma. AJR 143: 291–294

Cooperman RL (1976) Delayed opacification in congenital multicystic dysplastic kidney, an important roentgen sign. Radiology 121: 703–705

Cramer B, Green J, Harmett J et al. (1988) Sonographic and urographic correlation in Bardet Biedl syndrome (formally Laurence-Moon-Biedl syndrome). Urol Radiol 10: 176

Dunnick NR, Korobkin M, Clark WM (1984) CT demonstration of hyperdense renal carcinoma. J Comput Assist Tomogr 8: 1023–1024

Eilenberg SS, Lee JKT, Brown JJ, Mirowitz SA, Tartar VM (1990) Renal masses: evaluation with gradient echo GD-DTPA enhanced dynamic MR imaging. Radiology 176: 333–338

Elkin M, Bernstein J (1969) Cystic disease of the kidney - radiologic and pathological considerations. Clin Radiol 20: 65–82

Feiner HD, Katz LA, Gallo GR (1981) Acquired cystic disease of the kidney in chronic dialysis patients. Urology 17: 260–264

Feldberg MAM, Mali WPT (1980) An infected renal cyst. Mol Radiol 2: 47–49

Fill WL, Lamiell JM, Polk NO (1979) Radiographic manifestations of von Hippel-Lindau disease. Radiology 133: 289–295

Filling-Catz MR, Choyke PL, Patronas N et al. (1989) Radiologic screening for von Hippel-Lindau disease: the role of GD-DTPA enhanced MR imaging of the CNS. J Comput Assist Tomogr 13: 743–755

Finer HB, Catz LA, Gallo GR (1981) Acquired cystic disease of the kidney in chronic dialysis patients. Urology 17: 260–264

Fishman MC, Pollack HM, Arger PH, Banner MP (1983) High protein content: another cause of CT hyperdense benign renal cyst. J Comput Assist Tomogr 7: 1103–1106

Garel LA, Habib R, Pariente D et al. (1984) Juvenile nephronophthisis sonographic appearance in children with severe uremia. Radiology 151: 93–95

Gardner KB Jr (1976) Juvenile nephronophthisis in renal medullary cystic disease. In: Gardner KD Jr (ed) Cystic diseases of the kidney. Wiley, New York, pp 173–185

Glassberg AI, Filmer RB (1985) Renal dysplasia, renal hypoplasia and cystic disease of the kidney. In: Kelalis P (ed) Clinical pediatric urology, 2nd edn. W. B. Saunders, Philadelphia, pp 922–971

Glazer GM, Callen PW, Filly RA (1982) Medullary nephrocalcinosis: sonographic evaluation. AJR 138: 55–57

Gleason DC, McAlister WH, Kissane J (1967) Cystic disease of the kidneys in children. AJR 100: 135–146

Gross DM (1979) Diagnostic renal cyst puncture and percutaneous nephrostomy. Med Clin North Am 6: 409–424

Grossman H, Winchester BH, Chisari FV (1968) Roentgenographic classification of renal cystic disease. AJR 104: 319–331

Hartnett M, Bennett W (1976) Extrarenal manifestations of cystic kidney disease. In: Gardner KA (ed) Cystic disease of the kidney. Wiley, New York, pp 201–219

Hayden CK, Swischuk LE, Smith TH, Armstrong EA (1986) Renal cystic disease in childhood. Radiographics 6: 97–116

Hepler AB (1946) Experimental production of cysts in the kidney by fulguration of papilla of rabbit's kidney and ligation of posterior branch of renal artery. J Urol 44: 206–210

Hidalgo H, Dunnick MR, Rosenberg ER et al. (1982) Parapelvic cyst appearance on CT and sonography. AJR 138: 667–671

Howie JL, Nicholson RL (1980) CT evaluation of infantile polycystic disease. J Can Assoc Radiol 31: 202–203

Hricak H, Williams RD, Moon KL Jr, Moss AA (1983) Nuclear magnetic resonance imaging of the kidney: renal masses. Radiology 147: 765–772

Jackman RJ, Stevens GM (1974) Benign hemorrhagic renal cyst. Nephrotomography, renal arteriography and cyst puncture. Radiology 110: 7–13

Kier R, Taylor KJW, Feyock AL, Ramos IM (1990) Renal masses characterization with Doppler U.S. Radiology 176: 703–707

Kim WS, Goldman SM, Gatewood OMB, Marshall FF, Siegelman SS (1981) Computed tomography in calcified renal masses. J Comput Assist Tomogr 5: 855–860

Kuntz N (1988) Population studies. In: Gomez MR (ed) Tuberosclerosis, 2nd edn. Raven, New York, p 214

Lang EK (1966) The differential diagnosis of renal cysts and tumors. Cyst puncture, aspiration and analysis of cyst content for fat as diagnostic criteria for renal cysts. Radiology 87: 883–888

Lang EK (1971) Coexistence of cyst and tumor in the same kidney. Radiology 101: 7–16

Lang EK (1973) Roentgenographic assessment of asymptomatic renal lesions. Radiology 109: 257

Lang EK (1975) Roentgenologic assessment of medullary cysts. Semin Roentgenol 10: 145–154

Lang EK (1977) Renal cyst puncture and aspiration. A survey of complication. AJR 128: 723–727

Lang EK (1980) Roentgenologic approach to the diagnosis and management of cystic lesions of the kidney: Is cyst aspiration mandatory? Urol Clin North Am 7: 677–688

Lang EK (1984) Evaluation of renal mass lesions by imaging examination. In: Libertino JA (ed) Current concepts of uroradiology. Williams & Wilkins, Baltimore (International perspectives in urology, pp 86–101)

Lang EK (1986) Diagnosis and management of renal cyst. In: Lang EK (ed). Percutaneous and interventional urology and radiology. Springer, Heidelberg Berlin New York, pp 147–175

Lang EK (1987) Renal cyst puncture studies. Urol Clin North Am 14: 91–102

Lang EK, Gershanik JB (1978) Multicystic dysplastic kidney: diagnostic considerations and management. South Med J 71: 888–891

Larson TL, McClennan BL, Shirkhoda A (1978) Adult polycystic kidney disease: ultrasonographic and computed tomographic appearance. J Clin Ultrasound 6: 297–302

Leung AWL, Bydder GM, Steiner RE et al. (1984) Magnetic resonance imaging of the kidney. AJR 143: 1215–1227

Levine E, Grantham JJ (1985) High density renal cyst in autosomal dominant polycystic disease demonstrated by CT. Radiology 154: 477–482

Levine E, Grantham JJ (1987) Perinephric hemorrhage in autosomal dominant polycystic disease: CT and MR finding. J Comput Assist Tomogr 11: 108

Levine E, Grantham JJ, McDougall ML (1987) Spontaneous subcapsular and perinephric hemorrhage in end-stage kidney disease. Clinical and CT findings. AJR 148: 755–758

Levine E, Collins DL, Horton WA, Schimke RN (1982) CT screening of the abdomen in von Hippel-Lindau disease. AJR 139: 505–510

Levine E, Weigel JW, Collins DL (1983) Diagnosis and management of asymptomatic renal cell carcinoma in von Hippel-Lindau syndrome. Urology 21: 146–140

Levine E, Grantham JJ, Slusher SL et al. (1984) CT of acquired cystic kidney disease and renal tumors in long-term dialysis patients. AJR 142: 125–131

Levine E, Cook LT, Grantham JJ (1985) Liver cyst in autosomal dominant polycystic disease: clinical and computed tomographic study. AJR 145: 229–233

Lingard DA, Lawson TL (1979) Accuracy of ultrasound in predicting the nature of renal masses. J Urol 122: 724–727

Link DP, Hansen S, Palma J (1979) Hiddel's excretory urography in medullary cystic disease of the kidney. AJR 133: 303–305

LiPuma JP (1984) Magnetic resonance imaging of the kidney. Radiol Clin North Am 22: 925–941

Luisiri A, Sotelo-Abila C, Silverstein MJ et al. (1988) Sonography of the Zellweger syndrome. J Ultrasound Med 7: 169

Madewell JE, Hartman DS, Lichtenstein JE (1979) Radiologic pathologic correlation in cystic disease of the kidney. Radiol Clin North Am 17: 261–279

Marotti M, Hricak H, Fritsche P, Crooks LE, Hedgcock MW, Tanagho EA (1987) Complex and simple renal cysts: comparative evaluation with MR imaging. Radiology 162: 679–684

Mayer DB, Baron RL, Pollack HM (1982) Increase in CT attenuation values of peripelvic renal cyst after retrograde pyelography. AJR 139: 991–993

McAlister WH, Siegel WJ, Shackelford G et al. (1979) Glomerulocystic kidney. AJR 133: 536

McClennan BL, Stanley RJ, Melson GL et al. (1979) CT of the renal cyst: Is cyst aspiration necessary? AJR 133: 671–675

Mitnick JS, Bosniak MA, Hilton S et al. (1983) Cystic renal disease in tuberosclerosis. Radiology 147: 85–87

Moreno AJ, Parker AL, Spicer MJ, Brown TJ (1984) Scintigraphic and radiographic findings in Caroli's disease. Am J Gastroenterol 79: 299–303

Nakanuma Y, Terada T, Ohta G et al. (1982) Caroli's disease in congenital hepatic fibrosis and infantile polycystic disease. Liver 2: 346–354

Newhouse JH, Markisz JA, Kazam E (1986) Magnetic resonance imaging of the kidney. Cardiovasc Intervent Radiol 8: 351–366

Olsen A, Hojhus JH, Steffensen T (1988) Renal medullary cystic disease: findings of urography and ultrasonography. Acta Radiol 29: 527

Osathanondh B, Potter EL (1964) Pathogenesis of polycystic kidneys, type II due to inhibition of ampullary activity. Arch Pathol 77: 474–484

Palubinskas AJ (1961) Medullary sponge kidney. Radiology 76: 911–918

Parker DA, Skalko RG (1969) Congenital asymmetry: report of 10 cases with associated developmental abnormalities. Pediatrics 44: 589–599

Perez-Atayde AR, Iwaya S, Lack EE (1981) Angiomyolipomas and polycystic renal disease in tuberosclerosis. Urology 17: 607–610

Platt JF, Rubin JM, Ellis JH, DiPietro MA (1989) Duplex Doppler ultrasound of the kidney: differentiation of obstructive from nonobstructive dilatation. Radiology 171: 515–520

Pollack HM, Banner MP, Arger PH, Goldberg BB, Mulhern CB Jr (1979) Comparison of computed tomography and ultrasound in the diagnosis of renal masses. Clin Diagn Ultrasound 2: 25–72

Pollack HM, Banner MP, Arger PH et al. (1982) The accuracy of gray-scale renal ultrasonography in differentiating cystic neoplasms from benign cysts. Radiology 143: 741–745

Resnick JS, Siffon S, Vernier RL (1978) Tamm-Horsfall protein abnormal localization in renal disease. Lab Invest 38: 550–555

Sanders RC, Hartman DS (1984) The sonographic distinction between neonatal multicystic kidney and hydronephrosis. Radiology 151: 621–625

Saxton HM, Golding SJ, Chantler C et al. (1981) Diagnostic puncture in renal cystic dysplasia (multicystic kidney): evidence of etiology of cyst. Br J Radiol 54: 555–561

Scola FH, Cronan JJ, Schepps B (1989) Grade 1 hydronephrosis: pulsed Doppler ultrasound evaluation. Radiology 171: 519–524

Segal AJ, Spartaro RF (1982) Computed tomography of adult polycystic disease. J Comput Assist Tomogr 6: 777–780

Semelka RC, Hricak H, Tomei E, Floth A, Stoller M (1990) Obstructive nephropathy: evaluation with dynamic GD-DTPA enhanced MR imaging. Radiology 175: 797–804

Shanser JD, Hedgcock MW, Korobkin M (1978) Transit of contrast material into renal cysts following urography or arteriography. AJR 130: 584–586

Sherman JL, Hartman DS, Friedman AC et al. (1981) Angiomyolipoma computed tomographic-pathologic correlation of 17 cases. AJR 137: 1221–1226

Soffer O, Miller LR, Lichtman JB (1987) CT findings in complications of acquired renal cystic disease. J Comput Assist Tomogr 11: 905–911

Stella FJ, Massary SG, Kleeman CR (1976) Medullary sponge kidney associated with parathyroid adenoma: report of 2 cases. Nephron 10: 332–336

Stuck KG, Koff SA, Silver TM (1982) Ultrasonic features of multicystic dysplastic kidneys: expanded diagnostic criteria. Radiology 143: 217–221

Sussman S, Cochran St, Pagani JJ et al. (1984) Hyperdense renal masses: a CT manifestation of hemorrhagic renal cysts. Radiology 150: 207–211

Tada S, Yamagishi J, Kobayashi H et al. (1983) The incidence of simple renal cyst by computed tomography. Clin Radiol 34: 437–439

Takao R, Amamoto Y, Matsunaga N et al. (1980) Computed tomography of multicystic kidney. J Comput Assist Tomogr 4: 548–549

Vaziri ND, Darwish R, Martin DC, Hostetler J (1984) Acquired renal cystic disease in renal transplant recipients. Nephron 37: 203–205

Vinocur L, Slovis TL, Perlmutter AB, Watts FB Jr, Chang CH (1988) Follow-up studies of multicystic dysplastic kidneys. Radiology 167: 311–317

Weyman PJ, McClennan BL, Lee JKT et al. (1982) Computed tomography of calcified renal masses. AJR 138: 1095–1099

Worthington JL, Shackelford JD, Cole BR (1988) Sonographically detectable cyst in polycystic kidney disease in newborn and young infants. Pediatr Radiol 18: 287

Zirinsky K, Auh YH, Rubenstein WA et al. (1984) CT of the hyperdense renal cyst: sonographic correlation. AJR 143: 151–156

10 Malignant Renal Neoplasms

LUDOVICO DALLA-PALMA and ROBERTO POZZI-MUCELLI

CONTENTS

10.1 Sarcomas, Sarcomatoid Carcinoma,
      and Mixed Malignant Renal Tumors 251
10.1.1 Pathology 251
10.1.2 Clinical Findings 253
10.1.3 Diagnostic Imaging 253
10.1.3.1 Plain Radiograph 253
10.1.3.2 Intravenous Urography 253
10.1.3.3 Arteriography 253
10.1.3.4 Ultrasonography 253
10.1.3.5 Computed Tomography 255
10.1.4 Conclusion 256
10.2 Renal Metastases 256
10.2.1 Pathology 256
10.2.2 Clinical Findings 257
10.2.3 Diagnostic Imaging 258
10.2.3.1 Urography 258
10.2.3.2 Renal Angiography 258
10.2.3.3 Ultrasonography 258
10.2.3.4 Computed Tomography 259
10.2.4 Conclusion 261
10.3 Malignant Lymphomas 261
10.3.1 Pathology 261
10.3.2 Clinical Findings 262
10.3.3 Diagnostic Imaging 263
10.3.3.1 Computed Tomography 263
10.3.4 Conclusion 265
10.4 Carcinoma of the Renal Pelvis 265
10.4.1 Pathology 265
10.4.2 Clinical Findings 266
10.4.3 Diagnostic Imaging 266
10.4.3.1 Plain Radiographs 266
10.4.3.2 Urography and Retrograde Pyelography 266
10.4.3.3 Renal Angiography 267
10.4.3.4 Ultrasonography 267
10.4.3.5 Computed Tomography 269
        References 270

10.1 Sarcomas, Sarcomatoid Carcinoma, and Mixed Malignant Renal Tumors

10.1.1 Pathology

The kidney has a mesodermal origin and therefore different mesenchymal cells, such as connective tissue, osseous, adipose, and muscle cells, can be found. Different kinds of sarcomas may derive from these cells. Mesenchymal tumors may present as sarcomas, when a single cell type (connective tissue, adipose, or muscular) is found, or as sarcomatoid carcinomas, when epithelial cells are associated with mesenchymal cells.

Renal sarcomas have an incidence of 0.1% in autopsies (SHIRKODA and LEWIS 1987) of patients who have died of neoplastic disease and represent 2%-3% of primary malignant renal tumors (ELKIN 1980; FARROW et al. 1968; JENKINS et al. 1971; SAITOH et al. 1982; SRINIVAS et al. 1984; TOLIA et al. 1973).

Fibrosarcoma is an extremely rare tumor; it may arise from the parenchyma or, more commonly, from the renal capsule. Fibrosarcomas may reach large sizes. Hemorrhages and necroses are common within the mass (ELKIN 1980; LEDER et al. 1979).

Osteogenic sarcoma is also extremely rare and only a few cases have been reported in the literature (DAHLIN 1970; HAINING and POOLE 1936; HAMER and WISHARD 1948; HUDSON 1956; JOHNSON et al. 1970; SOTO et al. 1965). Their primary origin from the kidney is discussed; however, their incidence predominates after the fifth decade of life, while renal metastases from osteogenic sarcomas are typical of the first and second decades. Some authors (e.g., ELKIN 1980) consider these tumors as fibrosarcomas with osteoid metaplasia.

Osteogenic sarcomas may present as large masses, with extensive calcifications and ossifications. They infiltrate the renal parenchyma and give distant metastases to the liver and to the lungs.

Liposarcoma is also a rare tumor: by 1979 only 40 cases had been reported in the international literature (LEDER et al. 1979). Some authors (GRANMAYEH et al.; WILLIAMS and SAVAGE 1958) discuss whether this tumor arises from a benign tumor, such as a lipoma or an angiomyolipoma, or from undifferentiated mesenchymal cells. This last hypothesis is supported by the observation that liposarcomas frequently arise from the renal parenchyma or from the capsule, where adipose tissue is not represented (BENNINGTON and BECKWITH 1975; LIEN 1973).

LUDOVICO DALLA-PALMA, M.D., Professor and Chairman; ROBERTO POZZI-MUCELLI, M.D., Assistant Professor; Istituto di Radiologia dell' Università, Ospedale di Cattinara, Strada di Fiume, 34149 Trieste, Italy

Macroscopically liposarcomas have a subcapsular site and therefore are located at the periphery of the kidney (LIEN 1973; LEDER et al. 1979). They usually present as large, multinodular yellowish or gray masses; the cut surface shows adipose tissue with cystic areas.

Microscopically liposarcomas may present with different degrees of differentiation, varying from a proliferative lipoma to a sarcoma in which the recognition of the adipose nature may be difficult.

Leiomyosarcoma is the most common tumor among renal sarcomas (ADDISON and PERCH 1966; BENNINGTON and BECKWITH 1975; BONSIB et al. 1987; FARROW et al. 1968; LEDER et al. 1979; RAKOWSKY et al. 1987; SHIRKODA and LEWIS 1987): its incidence ranges from 33% (SAITOH et al. 1982) to 56% (FARROW et al. 1968). It arises from smooth muscle cells of the inner layer of the renal capsule, from the wall of the renal pelvis, or from vascular structures of the renal parenchma (SHIRKODA and LEWIS 1987).

The tumor is found in the adult age (GUPTA and DUBE 1971) and predominantly in women. Pathologically the tumor presents as a large mass; it has a multinodular appearance with firm areas associated with hyalinosis, necrosis, calcifications, focal hemorrhages, and cystic areas. A capsule is found in about half of the cases (FARROW et al. 1968); other times the tumor is invasive and tends to infiltrate the renal capsule, which represents an area of resistance to the extrarenal extension.

The tumor has a moderate degree of malignancy; however, local recurrences after surgery are reported. Distant metastases are also reported, more commonly to the liver, the peritoneum, and the lung (LEDER et al. 1979).

Rhabdomyosarcoma is the second histotype arising from muscle cells. Compared with leiomyosarcoma this tumor is extremely rare. Few primary rhabdomyosarcomas have been reported in the literature (FARROW et al. 1968; SEABURY 1967); however, according to some authors (COLABAWALLA 1972; ELKIN 1980) the rhabdomyosarcomas described in the literature may represent examples of Wilms' tumors in which the striated muscle cells are the dominant feature.

Tumors of vascular origin include angiosarcoma and malignant hemangiopericytoma.

Angiosarcoma is extremely rare so that its true renal origin is a matter of discussion (BENNINGTON and BECKWITH 1975; LEDER et al. 1979).

Malignant hemangiopericytoma ist less rare than angiosarcoma. The tumor has a multinodular appearance; a peripheral capsule may be present

(LEDER et al. 1979; WEISS et al. 1984). The tumor tends to occur at an eccentric location so it may be difficult to establish whether the tumor has a real renal origin or whether it is retroperitoneal.

Microscopically vascular areas and capillaries surrounded by tumor cells similar to pericytes are found. These tumors have a bad prognosis due to distant metastases and frequent local recurrences.

Sarcomatoid carcinoma results from a mixture of epithelial and mesenchymal cells. Unlike Wilms' tumor, the epithelial component contains renal carcinoma of the adult type; the mesenchymal component has morphologic features resembling those of a malignant fibrosarcoma, malignant fibrous histiocytoma (BONSIB et al. 1987; FARROW et al. 1968; RO et al. 1987). A consistent number of unclassified sarcomatoid cases have also been reported (RO et al. 1987). Less common features include hemangiopericytoma-like chondrosarcomatous and osteosarcomatous components. The proportion of carcinomatous to sarcomatous elements varies from case to case and may be divided into three categories (RO et al. 1987): category I, in which carcinomatous elements predominate, category II, in which carcinomatous and sarcomatous elements are roughly equal, and category III, in which sarcomatoid elements predominate. The interest in this distinction lies in the fact that category I tumors have a better prognosis than categories II and III.

Most of the cases reported by FARROW et al. (1968) and RO et al. (1987) occurred in the fifth decade of life.

Tumors present as palpable masses in most instances. The cut surface shows a multinodular appearance with yellowish, friable areas alternating with firm, fibrous areas. This appearance resembles that of renal carcinomas. The size of the tumor ranges from 4 to 20 cm. The site is usually parencyhmal; tumors are usually unencapsulated and invasive. In Farrow's series 31 cases had involvement of the renal pelvis by the tumor; thrombosis of the renal vein was present in 23 cases and the lymph nodes were involved in three cases.

Wilms' tumor in adults: The embryonal nephroblastoma characteristic of infancy and children is occasionally seen in adult age, with the same microscopic features of a mixed malignant tumor. This tumor, which is not encapsulated, arises in the renal parenchyma, which can be extensively destroyed (FARROW et al. 1968).

Finally, exceptional neurogenic tumors such as *neurofibrosarcoma* and *malignant schwannoma* may occur in the kidney (FARROW et al. 1968; FEIN and HAMM 1968).

10.1.2 Clinical Findings

Renal sarcomas may occur at all ages but typically occur in the last decades of life. The two kidneys are affected with the same incidence and there is no sex prevalence.

Symptoms and signs are similar to those of carcinomas although the finding of a palpable mass is reported more frequently in the literature in cases of sarcomas than adenocarcinomas, due to the large size of mesenchymal tumors. Hematuria is rare, due to the frequent capsular origin and site of these masses. Occasionally asymptomatic cases have been reported (MUCCI et al. 1987).

The prognosis of these tumors is poor, since they have a high degree of malignancy causing frequent local recurrences and distant metastases; liver, lung, and the skeleton are the most common sites of secondary lesions.

10.1.3 Diagnostic Imaging

Renal sarcomas, both in the pure and mixed forms, are extremely rare, so that most reports available from the radiologic literature deal with conventional modalities; up to now very few papers (MUCCI et al. 1987; SHIRKODA and LEWIS 1987) have dealt extensively with ultrasound (US) and computed tomographic (CT) findings of these tumors, and there are no reports on magnetic resonance imaging (MRI) findings.

10.1.3.1 Plain Radiograph

Three findings can be recognized on plain radiographs of the abdomen: (a) signs of mass, (b) calcifications, and (c) radiolucency.

The presence of a mass presenting as a focal or a diffuse enlargement of the kidney shadow is seen frequently in cases of sarcoma, since these tumors tend to be large. In these cases the kidney may be still recognizable but often there is loss of renal outlines or displacement of the kidney.

Calcifications are a relatively common finding: they are reported in 34% of cases of sarcoma and this incidence is greater than for carcinomas (MUCCI et al. 1987). Features of calcifications may be extremely variable, ranging from low to high intensity and from irregular to curvilinear or ovoid. Osteogenic sarcomas have calcifications of high intensity, greater than that of bones, with a "sunburst" appearance (TUTTLE et al. 1985).

The third finding that can be seen on plain radiographs is that of a radiolucency that is typical for liposarcomas with a large amount of fat; however, it should be remembered that this finding is also typical of large angiomyolipomas, which are more frequent than liposarcomas.

10.1.3.2 Intravenous Urography

The most common finding on intravenous urography and a frequent finding on nephrotomography is a mass associated with signs of displacement and infiltration of the pyelocalyceal system; less frequently a nonfunctioning kidney is seen (Fig. 10.6a). Occasionally urography may be normal (Fig. 10.3a).

10.1.3.3 Arteriography

The arteriographic literature deals with the most common histotypes, leiomyosarcomas, liposarcomas, and fibrosarcomas (GRANMAYEH et al. 1977; MYERSON et al. 1979; MUCCI et al. 1987; SHIRKODA and LEWIS 1987; WATSON 1968). There are not specific findings for each histotype but a number of common findings; different angiographic findings may be seen in the same histotype.

Renal sarcomas are predominantly hypovascular; encasement and vessel amputations are frequently seen, while findings such as tumor staining, pooling of contrast medium, and early venous filling are usually absent (Fig. 10.4b-d). However, examples of hypervascular tumors have been reported, mainly in cases of sarcomatoid carcinoma (SHIRKODA and LEWIS 1987), but also in a few cases of leiomyosarcoma and liposarcoma. These tumors simulate angiomyolipoma, which is usually hypervascular and has, as characteristic findings, small aneurysms and a sunburst appearance.

When sarcomas arise from the renal capsule, enlarged capsular arteries are seen (Fig. 10.4b). This sign, associated with the relatively hypovascularity of these masses (inferior in general to that of carcinomas) may suggest a diagnosis of renal sarcoma.

10.1.3.4 Ultrasonography

Ultrasound findings in five cases of renal sarcomas were reported by MUCCI et al. (1987): three cases demonstrated large solid masses, two of which had multiple complex echoes with acoustic shadowing

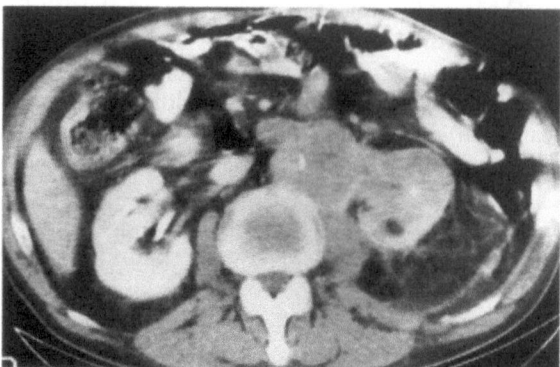

Fig. 10.1. Fibrosarcoma of the left kidney. Large, inhomogeneous, soft tissue mass with medial extension, invading the aorta and periaortic tissues

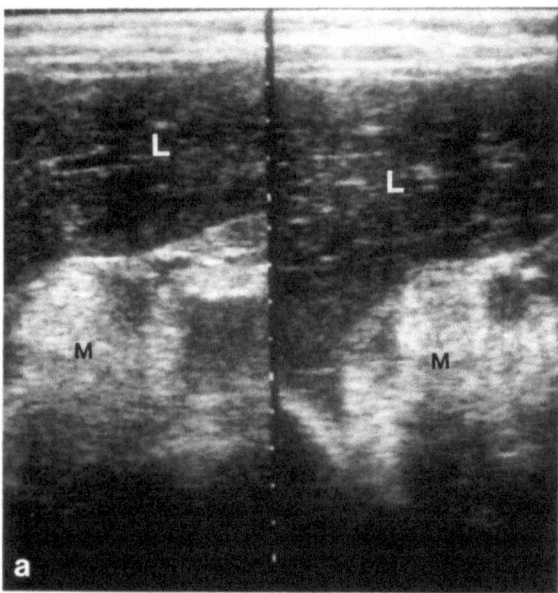

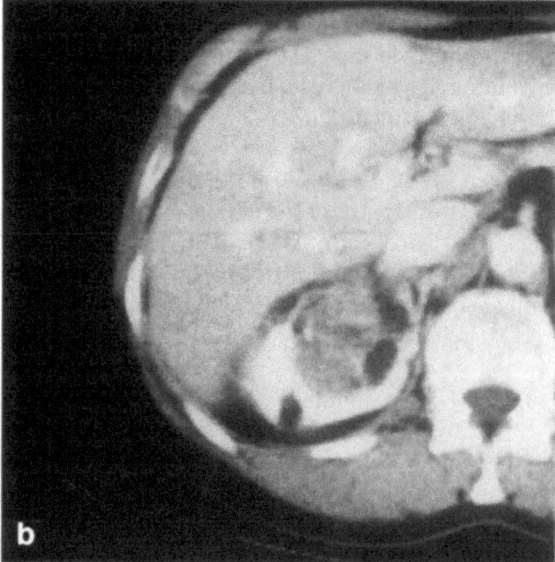

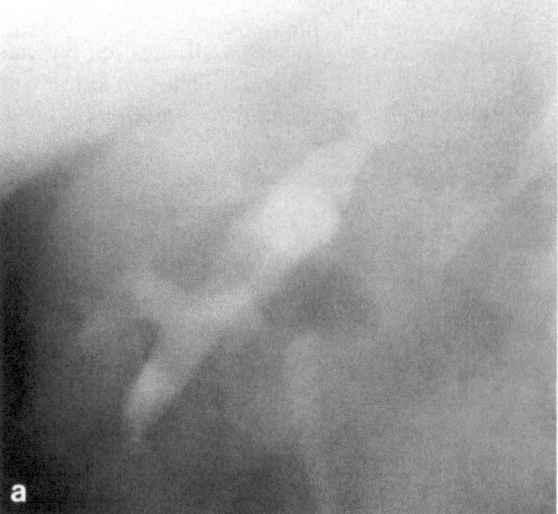

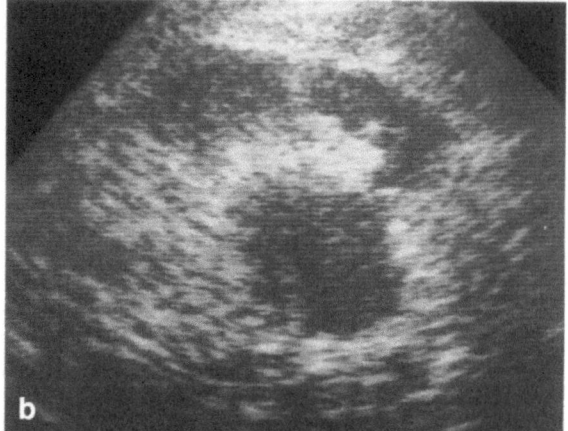

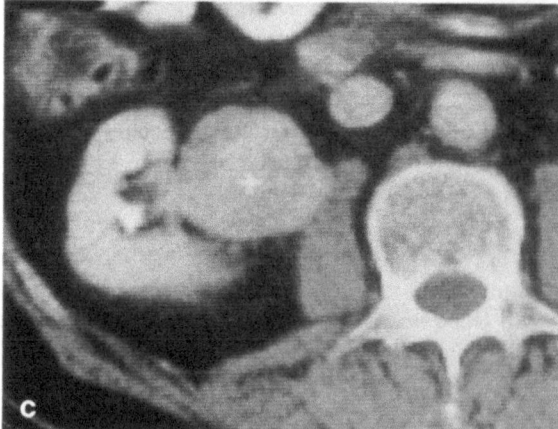

Fig. 10.3 a–c. Leiomyosarcoma of the right kidney. **a** IVU: normal. **b** US: round hypoechoic mass at the renal hilum. **c** CT: sharply demarcated, round soft tissue mass medial to the renal hilum

◁

Fig. 10.2 a, b. Liposarcoma of the right kidney. **a** US: hyperechogenic mass at the upper pole of the kidney. **b** CT: inhomogeneous mass showing fatty and soft tissue densities

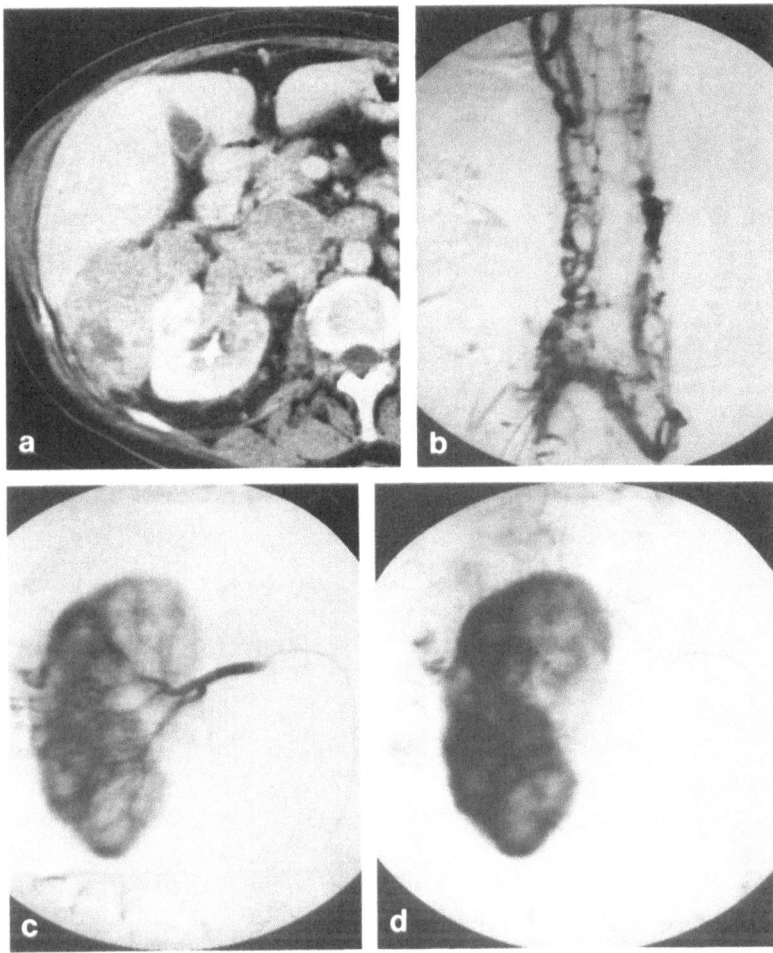

corresponding to calcified areas. Two had cystic areas associated with a mass: this finding was due to a dilated collecting system in one case. The solid masses may exhibit either a hypoechoic (Figs. 10.3 b, 10.6 b) or a hpyerechoic structure. These findings are not specific since adenocarcinomas also appear with different echogenicity. However, intense hyperechogenicity may be observed in cases of liposarcoma (Fig. 10.2 a) due to the intense reflectivity of fat. Once more, this finding cannot be considered specific, since it is also seen in angiomyolipomas.

10.1.3.5 Computed Tomography

Computed tomography can easily display the capsular (Fig. 10.4 a), sinusal (Fig. 10.3 c), or parenchymal origin (Figs. 10.1, 10.5, 10.6 c) of the mass (SHIR-KODA and LEWIS 1987). Tumors of sinusal origin cannot be differentiated against renal adenocarcinomas. In the cases with capsular origin, CT depicts the extraparenchymal location of the mass imping-

Fig. 10.4 a–d. Leiomyosarcoma of the right kidney. **a** CT: large, inhomogeneous, soft tissue mass, arising from the capsule with minimal impression on the lateral surface of the kidney. Thrombosis of the inferior vena cava is also shown. **b** Inferior cavography: extensive caval thrombosis with peri- and paravertebral collateral circulation. **c, d** Selective renal arteriography: hypovascular mass with some contrast pooling (**c**)

ing upon and displacing the kidney (Fig. 10.4 a). Density values of sarcomas are in the soft tissue range, with frequent hypodense areas due to necrosis (Figs. 10.1, 10.4 a). Liposarcomas show density ranges varying from fatty to soft tissue densities. Moreover, the tumor may enhance (Fig. 10.2 b). These findings may suggest the correct diagnosis of liposarcoma but in practice it may be difficult to differentiate these tumors from the more common angiomyolipoma.

Computed tomography can show the extension of the mass; lymph nodes are more commonly involved, mainly in cases of sarcomatoid carcinoma.

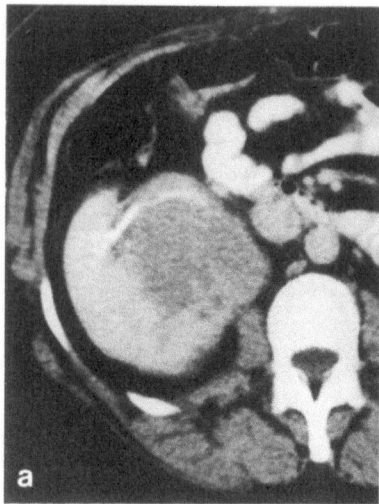
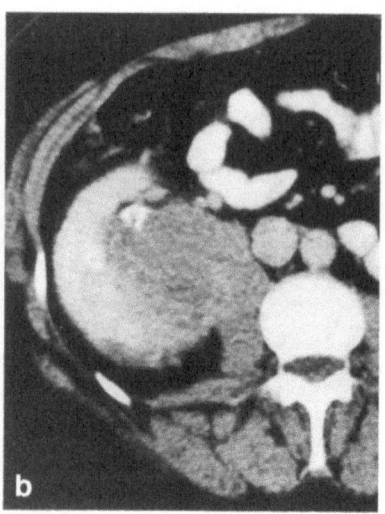

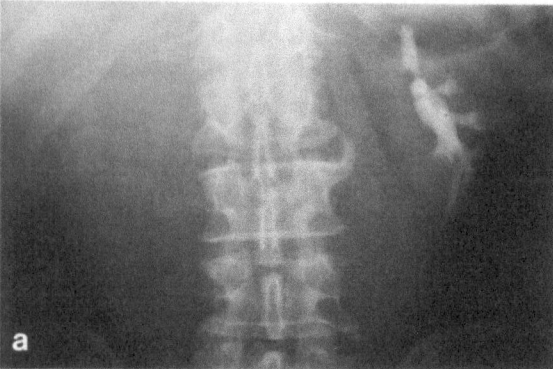
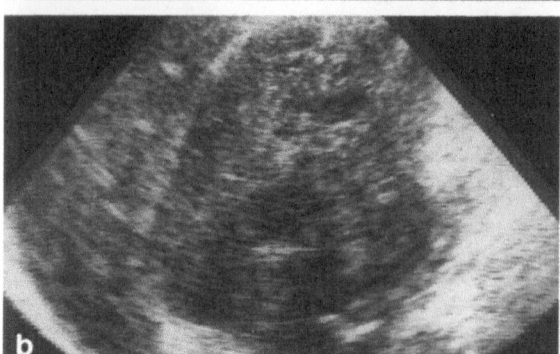
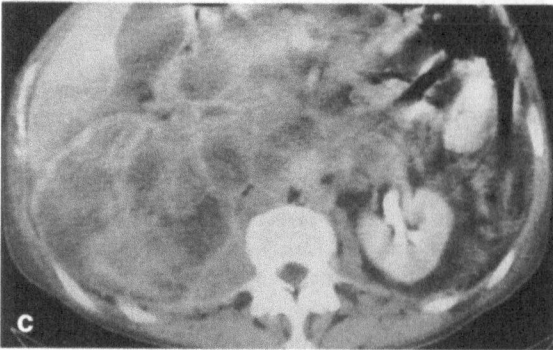

△

Fig. 10.5 a, b. Wilms' tumor in adults. CT shows a large homogeneous soft tissue mass invading pelvis and the psoas muscle

Fig. 10.6 a–c. Sarcomatoid carcinoma of the right kidney. **a** IVU: nonfunctioning right kidney. **b** US: large mass engulfing the right kidney. **c** CT: the lesion and its extension are better defined (v. cava and lymphnode involvement)

10.1.4 Conclusion

The accrued experience with diagnostic imaging modalities is still inadequate to permit a diagnosis of renal sarcoma.

The mesenchymal nature of the tumor can be suspected:

1. When the capsular or sinusal origin is revealed
2. When a fatty component is seen within a large mass
3. When arteriography shows a hypovascular mass, with capsular vessels, without venous filling

Computed tomography and arteriography are currently the most informative examinations. At present, experience with MRI is inadequate (see Fig. 10.7 for MRI findings in a fibrous histiocytoma).

10.2 Renal Metastases

10.2.1 Pathology

The frequency of renal metastases at autopsy is variable for different causes of death: it as about 2%

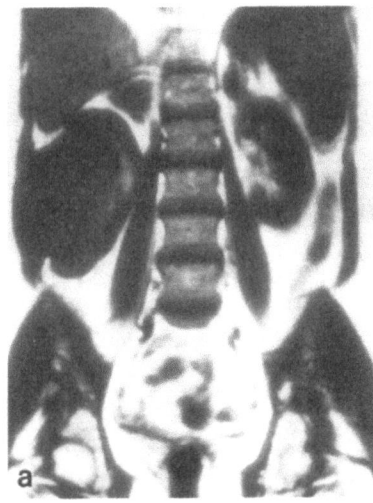

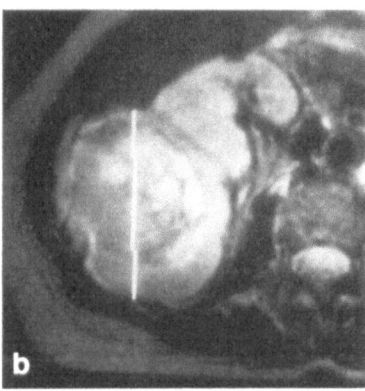

Fig. 10.7 a, b. Fibrous histiocytoma of the right kidney. **a** MRI: T1-weighted image (coronal plane) showing mass on the lateral surface of the kidney. **b** MRI: T2-weighted image on the axial plane showing the mass with inhomogeneous signal intensity (high and low intensity area compared to the kidney). The mass has a peripheral location and posterolateral extension; the kidney is anteriorly dislocated. (Courtesy of E. A. ZEHROUNI, Johns Hopkins Hospital, Baltimore, MD)

(KLINGER 1951) in nonselected autopsies and ranges between 6.5% and 12% in autopsies on cancer patients (ABRAMS et al. 1950). Renal metastases represent a rare clinical and surgical finding: 12 cases (5%) were described by BENOIT et al. (1983) out of 240 nephrectomies for renal tumor while eight cases out of 295 nephrectomies (3%) were reported by MAZEMAN et al. (1976).

In recent years, despite the greater accuracy of the new imaging modalities, diagnosis of these lesions "in vivo" (CHOYKE et al. 1987; THOMAS et al. 1982) has been quite rare.

The primary malignancies include carcinoma of the lung, which is the most common neoplasm to metastasize to the kidney (20%–30% of renal metastases), breast carcinoma, adenocarcinoma of the colon, malignant melanoma, and thyroid carcinoma

(ABRAMS et al. 1950; BECKER and SCHELLHAMMER 1986; BHATT et al. 1983; BRACKEN et al. 1979; CHOYKE et al. 1987; NISHITANI et al. 1984; OLSSON et al. 1971). In our material, including 139 cases of renal metastases, 76 (54%) were metastases from carcinoma of the lung, nine from carcinoma of the colon, five from carcinoma of the breast, three from carcinoma of the kidney, and three from melanoma.

In autopsy reports, renal metastases are generally multiple and bilateral (WILLIS 1952). However, they can also be unilateral (KLINGER 1951). Renal metastases are small in size, usually less than 2 cm. However, they can be exophytic and may have large dimensions (BOSNIAK et al. 1969; KLINGER 1951; EVANS and BOSNIAK 1971; PAGANI 1983); this aspect is more common in metastases of colon adenocarcinoma (CHOYKE et al. 1987).

Renal metastases are more frequently found in the cortex and preferably in the subcapsular region, because of the greater concentration of glomeruli. They may infiltrate the medulla and assume a radial appearance according to the architecture of the medullary rays. Veins and venules are frequently invaded.

Renal metastases may be found in the perirenal space (SHIRKODA 1986), mainly in patients with carcinoma of the lung or melanomas.

10.2.2 Clinical Findings

Clinically, renal metastases are usually asymptomatic: they become evident when the primary tumor has diffusely metastasized.

In the autopsy series of KLINGER (1951), azotemia was present in 17% of the cases and hematuria in 24%. In the 27 cases reported by CHOYKE et al. (1987), urine analyses were normal in nine (30%) and showed macroscopic hematuria in four (17%); minor and nonspecific changes such as microscopic hematuria (nine cases) and proteinuria (four cases) were also found.

Although clinical symptoms are rare and nonspecific, when they do occur they are an indication for radiologic examinations. Furthermore, it should be remembered that urinary cytology represents the best test to indicate or to confirm the diagnosis of renal metastasis in cases of squamous. cell carcinoma of the lung (CHOYKE et al. 1987).

10.2.3 Diagnostic Imaging

Before the introduction of US and CT, which significantly improved the diagnostic capabilities of imaging techniques, the diagnosis of renal metastases was based upon intravenous urography and arteriography.

We will analyze the contribution of each modality and will attempt to establish their respective roles.

10.2.3.1 Urography

Intravenous urography (IVU) and nephrotomography (NT) rarely show any abnormality, because of the small size and peripheral location of metastases. In a series of 24 cases, MASSELOT et al. (1973) reported a normal IVU in 15 (out of 25 investigations). Positive urographic findings are as follows: mass effect, nonfunctioning kidney, enlarged kidney, invasion of the pelvis and calyces, and, occasionally, disappearance of the renal capsule (best shown by NT). NT may show a mottled appearance (BOSNIAK et al. 1969).

In our experience, based upon eight cases diagnosed on US and CT, IVU was always negative. Therefore, IVU appears to have a low sensitivity and specificity.

10.2.3.2 Renal Angiography

Selective renal arteriography has a low specificity for renal metastases (LEMAITRE et al. 1975). The predominant finding is hypovascularity. There is a reduction in the number of parenchymal arterial branches; interlobular vessels may show stenoses, irregularities, encasements, and undulation.

Hypervascularity is extremely rare. Nonopacification of the renal vein was reported in two of seven cases by LEMAITRE et al. (1975); this finding was associated with dilatation of the peripheral veins attendant upon occlusion of the main renal vein (GRISE et al. 1987).

However, these findings are nonspecific. Different authors (IKEDA et al. 1968; LEMAITRE et al. 1975; TAKAYASU et al. 1968; LANG 1971 a, b) have stressed that vascularization of metastases depends on the primary tumor: the metastases from squamous cell carcinoma of the lung are hypovascular while the metastases from thyroid and breast carcinomas are generally hypervascular.

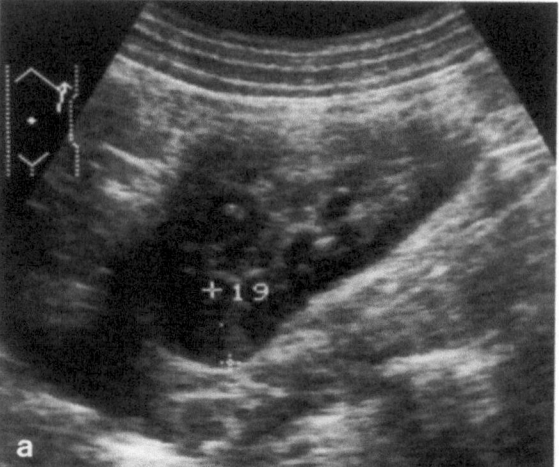

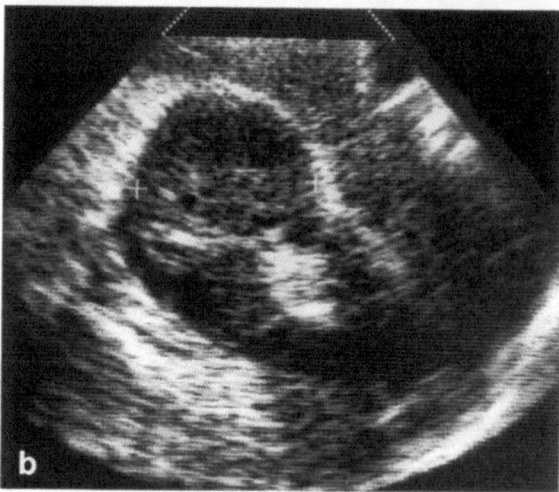

Fig. 10.8 a, b. US patterns of solitary renal metastases. **a** Small mass, mildly hyperechoic (19 mm in diameter), upper pole of the left kidney (primary: lung carcinoma). **b** Round and sharply demarcated mass, nearly isoechoic with normal renal parenchyma (primary: lung carcinoma)

10.2.3.3 Ultrasonography

In the literature the number of reports on US of renal metastases, excluding case reports, is relatively limited (CHOYKE et al. 1987; MITTY et al. 1987). The sensitivity of this technique is relatively high: US recognized eight of ten and four of six lesions in the most consistent series (CHOYKE et al. 1987; MITTY et al. 1987). However, it should be pointed out that US reveals a lower number of lesions than does CT (CHOYKE et al. 1987). There are two reasons for this discrepancy: the metastases may have the same echo structure as renal parenchyma, and they are small in size. In autopsy series, about one-tenth of metastases are larger than 3 cm while one-third have a diameter smaller than 1 cm.

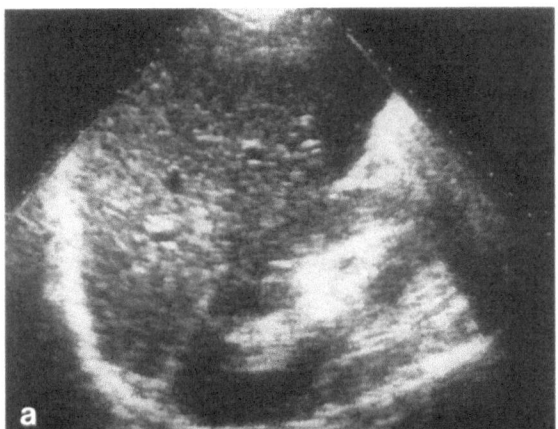

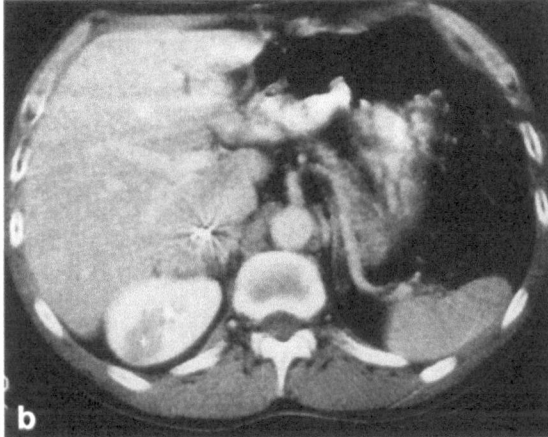

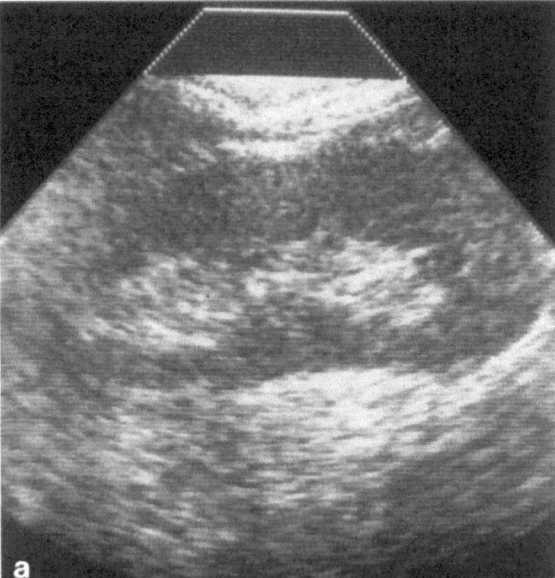

Fig. 10.9 a, b. Renal metastases undetected by US. **a** US: right longitudinal scan showing a normal kidney. **b** CT: irregularly marginated hypodense mass in the upper pole. Note also a recurrent right adrenal metastasis (primary: left renal adenocarcinoma)

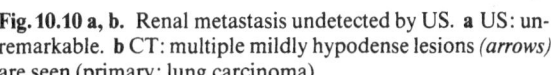

Fig. 10.10 a, b. Renal metastasis undetected by US. **a** US: unremarkable. **b** CT: multiple mildly hypodense lesions *(arrows)* are seen (primary: lung carcinoma)

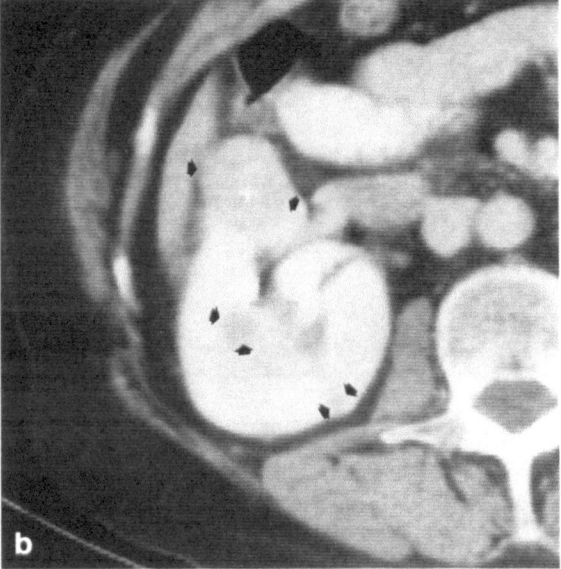

Renal metastases are homogeneously hypoechoic or may show a mixed echo pattern with areas of different degrees of echogenicity (MITTY et al. 1987).

In our material metastatic lesions were less echoic than the normal renal parenchyma; frequently, they were solitary round lesions varying in diameter from 2 to 9 cm (Fig. 10.8). Some lesions (both solitary and multiple) shown by CT were undetected by US (Figs. 10.9, 10.10).

10.2.3.4 Computed Tomography

The CT reports in the literature on the diagnosis of renal metastases are more numerous and detailed (BHATT et al. 1983; CHOYKE et al. 1987; MITNICK et al. 1985; HARTMAN et al. 1988; NISHITANI et al. 1984; PAGANI 1983; SHIRKODA 1986; THOMAS et al. 1982). Reasons for this are the extensive use of this technique for both staging and follow-up of these tumors. The technique is more sensitive due to the high contrast resolution and the good spatial resolution. The high sensitivity of CT is related also to the use of the intravenous contrast agents, which increase the density of normal renal parenchyma more than that of metastatic lesions.

The CT appearance of metastases, without contrast enhancement, is characterized by a mild hypodensity [20-40 Hounsfield units (HU)] compared to renal parenchyma. Few cases of hyperdense re-

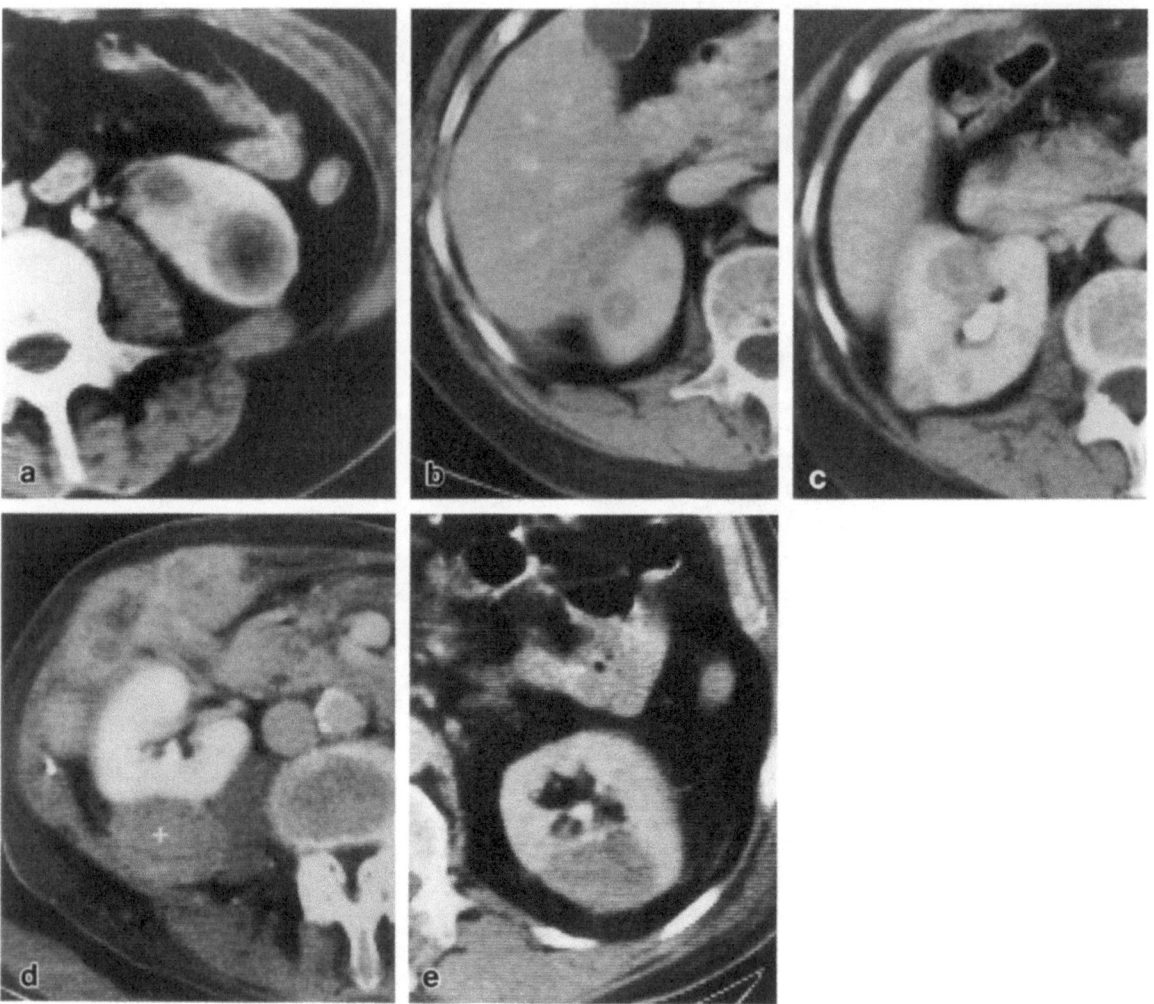

Fig. 10.11 a–e. CT pattern of renal metastases. **a** Hypodense lesions with central necrosis in the larger ones (primary: lung carcinoma). **b** Hypodense area with central hyperdensity (hypervascular metastases) (primary: left renal adenocarcinoma). **c** Hypodense area with central hyperdense ring (primary: left renal adenocarcinoma; same patient as in **b**). **d** Single large hypodense mass peripherally located (primary: colon carcinoma). **e** Wedge-shaped hypodense area resembling focal nephritis (primary: lung carcinoma)

nal metastases have been described (CHOYKE et al. 1987). Sometimes a central hypodensity (Fig. 10.11 a) or hyperdensity with a low density halo (Fig. 10.11 b) may be seen; a hyperdense ring within the lesion may be seen occasionally (Fig. 10.11 c).

Metastatic lesions are small, multiple, round, and bilateral (Fig. 10.12). These findings are more characteristic of carcinoma of the lung, breast, or head and neck, or of undifferentiated tumors. Metastases from colon carcinoma are relatively large and often

solitary; they appear as exophytic growth and therefore are similar to primary tumors of the kidney (Fig. 10.11 d).

Renal metastases may show a wedge-shaped appearance (Fig. 10.11 e); this finding is similar to that observed with renal infarcts or focal nephritis. The differential diagnosis in these cases will be based upon the clinical and laboratory findings, although it should be remembered that a patient with an advanced neoplasm may present with fever simulating an infection.

The renal cortex represents the most common site of metastases: this is related to the greater vascularity of glomeruli, where metastatic emboli are entrapped.

Perirenal metastases have also been reported (SHIRKODA 1986; CHOYKE et al. 1987) and are more commonly seen in patients with melanoma and lung carcinoma. The perirenal space has a rich vascular matrix formed by capsular arteries and veins,

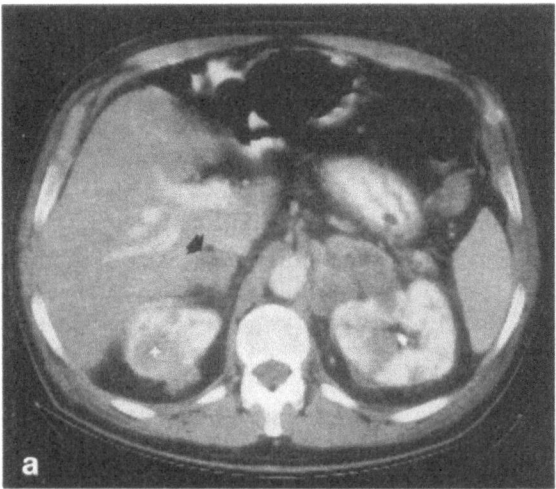

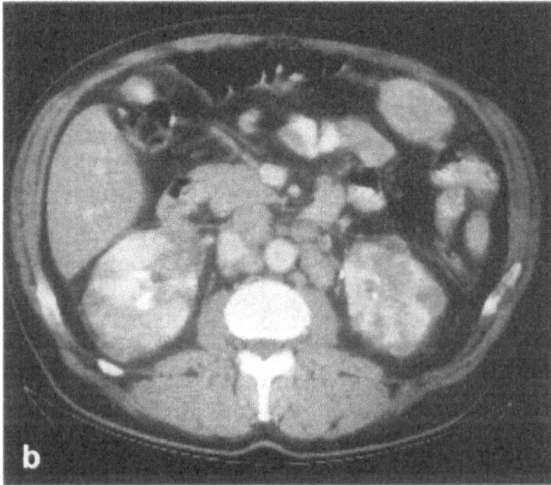

Fig. 10.12 a, b. CT patterns of renal metastases. Bilateral multiple hypodense round or oval metastases. *On the right* some metastases have an infiltrative appearance extending into the perirenal space. They are bilateral adrenal metastases and enlarged retroperitoneal nodes (primary: lung carcinoma)

perforating the perirenal fat, and two sets of lymphatic vessels, one superficial and one deep. The lesions do not necessarily involve the kidney in these cases.

10.2.4 Conclusion

The diagnosis of renal metastases was based in the past on conventional radiology, which could visualize only relatively large masses. Renal arteriography still maintains a limited role in the differential diagnosis of solitary masses (MITTY et al. 1987) where the problem of a primary renal tumor concomitant with a second primary in a different organ or a solitary renal metastasis exists.

A relatively high incidence of renal carcinomas (5/7) was reported by PAGANI (1983) in patients with a primary tumor in other organs. This incidence does not correspond to that observed by CHOYKE et al. (1987), who reported a 4:1 ratio between renal metastases and renal carcinomas concomitant with a second primary elsewhere.

A rich neovascularity may be shown by arteriography, in which case the diagnosis of renal carcinoma is extremely likely since renal metastases are almost always relatively hypovascular.

Today, the initial workup should commence with US and CT. The latter may be considered the technique of choice because of the greater sensitivity for staging neoplasms. However, US should be considered a valid alternative where CT is not available and for the follow-up of metastases treated by chemotherapy.

10.3 Malignant Lymphomas

10.3.1 Pathology

Malignant lymphomas represent a primary disease of the lymphatic system. Today malignant lymphomas are divided into two main groups, Hodgkin's lymphoma (HL) and non-Hodgkin's lymphomas (NHL). These two entities are very different pathologically, clinically, and in respect to prognosis. Parenchymal involvement is more frequent in NHL than in HL.

The genitourinary system and the kidneys may be involved by malignant lymphomas. The incidence of localization of lymphomas within the genitourinary system is variable. The limited number of cases and diverse classifications proposed by different authors make any comparison difficult (CUTLER 1935; JACKSON and PARKER 1947; RAPPAPORT et al. 1956; RICHMOND et al. 1962; SYMMERS 1948; WATSON et al. 1949). The contentions below are based largely on the paper by RICHMOND et al. (1962) for the pathological data and the paper by GILBERT and CASTELLINO (1986) for the clinicoradiologic data.

The frequency of involvement of the renal parenchyma in RICHMOND et al.'s series of 690 autopsy cases was 33.5%. Renal involvement depends on the type of lymphoma, being 13% in Hodgkin's disease, 63% in lymphosarcoma with marrow involvement, 38.5% in lymphosarcoma without marrow involvement, and 46% in reticulum cell sarcoma. The kidney is, after the lung, the most frequent organ involved by lymphomas (RICHMOND et al. 1962). Renal involvement may be unilateral (25%), but usually is bilateral (76%).

In a series of 225 patients with lymphoma studied by CT (HORII et al. 1983), renal involvement was recognized in 11 cases (4.9%). These 11 cases comprised four diffuse poorly differentiated lymphocytic, two diffuse histiocytic, one lymphocytic, one atypical lymphocytic, one pleomorphic histiocytic, and two mixed cell (histiocytic/lymphocytic) lymphomas. In the clinical series of GILBERT and CASTELLINO (1986), including 170 NHLs at the early stages of the disease, all examined with CT, renal involvement was present in ten cases (5.9%). The distribution of the cases was as follows: one poorly differentiated nodular lymphocytic lymphoma, one poorly differentiated diffuse lymphocytic lymphoma, five diffuse histiocytic lymphomas, and three immunoblastic lymphomas. None of the patients with HL examined with CT at an early stage of the disease exhibited renal involvement (GILBERT and CASTELLINO 1986). ·

Lymphomatous deposits are usually in the form of "multiple nodules," which were found in 61% of all affected kidneys by RICHMOND et al. (1962). Other kinds of infiltration were classified as "diffuse" (6%), "bulky single tumors" (7%), "solitary nodules" (7%), "invasion from perirenal disease" (11%), and that which could be detected only on microscopic examination (7%). The last type has been observed only in patients with lymphosarcoma and marrow involvement. The pathologic patterns of renal involvement appear to be similar in HL and NHL.

A different distribution of various kinds of lymphomatous deposits was reported by HARTMAN et al. (1982) in a series of 21 patients. All these patients underwent radiologic studies and histologic examination. In this series 48% had a solitary mass, 29% multiple nodules, and 19% almost complete parenchymal replacement by the tumor. These discrepant findings are probably best explained by different patient populations.

Because the kidney normally does not contain lymphoid tissue, primary lymphoma arising within the kidney is very rare. Whether the first neoplastic cells originate in the kidney and their progeny from the renal tumor, later escaping into the lymphoid system, or whether the first cells originate in the hematopoietic tissues and their progeny then migrate to the kidney is impossible to determine, but either origin is conceivable (KANDEL et al. 1987). Most frequently, renal lymphoma is secondary to hematogenous spread or results from contiguous extension of retroperitoneal lymphoma.

The gross morphology and consequent imaging aspects depend upon the mechanism of renal involvement. The hematogenous spread, at the early stage, leads to multiple, small nodules, with predominant location in the interstitium of the cortex where the tumor proliferates. In the early phase the nephrons, collecting ducts, and blood vessels are not involved but only displaced and compressed. As a result of this infiltrative growth, the tumor contour is irregular and a capsule or pseudocapsule is absent. In this phase, renal morphology and function are still normal. Subsequently, the growth becomes destructive and the tumor expansive. In cases of slow growing masses, the kidney may be enlarged with mild or no compression of the collecting system.

When the growth is rapid, nonuniform, and eccentric, the mass modifies the renal profile and displaces the collecting system, the findings being similar to those in cases of renal cell carcinoma.

10.3.2 Clinical Findings

The clinical and biochemical findings thought to be relevant in patients with renal involvement by lymphoma were reported by RICHMOND et al. (1962) in 142 patients who underwent autopsy. The clinical findings were as follows: (a) pain or tenderness or both, particularly in the loin or flank; (b) palpable mass in the renal area; (c) hypertension; (d) reduced urinary flow; (e) macroscopic hematuria; and (f) edema. The following biochemical changes were found: (a) albuminuria and/or cells or casts in the urinary sediment; (b) elevation of the blood urea nitrogen; (c) hypercalcemia; (d) hyperuricemia; and (e) hyperproteinemia.

The authors divided the 142 patients into two groups: in the first the clinical and biochemical changes were believed to have resulted from infiltration of the renal parenchyma (23% of the patients); the second comprised the remaining 77% of patients in whom the same features were in part ascribed to lesions other than renal infiltration, such as retroperitoneal masses with involvement of the genitourinary system. In patients with renal lymphoma, pain was present in 2.5%, palpable mass in 9%, hypertension in 8.5%, macroscopic hematuria and oliguria in 2%, albuminuria in 7.5%, elevated blood urea nitrogen in 12%, hyperuricemia in 5%, and hypercalcemia in 2%. Therefore, renal changes secondary to retroperitoneal lymphoma involving the genitourinary system should be considered when the above-mentioned clinical and biochemical findings are present.

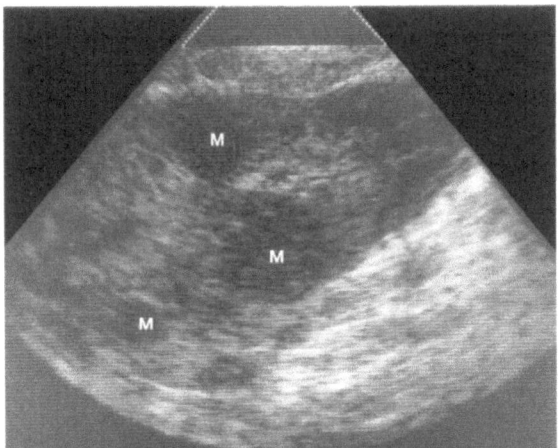

Fig. 10.13. US pattern of renal lymphoma. Multiple hypoechoic masses *(M)* reduced through transmission

10.3.3 Diagnostic Imaging

Diagnostic imaging modalities can show the renal involvement, with findings depending upon the pathologic features and the stage of the disease (HORII et al. 1983).

Specific US findings of American Burkitt's lymphoma have also been reported (SHAWKER et al. 1979). Burkitt's lymphoma, a malignancy endemic in tropical latitudes and in some regions of Africa, has been found with morphologically indistinguishable characteristics in American children (ARSENEAU et al. 1975; HERLITZKA et al. 1973). The American Burkitt's lymphoma is usually characterized by abdominal masses of varying size (often large) and by frequent renal complications caused by uric acid nephropathy or ureteric obstruction. US findings of renal involvement by this tumor consist of poorly defined peripheral hypoechoic masses (Fig. 10.13) within mildly enlarged kidneys; hydronephrosis may result from obstruction by pelvic or retroperitoneal tumors.

10.3.3.1 Computed Tomography

Numerous reports in the literature deal with the contribution of CT in the evaluation of lymphomas (AMBOS et al. 1977; CHILCOTE and BORKOWSKI 1983; HARTMAN et al. 1982; HORII et al. 1983; FELDBERG 1983; JAFRI et al. 1982; KANDEL et al. 1987; KRUDY et al. 1981; RUBIN 1979). Most series are in agreement that renal involvement occurs in the great majority of cases of NHL; the involvement is bilateral in about 50% of cases (JAFRI et al. 1984; CHILCOTE and BORKOWSKI 1983; HEIKEN et al. 1983).

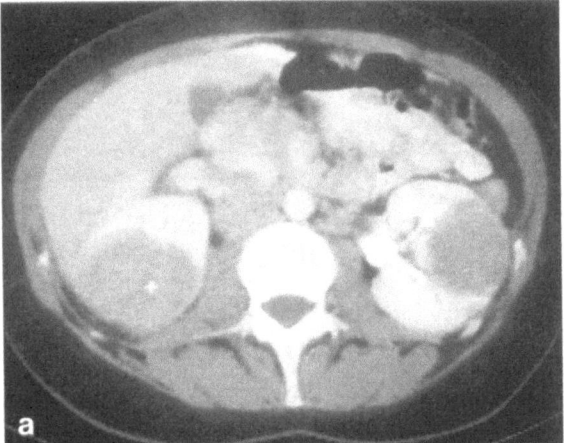

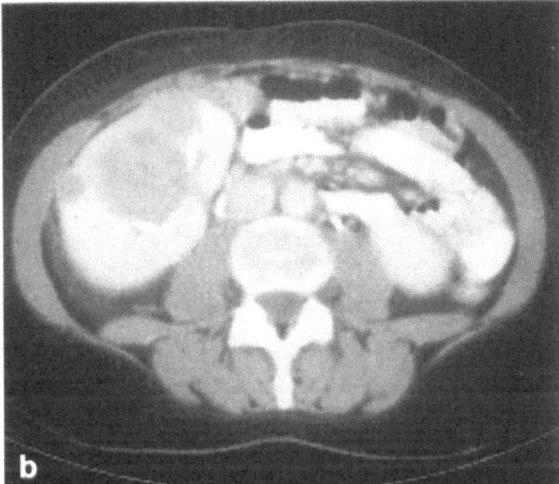

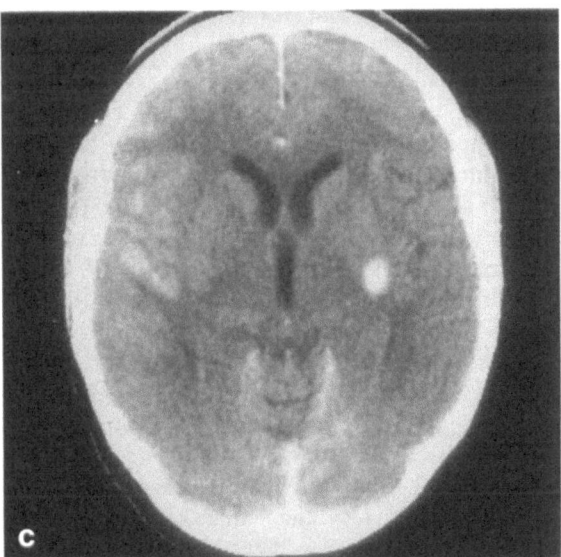

Fig. 10.14 a–c. CT patterns of renal lymphoma (non-Hodgkin's lymphoma). **a, b** Bilateral multiple round well-demarcated masses (type II lesions according to JAFRI et al.). **c** CT of brain showing enhancing lesion in the left hemisphere and diffuse enhancement in the right sylvian region

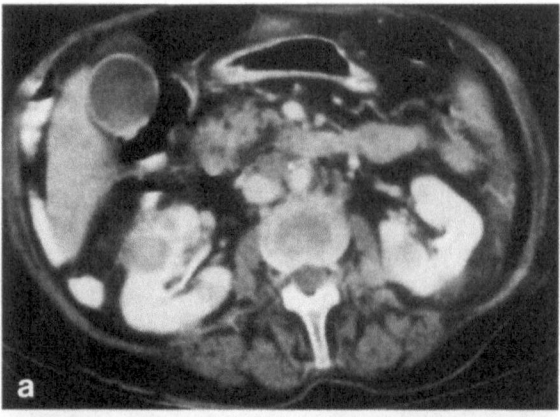

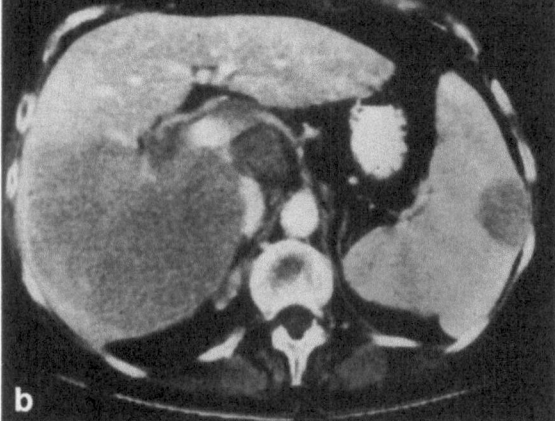

Fig. 10.15 a, b. CT patterns of renal lymphoma (non-Hodgkin's lymphoma). Bilateral hypodense masses (type II according to JAFRI et al.), one very well demarcated in the right kidney. Aortocaval node and extensive involvement of the liver and spleen are seen

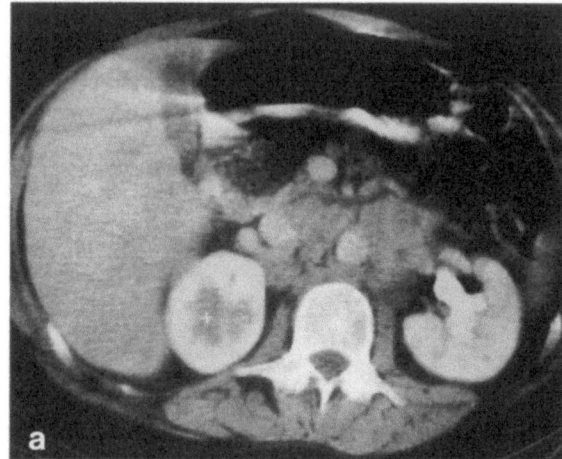

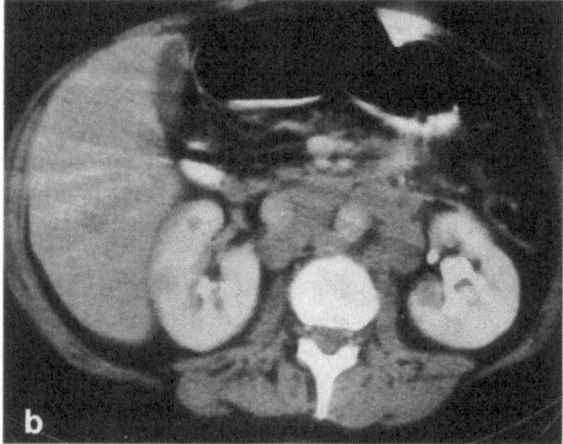

Fig. 10.16 a, b. CT patterns of renal lymphoma (non-Hodgkin's lymphoma). Infiltrative (a) and nodular (b) features coexist (type II according to JAFRI et al.)

Computed tomographic findings may be classified into four types, as suggested by AMBOS et al. (1977) and described by JAFRI et al. (1982); type I, solitary nudule; type II, multiple nodules; type III, infiltrative focal or diffuse lesion; type IV, kidney engulfed by contiguous retroperitoneal disease. Types I and II are the most common. Nodular masses range in size from 8 mm (JAFRI et al. 1982) to several centimeters. They may be hypodense or isodense, and rarely hyperdense, on non-contrast-enhanced scans. After contrast enhancement, lymphomatous lesions exhibit an increase in their density, which is less than that of normal renal parenchyma; therefore, detectability of lesions improves. For this reason in cases of suspected lymphoma, CT scans must always be obtained after contrast enhancement. The density is usually homogeneous and the contours are regular and sharply demarcated, giving the lesion a pseudocystic ap-

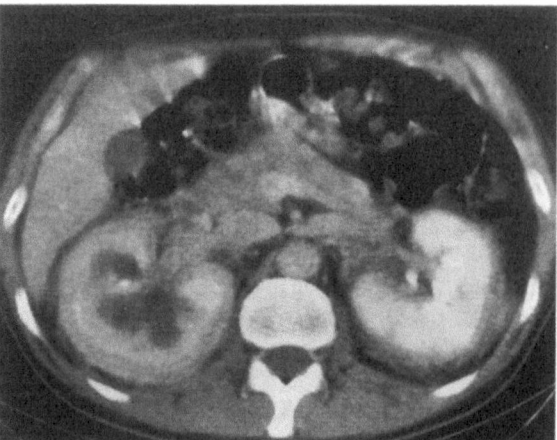

Fig. 10.17. Perirenal lymphoma. Both kidneys are enveloped by a soft tissue dense mass which involves the renal hilum as well. On the right, this causes obstructive nephropathy

pearance (GILBERT and CASTELLINO 1986). The nodular type (Figs. 10.14a, b, 10.15a), when multiple, may be difficult to differentiate from renal metastases and acute infection (diffuse nephritis); the correct diagnosis is based upon clinical findings and the presence of retroperitoneal adenopathy. These findings allow differentiation of a solitary nodule (type I) from a renal carcinoma. More difficult is differentiation from a primary renal lymphoma which presents as a solitary nodule (KANDEL et al. 1987).

The infiltrative type (type III) may appear as focal or diffuse lesion. In the focal type, a mild and small hypodensity with infiltration of the perirenal space is seen, while in the diffuse type (Fig. 10.16), the entire kidney is enlarged, hypodense, and replaced by tumor. In type IV (Fig. 10.17), the kidney is involved by contiguous invasion from retroperitoneal masses. The invasion differentiates a renal lymphoma from a primary retroperitoneal tumor which displaces rather than invades the kidney. In this instance, an irregular ureteral stenosis or an obstruction of the ureter with hydronephrosis or nonvisualized excretory system are frequently observed.

Thickening of Gerota's fascia and small curvilinear densities in the perirenal space have also been reported (JAFRI et al. 1982; FELDBERG 1983).

Finally, American Burkitt's lymphoma may present as diffuse infiltration with renomegaly and a slight increase in density before contrast enhancement; dense nephrography after contrast enhancement consistent with urate nephropathy may be observed (KRUDY et al. 1981).

10.3.4 Conclusion

Diagnostic imaging of renal lymphomas is based today upon US and CT. Conventional IVU is no longer justified because of a high false-negative rate.

The different aspects of the renal involvement by lymphoma are best visualized by CT, which is also indicated for the staging of lymphomas. CT makes possible correct definition of the different types of lesion and the extrarenal manifestations of lymphoma.

10.4 Carcinoma of the Renal Pelvis

10.4.1 Pathology

Carcinoma of the renal pelvis is a relatively rare tumor of the kidney: its incidence is reported to be between 5% and 12% of all malignant tumors of the kidney (BLOOM et al. 1970; GRABSTALD et al. 1971; LEDER et al. 1979; NOCKS et al. 1982), or 5% of all urothelial tumors (NOCKS et al. 1982). It is commonly seen in older patients, usually between the sixth and the eight decade of life. The incidence in men exceeds that in women. The usual sex ratio is between 2:1 and 4:1 (NOCKS et al. 1982).

This tumor is characteristically multiple, affecting the pelvis, the ureter and the bladder at the same time. The multiplicity of site may be synchronous or metachronous (YOUSEM et al. 1988).

The synchronous incidence ranges between 30%-40% (NOCKS et al. 1982) and 50% (GRABSTALD et al. 1971). It is thought to be related to the diffuse potential tumorigenesis of the urothelium (GRABSTALD et al. 1971).

The incidence of metachronous tumors of the urothelium is much higher for tumors originating in the renal pelvis (23%-40%) than for those originating in the bladder (0%-6.4%) (YOUSEM et al. 1988).

Transitional and squamous cell carcinoma of the renal pelvis may be experimentally induced by several agents, e.g., dibenzanthracene, methylcholanthrene, benzopyrene, the metabolites of benzidine, and lead salts. Associations have been observed with some RNA viruses. A relationship between these tumors and Thorotrast (LEDER et al. 1979), used for retrograde pyelography, phenacetin (BENGTSSON et al. 1968; JOHANSSON et al. 1974), and tobacco smoke (BENNINGTON and BECKWITH 1975; MORRISON 1984) has been shown. Other factors include artificial sweeteners (e.g., saccharin), hair dye, diet (low intake of vitamin A), drugs (chloraphazine, cyclophosphamide), and bladder infections (MORRISON 1974). The relationship between coffee drinking and urothelial cancer is a matter of controversy. Carcinoma of the renal pelvis includes the following histologic types (GRABSTALD et al. 1971): transitional cell carcinoma, epidermoid carcinoma, adenocarcinoma, and undifferentiated carcinoma.

Transitional cell carcinoma shows a papillary configuration. The tumor may present in this fashion or may develop as a result of malignant evolution of a papilloma. Transitional cell carcinomas may show infiltrative characteristics and are prone to necrosis. In some cases, focal areas of squamous cell or glandular epithelium may coexist (LANZA 1969; LEDER et al. 1979; GRABSTALD et al. 1971; BENNINGTON and BECKWITH 1975). Transitional cell carcinomas tend to be multicentric more often than other histological types.

Epidermoid carcinoma (squamous epithelial carcinoma) is rare and occurs in patients with a long previous history of stones, urinary tract infections, and hematuria (DEL REGATO and SPJUT 1977; LEDER et al. 1979). This tumor has a rapid growth. It infiltrates and invades the ureter, the perirenal fat, and the lymph nodes and also metastasizes early. Macroscopically the tumor presents as a mass inside the lumen, infiltrating both the wall and the renal parenchyma. The tumor is rarely multicentric. However, due to its greater aggressiveness, the prognosis is poor (AKAZA et al. 1987).

Adenocarcinoma of the renal pelvis is still less common than other histologic types, and, as in the case of epidermoid carcinoma, is associated with a history of stones and urinary tract infections (DEL REGATO and SPJUT 1977; LEDER et al. 1979). It has been suggested that adenocarcinoma may originate from the glandular metaplasia following chronic irritation and repeated inflammatory disease.

Undifferentiated carcinoma has a histologic pattern which differs from case to case (BENNINGTON and BECKWITH 1975). Some cases resemble small cell carcinoma of the lung; in others the degree of anaplasia is so high that classification is not possible.

As far as staging is concerned, RUBENSTEIN et al. (1978) proposed the following classification for tumors of the renal pelvis:

Stage A: tumors limited to the mucosa and submucosa of the renal pelvis
Stage B: tumors invading the pelvis wall and the renal parenchyma, but confined to the kidney
Stage C: tumors penetrating the peripelvic fat, without metastases
Stage D: tumors with distant metastases

10.4.2 Clinical Findings

In a series of 460 patients (AKAZA et al. 1987), the chief complaint was gross hematuria (76.3%); abdominal pain and palpable tumor mass were observed with frequencies of 10.9% and 1.1% respectively. Hematuria may also be intermittent and sometimes microscopic. However, these tumors may also be asymptomatic and diagnosed incidentally during urographic examination performed for other clinical symptoms (NOCKS et al. 1982). In some cases, the clinical presentation may be that of urinary retention following obstruction by clots.

In about 10%–15% of cases, predisposing factors like cystitis, urethritis, calculi, and pyelonephritis may exist (GRABSTALD et al. 1971).

The prognosis depends on various factors: histologic grade, stage, tumor size, and number of lesions.

Patients with squamous cell carcinoma show a significantly poorer prognosis than those with transitional cell carcinoma (AKAZA et al. 1987).

MAZEMAN and WEMEAU (1975) reported tumor recurrence to be highest for tumor of the renal pelvis in a multicenter series of 1118 urothelial tumors managed by surgery.

10.4.3 Diagnostic Imaging

10.4.3.1 Plain Radiographs

Plain radiographs of the abdomen occasionally show enlargement of the affected kidney (LOWE and ROYLANCE 1976) and rarely calcifications (BRABAND 1961; FERRIS and O'CONNORS 1965; DANIEL et al. 1972; DINSMORE et al. 1988), which have a coarse, punctuated linear and granular appearance (DINSMORE et al. 1988). This may lead to confusion with medullary sponge kidney or small renal calculi, but the irregular aspect and indistinct border of the calcifications should suggest transitional cell carcinoma. The calcifications can be located peripherally in the kidney, simulating other benign or malignant lesions, such as renal abscess, the calcified shell of pyonephrosis, tuberculosis, and leukoplakia (DINSMORE et al. 1988).

The radiographic pattern coupled with the pyelographic findings and clinical data should narrow the differential diagnosis. As in the case of bladder tumors, the calcifications may be influenced by local ischemia, infection, or urinary pH (calcium phosphate deposition in necrotic tissue is potentiated when the urine is alkaline) (POLLACK et al. 1981; MILLER and PFISTER 1974).

10.4.3.2 Urography and Retrograde Pyelography

High quality urograms are essential for an accurate diagnosis. Nonionic contrast media are said to improve opacity and therefore the quality of the pyelogram (STACUL et al. 1987). According to LOWE and ROYLANCE (1976), five distinct groups of findings are definable on the basis of urography:

1. Discrete sharply marginated filling defects causing obliteration of the adjoining collecting system (Fig. 10.19a).
2. Filling defects within distended calyces with obstruction of the adjoining calyces (Fig. 10.19b, c).
3. Calyceal obliteration with involvement of some or all calyces. Nodular filling defects can be seen in

the pelvis. The pattern may be better defined with retrograde pyelography.

4. Hydronephrosis with renal enlargement (Fig. 10.18).
5. Reduced function without renal enlargement. The absence of visualization can be the results of retropelvic obstruction and is not necessarily due to parenchymal invasion (GRABSTALD et al. 1971). The nephrogram may be irregular or can be absent.

The retrograde pyelogram is important for demonstrating involved (or potentially involved) mucosal surfaces in great detail, for visualizing bulky intrapelvic lesions in poorly excreting, hydronephrotic kidneys, and for providing an avenue for brush biopsy (DINSMORE et al. 1988; LANG et al. 1978). Retrograde pyelography is contraindicated in the presence of gross hydronephrosis (WILSON et al. 1968). Antegrade pyelography using a percutaneous translumbar approach may be used in nonfunctioning kidneys. This can be combined with brush biopsy. A sheath advanced to the posterior renal fascia is used to protect against tumor seeding along the tract (LANG et al. 1978) (Fig. 10.19b, see p. 268).

Thanks to complete visualization of the excretory pathways and good resolution, urography is the method of choice for the recognition of even very small lesions in the pelvis, calyces, ureter, and bladder (Fig. 10.18). Morphology usually indicates histopathology; therefore, no further radiologic investigations are required in most cases. However, in some cases, the differential diagnosis of radiolucent calculi, blood clots, and lesions of the urothelial mucosa (such as pyelitis cystica and fibroepithelial polyps) must be considered (LOWE and ROYLANCE 1976). Vascular impressions should be differentiable on the basis of location and morphology. Finally pelvic and ureteral metastases from renal carcinoma may present in a similar fashion (MITTI et al. 1987).

Ultrasound and CT are extremely useful in those cases in which the urothelial tumors present as nonfunctioning kidney or with hydronephrosis (Fig. 10.23).

10.4.3.3 Renal Angiography

Selective renal arteriography has been performed in the past to evaluate the origin and extension of the tumor and to distinguish carcinoma of the renal pelvis from renal cell carcinoma (ELKIN 1980; MICHEL et al. 1975). Today US and CT can define these aspects noninvasively.

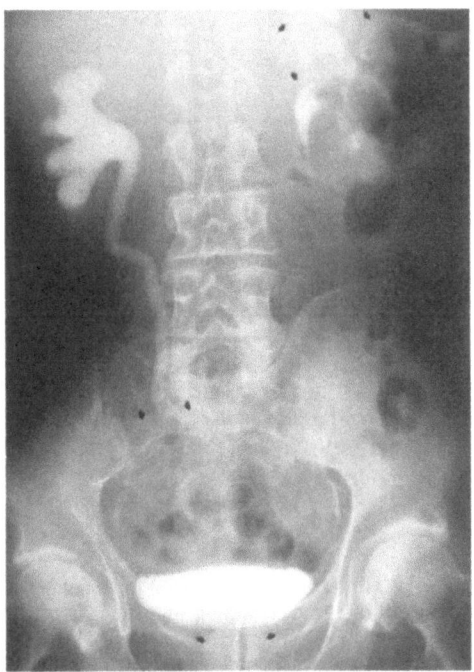

Fig. 10.18. IVU findings in urothelial tumors. Multiple filling defects *(arrows)* are seen in the upper calyces of the left kidney, the right ureter, and the bladder

In extensive neoplasms, arteriography may be useful to define the origin. Tumors of the renal pelvis are hypovascular; they may show few irregular malignant vessels and encasement of the main renal artery or of its segmental branches but without infiltration into the renal parenchyma. The urothelial origin of hypervascular tumors may be suspected if enlargement of the pelvic artery and widened and tortuous ureteropelvic arteries are present (ELKIN 1980).

10.4.3.4 Ultrasonography

While a few years ago the recognition of tumors of the renal pelvis was difficult by US (LANTZ and HATTERY 1984), today's improved equipment makes possible recognition in a high percentage of cases, unless they are small in size or have an infiltrative character. In a personal series of 33 cases, seven neoplasms with this pattern remained undetected (DALLA PALMA et al. 1984).

A hypoechoic area inside the renal sinus is the most common ultrasonographic feature (ARGER et al. 1979; CUNNINGHAM 1982; DALLA PALMA et al. 1984; GRAEB and UHRICH 1980; GRANT et al. 1986; HOMER and KLEIN 1975; MULHOLLAND et al. 1979; OSTROWSKY et al. 1985; ROSENFIELD et al. 1978,

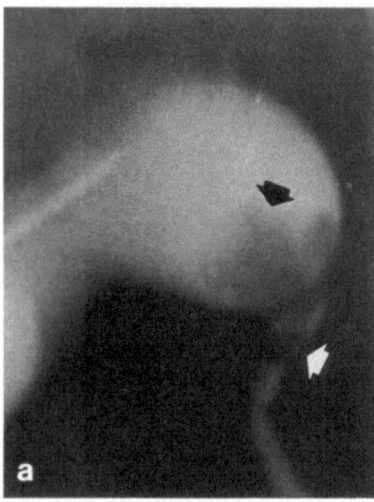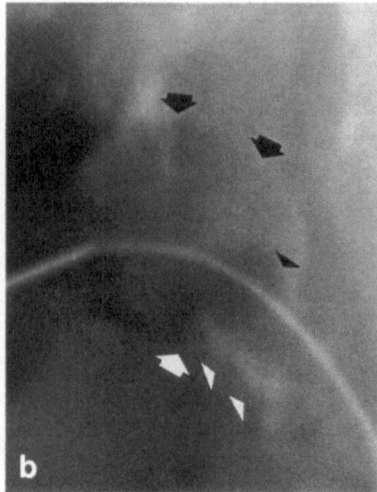

△

Fig. 10.19 a, b. IVU findings in carcinoma of the renal pelvis. **a** Antegrade pyelogram demonstrating lobulated defects at the ureteropelvic junction and in the upper right ureter *(arrows)*. The collecting system is moderately hydronephrotic. **b** A brush element has been introduced through the 18T needle. The brush biopsy is performed under double contrast guidance. A 16T sheath is advanced to the level of the posterior renal fascia. The 18T needle introduced into the calyceal system is advanced through this sheath. The double sheath technique safeguards against seeding of malignant cells along the tract when retracting the brush and 18T needle. (LANG et al. 1978)

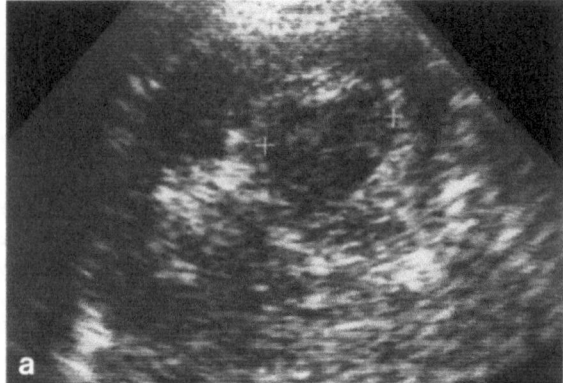

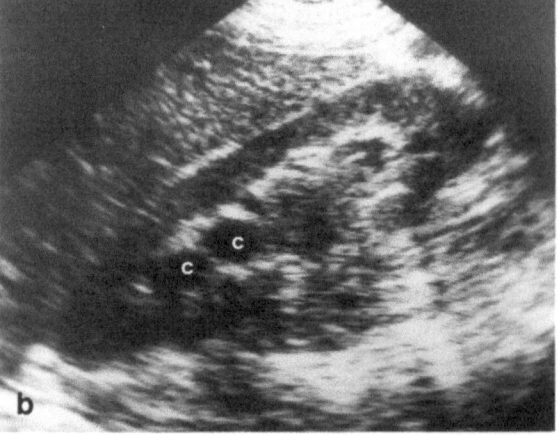

Fig. 10.20 a, b. US patterns in carcinoma of the renal pelvis. **a** Round, sinus mass isoechogenic with the renal parenchyma. **b** Sinus hyperechoic mass with ill-defined contours, well demarcated against normal parenchyma. Some dilated calyces *(C)* are also seen

1979; SUBRAMANYAM et al. 1982; WIMBISH et al. 1983). The echogenicity is generally similar to that of the renal parenchyma (Figs. 10.20 a, 10.21), but in a small number of cases the lesion appears hypo- or hyperechoic (Fig. 10.20 b) compared with the renal parenchyma (DALLA PALMA et al. 1984; GRANT et al. 1986).

The lesion in the dilated calyx is generally surrounded by the echogenic renal sinus. However, it should be kept in mind that US findings are not specific. The differential diagnosis includes clots, hydrocalyces, and small cysts in the renal sinus.

Multiple cysts in the renal sinus, when abutting each other, cause acoustic effects simulating a solid lesion. This effect also may be produced by the normal structures of the sinus, mainly the vessels.

Clots in the renal pelvis may be differentiated on the basis of changes in size and echo structure on serial scans.

Ultrasonography has a lower sensitivity and specificity than IVU. It is ancillary to IVU in the following situations (DALLA PALMA et al. 1984):

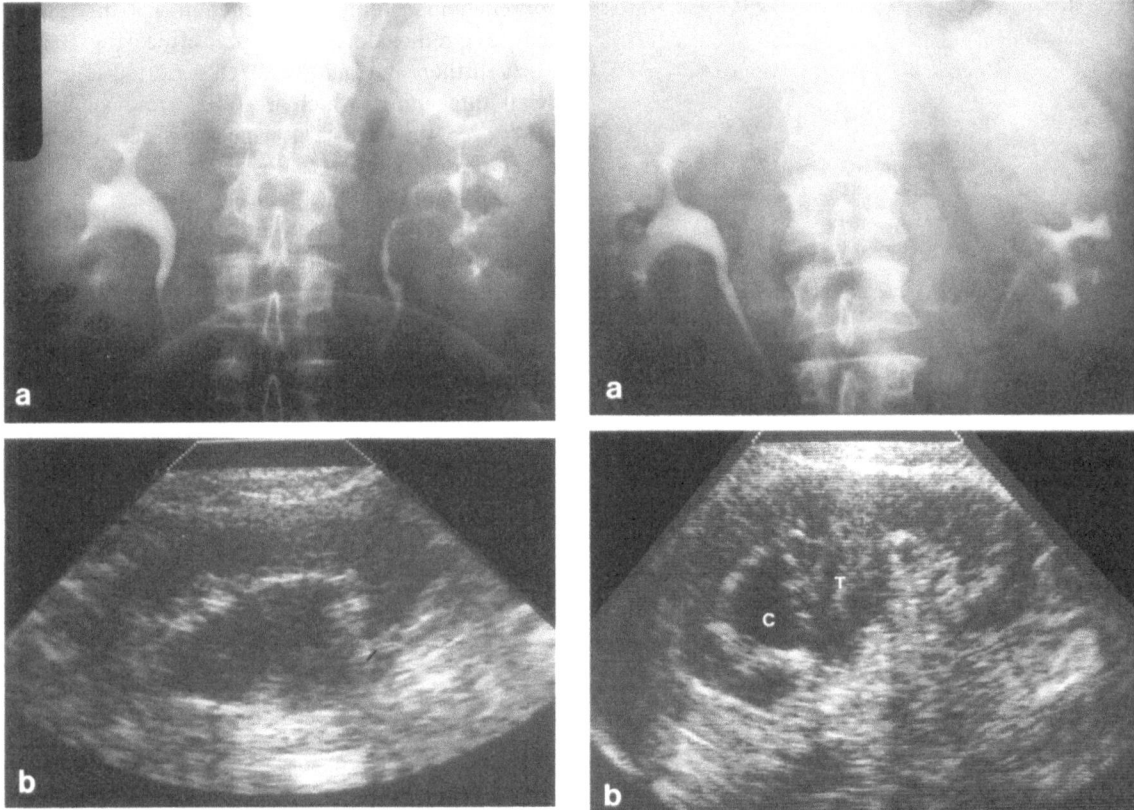

Fig. 10.21 a, b. IVU and US in carcinoma of the renal pelvis. **a** IVU: extensive invasion of calyces, pelvis, and upper ureter. **b** US: large mass isoechoic with renal parenchyma located in the sinus. The mass is separated from the renal parenchyma by an echogenic rim

Fig. 10.22. a IVU: obstruction of the superior infundibulum and dilatation of superior calyces; increased nephrogram of the superior half of the kidney. IVU cannot distinguish a tumor of the renal pelvis from a parenchymal tumor. **b** US: solid mass *(T)* within the sinus. Dilated calyces *(C)* superiorly. US findings are consistent with a tumor originating in the renal sinus

1. In the case of a nonvisualized kidney (US may reveal the lesion)
2. When the nature of a urographic filling defect is doubtful [US may make possible differentiation against a radiolucent stone (shadowing) or a clot (changes on serial examinations)]
3. When urography does not differentiate the pyelic or parenchymal origin of the tumor (Fig. 10.22).

Ultrasonography is superior in defining the tumor extension, which can be greater than that observed on the pyelogram (GRANT et al. 1986).

10.4.3.5 Computed Tomography

Computed tomography may complement IVU and US in the evaluation of carcinomas of the renal pelvis in two ways (McCLENNAN and LEE 1983): (a) to solve the diagnostic problems of a radiolucent filling defect in the renal pelvis or ureter seen on IVU and (b) to delineate the tumor extent for preoperative staging.

In cases of carcinoma of the renal pelvis, CT findings include demonstration of mass, concentric or eccentric ureteral wall thickening, and a large infiltrating mass (Fig. 10.23) (BARON et al. 1982; GATEWOOD et al. 1982; HARTMAN et al. 1988; LANTZ and HATTERY 1984; McCLENNAN and LEE 1983; PARIENTY et al. 1982; POLLACK et al. 1981; SCHWARTZ et al. 1988; WIMBISH et al. 1983). Rarely calcifications may be seen associated with transitional cell carcinoma (DINSMORE et al. 1988).

The intraluminal mass is the most frequent finding; precontrast attenuation values are in the range of 20–40 HU (PARIENTY et al. 1982; POLLACK et al. 1981). The mass may appear inhomogeneous.

After contrast enhancement, there is only a mini-

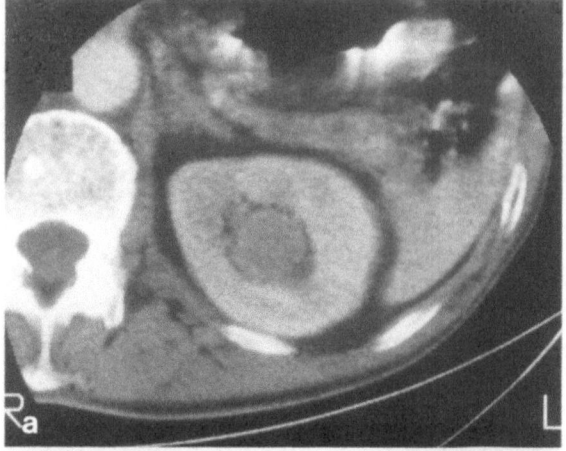

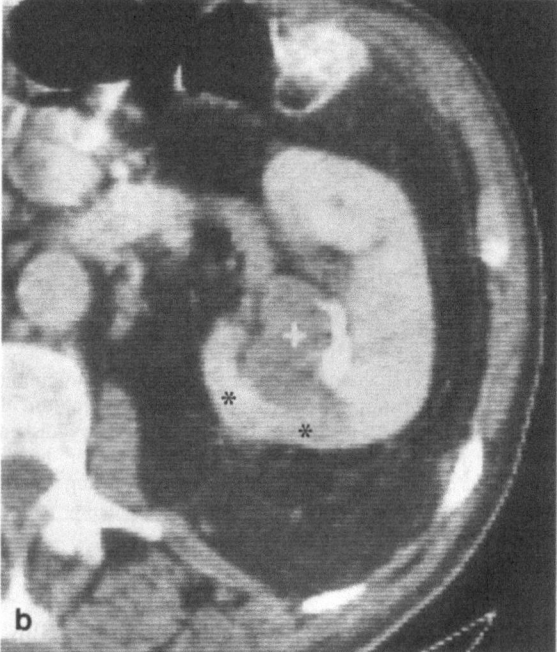

Fig. 10.23 a, b. CT patterns of carcinoma of the renal pelvis. **a** Marginated round soft tissue mass within the sinus, well separated against renal parenchyma by a complete rim of fat. **b** Soft tissue mass in posterior calyx infiltrating the posterior parenchymal lip

mal increase in density. In this phase density values are in the range of 40–70 HU (MCCLENNAN and LEE 1983; RAYAN et al. 1979) and depend on the degree of vascularity and the amount of contrast agent. However, in most cases the mass is hypovascular; this makes possible differentiation against renal cell carcinoma, which is hypervascular in almost all cases (LANG 1984).

Pelvic masses with infiltrative characteristics may extend beyond the wall into the renal parenchyma and consequently become indistinguishable from a parenchymal tumor. Obstruction by the tumors causes a reduced nephrographic effect (Fig. 10.23 b).

A further sign that has been reported is ureteral wall thickening, which is diffuse and symmetric. However, this sign is nonspecific since it has also been reported in tuberculosis, lymphoma, and amyloidosis (BARON et al. 1982).

Extrarenal extension alters the normal transparency of perirenal fat. CT is primarily useful to determine the nature of an undetermined urographic filling defect or to ascertain the presence of faint tumor calcifications (Fig. 10.24, see p. 271). (DINSMORE 1988; ZINCKE and NEVES 1984).

References

Abrams HL, Spiro R, Goldstein N (1950) Metastases in carcinoma. Analysis of 1000 autopsied cases. Cancer 3: 75–85

Addison NW, Perch B (1966) Smooth muscle tumors of the kidney. Report of two cases. Br J Urol 38: 382–387

Akaza H, Koiso K, Niijima T (1987) Clinical evaluation of urothelial tumors of the renal pelvis and ureter based on a new classification system. Cancer 59: 1369–1375

Ambos MA, Bosniak MA, Madayag MA, Leffeur RS (1977) Infiltrating neoplasms of the kidney. AJR 129: 859–864

Arger P, Mulhern C, Pollack H, Banner M, Wein A (1979) Ultrasound assesment of renal transitional cell carcinoma: preliminary report. AJR 132: 407–411

Arseneau JC, Canellos GP, Banks PM (1975) American Burkitt's lymphoma: a clinicopathologic study of 30 cases. Clinical findings. Am J Med 58: 314–316

Baron RL, McClennan BL, Lee JKT, Lawson TL (1982) Computed tomography of transitional-cell carcinoma of the renal pelvis and ureter. Radiology 144: 125–130

Becker WE, Schellhammer PF (1986) Renal metastases from carcinoma of the lung. Br J Urol 58: 494–498

Bengtsson U, Angervall L, Ekman H, Lehmann L (1968) Transitional cell tumors of the renal pelvis in analgesic abusers. Scand J Urol Nephrol 2: 145–150

Bennington G, Beckwith J (1975) Atlas of tumor pathology. Armed Forces Institute of Pathology, Washington DC

Benoit G, Boccon-Gibod L, Evrard P, Stag A (1983) Tumerus secondaires du rein. Sem Hop Paris 59: 3127–3129

Bhatt GM, Bernardino MB, Graham SD Jr (1983) CT diagnosis of renal metastases. J Comput Assist Tomogr 7: 1032–1034

Bloom NA, Vidone RA, Lytton B (1970) Primary carcinoma of the ureter, a report of 102 new cases. J Urol 103: 590–594

Bonsib SM, Fisher J, Plattner S, Fallon B (1987) Sarcomatoid renal tumors. Clinicopathologic correlation of three cases. Cancer 59: 527–532

Bosniak MA, Stern W, Lopez F, Tehranian N, O'Connor J (1969) Metastatic neoplasm to the kidney. Radiology 92: 989–993

Braband H (1961) Incidence of urographic findings in tumors of the urinary bladder. Br J Radiol 30: 51–66

Bracken RB, Chika G, Johnson DE, Luna M (1979) Secondary renal neoplasms: an autopsy study. South Med J 72: 806–807

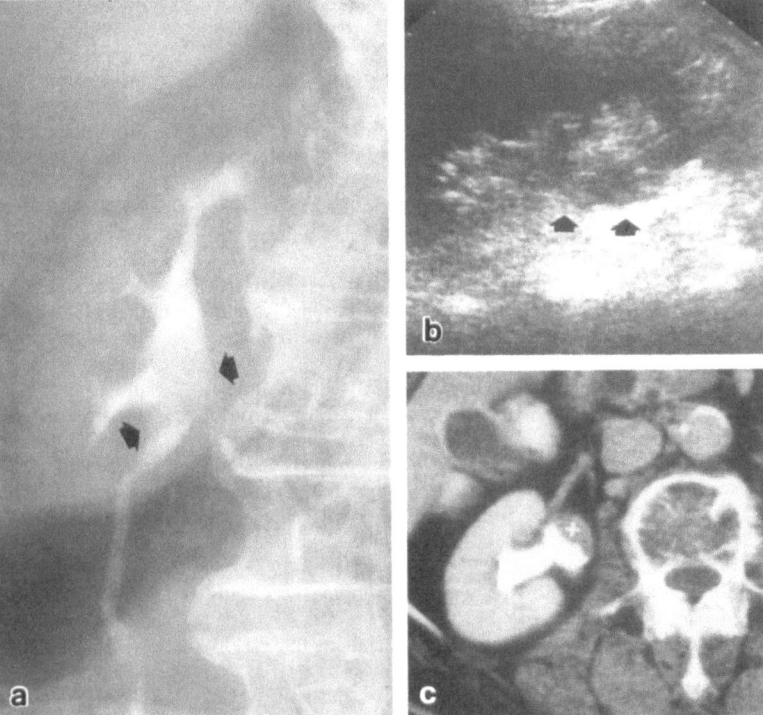

Fig. 10.24. a IVU: lobulated filling defect in the renal pelvis *(arrows)*. **b** US: solid mass *(arrows)* in the renal hilum. **c** CT: small soft tissue mass (+) in the renal pelvis without extension beyond the pelvis

Carrol BA, Ta HN (1980) The ultrasonic appearance of extranodal abdominal lymphoma. Radiology 136: 419–425

Chilcote WA, Borkowski GP (1983) Computed tomography in renal lymphoma. J Comput Assist Tomogr 7: 439–443

Choyke PL, White EM, Zeman RK, Jaffe MH, Clark LR (1987) Renal metastases: clinicopathologic and radiologic correlation. Radiology 162: 359–363

Colabawalla BN (1972) Renal hamartoma. Br J Urol 44: 112–116

Cunningham J (1982) Ultrasonic demonstration of renal collecting system invasion by transitional cell cancer. J Clin Ultrasound 10: 339–341

Cutler M (1935) Lymphosarcoma. Arch Surg 30: 405–412

Dahlin DC (1970) Bone tumors. Thomas, Springfield Ill.

Dalla Palma L, Bazzocchi M, Pozzi-Mucelli RS, Rossi M, Stacul F, Agostini R, Maffessanti M (1984) The role of ultrasonography in the diagosis of tumors of the renal pelvis. Eur J Radiol 4: 156–160

Daniel WW, Hartman GW, Witter DM, Farrow GM, Ketalis PP (1972) Calcified renal masses: a review of ten years' experience at the Mayo Clinic. Radiology 103: 503–508

Del Regato JA, Spjut HJ (1977) Cancer. Diagnosi, treatment and prognosis. Mosby, St. Louis

Dinsmore BJ, Pollack HM, Banner MP (1988) Calcified transitional cell carcinoma of the renal pelvis. Radiology 167: 401–404

Elkin M (1980) Radiology of the urinary system. Little, Brown & Co., Boston

Evans JA, Bosniak MA (1971) The kidney. Year Book Medical Publishers, Chicago

Falappa P, Trodella L, Maresca G (1980) Lymphomatous involvement of the kidneys: computed tomography and ultrasound demonstration. Diagn Imaging 49: 266–268

Farrow GM, Harrison EG, Utz D, Remine WH (1968) Sarcomas and sarcomatoid and mixed malignant tumors of the kidney in adults. Cancer 22: 545–563

Fein RL, Hamm FC (1968) Malignant schwannoma of renal pelvis: a review of the literature of a case report. J Urol 94: 356–361

Feldberg MAM (1983) Computed tomography of the retroperitoneum. Martinus Nijhoff, Boston

Ferris EJ, O'Connors ST (1965) Calcification in urinary bladder tumors. AJR 95: 447–449

Gatewood OM, Goldman SM, Marshall FF, Siegelman SS (1982) Computed tomography in the diagnosis of transitional cell carcinoma of the kidney. J Urol 127: 876–877

Geerdsen J (1979) Tumors of the renal pelvis and ureter. Scand J Urol Nephrol 13: 287–290

Gilbert TG, Castellino RA (1986) Linfomi maligni dell'apparato genito-urinario. In: Dalla Palma L (ed) Progressi in Radiologia - Radiourologia 1986, Lint, Trieste, pp 265–280

Grabstald H, Whitmore WF, Melamed MR (1971) Renal pelvic tumors. JAMA 218: 845–854

Graeb D, Uhrich P (1980) Diffuse renal transitional cell carcinoma and hydronephrosis. AJR 135: 620–621

Granmayeh M, Wallace S, Barrett AF, Fisher R, Hesplep JH (1977) Sarcoma of the kidney: angiographic features. AJR 129: 107–112

Grant DC, Dee GJ, Yoderi IC, Newhouse JH (1986) Sonography in transitional cell carcinoma of the renal pelvis. Urol Radiol 8: 1–5

Gregory A, Behan M (1981) Lymphoma of the kidneys: unusual ultrasound appearance due to infiltration of the renal sinus. J Clin Ultrasound 9: 343–345

Grise P, Botto H, Camey M (1987) Esophageal cancer metastatic to kidney: report of 2 cases. J Urol 137: 274–276

Gupta OP, Dube MK (1971) Rare primary renal sarcoma. Br J Urol 43: 546–551

Haining RB, Poole FE (1936) Osteoblastoma of the kidney, histologically identical with osteogenic sarcoma. Arch Pathol 21: 44-54

Hamer HG, Wishard WN (1948) Osteogenic sarcoma involving the right kidney. J Urol 60: 10-17

Hartman DS, Davis CJ Jr, Goldman SM, Friedman AC, Fritzsche P (1982) Renal lymphoma: radiologic-pathologic correlation of 21 cases. Radiology 144: 759-766

Hartman DS, Davidson AJ, Davius CJ, Goldman SM (1988) Infiltrative renal lesions: CT-sonographic-pathologic correlations. AJR 150: 1061-1064

Heiken JP, Palmer Gold R, Schnur MJ, King DL, Bashist B, Glazer HS (1983) Computed tomography of renal lymphoma with ultrasound correlation. J Comput Assist Tomogr 7: 245-250

Herlitzka AJ, Babruddoja M, Dube VE (1973) Clinical and pathological features of Burkitt's lymphoma. Surg Gynecol Obstet 136: 81-86

Homer MJ, Klein LA (1975) Ultrasonography B-mode scanning for invasive transitional cell carcinoma of kidney. Urology 6: 650-652

Horii SC, Bosniak MA, Megibow AJ, Raghavendra BN, Subramanyam BR, Rothberg M (1983) Correlation of CT and ultrasound in the evaluation of renal lymphoma. Urol Radiol 5: 69-76

Hudson HC (1956) Osteogenic sarcoma involving the left kidney. J Urol 75: 21-24

Ikeda M, Neyazaky T, Chiba S, Yobbetti M, Susuki C (1968) Bronchial vascular pattern of various pulmonary diseases, with particular emphasis on its diagnostic value in pulmonary cancer. J Thorac Cardiovasc Surg 55: 642-652

Jackson H, Parker F (1947) Hodgkin's disease and allied disorders. Oxford University Press, New York

Jafri SZH, Bree RL, Amendola MA, Glazer GM, Schwab RE, Francis IR, Borlaza G (1982) CT of renal and perirenal non-Hodgkin lymphoma. AJR 138: 1101-1105

Jafri SZH, Amendola MA, Brady TM, Cho KJ, Hoskins PA, Ellword RA (1984) Angiographic patterns of involvement in renal and perirenal lymphoma. Urol Radiol 6: 14-19

Jenkins JD, Chir M, Anderson CK, Williams E (1971) Renal sarcoma. Br J Urol 43: 263-267

Johansson S, Angerwall L, Bengtsson W, Wahlquist L (1974) Urothelial tumors of the renal pelvis associated with abuse of phenacetin-containing analgesic. Cancer 33: 743-753

Johnson LA, Ancona VC, Johnson T, Pineda NB (1970) Primary osteogenic sarcoma of the kidney. J Urol 104: 528-531

Kandel LB, McCollough DC, Harrison LH, Woodruff RD, Ahl E Jr, Munitz A (1987) Primary renal lymphoma. Does it exist? Cancer 60: 386-391

Kaude JV, Lacy GD (1978) Ultrasound in renal lymphoma. J Clin Ultrasound 6: 321-323

Klapproth HJ (1972) Renal angiomyolipoma. Arch Pathol 67: 400-411

Klinger ME (1951) Secondary tumors of the genito-urinary tract. J Urol 65: 144-155

Krudy AG, Dunnick NR, Magrath IT, Shawker TH, Doppman JL, Spiegel R (1981) CT of American Burkitt's lymphoma. AJR 136: 747-754

Kyaw M, Koehlor PR (1969) Renal and perirenal lymphoma: arteriographic findings. Radiology 93: 1055-1058

Kursh ED, Persky L (1971) Selective renal arteriography in renal lymphoma. J Urol 105: 772-775

Lanza G (1969) Manuale di anatomia patologica. Piccin, Padua

Lang EK (1971a) The accuracy of roentgenographic techniques in the diagnosis of the renal mass lesions. Radiology 98: 119-128

Lang EK (1971b) The roentgenographic diagnosis of renal mass lesions. WH Green, St. Louis, Missouri

Lang EK (1984) Staging of renal cell carcinoma: concepts of uroradiology staging of renal cell carcinoma. Williams & Wilkins, Baltimore

Lang EK, Alexander R, Barnett T, Palomar J, Hamway S (1978) Brush biopsy of pyelocalyceal lesions via a percutaneous approach. Radiology 129: 623-627

Lantz EJ, Hattery RR (1984) Diagnostic imaging of urothelial cancer. Urol Clin North Am 11: 567-583

Lathan HS, Kay S (1974) Malignant tumors of the renal pelvis. Surg Gynecol Obstet 138: 613-622

Leder LD, Richter HJ, Stambolis C (1979) Pathology of renal and adrenal neoplasm. In: Lohr E (ed) Renal and adrenal tumors. Springer, Berlin, Heidelberg, New York, pp 1-68

Lemaitre G, Dehaene JL, Remy J, Maillard JP (1975) Aspects radiologiques des metastases renales. A propos de 9 observations. J Radiol Electrol 56: 505-512

Leong CG, Lim TK, Wong KK, Ong GB (1976) Carcinoma of the renal pelvis: an analysis of the diagnostic problems in 23 cases. Br J Surg 63: 102-106

Lien WM (1973) Liposarcoma of the kidney. Postgrad Med J 49: 660-663

Lowe PP, Roylance J (1976) Transitional cell carcinoma of the kidney. Clin Radiol 27: 503-512

Lucke B, Schulumbeerger HG (1957) Tumors of the kidney, renal pelvis and ureter. Armed Forces Institute of Pathology, Washington DC

Masselot J, Baudet P, Bergiron C, Blache R, Rouesse J, Markovits P (1973) Semiologie radiologique (arteriographie exclue) de metastases renales des tumeurs solides. J Radiol 54: 477-483

Mazeman E, Wemeau L (1975) Les limites du traitement chirugical du cancer du rein. J Urol Nephrol 80: 82-89

Mazeman E, Wemean L, Lemaitre G, Koryreff P (1976) Les tumeurs secondaires due rein. J Urol Nephrol 3: 145-160

McClennan BL, Lee JKT (1983) Kidney. In: Lee JKT, Sagel SS, Stanley RJ (eds) Computed body tomography. Raven, New York, pp 341-378

Michel JR, Vital JL, Moreau JF, Affre J (1975) La diagnostic radiologique des tumeurs pielocaliciells. Accent mis sur l'interet de l'arteriographie, sur on apres epreuve a l'angiotensine. J Radiol Electrol 56: 875-886

Miller SW, Pfister RC (1974) Calcification in uroepithelial tumors of the bladder. AJR 121: 827-944

Mintz ER (1937) Sarcomas of the kidney in adults. Ann Surg 105: 52-61

Mitnick JS, Bosniak MA, Rothberg M, Megibow AJ, Raghavendra BN, Subramanyam BR (1985) Metastatic neoplasm to the kidney studied by computed tomography and sonography. J Comput Assist Tomogr 9: 43-49

Mitty HA, Droller MJ, Dikmas SJ (1987) Ureteral and renal pelvic metastases from renal cell carcinoma. Urol Radiol 9: 16-20

Morrison AS (1984) Advances in etiology of urothelial cancer. Urol Clin North Am 11: 557-566

Mucci B, Lewi HJI, Fleming S (1987) The radiology of sarcomas and sarcomatoid carcinomas of the kidney. Clin Radiol 38: 249-254

Mulholland SG, Arger PH, Goldberg BB, Pollack HM (1979) Ultrasonic differentiation of renal pelvis filling defects. J Urol 122: 14-16

Myerson D, Rosenfield AT, Itzchak Y (1979) Renal capsular tumors: the angiographic features. J Urol 121: 238-241

National Cancer Institute Sponsored Study of Classifications of Non-Hodgkin's Lymphomas (1982) Cancer 49: 2112-2135

Nishitani H, Onitsuka H, Kawahire K, Ono M, Jinnouchi Y, Ohba T, Marsuura K (1984) Computed tomography of renal metastases. J Comput Assist Tomogr 8: 727-730

Nocks BN, Heney NM, Daly JJ, Perrons TA, Griffin PP, Prout GR (1982) Transitional cell carcinoma of the renal pelvis. Urology 19: 472-477

Olsson CA, Moyer JD, Laferte RO (1971) Pulmonary cancer metastatic to the kidney: a common renal neoplasm. J Urol 105: 492-496

Ostrowsky PD, Carr L, Goodman J (1985) Ultrasound of transitional cell carcinoma. J Clin Ultrasound 13: 35-36

Pagani JJ (1983) Solid renal mass in the cancer patient: second primary renal cell carcinoma versus renal metastasis. J Comput Assist Tomogr 7: 444-448

Parienty RA, Ducellier R, Pradel J, Lubrano JM, Coquille F, Richard F (1982) Diagnostic value of CT numbers in pelvocalyceal filling defects. Radiology 145: 743-747

Pick RA, Castellino RA, Seltzer RA (1971) Arteriographic findings in renal lymphoma. AJR 111: 530-534

Pollack HM, Arger PH, Banner MP, Mulhern CB, Coleman BG (1981) Computed tomogrpahy of renal pelvic filling defect. Radiology 138: 645-651

Pollack HM, Banner MP, Martinez LO, Hodson CJ (1986) Diagnostic considerations in urinary bladder wall calcifications. AJR 136: 827-831

Rakowsky E, Barzilay J, Schujman E, Servadio C (1987) Leiomyosarcoma of the kidney. Urology 29: 68-70

Rappaport H, Winter WJ, Hicks EB (1956) Follicular lymphoma: a reevaluation of its position in the scheme of malignant lymphoma based on a survey of 253 cases. Cancer 9: 792-821

Rayan KG, Hoch WH, Graven RM (1979) Intraureteral tumor demonstrated by computed tomography. J Comput Assist Tomogr 3: 759-764

Richmond J, Sherman RS, Diamond HD, Craver LF (1962) Renal lesions associated with malignant lymphomas. Am J Med 32: 184-207

Ro JY, Ayala A, Sella A, Samuels ML, Swanson DA (1987) Sarcomatoid renal cell carcinoma: clinicopathologic. A study of 42 cases. Cancer 59: 516-526

Rosenfield AT, Taylor J, Crade M, Degraaf CJ (1978) Anatomy and pathology of the kidney by gray scale ultrasound. Radiology 128: 737-744

Rosenfield AT, Taylor J, Dembner AG, Jacobson P (1979) Ultrasound of renal sinus: a new observation. AJR 133: 441-448

Rubenstein MA, Walz BJ, Bucy JC (1978) Transitional cell carcinoma of the kidney: 25 year experience. J Urol 119: 594-597

Rubin BE (1979) Computed tomography in the evaluation of renal lymphoma. J Comput Assist Tomogr 3: 759-764

Saitoh H, Shimbo T, Akabayashi T, Takeda M, Ogishima K (1982) Metastasis of renal sarcoma. Tokai Exp Clin Med 7: 365-369

Say CC (1974) Transitional cell carcinoma of the renal pelvis. Experience from 1940 to 1972 and literature review. J Urol 112: 439-446

Schwartz JM, Bosniak MA, Hulnick DH, Megibow AJ (1988) The use of computed tomography in the diagnosis of carcinoma of the renal pelvis causing ureteropelvic junction obstruction. Urol Radiol 9: 204-209

Seabury JC (1967) Renal rhabdomyosarcoma. JAMA 201: 1043-1044

Sella A, Ro JY (1987) Renal cell cancer: best recipient of tumor-to-tumor metastasis. Urology 30: 35-38

Seltzer RA, Wenlund DE (1967) Renal lymphoma arteriographic studies. AJR 101: 692-695

Shawker TH, Dunnick NR, Head GL, Magrath IT (1979) Ultrasound evaluation of American Burkitt's lymphoma. J Clin Ultrasound 9: 279-283

Shirkoda A (1986) Computed tomography of perirenal metastases. J Comput Assist Tomogr 10: 435-438

Shirkoda A, Lewis E (1987) Renal sarcoma and sarcomaotid renal cell carcinoma: CT and angiographic features. Radiology 162: 353-357

Shirkoda A, Staab EV, Mitteltaedt CA (1980) Renal lymphoma imaged by ultrasound and gallium-67. Radiology 137: 175-180

Soto PJ, Radler ES, Martin JM, Gregowicz A (1965) Osteogenic sarcoma of the kidney: report of a case. J Urol 94: 532-535

Srinivas V, Sogani PC, Haidu SI, Whitermore JR (1984) Sarcoma of the kidney. J Urol 132: 13-16

Stacul F, Carraro M, Magnaldi S, Faccini L, Guarnieri G, Dalla Palma L (1987) Contrast agent nephrotoxicity: comparison of ionic and non ionic contrast agents. AJR 149: 1287-1289

Subramanyam B, Raghavendra B, Madambra R (1982) Renal transitional cell carcinoma: sonographic and pathologic correlation. J Clin Ultrasound 10: 203-210

Symmers D (1948) Lymphoid diseases. Arch Pathol 45: 73-79

Takayasu H, Kumamoto Y, Terewak Y, Ueno A (1968) A case of bilateral metastatic tumor originating from a thyroid carcinoma. J Urol 100: 717-719

Thomas JL, Barnes PA, Bernardino ME, Lewis E (1982) Diagnostic approaches to adrenal and renal metastases. Radiol Clin North Am 20: 531-544

Thomas ML, Lamb HR (1978) Angiographic features of primary leiomyosarcoma of the kidney. Aust Radiol 22: 155-157

Tolia BM, Hajdu SI, Whitemore WF (1973) Leiomyosarcoma of the renal pelvis. J Urol 109: 974-976

Tomero KV, Farrow GM, Lieber MM (1983) Sarcomatoid renal carcinoma. J Urol 130: 657-659

Tuttle RJ, Salama S, Matthews WR (1985) Primary osteosarcoma of kidney with liposarcomatous elements. J Can Assoc Radiol 36: 76-78

Watson RC (1968) Arteriography in the diagnosis of renal carcinoma. Review of 100 cases. Radiology 91: 888-897

Watson EM, Sauer HR, Sadugor MG (1949) Manifestation of the lymphoblastoma in the genitourinary tract. J Urol 61: 626-634

Weiss JP, Pollack HM, McCormick JF, Malloy TM, Hanno PM, Carpiniello VL (1984) Renal hemangiopericytoma: surgical, radiological and pathological implications. J Urol 132: 337-339

White A, Palubinskas AJ (1970) Renal Hodgkin's disease. Arteriography demonstration. Radiology 96: 551-552

Williams CB, Mitchell JP (1973) Carcinoma of the ureter. A review of 54 cases. Br J Urol 45: 377-387

Williams JP, Savage PS (1958) Liposarcoma of the kidney. Br J Surg 46: 225-238

Williams LH, Anastopulos HP, Prasant CA (1969) Selective renal arteriography in Hodgkin's disease of the kidney. Radiology 93: 1059-1060

Willis RA (1952) The spread of tumors in the human body. Butterworths, London

Wimbish KJ, Sanders MM, Samuels BI, Francis IR (1983) Squamous cell carcinoma of the renal pelvis: case report emphasizing sonographic and CT appearance. Urol Radiol 5: 267-269

Wilson MC, Wilson CL, Mendelsohn EA, Crow NE, Snider JR (1968) Selected adjuncts to urography. JAMA 204: 1057-1080

Yousem DM, Gatewood OMB, Goldman SM, Marshall FF (1988) Synchronous and metachronous transitional cell carcinoma of the urinary tract: prevalence, incidence, and radiographic detection. Radiology 167: 613-618

Zincke H, Neves RJ (1984) Feasibility of conservative surgery for transitional cell cancer of the upper urinary tract. Urol Clin North Am 11: 717-724

11 Renal Cell Carcinoma

ALAN C. WINFIELD and W. SCOTT McDOUGAL

CONTENTS

11.1 Introduction 275
11.2 Etiology 275
11.3 Symptoms 275
11.4 Pathology 276
11.5 Staging 277
11.6 Renal Cancer Invading the Vena Cava 278
11.7 Radiologic Imaging 279
11.7.1 Excretory Urography 279
11.7.2 Computed Tomography 280
11.7.3 Ultrasound 285
11.7.4 Angiography and Venography 287
11.7.5 Magnetic Resonance Imaging 288
11.7.6 Evaluation for Distant Metastases 291
11.8 Therapy 291
      References 292

11.1 Introduction

Renal adenocarcinoma is a disease with protean manifestations involving approximately 15000 individuals in the United States annually. The incidence doubled in males and slightly increased in females over the period from 1930 to 1967. Currently, about 5000–7000 patients die of this disease annually. The incidence of renal adenocarcinoma increases steadily after the age of 30. In men, the tumor is most prevalent in the sixth decade and in women, in the seventh decade. The average age at the time of diagnosis is 57 years. It is rarely found in children, having been reported somewhat less than 100 times in infancy and childhood.

11.2 Etiology

Renal adenocarcinoma is thought to arise from the proximal renal tubule. Its origin from the renal tubule was originally described by SUDECK in 1893.

ALAN C. WINFIELD, M.D., Professor of Radiology; Department of Radiology and Radiological Sciences; W. SCOTT McDOUGAL, M.D., Professor and Chairman; Department of Urology, Vanderbilt University School of Medicine, Nashville, TN 37232-2730, USA

Evidence for a proximal tubule origin includes electron microscopic observations which demonstrate a histologic similarity with cells of the proximal convoluted tubule (OBERLING et al. 1960) and antibody experiments which reveal that antigens specific for the proximal tubule are located in these tumors as well (WALLACE and NAIRN 1972).

Several environmental carcinogens have been implicated, including tobacco, cadmium, and petroleum by-products; however, a specific relationship has not been established. The disease is more common in patients with certain HLA haplotypes, patients with specific chromosomal abnormalities, and those with von Hippel-Lindau disease (COHEN et al. 1979). A familial incidence has also been described. Adult polycystic disease, horseshoe kidneys, and acquired renal cystic disease of dialysis are also associated with an increased incidence of renal adenocarcinoma (Fig. 11.1). The incidence of acquired renal cystic disease, secondary to end-stage renal failure and long-term hemodialysis, has been reputed to range from 30% to 95% (BASILE et al. 1988). Neoplasm has been demonstrated more frequently in these patients.

11.3 Symptoms

Unfortunately, many patients who harbor renal adenocarcinoma are asymptomatic, thus delaying the diagnosis. The tumor often produces symptoms only after it achieves a significant size or metastasizes. At the time of initial diagnosis, 30% of patients have metastatic disease (WATERS and RICHIE 1979). At the time of discovery, 60% of patients will have hematuria, 50% will have flank pain, and 33% will have a mass; however, the triad of flank pain, hematuria, and mass occurs in only 10%–15% of patients. Malaise, fever, and weight loss are more common occurrences. Other symptoms include an acute varicocele due to obstruction of the gonadal vessel and high output cardiac failure resulting from large arteriovenous fistulae within the tumor. There are also many endocrine abnormalities which occasion-

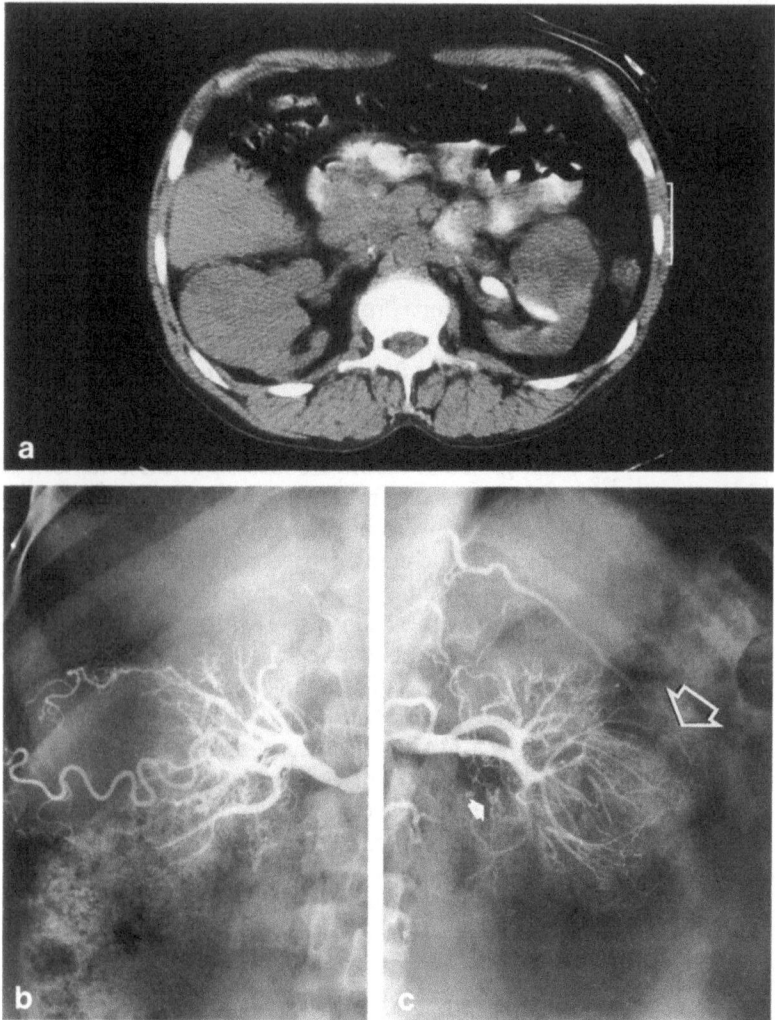

Fig. 11.1a–c. Renal cell carcinomas associated with end-stage renal disease. **a** CT. Both kidneys are enlarged and irregular in contour, due to the presence of bilateral renal cell carcinomas. **b** Selective renal angiogram, *right*, demonstrates neovascularity, as well as vascular extension reflecting tumor extending beyond the renal capsule. Uninvolved portions of the kidney reveal pruned and withered appearance of chronic renal disease. **c** Selective renal angiogram, *left*. Hypovascular mass *(open arrow)* extending laterally. Vascular pattern deformed by mass effect. Neovascularity *(arrow)* reflects medial extension of tumor

ally occur in this disease, including erythrocytosis, hypertension, hypercalcemia, enteropathy, excessive gonadotropin production, hyperpyrexia, anemia, hepatopathy (Stauffer's syndrome), amyloidosis, and neuromyopathy (RUBIN et al. 1975). At the time of initial presentation, 30%–45% of patients have no symptoms directly related to the primary tumor. Oftentimes the earliest symptoms are weight loss,

weakness, and anemia, which occur in approximately one-third of patients. Sixty percent have vague abdominal pain or other gastrointestinal complaints.

11.4 Pathology

Tumors of the kidney may be divided into those of embryonal origin (including nephroblastoma, congenital mesoblastic nephroma, and solitary multilocular cyst; renal adenocarcinoma, which is the subject of this chapter; and mesenchymal tumors) and tumors of the renal pelvis, which are epithelial or mesodermal in origin. Renal adenocarcinoma pathologically can be subclassified into clear cell, granular cell, sarcomatoid, and papillary. It is important to note that papillary renal adenocarcinomas are often hypovascular and may give this appearance angiographically.

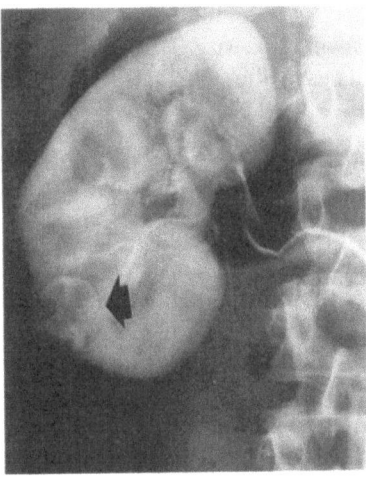

Fig. 11.2. Selective renal angiography. Small, 2 cm minimally hypervascular carcinoma *(arrow)* in parenchyma. Excretory urogram was perfectly normal

Table 11.1. Sites of metastases for renal adenocarcinoma

Site	%
Lung	50–60
Lymph nodes	30–40
Liver	30–40
Bone	30–40
Adrenal	20
Opposite kidney	10
Brain	5

Table 11.2. Comparison of modified ROBSON and TNM staging systems for renal adenocarcinoma

Modified Robson stage	T	N	M
I - Confined by renal capsule	T_1 – small T_2 – large	N_0	M_0
II - Through renal capsule confined by Gerota's fascia	T_{3a}	N_0	M_0
IIIa - Renal vein involvement	T_{3b}	N_0	M_0
IIIb - Lymphatic involvement	T_{1-3b}	N_{1-4}	M_0
IV - Contiguous organ involvement or	T_{1-3b}	N_{0-4}	M_0
Metastatic spread	T_{1-3b}	N_{0-4}	M_1

Approximately 85% of renal parenchymal tumors are adenocarcinomas, with 4% of patients with renal cancer having bilateral disease - either simultaneous or metachronous. Since the size of the tumor is directly related to the incidence of metastases, it has been suggested that a differentiation between adenoma and adenocarcinoma be made based on size. Proponents of this classification suggest that cortical tumors of less than 3 cm in diameter be classified as benign adenomas since small tumors are rarely metastatic (Fig. 11.2). Conversely, patients with tumors greater than 10 cm have an 80% chance of metastatic disease. It seems arbitrary to subclassify these tumors as adenoma or adenocarcinoma depending upon size since all sizes of tumors have demonstrated metastatic spread - only the incidence varies. It is our preference not to subclassify these tumors as adenomas, but rather to consider them all as malignancies irrespective of size. Renal adenocarcinoma may be graded histologically, and there is some correlation between survival and grade, those of higher grade usually having metastases (FUHRMAN et al. 1982).

Renal adenocarcinoma spreads hematogenously as well as via the lymphatics. The sites of metastases in order of frequency are listed in Table 11.1, the most common sites being lung, lymph nodes, liver, and bone. The lymphatic drainage of the kidney is variable and unfortunately is not always to the ipsilateral hilum. Solitary lymph node metastases have been reported in the iliac, hilar, intraaortocaval, supraclavicular, and subdiaphragmatic areas. In 10%–20% of patients, the tumor involves the ipsilateral renal vein, and in 8%–10% of patients, a tumor thrombus involves the inferior vena cava. Since approximately a third of patients will have metastases at the time of initial presentation, the prognosis of this tumor is often grave. The prognosis is better if the metastasis is solitary: 1.5%–3.5% of patients with renal adenocarcinoma will have solitary metastases which are amenable to surgical therapy. Patients who have their solitary metastases and primary tumor removed have a 5-year survival between 34% and 59% (TOBIA and WHITHMORE 1975; O'DEA et al. 1978).

11.5 Staging

There are two staging systems which are in common use: the TNM system, which has the advantage of being more specific but the disadvantage of being cumbersome, and a modification of the Robson staging system, which has more practicality and is more widely used in this country. Table 11.2 illustrates both staging systems. The prognosis and survival are clearly dependent upon the stage of the disease. For stage I tumors, 60%–70% 5-year survivals are reported; for stage II, 50%–65%; and for stage III A or those with only renal vein involvement, 50%–60%, provided the extension in the renal vein is not into the inferior vena cava. Patients with extension into the inferior vena cava but not above the diaphragm have a 25%–35% 5-year survival. When the tumor thrombus extends above the diaphragm into the atrium, the survival is limited. Stage III B patients or those with node disease have a 15% 5-year survival; however, if only several nodes are involved with microscopic disease and these are resected, the 5-year survival is much better (PETERS and BROWN 1980; GIULIANO et al. 1983; deKERNION 1980). Stage IV disease has a 0%–5% 5-year survival. The prognosis is most dependent on the presence of distant metastases or nodal involvement, with a lesser dependence on the tumor size, its grade, sex of the individual, and whether or not the renal veins are involved. If adjacent organs are involved, the survival is markedly reduced and approximates 10%. The natural history of renal cancer in the solitary kidney or when both kidneys are involved with tumor is the same stage for stage as described above. In the solitary kidney, if surgery is not performed there is approximately a 27% survival; with bilateral involvement there is no survival at 2 years. With therapy for either solitary tumors or bilateral tumors the survival is markedly improved and is dependent upon complete excision of the tumor (PALMER 1983).

Since there is very little alternative therapy to offer patients with renal cell carcinoma, in that chemotherapy and radiotherapy are relatively ineffective, surgery plays a dominant role in the therapy for the disease. A radical nephrectomy should be performed for all renal adenocarcinomas which are confined, i.e., stages I and II. A radical nephrectomy includes Gerota's fascia, the ipsilateral adrenal, and the hilar, periaortic, and intraaortocaval lymph nodes. Whether lymphadenectomy is beneficial or not is unclear (GIULIANO et al. 1983; deKERNION 1980). Certainly for stage A and B disease it has no therapeutic benefit. However, others report that stage C disease with lymphadenectomy carries a 44% 5-year survival, whereas without lymphadenectomy a 26% 5-year survival is obtained (PETERS and BROWN 1980). ROBSON (1982) and GIULIANO et al. (1983) also reported an increased survival in patients with node disease who underwent lymphadenectomy. These data, however, have not been confirmed by others, and the therapeutic benefit of lymphadenectomy remains controversial (deKERNION 1980). It is likely, nevertheless, that if one or two microscopic foci are found there is a therapeutic advantage to lymphadenectomy, increasing the 5-year survival in those with node-positive disease from 0% to 17%–30%. Patients with inferior vena caval extension also benefit from removal of the tumor thrombus as well as the primary tumor. When the tumor thrombus extends only into the renal vein, the survival is comparable to that in patients with stage I or II disease. However, if it extends into the vena cava, the survival is reduced.

11.6 Renal Cancer Invading the Vena Cava

The average age of patients with renal cancer invading the vena cava is 58, with a male to female ratio of 1.5:1. The primary tumor is more often on the right, occurring in that location approximately 69%–88% of the time. When the vena cava is involved there is generally invasion around the entrance of the renal vein. Upon exploration, unsuspected metastases are noted in approximately 45% of patients (KEARNEY et al. 1981). Signs of vena cava obstruction occur in 7%–36% of patients and include: edema, abdominal distention with ascites, liver dysfunction, nephrotic syndrome, venous collaterals on the abdominal wall, varicocele, malabsorption, pulmonary embolus, and jugular venous distention. When the vena cava is occluded a number of collaterals occur through which the blood returning from the lower extremities gains access to the right heart. The most prominent collaterals are the hemiazygos and azygos systems, and to a lesser degree the veins of the anterior abdominal wall and the mesenteric venous system (DUCKETT et al. 1973). Vena cava tumor thrombus is classified into one of two groups according to location: supradiaphragmatic, which is subclassified into intracardiac or intrapericardial, and infradiaphragmatic, which includes suprahepatic or infrahepatic (LIBERTINO et al. 1987; BISSADA et al. 1977). The survival in these patients is dependent upon whether or not there are positive nodes. If, in fact, the nodes are positive, there is no 5-year survival, and if there are distinct metastases, again there is no 5-year survival. With patients who have the tumor extracted and the tumor involves the infrahepatic vena cava, there is a 42%–53% 5-year survival (CHERRIE et al. 1982). If the tumor thrombus is above the diaphragm, the survival is limited.

Occasionally, the vena cava requires resection. In these patients, approximately one-quarter to one-third require dialysis after the resection (KEARNEY et al. 1981). One must preserve the drainage of the renal vein. On the right the renal vein may be anastomosed to the portal vein, and on the left it may be anastomosed to the inferior mesenteric vein. There is, however, no evidence that vena cava resection improves survival over a mere venacavotomy. The complications which follow cancer invading the vena cava include pulmonary embolus, which is often fatal, elevated bilirubin in 36%, renal dysfunc-

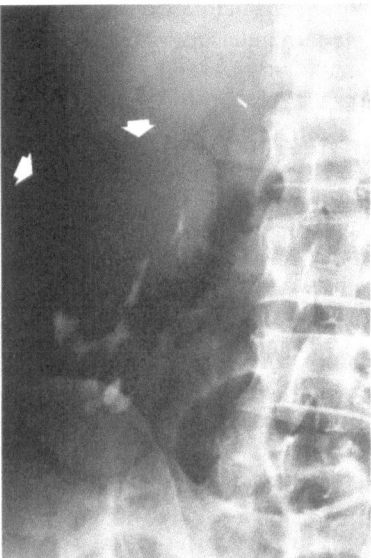

Fig. 11.3. Excretory urogram. Mass lesion in upper pole, right kidney. Parenchymal contour is effaced *(arrows)*. Collecting system is displaced inferiorly and medially by the mass lesion

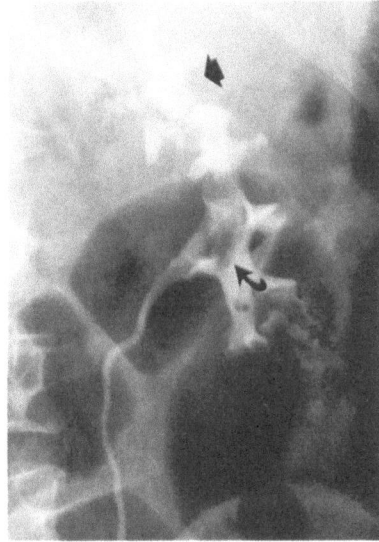

Fig. 11.4. Excretory urogram, renal cell carcinoma. Irregularity and distortion of the collecting system in the upper pole. Contrast collecting within parenchyma reflects ulceration and necrosis within tumor *(arrow)*. Filling defect in renal pelvis proved to be invasion by the tumor mass *(curved arrow)*

tion in 20%, pulmonary insufficiency in 12%, and adrenal insufficiency (NEVES and ZINCKE 1987; PRITCHETT et al. 1986). Not infrequently, patients with supradiaphragmatic thrombus will have a Budd-Chiari type syndrome in which severe liver dysfunction occurs.

11.7 Radiologic Imaging

11.7.1 Excretory Urography

Although numerous imaging modalities are utilized to discover and characterize renal cell carcinoma, the investigation usually begins with excretory urography in the assessment of hematuria, flank pain, weight loss, etc. Many renal cell carcinomas are detected coincidentally; about 30% are first observed during urography performed for other reasons. The sensitivity of excretory urography for detection of renal masses may not compare to that of other available imaging techniques, but is enhanced by utilization of meticulous technique. As a matter of fact, only one-third of all small tumors (less than 3 cm in diameter) will be discovered initially by excretory urography (CURRY et al. 1986) (Fig. 11.2). Careful examination of the preliminary film may reveal abnormalities suggestive of tumor. Focal bulging and irregular contour may be detected and suggest the presence of a renal mass (Figs. II.3, II.4). Local en-

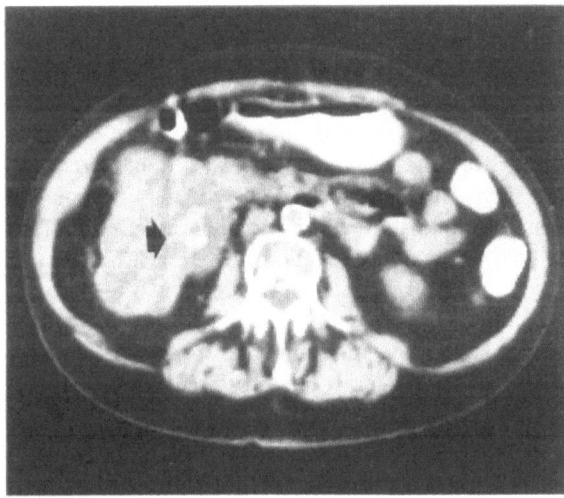

Fig. 11.5. CT; renal cell carcinoma. Large irregular mass containing amorphous deposit of calcification *(arrow)*

largement in either the longitudinal or the transverse axis may be recognized. If the neoplasm diffusely infiltrates the kidney, global enlargement of the kidney may be manifested. A proper examination should insure that the entire renal contour be evaluated. Loss of normal contour is easily overlooked but may reflect the presence of a peripherally placed tumor. Calcification may be present within the confines of a neoplasm (Fig. 11.5). Indeed, about 5% of renal cell carcinomas demonstrate dystrophic calci-

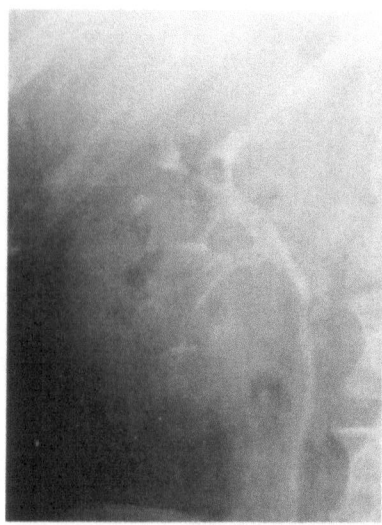

Fig. 11.6. Excretory urogram; renal cell carcinoma. Renal outline normal; collecting system shows no displacement. Soft tissue defect filling the collecting system reflects blood clot and tumor invading the renal pelvis

fication, the appearance of which is neither specific nor distinctive. Calcific deposits may also be found in tuberculosis, xanthogranulomatous pyelonephritis, cyst, aneurysm, and occasionally hamartomatous masses. The presence of calcification within a renal mass, however, requires further investigation to exclude the existence of carcinoma.

Distortion of the pelvicalyceal system is frequently seen. Infundibula and calyces may be splayed, displaced, distorted, or irregular in contour (Fig. 11.4). Calyceal amputation may reflect obstruction by the tumor mass. Appreciation of these abnormalities requires optimal visualization of the collecting system. Adequate amounts of contrast and utilization of ureteral compression are helpful to enhance pelvicalyceal filling. Mass lesions frequently alter the axis of the intrarenal collecting system, which normally aligns from superomedial to inferolateral in direction. Such distortion of the normal axis is more often due to masses in either the upper or the lower pole of the kidney. The presence of filling defects within the calyces or pelvis may be noted and can be the result of blood clots within the collecting system when the tumor causes hematuria (Fig. 11.6). At times, however, the parenchymal tumor will invade the collecting system, resulting in filling defects. Such invasion may also obstruct infundibula or calyces and result in focal dilatation of parts of the intrarenal collecting system.

On occasion one may encounter nonvisualization of the collecting system. This is generally the result of occlusion of the renal vein, commonly a reflection of neoplastic extension. The kidney outline may be enlarged and is often irregular because of the associated intrarenal mass. On occasion serpiginous irregular soft tissue structures may be identified in the perirenal fat. These reflect enlarged collateral venous vessels and are not specific, occasionally being the result of increased blood flow secondary to the often accompanying hypervascularity of the tumor. Such a finding is more readily appreciated by computed tomography. The existence of venous collaterals secondary to renal vein occlusion is at times also manifested by ureteral notching, the result of extensive periureteral collateral venous drainage.

11.7.2 Computed Tomography

Although excretory urography is a reasonable screening tool for the presence of renal masses, computed tomography (CT) is more sensitive and yields considerably more information regarding a mass already discovered (LEVINE et al. 1980). CT is currently the primary technique for evaluation of mass definition, size, extension, spread, and tissue characterization.

The combination of state-of-the-art equipment and meticulous technique is necessary for optimal evaluation of the kidneys. The examination should begin with scanning at 1-cm cuts without use of contrast. Normal renal parenchyma will demonstrated density of 30–60 Hounsfield units (depending upon state of hydration, level of hematocrit, technology of the scanner, etc.). Although the corticomedullary junction will be identifiable, its definition will be enhanced by use of iodinated contrast. The presence of calcification should be noted and may be obscured by the subsequent use of contrast. Both pre- and postcontrast scans are necessary components of the examination. The contrast may be delivered in bolus fashion or by infusion; some examiners will use both techniques. Dosage of contrast so as to deliver 20–40 Gm iodine is usually ample. On occasion it is quite helpful to employ rapid sequence filming at some levels after the bolus injection of contrast, so-called dynamic CT, to answer specific questions as regards the vascular distribution (LANG 1983, 1984a, b).

The presence of a renal mass is characterized by alteration of the normal renal outline and distortion of parapelvic fat, collecting system, and/or renal capsule. The most common renal mass is a simple cyst, and the differentiation of cyst from solid tumor, especially renal cell carcinoma, is critical. The ability to differentiate cyst from neoplasm by CT is in the neighborhood of 95% (McCLENNAN et al. 1979).

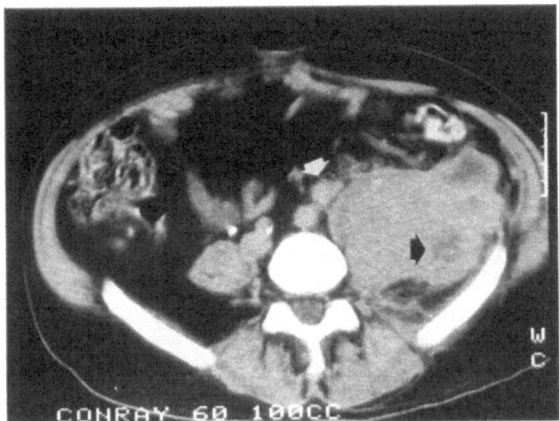

Fig. 11.7. CT, enhanced; renal cell carcinoma. Very large, irregularly shaped tumor, extending beyond perirenal space anteriorly. Low density zone reflects tumor necrosis *(black arrow)*. Extension to hilar lymph node noted *(white arrow)*

The CT diagnosis of simple renal cyst must be based on the presence of thin wall, homogeneous attenuation of water-like density, and lack of enhancement after injection of contrast. Failure to note any of these characteristics increases the level of suspicion for tumor and warrants further investigation. Evidence of any fatty tissue within the mass makes the diagnosis of angiomyolipoma (hamartoma) very likely (BOSNIAK et al. 1988). There are times when the only indication of the presence of a small renal cell tumor is the presence of a spontaneous subcapsular hematoma (HILTON et al. 1981). CT is a valuable tool in such a discovery.

The mass of renal cell carcinoma is usually irregular in outline and heterogeneous in density (Figs. 11.7, 11.8). Areas of reduced attenuation often reflect necrosis within the tumor mass (Fig. 11.9). Such necrosis could give a cystic appearance to the mass (Fig. 11.7). However, the wall would be thick and irregular. Characteristic patterns for cystic renal cell carcinoma include a cyst greater than 10 cm in diameter, localized wall thickening, focal enhancement of the cyst wall, and irregularity of the cyst-kidney interface (PARIENTY et al. 1985). The presence of calcification within the mass is strong evidence for a neoplasm (Fig. 11.5), although some inflammatory lesions may exhibit a similar finding. If the calcification is curvilinear and peripheral, a simple cyst is more likely (DAVIDSON 1985). Renal cell carcinomas will generally enhance after the injection of contrast, although the enhancement may be patchy and irregular due to areas of necrosis. Most carcinomas demonstrate a hypodense attenuation pattern when compared to the surrounding normal renal parenchyma, and this is exaggerated after the administra-

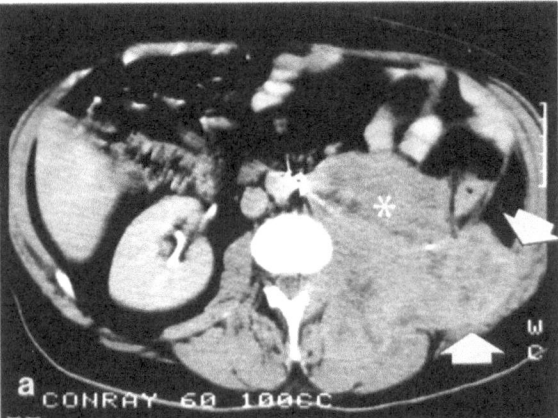

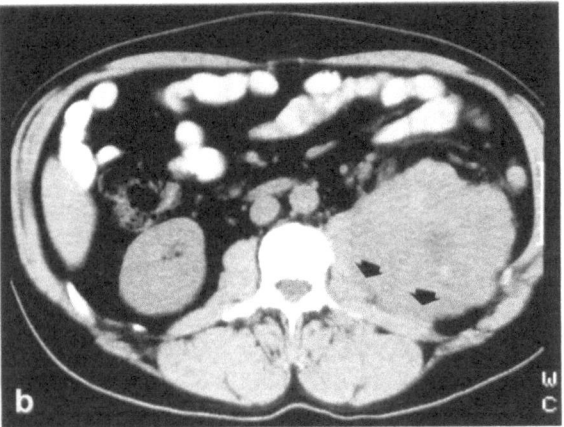

Fig. 11.8a, b. CT; recurrent renal cell carcinoma. a There is extensive extension of the tumor into the paravertebral and flank muscles *(arrows)* as well as the anterior pararenal space *(asterisk)*. b Posterior extension through posterior pararenal space and into adjacent muscle

tion of iodinated contrast material. However, occasionally one will encounter a carcinoma with a hyperdense pattern. Such an attenuation pattern may become isodense to the renal tissue when contrast enhancement is employed (Fig. 11.10).

Computed tomography is effective in the search for evidence of extension of the tumor (WEYMAN et al. 1980; LANG 1984a, b). Gerota's fascia is usually well seen and the presence of tumor beyond the fascia can sometimes be appreciated (Figs. 11.7–11.9). It should be noted that localized thickening of Gerota's fascia is a frequent finding and does not necessarily indicate tumor extension into the perinephric space (MCCLENNAN and LEE 1982). Further, the modality is not overly sensitive in detecting the presence of perinephric spread. One series demonstrated only a 46% sensitivity, although the observation was specific for invasion in 98% of cases (JOHNSON et al. 1986). Identification of blood in the perinephric space is sometimes helpful. Extension

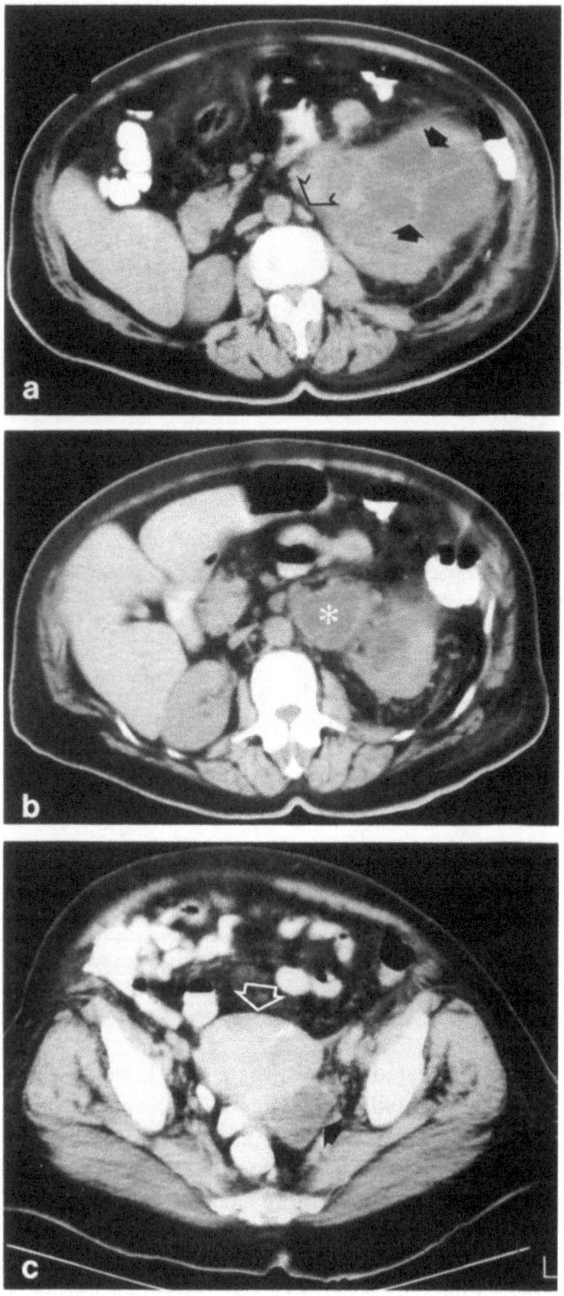

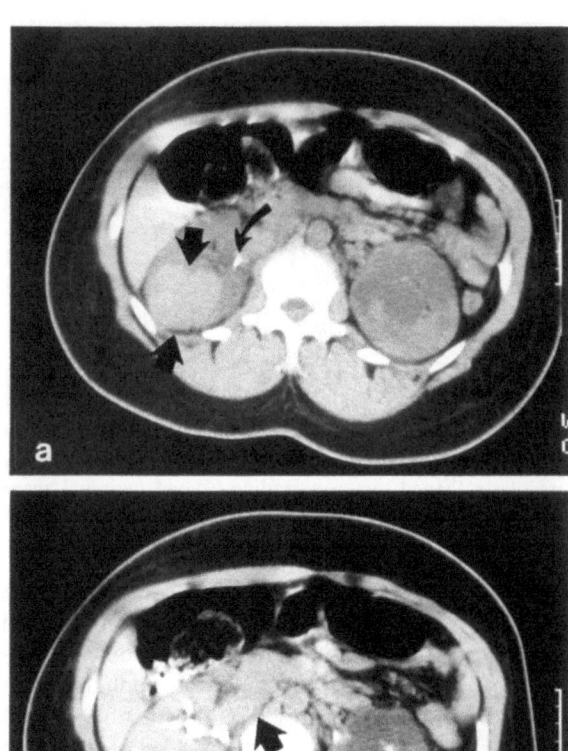

Fig. 11.9 a–c. CT, enhanced; renal cell carcinoma. Very extensive local extension of tumor. **a** Tumor extends into perirenal and anterior pararenal space. Numerous large foci of necrosis *(arrows)*. Small tumor-laden lymph node in hilum *(open arrow)*. **b** Large tumor thrombus filling and expanding the renal vein *(asterisk)*. **c** Direct extension of tumor *(arrow)* inferiorly into pelvis, adjacent to coincidentally enlarged uterus *(open arrow)*

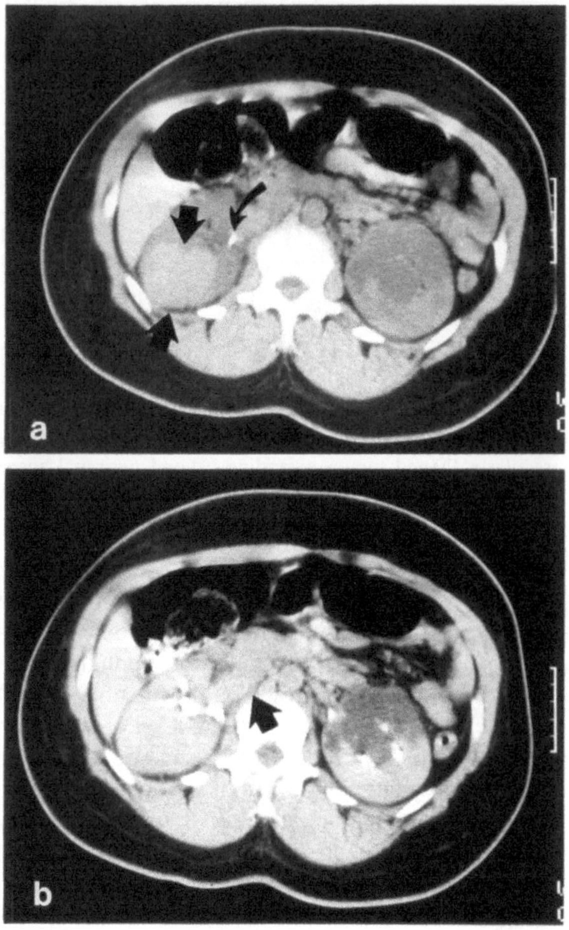

Fig. 11.10 a, b. CT, with and without contrast enhancement. **a** Without contrast. Renal cell carcinoma *(arrows)* in right kidney presenting as a mass with greater attenuation than the surrounding normal parenchyma. There is a ureteral stent in the right renal collecting system *(curved arrow)*. Note the several large lymph nodes in the renal hilum *(curved arrow)*. Incidental occurrence of segmental multicystic mass in left kidney. **b** The mass, hyperdense on the unenhanced scan, is now seen to be isodense after contrast. Such a lesion could be overlooked completely if the examination were limited to an enhanced scan only.

of tumor mass beyond the perinephric space is often seen as a reflection of invasion of the body wall or neighboring bones. Frequently, it is very difficult to ascertain the presence of liver invasion by a renal cell carcinoma involving the superior portion of the right kidney. CT may be unable to define the tissue plane between these two organs, resulting in a false impression of liver invasion.

The propensity of the dynamic computed tomogram to demonstrate tissues during the phase of capillary transit of contrast medium is useful for identification of hypervascular renal cell carcinomas.

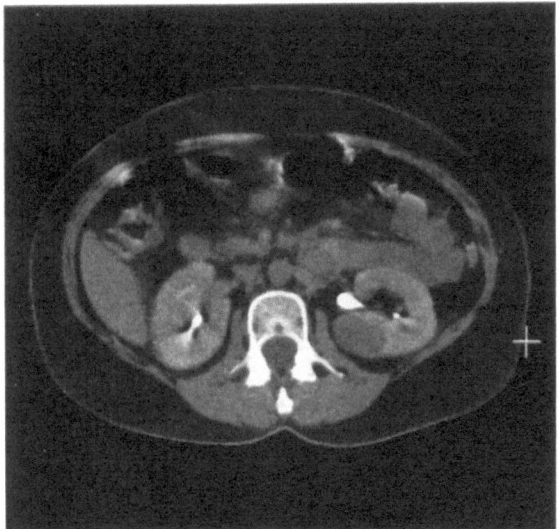

Fig. 11.11. Conventional postenhancement CT suggesting that the neoplasm is confined to the kidney. (LANG 1984b)

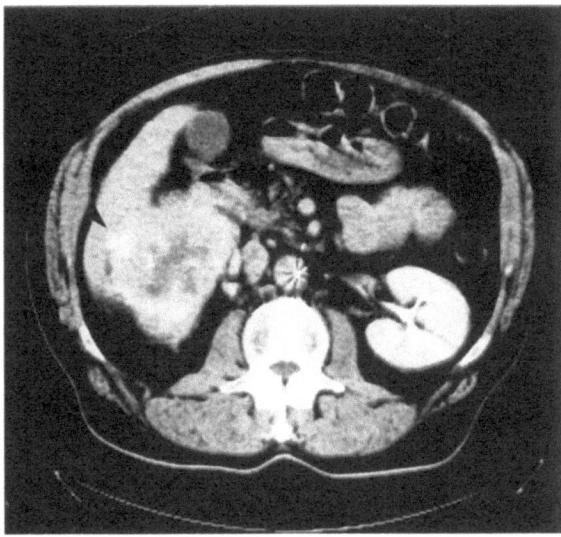

Fig. 11.13. Angio CT demonstrating contiguous extension of a hypervascular tumor component into the right liver lobe. (LANG 1986b)

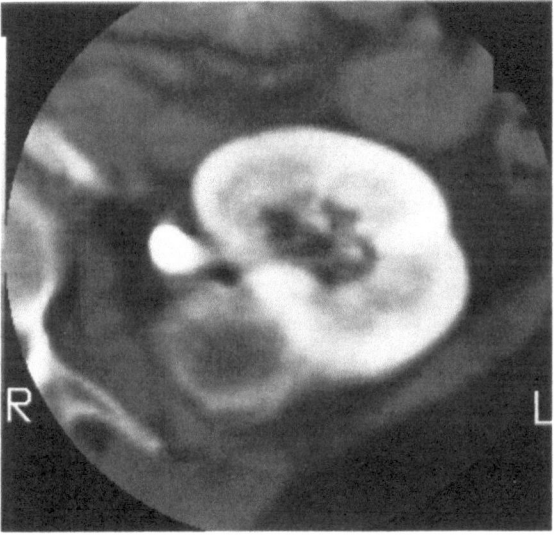

Fig. 11.12. Dynamic CT clearly demonstrating extension of hypervascular neoplasm into the perinephric space in the same patient as in Fig. 11.11. (LANG 1983)

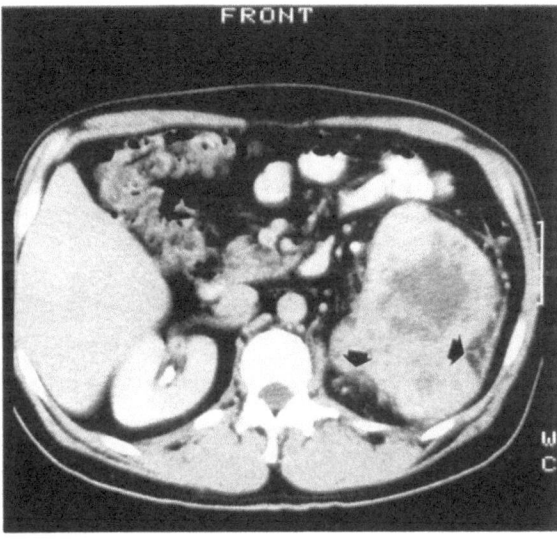

Fig. 11.14. CT, enhanced. Large necrotic tumor filling and expanding the perirenal space. Several small nodular densities, circular and linear *(arrows)*, reflect collateral venous pathways, in this case a reflection of renal vein tumor thrombosis

Extension of hypervascular tumor elements into the perirenal space or through anterior or posterior renal fascia is convincingly demonstrated on such studies (Figs. 11.11, 11.12) (LANG 1983, 1984a, b). Angio CT, a technique recording computed tomograms during and immediately after infusion of a relatively small amount of contrast medium through a catheter placed in the respective renal artery, offers even further improvement of detail. The latter technique has been advocated for resolving the often difficult question of contiguous tumor extension into an adjacent organ (Fig. 11.13).

The presence of lymph nodes, particularly in the area of the renal hilus, should be noted (Figs. 11.7, 11.9, 11.10). Nodes less than 1 cm in diameter are probably of no significance and are considered within limits of normal. Larger nodes, on the other hand, are likely a reflection of tumor spread. Rarely they may be reactive in nature.

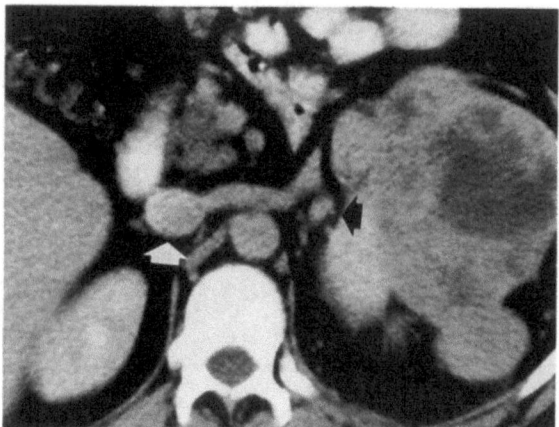

Fig. 11.15. CT, enhanced. Large renal vein secondary to tumor thrombus. Low density zone in inferior vena cava *(white arrow)* is due to extension of thrombus. An enlarged lymph node is also noted in hilar area *(black arrow)*

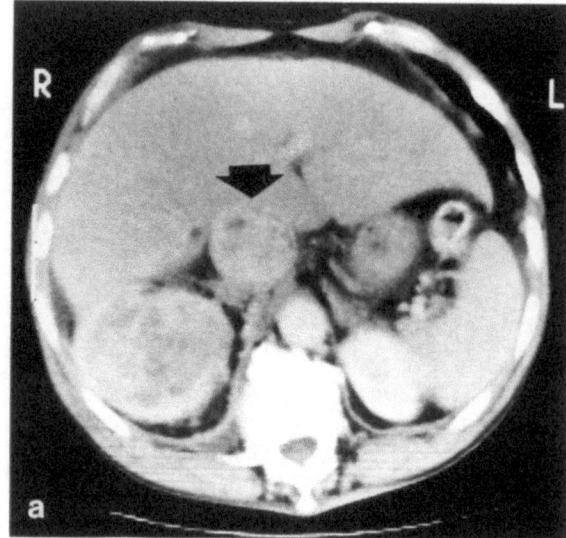

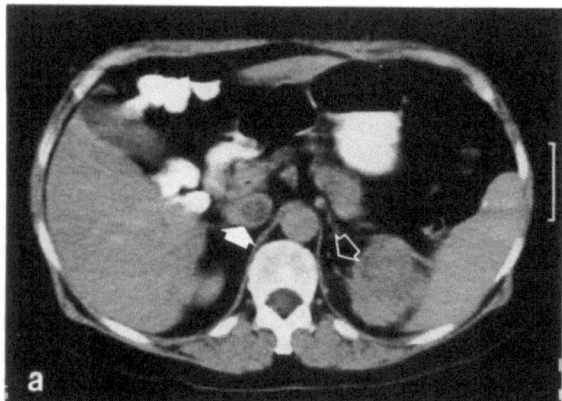

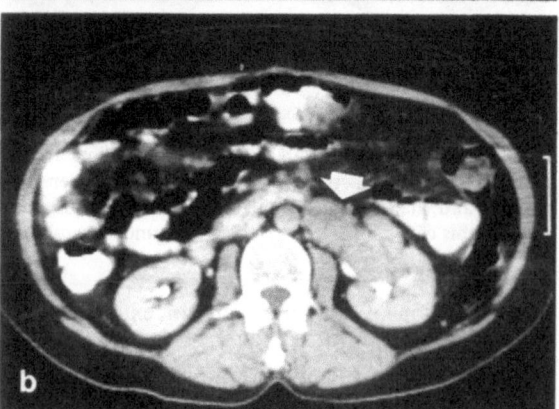

Fig. 11.16a, b. CT; renal cell carcinoma. **a** Large irregular mass of variable density in upper pole of left kidney. Collateral veins, secondary to renal vein occlusion, noted medial to tumor *(open arrow)*. Low density tumor thrombus noted in lumen of inferior vena cava *(white arrow)*. **b** Lower level. Enhanced scan. Renal vein dilated and irregular because of extensive tumor thrombus *(arrow)*

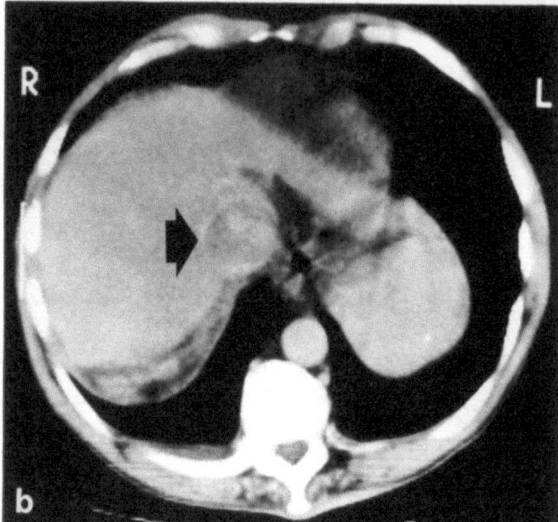

Fig. 11.17a, b. CT, enhanced; renal cell carcinoma. **a** Large necrotic tumor mass in right kidney. Inferior vena cava is markedly dilated and contains laminated and irregular tumor thrombus *(arrow)*. **b** More cephalad level. Intrahepatic portion of vena cava shows extension of tumor thrombus *(arrow)*

The propensity for neoplastic extension into the renal vein and beyond mandates evaluation of the vascular structures. Although CT is not as sensitive as either magnetic resonance imaging (MRI) or venography, it frequently enables the diagnosis of vascular extension to be established (Figs. 11.14–11.16). Enlargement of the renal vein, particularly when associated on contrast studies with a low density filling defect due to thrombus, is convincing evidence. Often there are abundant collateral vessels in the perinephric space, seen as serpiginous, spidery structures (Fig. 11.14). Although such an appearance often signifies obstruction of the renal vein with engorged collaterals, their presence may merely be a reflection of marked hypervascularity and increased blood flow through the renal circulation, tumor extension, or inflammatory change. It is important to evaluate the diameter of the inferior vena cava and to search for thrombus within its lumen on contrasted studies (Figs. 11.14, 11.16, 11.17). Bolus injections via the veins of the lower extremity were at one time advocated to help in this assessment. Such a technique may, however, result in false appearance of thrombus due to streaming phenomenon and poor mixing of contrast and uncontrasted blood in the vena cava. Cephalad extension of tumor thrombus in the inferior vena cava may be seen (Fig. 11.17) but is far better evaluated by venography or MRI.

Dynamic CT, once again, is useful for identification of tumor thrombus in the renal vein and inferior vena cava. The propensity of tumor thrombi to show opacification of giant capillaries within such thrombi during the phase of capillary enhancement facilitates their visualization by this technique (Figs. 11.18, 11.19) (LANG 1986b).

Finally, it should be noted that CT is valuable in detecting evidence of distant metastases. Examination of the patient with established or suspected renal cell carcinoma should always include study of the liver and adrenals. Evaluation of metastatic disease to lungs and bone is also necessary, but other modalities are usually employed. Obtaining a simultaneous scan of the chest and abdomen may be more efficient – if obtained it only requires the addition of a bone scan to complete the metastatic workup.

11.7.3 Ultrasound

The role of ultrasound in the diagnosis of renal cell carcinoma is limited. In the initial evaluation of an undefined renal mass, ultrasound is often the first imaging technique employed and is quite effective in differentiating a simple renal cyst from a solid tumor (Fig. 11.20). Indeed, if the rigid criteria of cyst (sonolucent mass with no internal acoustic echoes, sharp margins, far wall enhancement) are met, neoplasm can be excluded with reasonable assurance. However, determinations of mass margins, tumor extension, and vascularity are sometimes less well defined with ultrasound than with CT.

Sonography may be helpful in the search for renal vein and inferior vena cava extension. Echogenic pattern within these vascular structures may reflect tumor thrombus.

The role of Doppler ultrasound in the evaluation of renal cell carcinoma has not yet been established.

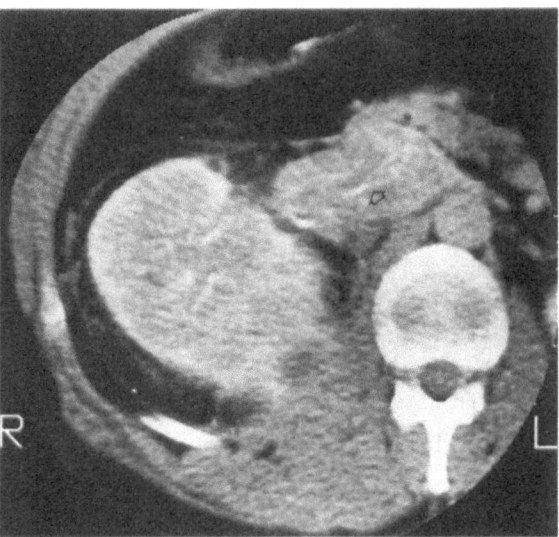

Fig. 11.18. Dynamic CT demonstrating opacification of giant capillaries in a tumor thrombus in the renal vein *(open arrow)* during the phase of capillary transit of contrast medium. (LANG 1987)

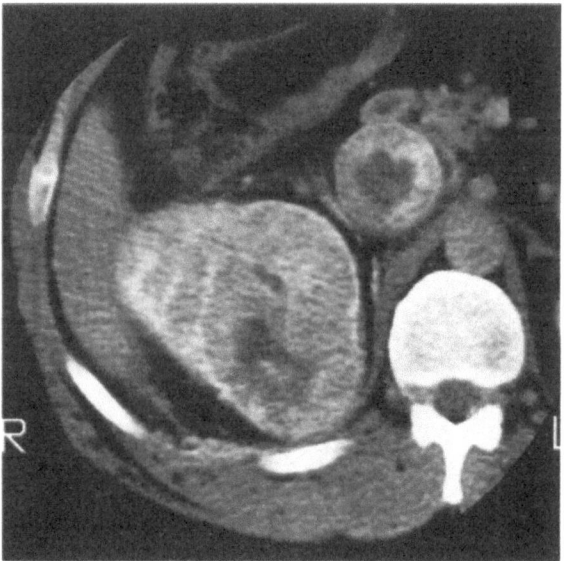

Fig. 11.19. Dynamic CT in the same patient as in Fig. 11.18, demonstrating dense capillary enhancement of a tumor thrombus adherent to the wall of the inferior vena cava. Note the presence of a patent central lumen. (LANG 1986b)

DUBBINS has demonstrated that at least three flow patterns may be seen with these tumors and suggests that this technology may play a role in the preliminary investigation of some renal masses (DUBBINS and WELLS 1986). Its ultimate role has not yet been determined.

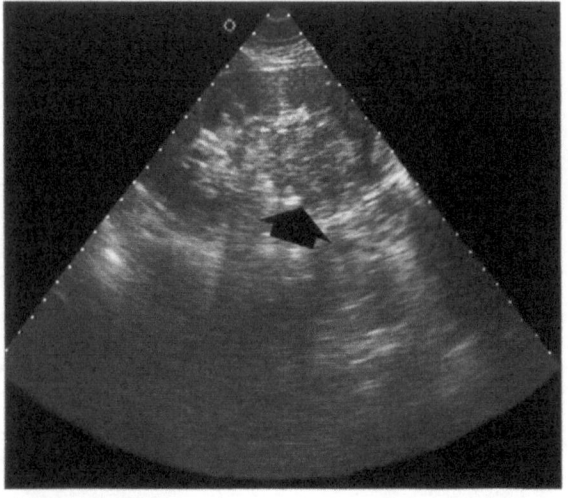

Fig. 11.20. Ultrasound. Irregular echogenic mass *(arrow)* in mid-zone of kidney, reflecting a solid mass and consistent with renal cell carcinoma. (Courtesy of A. C. FLEISCHER, M. D., Nashville, TN)

Fig. 11.22. Selective renal angiography; hypervascular carcinoma. Vessels distorted, crowded, and increased in number with disruption of the normal architecture

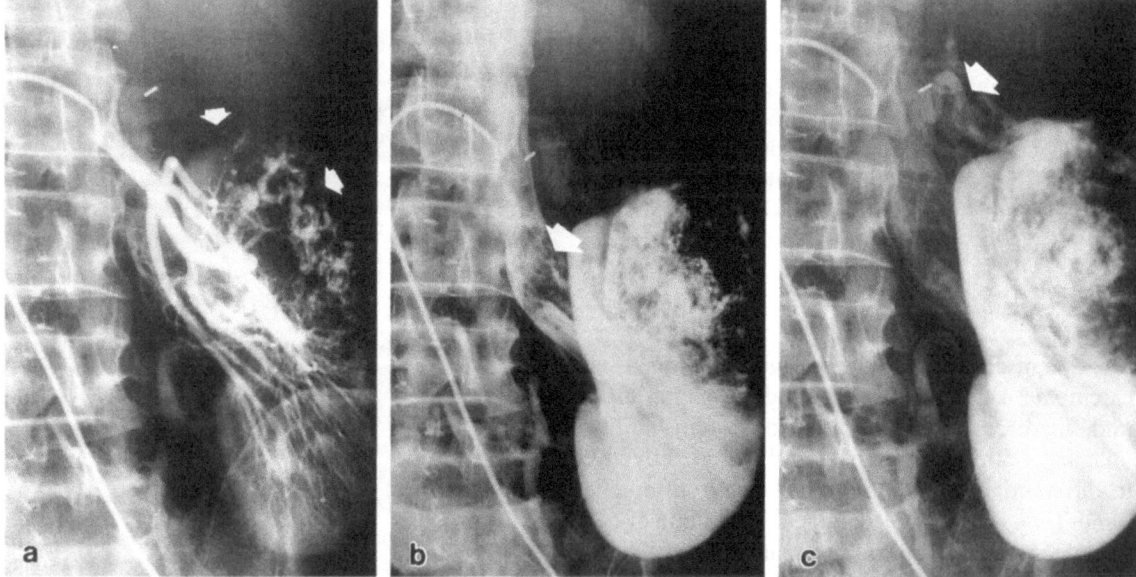

Fig. 11.21 a–c. Selective renal arteriography; renal cell carcinoma. **a** Arterial phase. Large irregular, hypervascular mass in upper pole of right kidney *(arrows)*. Neovascularity, puddling, and arteriovenous shunting is noted. **b** Hypervascular mass is better defined. Left renal vein is filled. Note the large throm- bus occluding the lumen of the vein *(arrow)*. **c** Venous collateral is noted *(arrow)*. This may be due either to the increased vascular flow, the venous occlusion, or a combination of both factors

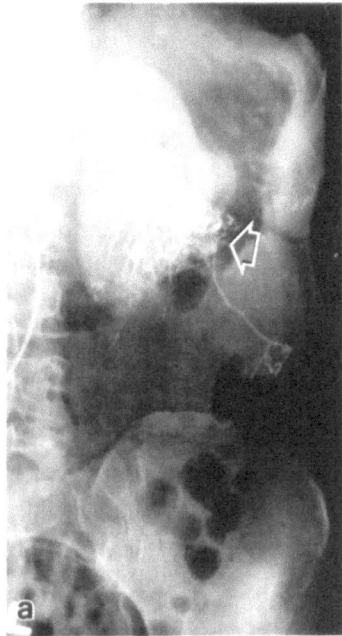 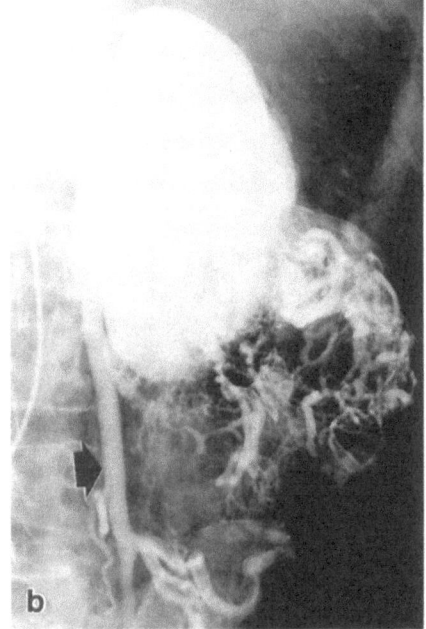

△

Fig. 11.23a, b. Selective renal angiography; hypervascular carcinoma. **a** Large, very vascular tumor in lower pole of left kidney. Note bizarre appearance of primitive-appearing vasculature *(open arrow).* **b** Parasitization. A significant contribution to the blood supply of this tumor is derived from the superior mesenteric artery *(arrow).* Tumor is seen to extend far beyond the confines of the renal capsule

11.7.4 Angiography and Venography

Evaluation of the vascular renal structures plays an important role in the diagnosis and staging of renal cell carcinoma. Most adenocarcinomas of the kidney are quite vascular and characterized by the angiographic appearance of neovascularity, arteriovenous shunting with early vein filling, vascular puddling of contrast, tumor staining, and vascular extension often beyond the confines of the kidney (Figs. 11.21–11.24) (LANG 1973).

A minority of these tumors will be hypovascular and pose a distinct diagnostic problem. They may still, however, demonstrate focal areas of arteriovenous shunting or neovascularity. Irregularity of the caliber of the vessels may reflect encasement by infiltrating tumor (Fig. 11.25). Such hypovascularity within the tumor often denotes papillary adenocarcinoma (BARD et al. 1982). Zones of hypovascularity within a tumor may be a reflection of necrosis and cavitation. Search for zones of neovascularity in a hypovascular mass may be aided by the utilization of 5–10 µg epinephrine injected selectively into the renal artery 30–60 s prior to selective angiography

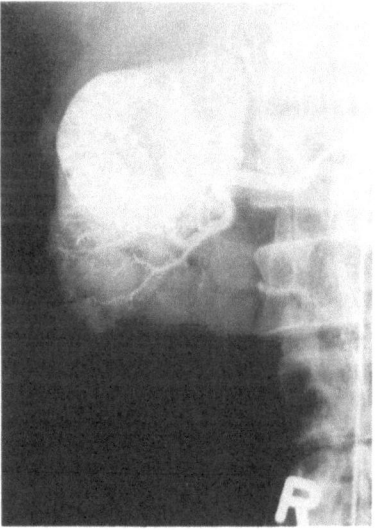

Fig. 11.24. Selective renal angiography; well-demarcated carcinoma. A large, very vascular, but sharply marginated renal cell carcinoma. The pattern is somewhat suggestive of that seen with oncocytoma

(Fig. 11.25). Epinephrine will cause profound vasoconstriction of normal vessels and the vessels associated with inflammatory change but has little or no effect on tumor neovascularity.

Not all hypervascular renal masses are due to adenocarcinoma. Indeed, inflammatory masses may present with increased blood supply and contrast staining. Characteristically, this increased vascularity consists of an increase in normal appearing,

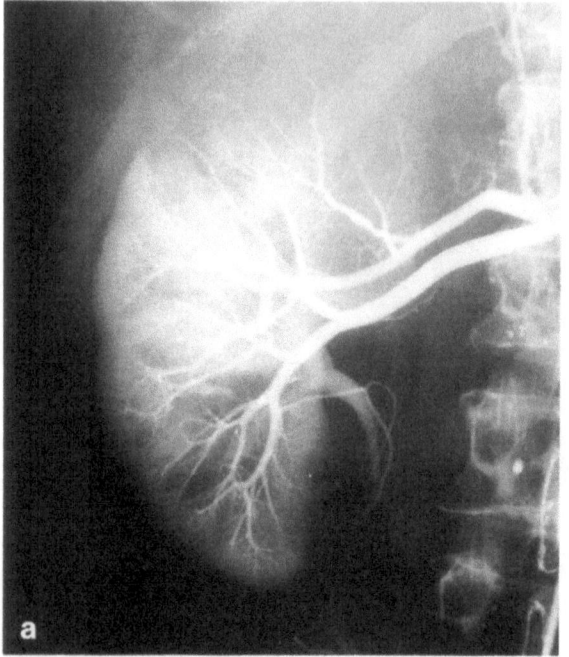

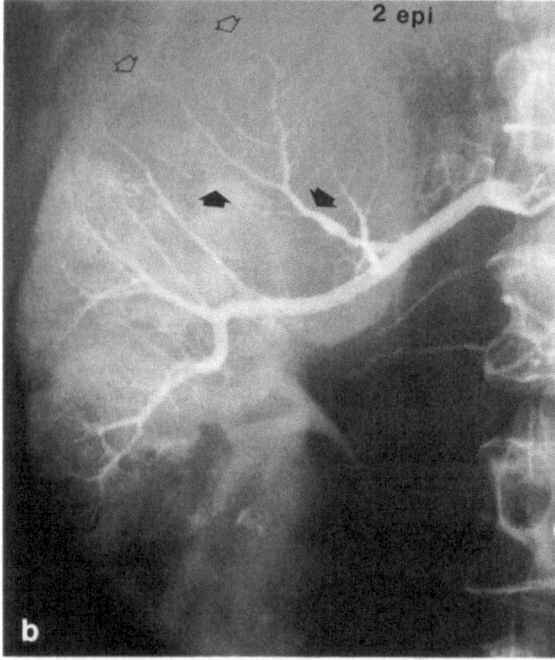

Fig. 11.25 a, b. Selective renal angiography; hypovascular renal cell carcinoma. **a** Large, relatively hypovascular mass in upper pole of right kidney. **b** Intraarterial administration of epinephrine followed by selective angiography confirms the hypovascular nature of the lesion. However, the vessels are seen to be distorted with encasement in several locations due to the infiltrating neoplasm *(arrows)*

relatively orderly vessels. Encasement, puddling, arteriovenous shunting, and neovascularity are cited as being indicative of neoplasm (ELKIN 1980). However, LEVIN et al. (1976) demonstrated the nonspecificity of increased vascularity and the extreme difficulty in differentiating some inflammatory masses from adenocarcinoma.

Extension of the tumor into the renal vein is often detected by angiography. The kidney is enlarged, there is visualization of a dilated renal vein, and collateral venous structures may be identified in the perirenal and periureteral spaces (Fig. 11.21). Filling of the collecting system may be absent or delayed. Venography is, in fact, a more accurate technique to assess venous tumor thrombus. It not only identifies renal vein involvement but also assesses the extent of thrombus into the inferior vena cava (Figs. 11.26, 11.27). Such information is necessary for proper surgical planning. Selective renal venography is accurate in detecting renal vein involvement. Although it carries a theoretical risk of tumor embolus if tumor thrombus exists, there is little evidence to suggest that such an occurrence is likely.

Evidence is accumulating that contrast CT approaches venacavography in assessing caval involvement (CRONAN et al. 1988). It would appear that MRI may be the technique of choice to study tumor extension into the venous system. Initial reports are quite favorable in this regard, and it seems likely that, when available, this may be the technique of choice to search for tumor thrombus in renal vein and vena cava.

11.7.5 Magnetic Resonance Imaging

The role of MRI in the diagnosis of renal cell carcinoma is as yet uncertain. Although it was hoped that MRI would demonstrate the ability to differentiate benign from malignant tumors, most studies reveal a wide range of values for calculated T1 and T2 in the assessment of solid renal masses (Figs. 11.28, 11.29) (PATEL et al. 1987). HRICAK has demonstrated, however, that calculated T1 and T2 measurements are usually higher than the surrounding parenchyma (HRICAK et al. 1985). Generally, T1-weighted images of renal masses will permit differentiation of cyst and solid mass. This is, however, not consistent. Cysts, as well as solid mass lesions, show a wide range of signal intensity. Further, both solid masses and cysts may appear very intense of T2-weighted images (PATEL et al. 1987). Fortunately, CT and ultrasound have permitted the differentiation of these lesions with 95%–97% accuracy (McCLENNAN

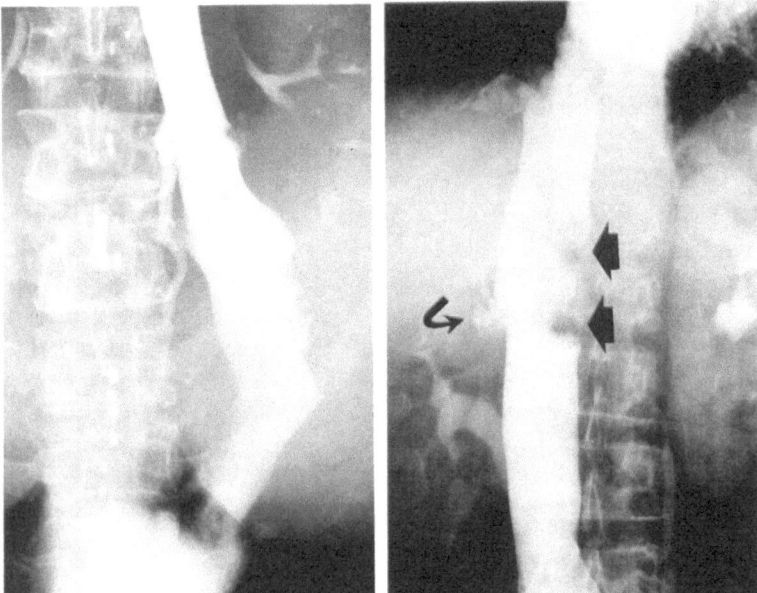

△
Fig. 11.26 *(left)*. Venacavogram. Long segment of tumor thrombus extending into vena cava from right renal vein. Occluded renal vein not opacified

Fig. 11.27 *(right)*. Inferior venacavogram. Irregular tumor thrombus extending into vena cava *(arrows)* from left renal vein. Note reflux of contrast into patent right renal vein *(curved arrow)*

et al. 1979; BALFE et al. 1982). The relatively slow image acquisition times needed in MRI tend to degrade image sharpness and are detrimental in evaluating extent of involvement. The technical advances in this arena are, however, occurring with such rapidity that these qualifications may not be valid in the very near future. Detection of lymph node enlargement is currently no better than with CT, and the technology is as yet unable to identify the small, tumor-laden node. MRI does, however, have the capability to evaluate the venous anatomy, even without utilization of intravascular contrast media (Figs. 11.29, 11.30). This vascular imaging has been extremely valuable and has, in our institution, tended to replace venacavography for the assessment of tumor thrombi in renal vein and inferior vena cava. Identification of thrombus in these vascular structures may be accomplished without the need to revert to invasive procedures such as cavography. Further, evidence is accumulating to suggest that one can differentiate tumor thrombus from bland, nontumor thrombus, which frequently is present at the margins of the tumor thrombus, by use of gadolinium-DTPA labeling (FALKE et al. 1988). In addition, the ability to obtain images at any body

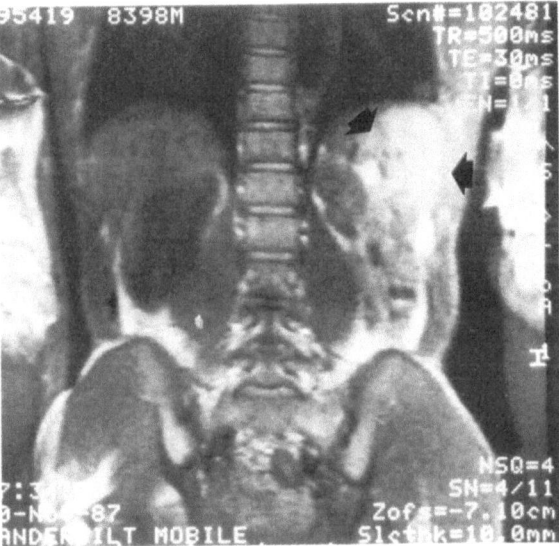

Fig. 11.28. MRI, renal cell carcinoma. T1-weighted image. Large mass arising from upper pole of left kidney and extending widely beyond perirenal space *(arrows)*

plane without degradation of detail is helpful in obtaining optimal venous depiction. There is evidence that MRI may, in fact, be superior to CT in assessing the presence of invasion of the liver by an adjacent right renal cell carcinoma (HRICAK et al. 1985). Currently, MRI would seem to offer promise as a valuable tool in the staging of renal cell carcinoma.

Some limitations to utilization of MRI should be mentioned. Claustrophobic reactions by a small number of patients can, at times, obviate the exam-

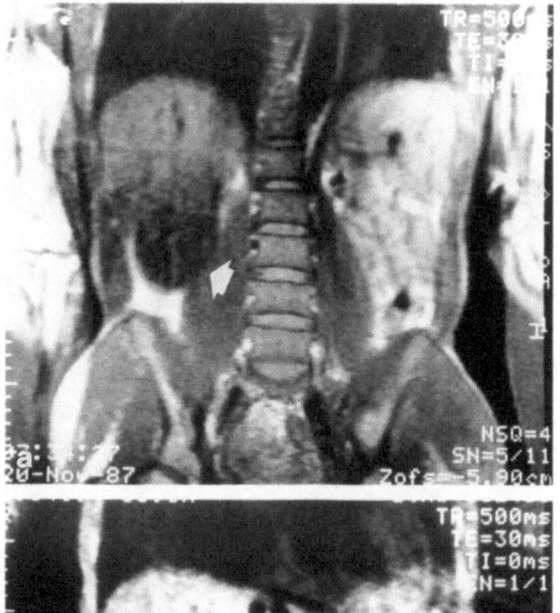

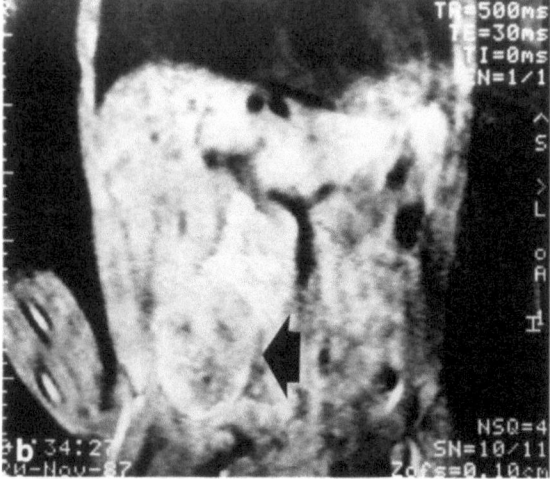

Fig. 11.29 a, b. MRI, coronal view. Renal cell carcinoma in patient with end-stage renal disease and renal allograft. **a** T1-weighted image. Large irregular mass with low signal intensity in lower pole of right kidney *(arrow)*. **b** More anterior image. Inferior vena cava caudal to level of renal veins is occluded by tumor thrombus and is not visualized. More cephalad portion of vena cava and the aorta are well defined. Note the allograft in the right iliac fossa *(black arrow)*

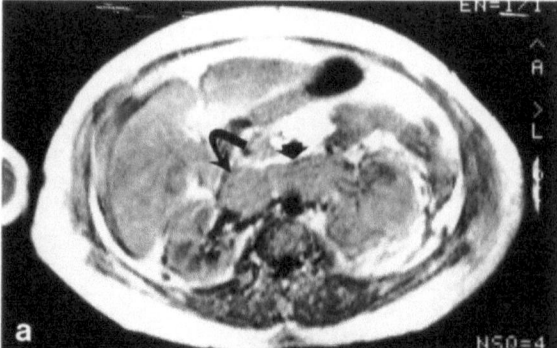

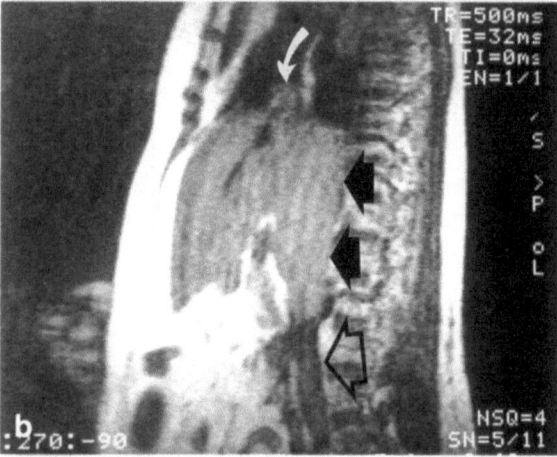

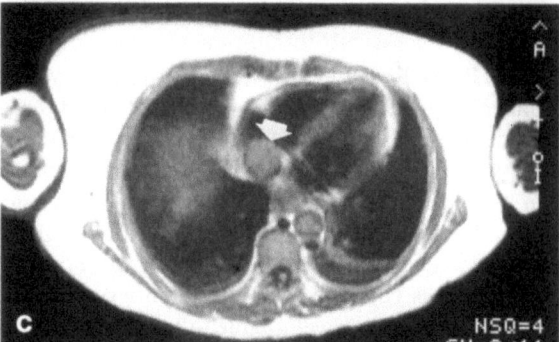

Fig. 11.30 a–c. MRI, renal cell carcinoma. Excellent example of delineation of tumor thrombus propagating through renal vein and inferior vena cava cephalad to right atrium. **a** Transverse section through renal vein. Absence of signal defect in left renal vein *(arrow)* and vena cava *(curved arrow)* reflects tumor thrombus. **b** Sagittal plane through vena cava. Tumor thrombus fills and distends vena cava *(black arrow)*. Tumor extends above diaphragm into right atrium *(curved arrow)*. Caudal portion of cava is spared *(open arrow)*. **c** Transverse section through heart. Obvious extension of thrombus into right atrium *(arrow)*. (Courtesy of M. MAZER, M. D., Nashville, TN)

ination. The presence of metallic foreign bodies (e.g., cardiac pacemakers) contraindicates the procedure. The slow imaging acquisition, as mentioned above, still results in some loss of detail when compared to rapid-imaging CT. Respiratory gating and larger magnets have already begun to correct this latter problem. It is likely that the role of MRI in diagnosis and staging of renal cell carcinoma will increase dramatically in the very near future.

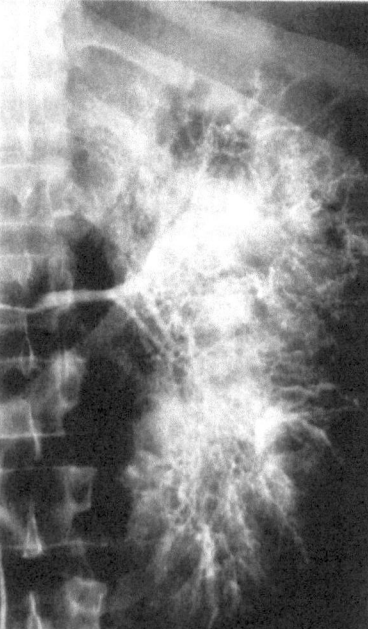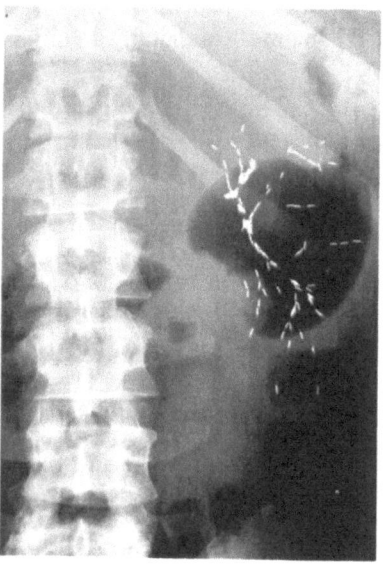

△

Fig. 11.31 *(left).* Arteriogram showing extensive neovascularity of renal cell carcinoma throughout the right kidney. (LANG 1988)

Fig. 11.32 *(right).* Iodine 125 particles have been seated in the neoplasm using a transcatheter embolization technique. There is satisfactory distribution of particles throughout the neoplasm to achieve a dose of 95 gyn

11.7.6 Evaluation for Distant Metastases

The role of imaging modalities in the preoperative evaluation for distant metastases will vary from center to center. Investigation for pulmonary metastases will be sought with CT or conventional tomography. CT is frequently performed to evaluate for hepatic involvement, although some contend that liver function studies are equally sensitive. The role of isotope bone scans is also unsettled. Although they are advocated by some, LINDNER has suggested that, in the patient without bone symptoms, alkaline phosphatase levels may be sufficient, and isotope investigations are not cost-effective on a routine basis (LINDNER et al. 1983). However, it is less cost-effective to subject a patient with metastatic disease to surgery. It is, therefore, our practice to obtain bone scans in all patients for whom therapy would be altered significantly if the scans were positive.

11.8 Therapy

The role of chemotherapy, immunotherapy, hormonal therapy, and radiation therapy is rather limited in this disease. Although local reduction in size may be achieved with radiation therapy, cure does not appear to be within the realm of this modality. Its use for palliation of bony metastases is its main role in this disease. Treatment by interstitial radiation therapy with iodine 125 permits delivery of a large dose in the range of 80–160 gyn to the tumor-bearing area with only a minimal integral dose to the host. The vascular bed of tumors has been a ready recipient for transcatheter embolization with iodine 125 particles to create such an interstitial infarct implant (LANG 1988). The method has been lauded for prolongation of life, reduction of tumor volume, creation of remission of activities, and curtailment of manifestations such as hematuria and pain (Figs. 11.31, 11.32). Despite attaining high dose level to the tumor-bearing area, cures have not resulted from this type of therapy. Chemotherapy is relatively limited. Progestational agents originally showed some promise, but more recent evidence suggests they have little benefit. Vinblastine has shown some promise in selected cases, but generally its effect is relatively modest. Immune RNA immunotherapy, interleukin, interferon, and activated killer lymphocyte therapy have also been used with limited and variable success. At this time there is no chemotherapy which is uniformly successful for the majority of patients. Thus, surgery continues to be the mainstay of therapy in this disease.

References

Balfe DM, McClennan BL, Stanley RJ et al. (1982) Evaluation of renal masses considered indeterminate on computed tomography. Radiology 142: 421–428

Bard RH, Lord B, Fromowitz F (1982) Papillary adenocarcinoma of kidney II. Radiographic and biologic characteristics. Urology 19: 16–19

Basile JJ, McCullough DL, Harrison LH, Dyer RB (1988) End stage renal disease associated with acquired cystic disease and neoplasia. Urology 140: 938–943

Bissada NK, Finkbeiner AE, Williams JD et al. (1977) Successful extraction of intracardiac tumor thrombus of renal carcinoma. J Urol 118: 474–475

Bosniak MA, Megibow AJ, Hulnick DH et al. (1988) CT diagnosis of renal angiomyolipoma: the importance of detecting small amounts of fat. AJR 151: 497–502

Cherrie RJ, Goldman DG, Lindner A, DeKernion JB (1982) Prognostic implications of vena caval extension of renal cell carcinoma. J Urol 128: 910–912

Cohen AJ, Li FP, Berg S et al. (1979) Hereditary RCC associated with chromosomal translocation. N Engl J Med 301: 592–595

Cronan JJ, Ridlen MS, Dorfman GS et al. (1988) Renal cell carcinoma: Can CT actually stage the IVC? AJR 151: 208

Curry NS, Schabel SI, Betsill WL (1986) Small renal neoplasms: diagnostic imaging, pathologic features and clinical course. Radiology 158: 113–117

Davidson AJ (1985) Radiology of the kidney. W. B. Saunders, Philadelphia, pp 329–394

deKernion J (1980) Lymphadenectomy for renal cell carcinoma, therapeutic complications. Urol Clin North Am 7: 697–703

Dubbins PA, Wells I (1986) Renal carcinoma: Duplex dropper evaluation. Br J Radiol 59: 231–236

Duckett JW Jr, Lifland JH, Peters PC (1973) Resection of the inferior vena cava for adjacent malignant diseases. Surg Gynecol Obstet 136: 711–716

Elkin M (1980) Radiology of the urinary system. Little, Brown, and Co., Boston, pp 299–327

Falke THM, Peetom JJ, van de Velde CJH et al. (1988) Gadolinium-DTPA enhanced MR imaging of intravenous extension of adrenocortical carcinoma. J Comput Assist Tomogr 12: 331–334

Fuhrman SA, Lasky LC, Limas C (1982) Prognostic significance of morphologic parameters in renal cell carcinoma. Am J Surg Pathol 6: 655–663

Giuliani L, Gilberti C, Ruggiero LM et al. (1983) Results of radical nephrectomy and extensive lymphadenectomy for renal cell carcinoma. J Urol 130: 664–668

Hilton S, Bosniak MA, Megibow AJ (1981) Computed tomographic demonstration of a spontaneous subcapsular hematoma due to a small renal cell carcinoma. Radiology 141: 743–744

Hricak H, Demas B, Williams R et al. (1985) Magnetic resonance imaging in the diagnosis and staging of renal and perirenal neoplasms. Radiology 154: 709–715

Johnson CD, Dunnick NR, Cohan RH et al. (1986) Renal adenocarcinoma: CT staging of 100 tumors. AJR 148: 59–63

Kearney GP, Waters WB, Klein LA, Richie JP, Gittes RF (1981) Results of inferior vena cava resection for renal cell carcinoma. J Urol 125: 769–773

Lang EK (1973) Arteriography in the diagnosis and staging of hypernephromas. Cancer 32: 1043–1052

Lang EK (1984a) Angio-computed tomography and dynamic computed tomography in staging of renal cell carcinoma. Radiology 151: 149–155

Lang EK (1984b) Comparison of dynamic and conventional computed tomography, angiography and ultrasonography in the staging of renal cell carcinoma. Cancer 54: 2205–2214

Lang EK (1986a) An algorithmic approach to the diagnosis and staging of renal neoplasms. Interventional uroradiology. W. B. Saunders, Philadelphia, pp 683–694

Lang EK (1986b) Percutaneous and interventional urology and radiology. Springer, Berlin Heidelberg New York

Lang EK (1988) Management of primary and metastatic renal cell carcinoma by transcatheter embolization with I-125. Cancer 62: 274–282

Levin DC, Gordon D, Kinkhabwala M et al. (1976) Reticular neovascularity in malignant and inflammatory renal masses. Radiology 120: 61–66

Levine E, Maklad NF, Rosenthall JJ et al. (1980) Comparison of computed tomography and ultrasound in abdominal staging of renal cancer. Urology 161: 317–322

Libertino JH, Zinman L, Watkins E Jr (1987) Long-term results of resection of renal cell cancer with extension into inferior vena cava. J Urol 137: 21–24

Lindner A, Goldman DG, deKernion JB (1983) Cost effective analysis of prenephrectomy radioisotope scans in renal cell carcinoma. Urology 22: 127–129

McClennan BL, Lee JKT (1982) Kidneys. In: Lee JKT, Sagel SS, Stanley RJ (eds) Computed body tomography. Raven, New York

McClennan BL, Stanley RJ, Weyman PJ et al. (1979) CT of the renal cyst: Is cyst aspiration necessary? AJR 133: 671–675

Neves RJ, Zincke H (1987) Surgical treatment of renal cancer with vena cava extension. Br J Urol 59: 390–395

Oberling C, Riviere M, Haguenau F (1960) Ultrastructure of the clear cells in renal carcinoma and its importance for the demonstration of their renal origin. Nature 186: 402–403

O'Dea MJ, Zincke H, Utz DC, Bernatz PE (1978) The treatment of renal cell carcinoma with solitary metastases. J Urol 120: 540–542

Palmer JM (1983) Role of partial nephrectomy in solitary or bilateral renal tumors. JAMA 249: 2357–2361

Parienty RA, Pradel J, Parienty I (1985) Cystic renal cancers: CT characteristics. Radiology 157: 741–744

Patel SK, Stack CM, Turner DA (1987) Magnetic resonance imaging in staging of renal cell carcinoma. Radiographics 7: 703–728

Peters PC, Brown GL (1980) The role of lymphadenectomy in the management of renal cell carcinoma. Urol Clin North Am 7: 705–709

Pritchett TR, Lieskovsky G, Skinner DG (1986) Extension of renal cell carcinoma into the vena cava: clinical review and surgical approach. J Urol 135: 460–464

Robson CJ (1982) Results of radical thoracoabdominal nephrectomy in the treatment of renal cell carcinoma. In: Kuss R, Murphy GP, Khoury S, Karr JP (eds) Renal tumors: proceedings of the first international symposium on kidney tumors. Alan R. Liss, New York, p 481

Rubin AL, Cheigh JS, Stenzel KH (1975) Symposium on endocrine functions of the kidney. Foreword. Am J Med 58: 1

Skinner DG, Pfister RF, Colvin R (1972) Extension of renal cell carcinoma into the vena cava; the rationale for aggressive surgical management. J Urol 107: 711–716

Sudeck P (1893) Zwei Fälle von Adenosarcom der Niere. Virchows Arch [A] 133: 558–562

Tobia BM, Whitmore WF Jr (1975) Solitary metastases from renal cell carcinoma. J Urol 114: 836–838

Wallace AC, Nairn RC (1972) Renal tubular antigens in kidney tumors. Cancer 29: 977–981

Waters WB, Richie JP (1979) Aggressive surgical approach to renal cell carcinoma: review of 130 cases. J Urol 122: 306–309

Weyman PJ, McClennan BL, Stanley RJ et al. (1980) Comparison of computed tomography and angiography in the evaluation of renal cell carcinoma. Radiology 137: 417–424

12 Renovascular Hypertension

Leif Ekelund and Sven-Ola Hietala

CONTENTS

12.1   Introduction 295
12.2   Etiology and Pathophysiology 295
12.3   Clinical Diagnosis 296
12.4   Radiologic Screening Methods 296
12.4.1 Urography 296
12.4.2 Nuclear Medicine 297
12.4.3 Doppler Ultrasonography 297
12.4.4 Intravenous Digital Subtraction Angiography . 298
12.4.5 Renal Angiography 298
12.4.5.1 Technique 299
12.4.5.2 Findings 299
12.4.5.3 Complications 300
12.5   Radiologic Appearances According to Etiology 300
12.5.1 Atherosclerosis 300
12.5.2 Fibromuscular Hyperplasia 301
12.5.3 Renal Artery Aneurysms 301
12.5.4 Arteriovenous Communications 302
12.5.5 Collagenous Disease of the Kidney 302
12.5.6 Embolization of the Renal Artery 303
12.5.7 Neurofibromatosis 303
12.5.8 Page Kidney 304
12.5.9 Hypertension Following Renal Transplantation 304
12.6   Imaging Following Revascularization
       Procedures 305
12.7   Radiologic Intervention
       in Renovascular Hypertension 306
12.7.1 Percutaneous Transluminal Renal Angioplasty 306
12.7.1.1 Technique 306
12.7.1.2 Results 307
12.7.1.3 Complications 307
12.7.2 Transcatheter Embolization
       of Renovascular Malformations 308
       References 308

12.1 Introduction

Hypertension may be defined as a blood pressure of 160/95 mm Hg or more. The great majority of hypertensive patients have essential hypertension and require lifelong medical therapy. Individuals with renovascular hypertension represent a small but important group of hypertensives as revasculari-

zation may cure these patients. The prevalence of renovascular hypertension was reported to range between 2% and 6% by HUNT and STRONG (1973). Significantly lower figures were reported from the Mayo Clinic, with a prevalence of 0.18% among hypertensives with a diastolic blood pressure ≥ 95 mm Hg (TUCKER and LABARTHE 1977). The "true" frequency is difficult to establish but a common opinion is that it is approximately 1% in unselected patients with hypertension (BECH and HILDEN 1975).

The purpose of this chapter is to briefly review the etiology and pathophysiology of renovascular hypertension, to indicate the role of various imaging procedures in diagnosis, and finally to describe interventional radiologic techniques for the management of renovascular hypertension.

12.2 Etiology and Pathophysiology

The term *renovascular hypertension* is reserved for those cases where the successful treatment of disease results in the amelioration or cure of blood pressure elevation. Atherosclerosis, fibromuscular lesions, thrombosis, embolism, arteritis, aneurysms, and dissections of the renal arteries all cause renovascular hypertension. In the Cooperative Study of renovascular hypertension, atherosclerosis accounted for 63% and fibromuscular hyperplasia for 32% of the cases of renovascular hypertension (SIMON et al. 1972).

Alteration in renal hemodynamics resulting in reduction of pulse and perfusion pressure stimulates the juxtaglomerular cells to produce the enzyme renin. Released in the circulation, renin hydrolyzes the liver-produced peptide angiotensinogen, forming the mildly vasoactive decapeptide angiotensin I, which is converted to the highly vasoactive octapeptide, angiotensin II. This acts upon systemic resistance vessels and, together with its stimulation of the adrenal gland to secrete aldosterone, serves to produce blood pressure elevation.

LEIF EKELUND, M.D. PhD., Professor and Chairman; SVEN-OLA HIETALA, M.D. PhD., Associate Professor of Diagnostic Radiology; Department of Diagnostic Radiology, University Hospital, 90185 Umeå, Sweden

12.3 Clinical Diagnosis

It is difficult to separate on a clinical basis patients with renovascular from those with essential hypertension. Heredity for hypertension is more common with the essential type. Some helpful clues to renovascular hypertension include:

1. Short duration of hypertension
2. Young patients
3. Onset after age 50
4. Abdominal bruit
5. Grade 3 or 4 fundoscopic changes

And perhaps more clinically relevant:

6. Moderate to severe, accelerated or malignant hypertension
7. Hypertension poorly responsive to maximal medical therapy
8. Reduced renal function

Examination of the peripheral plasma renin activity (PRA) has been used as a test for diagnosing renovascular hypertension. However, diet, posture, and drugs cause wide variations in PRA, and false-negative and false-positive results occur (KAUFMAN 1979). Saralasin, an angiotensin II antagonist, has been used for detecting renin-dependent hypertension, but although the initial studies were very encouraging, subsequent studies have shown the test to be positive in only 63% of proven cases (HORNE et al. 1979). Captopril, an angiotensin converting enzyme inhibitor, increases both sensitivity and specificity in the evaluation of PRA (MULLER et al. 1986). However, patients should discontinue antihypertensive medication 2 or preferably 4 weeks before testing, which may be practically impossible. The present opinion is that PRA analysis in peripheral blood is of limited value as a screening method owing to difficulties in standardization.

12.4 Radiologic Screening Methods

Only patients with a careful clinical evaluation indicating the possibility of renovascular etiology should be further studied by radiologic techniques.

12.4.1 Urography

Certain urographic abnormalities have long been recognized as indicative of renovascular disease. Rapid sequence urography (MAXWELL et al. 1964) provides several criteria that might indicate renovascular hypertension:

1. Difference in renal size (a right kidney 1.0 cm or a left kidney 1.5 cm smaller than the contralateral kidney)
2. Difference in nephrographic intensity
3. Delayed filling of collecting structures on the affected side
4. Hyperconcentration of the contrast medium in collecting structures of the affected side
5. Smaller collecting system on the affected side
6. Ureteral notching secondary to collateral circulation

At urography other abnormalities that may cause hypertension may also be demonstrated, such as calcified aneurysms, compression of renal parenchyma secondary to tumor or subcapsular hematoma, and chronic pyelonephritis. Occasionally, an unsuspected pheochromocytoma may be diagnosed while performing urography in a hypertensive patient. The Cooperative Study on Renovascular Hypertension (BOOKSTEIN et al. 1972a) found that the most useful sign was that of asymmetric pyelocalyceal appearance of contrast medium (Fig. 12.1). This was present in 59% of patients with renovascular disease. The false-positive rate was only 2%. Overall, urography correctly identified 83% of individuals with significant unilateral renal artery stenosis and 71% of those with bilateral disease. The specificity was 89%. However, the more recent study by THORNBURY et al. (1982) showed less favorable results: Positive urography was seen in only 60% of cases with renal artery stenosis causing hypertension, and the false-negative rate was thus 40%. Reanalysis of the Cooperative Study data showed that the false-negative rate for screening is at least 21.8%, rather than 1.7% (THORNBURY et al. 1982). These figures obviously indicate a significant degree of unreliability.

Modifications of rapid sequence urography using such diuretics as furosemide and urea to accentuate physiologic differences have been advocated as providing a more sensitive test of the presence and significance of a renal artery stenosis (WOLF 1973). However, more extensive experience with these techniques has not confirmed their utility (TALNER et al. 1978).

Realizing these limitations, several hypertensive centers have ceased accepting referrals for rapid sequence urography for the isolated indication of hypertension and instead perform delayed digital urograms as an adjunct to the intravenous digital subtraction angiogram (HILLMAN 1983).

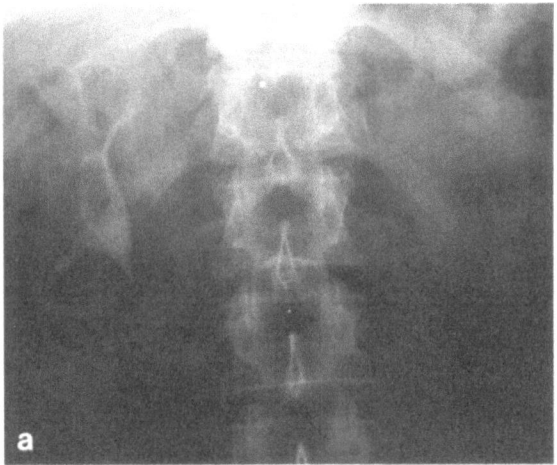

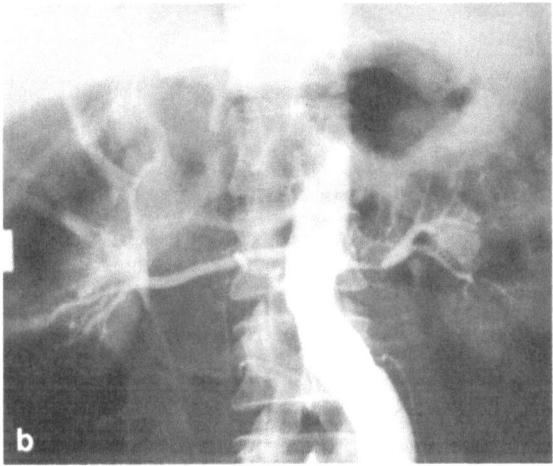

Fig. 12.1. a Delayed contrast excretion on the left side at urography. **b** Abdominal aortogram in the same patient demonstrating marked stenosis of the left renal artery. (The right kidney is supplied by two arteries.)

12.4.2 Nuclear Medicine

Radionuclide studies, i.e., hippuran renography, and different Tc99m-labeled renal agents (e.g., DTPA) have generated considerable interest as means of identifying patients with renovascular hypertension and assessing the change in renal perfusion and function following revascularization. The role of nuclear medicine in the differential diagnosis of renovascular hypertension has been somewhat controversial. However, renography is safe and easily performed and allows differentiation between normal renal function and asymmetric renal disease. Experience has shown that the true-positive rate is approximately 80%-90%, which implies that about 10%-20% of patients with renovascular hypertension will be missed by renal scintigraphy (BLAUFOX and FREEMAN 1988). The false-positive

rate for detection of renovascular hypertension is approximately 10%-15% (SFAKIANAKIS et al. 1985), which is not acceptable. Under these circumstances and with a disease of low prevalence such as renovascular hypertension, a large number of patients will go on to undergo more invasive examinations. In spite of this, renography has been mistakenly overlooked as a useful test in renovascular disease. In fact, if patients are regularly screened for renovascular disease with renography, the cost-effectiveness of the test is far greater than if all suspected patients are initially screened with more expensive examinations such as digital subtraction angiography.

The introduction of captopril renography (BLYTHE 1983) promises to improve greatly the efficiency of renography in the diagnosis of renovascular hypertension. The test is based on the fact that renal function appears to be maintained in renovascular hypertension through the renin-angiotensin system. The administration of captopril blocks angiotensin converting enzyme activity and thereby angiotensin II levels. Consequently, renal function on the side of the arterial stenosis is further decreased after captopril. The administration of captopril to patients in whom renography is abnormal can help to differentiate true-positive from false-positive findings. It has also been suggested as a way of increasing the sensitivity of screening, although its value in this respect is more doubtful (GEYSHES et al. 1986).

At the present time insufficient data are available to define the specificity and accuracy of renography with captopril in renovascular hypertension. A number of conditions which may present as renovascular hypertension and asymmetric renal disease resulting from renal nephrosclerosis need to be further evaluated to define the reliability of this test.

12.4.3 Doppler Ultrasonography

Doppler ultrasonography can be used in the diagnosis of renal artery or vein occlusion. This technique has also been evaluated in the investigation of renal artery stenosis. AVASTHI et al. (1984) studied 68 patients for renal artery disease with Doppler ultrasonography. Eleven patients (16%) had technically inadequate studies. Twenty-six patients were subjected to arteriography. The presence of one or more of the following hemodynamic abnormalities observed by Doppler examination was used to diagnose stenosis: peak blood velocity of 100 cm/s, absence of blood velocity during diastole, absence of any detectable blood velocity indicating occlusion, and broad-band Doppler frequency spectra caused by focal blood velocity disturbances. The sensitivity for renal artery stenosis was 89%, with a specificity of 73%.

In 1986, KOHLER et al. reported using the ratio of peak renal artery velocity to aortic velocity to distinguish stenotic (>60% diameter reduction) from nonstenotic renal arteries in a retrospective study. Ninety percent of the Doppler examinations were technically adequate, and arteriographic correlation was available for 43 renal arteries. With a ratio of greater than 3.5 taken to indicate a stenotic lesion, this method had a sensitivity of 91% and a specificity of 95%. Whether Doppler ultrasonography will be useful for screening purposes remains unclear. The results appear encouraging, but further clinical investigation in prospective studies is required.

12.4.4 Intravenous Digital Subtraction Angiography

Many different techniques have been attempted for intravenous digital subtraction angiography (IVDSA). To assess the practical aspects of IVDSA, ESKRIDGE et al. (1983) performed a study on 75 patients and concluded that superior studies were obtained by utilizing a central venous injection. HILLMAN (1983) advocated central venous catheterization by way of an antecubital vein puncture, using a 6-French pigtail catheter. One to three injections of contrast medium, in different projections, are required to demonstrate the major circulation. Between 40 and 50 ml of contrast medium, injected at a rate of 20–25 ml/s, is typically used. Immediately upon injection, exposures are obtained at a rate of one image per second for 20 s. Digital reconstructed images exposed before the arrival of contrast medium in the abdominal circulation are subtracted from those containing intraarterial contrast medium to produce diagnostic subtraction images (Fig. 12.2). In a comparative study performed by BUONOCORE et al. (1981) the overall accuracy of IVDSA was 71% (50/70), with a sensitivity of 93% and specificity of 91.5%. HILLMAN achieved 90% accuracy (including technically unsuccessful examinations) of diagnosis in nearly 100 cases in which the indication was hypertension. Similar results were reported by WILMS et al. in 1986. The ability of IVDSA to demonstrate the degree of renal artery stenosis was compared with that of intraarterial angiography in 45 patients and 92 arteries. There was agreement about the degree of stenosis in 90% of the cases. IVDSA grading was correct in 94% of atheromatous lesions but in only 56% of the fibromuscular hyper-

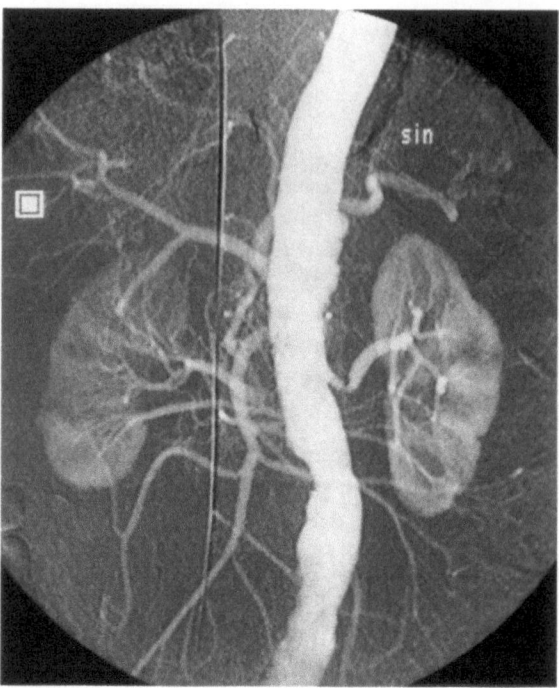

Fig. 12.2. IVDSA showing atherosclerotic stenosis of the left renal artery. Contrast medium injected through catheter placed in the inferior vena cava via the femoral vein approach

plastic stenoses. In the high grade atheromatous lesions, the degree of stenosis was slightly overestimated on IVDSA studies in 22.5% of the cases. In fibromuscular hyperplasia, stenosis was underestimated in 33%.

A unique advantage of IVDSA in patients with suspected renovascular hypertension is that selected renal vein renin samples can be obtained at the time of the imaging study. Urography, using the contrast medium injected for the DSA examination, may be performed adjunctively. However, bowel gas often degrades the arterial morphologic detail. Several methods have been tried to reduce bowel gas artifact, including abdominal compression, intravenous glucagon, and prone positioning. Unfortunately, a consistent solution to this problem is not currently available. However, intraarterial DSA may be added in any situation in which conventional arteriography is warranted.

12.4.5 Renal Angiography

Renal angiography is the definitive study, but it is invasive and should be performed only in patients who are candidates for revascularization procedures, percutaneous or surgical. Indications for renal angiography in suspected renovascular hypertension include:

1. Young patients
2. Severe hypertension, refractory to medical treatment in patients below 60–65 years of age
3. Abdominal bruit
4. Malignant or accelerating hypertension
5. Abnormal urography or renography

12.4.5.1 Technique

Aortography is first performed, using a pigtail catheter introduced by the Seldinger technique. Forty ml of contrast medium is injected at a rate of 20 ml/s. Modern, low osmolar contrast media are preferred. Oblique projections are often necessary in order to demonstrate the origin of the renal arteries optimally. Selective renal angiography is often indicated in order to better define the extent of the vascular lesion or when a peripheral renal artery stenosis is suspected. However, selective catheterization should be avoided in cases of very tight stenoses because of the risk of intimal damage.

12.4.5.2 Findings

Good technical quality and thorough knowledge of the anatomy of the renal vessels are essential as the abnormalities are not always conspicuous. Practically always the dorsal renal artery can be identified in an anteroposterior projection by its characteristic course in the sinus where it crosses the branches of the ventral artery (BOIJSEN 1959). It is important to observe the absence of crossing arteries in part of the kidney, which may be the only indication of a branch occlusion when no collateral circulation is visible (ANDERSSON 1976).

Angiographic criteria (BOOKSTEIN 1966) that may be important in the evaluation of the hemodynamic significance of a *renal artery stenosis* are:

1. Lumen < 1.5 mm
2. Collateral circulation
3. Poststenotic dilatation

Collateral circulation (Fig. 12.3) is more often seen in patients below the age of 50 and, when present, predicts a good prognosis of revascularization procedures. The poststenotic dilatation is a hemodynamic effect that may be found even with a 50% stenosis and consequently is not very discriminating.

The procedure that has best predicted successful invasive therapy is the selective sampling of renal

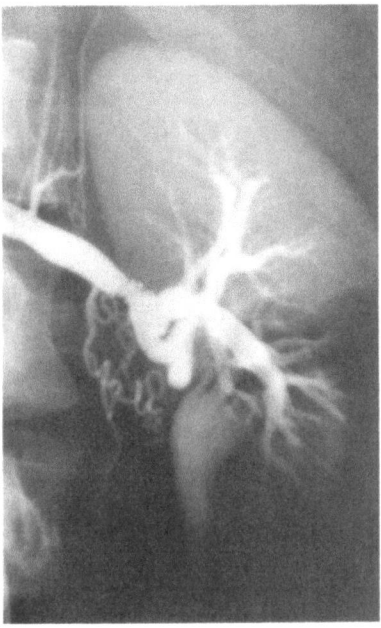

Fig. 12.3. Selective angiography of the left kidney demonstrating short fibromuscular lesion in the distal part of the main renal artery with collateral circulation from widened pelviureteric arteries. (The lower pole of the kidney was supplied by a supplementary artery.)

venous blood for renin analysis. A ratio of ≥ 1.5 between the stenotic and the contralateral kidney suggests significant stenosis. However, factors such as the spontaneous variation in renin secretion, patient posture, antihypertensive medication, improper patient preparation, and sampling technique have resulted in a high rate of false-negative results (MARKS and MAXWELL 1975). The decision whether or not to correct a renal artery stenosis has to be individualized on several bases such as clinical aspects, arteriographic findings, and the results of renal vein renin analysis.

The angiographic findings are decisive for the choice of therapy. The following lesions causing renovascular hypertension can be identified by angiography:

1. *Primary vascular lesions*
   a) Atherosclerosis
   b) Fibromuscular hyperplasia
   c) Aneurysm
   d) Arteriovenous malformation
   e) Thrombosis or embolus
   f) Arteritis

2. *Secondary vascular lesions*
   a) Lumbar aorta
      - atherosclerosis
      - dissecting aneurysm

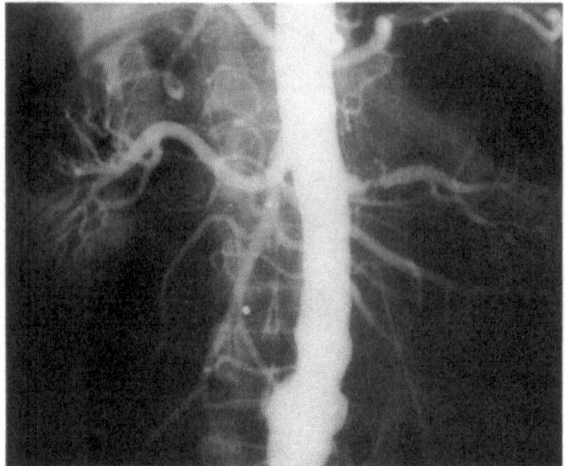

Fig. 12.4. Abdominal aortogram showing the typical appearance of an atherosclerotic renal artery stenosis on the left side. Note aneurysm in lower part of abdominal aorta

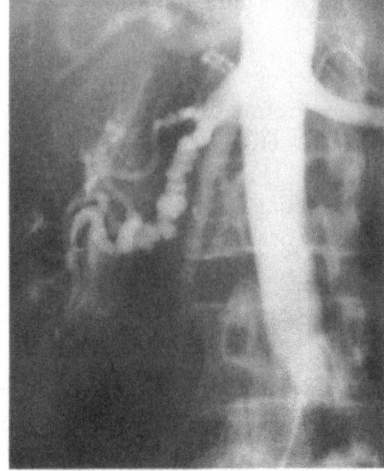

Fig. 12.5. Typical "string of beads" appearance caused by fibromuscular hyperplasia in the right renal artery

- arteritis
- coarctation
b) Trauma
- arteriovenous fistula
- thrombosis, occlusion
- compression
c) Tumors
- arterial encasement
- compression
- reninoma
d) Fibrous bands
- neurofibromatosis

12.4.5.3 Complications

The *complication rate* of renal angiography in hypertension is higher than in normotensive patients. The mortality in the well-known Cooperative Study was 0.11% (2719 examinations) and significant complications were found in no less than 1.2%, e.g., major hemorrhage, thrombosis, or neurologic symptoms (BOOKSTEIN et al. 1972b). Lower complication rates have also been reported (e.g., FOSTER et al. 1973: 0.4%).

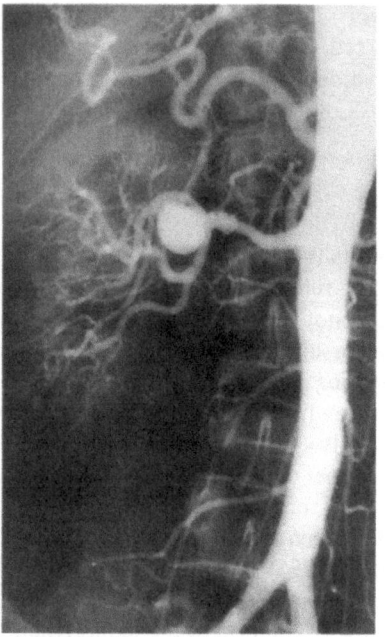

Fig. 12.6. Abdominal aortogram showing fibromuscular hyperplasia in the distal portion of the right renal artery and a large aneurysm in the bifurcation

12.5 Radiologic Appearances According to Etiology

12.5.1 Atherosclerosis

In atherosclerosis the stenosis is usually situated in the proximal third of the renal artery and accompanied by atherosclerotic changes in the wall of the abdominal aorta (Fig. 12.4). Lesions may be focal or extend eccentrically to involve the entire circumference of the wall. This type of renal artery stenosis is usually seen in individuals over 50 years of age and accounts for about two-thirds of all renal artery stenoses.

12.5.2 Fibromuscular Hyperplasia

Fibromuscular hyperplasia has been called a disease of young women (20–40 years). However, in a review of 100 cases with this entity, 83% were women, with a peak incidence between 40 and 60 years (EKELUND et al. 1978a). This disease, which acconts for about one-third of all renal artery stenoses, occurs in several forms, which can be classified as medial, intimal, and subadventitial (HUNT et al. 1962). In their review of the angiographic appearances EKELUND et al. found a typical "string of beads" appearance in 73%, while a short membranous stenosis was the only abnormality in five patients (Fig. 12.5). Bilateral involvement of the renal arteries was demonstrated in 67%. Out of the 33 cases with unilateral disease, 31 were found on the right side. The middle and distal thirds of the main stem of the renal artery were involved in 93%. Segmental arterial involvement was found to a varying degree in 60%. Aneurysms were seen in 9% (Figs. 12.6, 12.7). Extrarenal manifestation of the disease was observed in 12 patients, all of whom also had involvement of the renal artery (Fig. 12.8).

12.5.3 Renal Artery Aneurysms

Renal artery aneurysms are often situated in the hilar region of the kidney and may cause filling defects of the renal pelvis, creating differential diagnostic problems (Fig. 12.9). The occurrence of renal artery aneurysms varies between 0.3% and 1% (EDSMAN 1957; DE BAKEY et al. 1973; THAM et al. 1983). One of the most common indications for renal angiography is suspected renovascular hypertension. Therefore, it is not surprising that a large number of patients with renal artery aneurysms have hypertension. In one series of 100 patients with fibromuscular hyperplasia of the renal artery, aneurysms occurred in 9% (EKELUND et al. 1978a). In a careful study, CUMMINGS et al. (1973) demonstrated that those patients with renal artery aneurysm combined

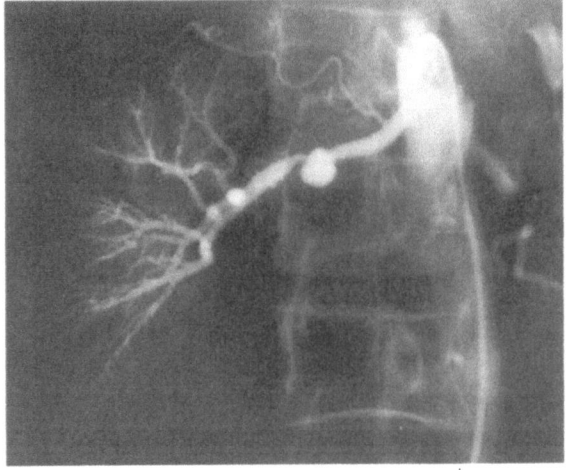

Fig. 12.7. Aortogram demonstrating an aneurysm in the middle part of the right renal artery, followed by a tight stenosis and fibromuscular changes in the distal third of the artery

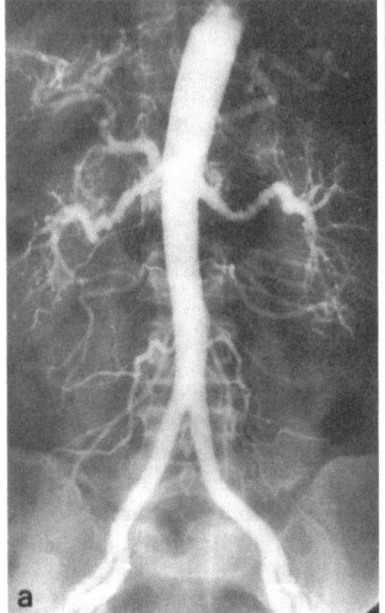

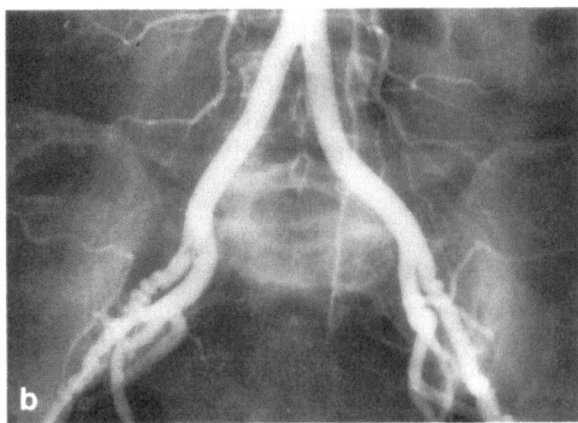

Fig. 12.8. a Aortogram showing fibromuscular hyperplasia in both renal arteries. **b** Pelvic angiography in the same patient revealing similar changes in the external iliac arteries, especially on the right side

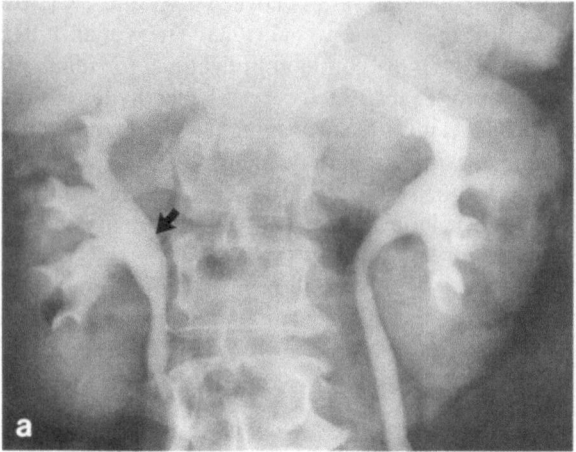

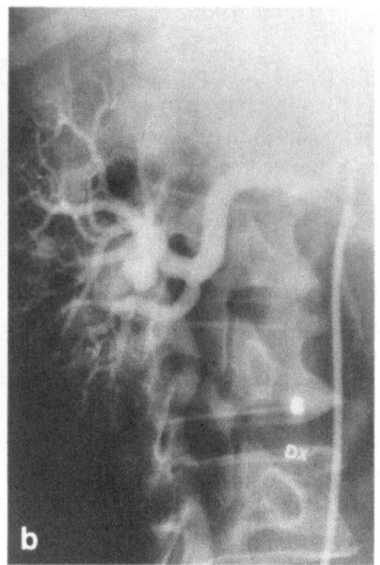

△

Fig. 12.9. a Urography. Contrast defect in the right renal pelvis suggesting tumor (*arrow*). **b** Selective angiography of the right kidney in the RAO projection clearly demonstrates the aneurysm

Fig. 12.10. Arteriovenous fistula following renal biopsy

with a hemodynamically significant stenosis, as verified with renal renin studies, could be cured by surgery. In contrast, those without evidence of stenosis, and with negative renin studies, remained hypertensive even after a technically successful reconstruction. Also in the series presented by THAM et al., most of the patients with renal artery aneurysm and hypertension remained hypertensive after surgery. Therefore, hypertension alone in a patient with a renal artery aneurysm is not an indication for surgery. The risk for rupture of a renal artery aneurysm is very small (THAM et al. 1983).

12.5.4 Arteriovenous Communications

Arteriovenous communications, whether congenital or acquired, may cause renovascular hypertension by making ischemic the parenchyma peripheral to the shunting. Depending on the size of the fistula and the time for which it has been present, patients present with hypertension, hematuria, or even congestive heart failure. Primary arteriovenous communications are usually hemangiomas while the most common acquired type is posttraumatic and often secondary to renal biopsy (EKELUND and LINDHOLM 1971, LANG 1975) (Fig. 12.10).

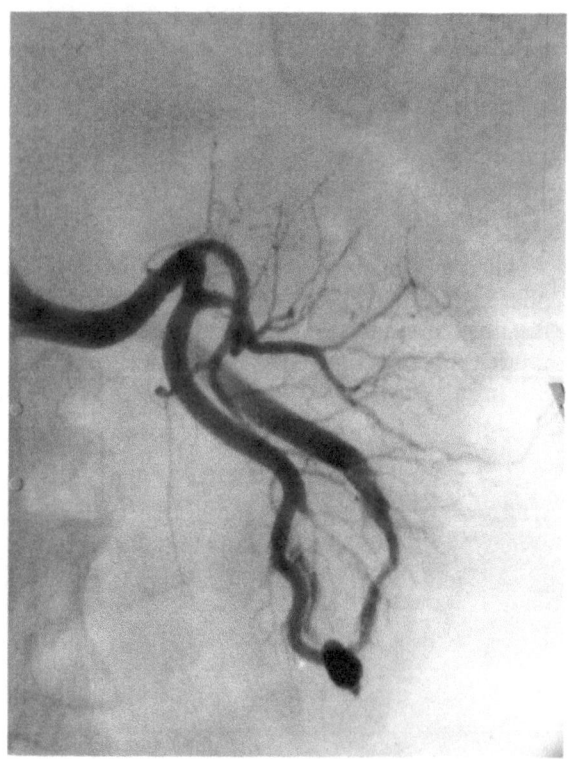

12.5.5 Collagenous Disease of the Kidney

Renal vascular lesions in collagenous disease of the kidney, such as polyarteritis nodosa or scleroderma, may lead to arterial occlusions and subsequent infarctions of the kidneys, resulting in hypertension. Polyarteritis nodosa is a systemic disease characterized by fibrinoid necrosis of the vessel walls.

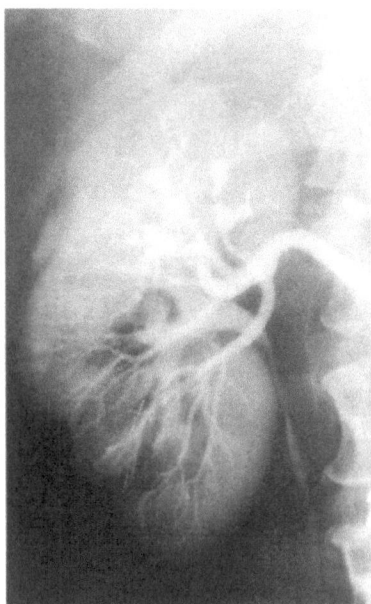

Fig. 12.11. Appearance in a patient with polyarteritis nodosa and multiple aneurysms in the upper half of the right kidney

Renal involvement is reported in about 80% of the cases (ROSE 1957). Multiple aneurysms of intrarenal arteries (Fig. 12.11) have been described by several investigators and these aneurysms may be transitory in nature (ROBINS and BOOKSTEIN 1972). Progressive lesions with arterial irregularities and occlusions with ensuing infarctions of the kidneys have also been reported (EKELUND and LINDHOLM 1974). These authors also described irregular arterial narrowing, tortuosity of intrarenal arteries, prolonged circulation time, and poor nephrographic effect in a kidney involved by scleroderma.

12.5.6 Embolization of the Renal Artery

Embolization of the renal artery or its tributaries may be seen in patients with mitral stenosis and left atrial or left ventricular thrombi as a consequence of myocardial infarction. This may result in renal colic and sudden onset of hypertension. Infarction of renal parenchyma can be demonstrated by computed tomography and subsequent angiography will show the extent of the vascular occlusion (Fig. 12.12).

12.5.7 Neurofibromatosis

In childhood and adolescents, lesions related to neurofibromatosis, Takayasu's arteritis, and

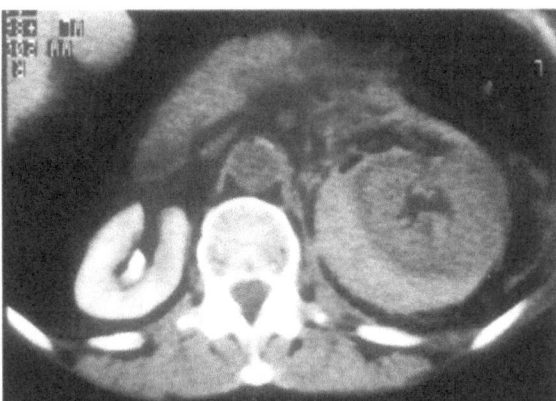

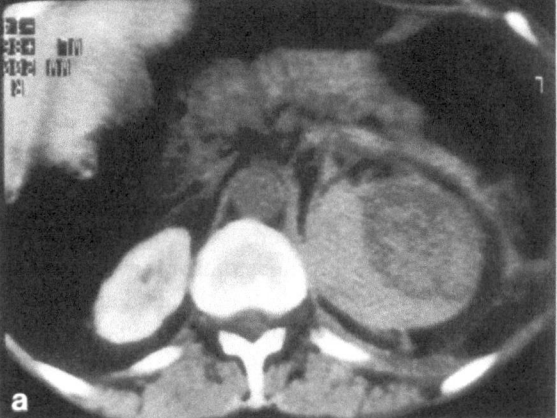

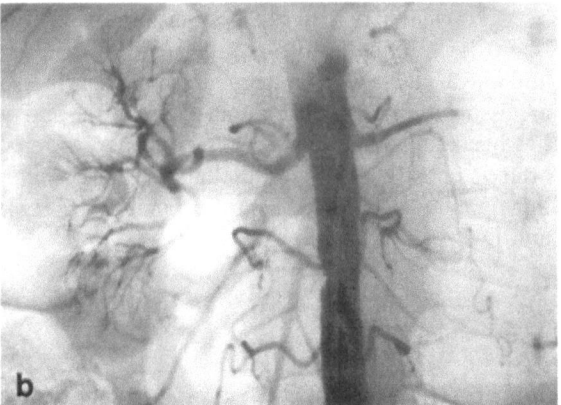

Fig. 12.12. a Contrast-enhanced CT scans showing nonopacification of the left kidney and subcapsular hematoma in a 70-year-old female with mitral stenosis and sudden onset of left renal colic. **b** Abdominal aortogram (photographic subtraction) demonstrates embolic occlusion of the distal part of the main stem of the left renal artery

stenoses associated with abdominal aortic coarctation are more commonly located at or near renal artery origins (CLAYMAN and BOOKSTEIN 1973; STANLEY et al. 1978). Renal artery stenosis occurring in neurofibromatosis has been associated with pheochromocytoma.

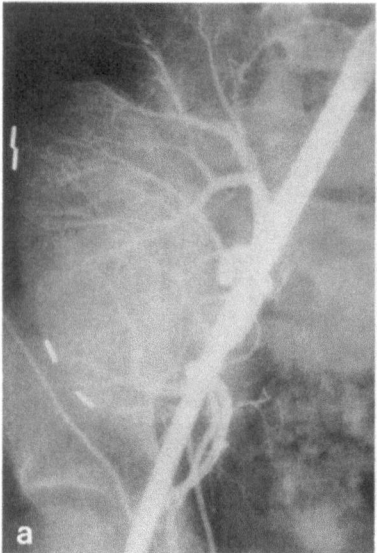 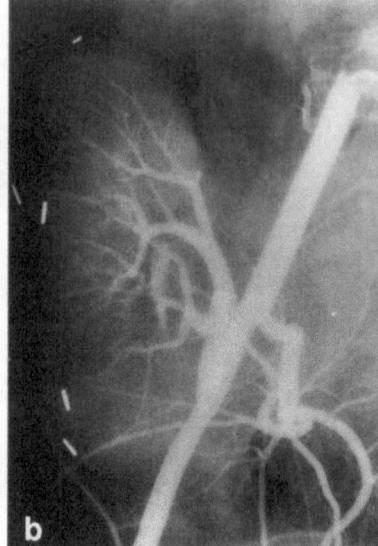 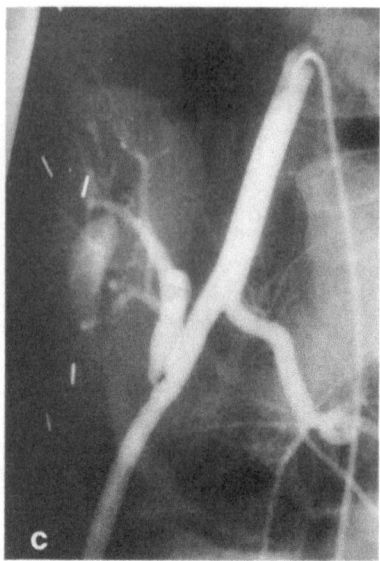

In children, neurofibromatosis is thought to be the cause of hypertension seven times more frequently than pheochromocytoma. Moreover, the response in such patients to transluminal angioplasty tends to be delayed (GARDINER et al. 1988).

According to TILFORD and KELSCH (1973), renal lesions do not occur in the absence of skin café au lait lesions. The stenoses of neurofibromatosis may be perivascular or caused by transmural intrinsic sclerosis. Arteriographically, the stenoses are short and may be associated with aneurysms. There is also an association with abdominal coarctation and it has been suggested that the observed triad of renal artery stenosis, aneurysms, and abdominal coarctation is characteristic of neurofibromatosis (ALLAN and DAVIES 1970).

12.5.8 Page Kidney

Subcapsular hematomas compressing renal parenchyma may produce hypertension and this effect has been called the Page kidney. In a series of patients with a Page kidney, 78% of cases could be attributed to trauma, whereas the remainder were associated with such conditions as polyarteritis nodosa, vascular masses, and coagulopathies. The subcapsular collection was predominantly blood in 85% and urine in the remainder (SONDA et al. 1982).

Fig. 12.13a–c. 35-year-old male with sudden onset of hypertension following renal transplantation. **a** Common iliac arteriogram in the AP projection is nondiagnostic. **b** Repeat study in the RPO projection does not show the anastomosis between the renal artery and the right external iliac artery. **c** With the patient in a steep RPO projection the tight stenosis at the anastomosis could be demonstrated

12.5.9 Hypertension Following Renal Transplantation

Suspected renal artery stenosis today is the main indication for angiography in renal transplants. In larger patient groups the prevalence of hypertension caused by renal artery stenosis in a kidney transplant recipient has been reported to be 10%–12% (BARTH et al. 1989; DOYLE et al. 1975; MUNDA et al. 1977; LACOMBE 1980). It is important to identify transplant renal artery stenosis as a cause of hypertension since it responds poorly to medical treatment. Focal stenosis at the site of the anastomosis is usually caused by poor adaptation of the intima or fibrotic scarring of the suture line due to local reaction to the sutures or trauma to the donor or recipient artery (LACOMBE 1975; SMITH et al. 1976; MUNDA et al. 1977; RICOTTA et al. 1978). Other causative factors include intimal hyperplasia and fibrosis, probably the result of immunologic factors or hemodynamic disturbances (MORRIS et al. 1971; O'CONNELL and MOWBRAY 1973).

Catheterization is usually performed from the contralateral femoral artery and ipsilateral common iliac arteriograms are then obtained. Low osmolar contrast media are recommended in order to min-

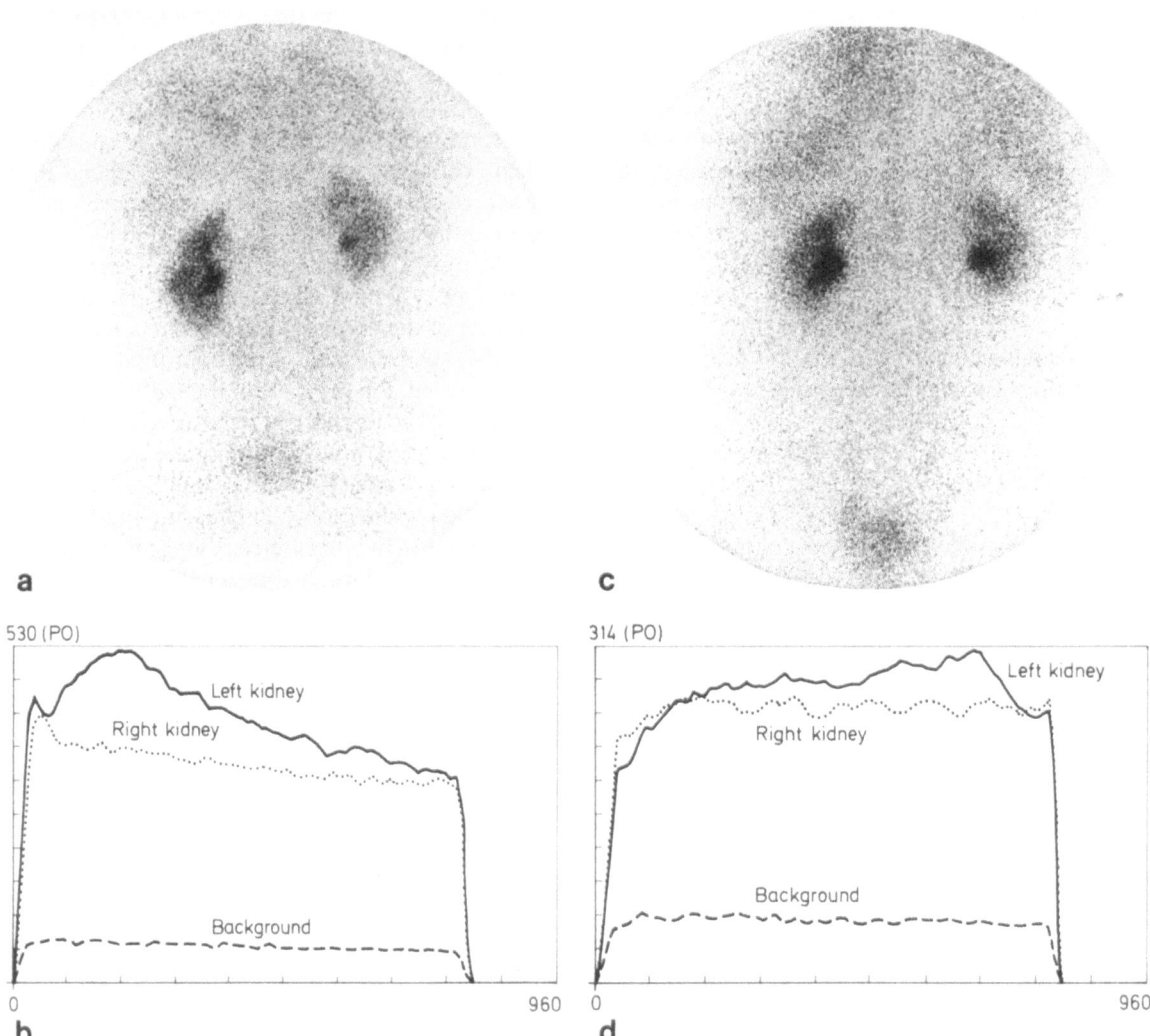

Fig. 12.14 a–d. 48-year-old hypertensive man with a right renal artery stenosis. **a** Radionuclide scan in PA projection after injection of Tc99m DTPA showing somewhat reduced activity in the right kidney compared to the left before PTRA. **b** The renographic curves are asymmetric with a somewhat diminished renographic phase on the right side. These findings are suggestive of right renal artery stenosis. **c** The radionuclide scan 6 months after PTRA shows equal bilateral activity levels in both kidneys; symmetric renographic curves are now seen (**d**)

imize nephrotoxicity. Positioning of the patient is extremely important in order to demonstrate relevant arterial anatomy and often several projections with the patient in different degrees of obliquity are necessary to demonstrate the arterial stenosis (Fig. 12.13).

12.6 Imaging Following Revascularization Procedures

Renal scintigraphy is a useful technique to evaluate the renal circulation following corrective treatment for renovascular hypertension, either surgical or percutaneous (Fig. 12.14). Thrombosis of the renal artery or the graft may be diagnosed and the presence of residual stenosis or diminished parenchymal function can be suggested. Renal Doppler ultrasonography is noninvasive and therefore well suited for following patients after revascularization or angioplasty.

Both conventional arteriography and DSA provide definitive information about the postoperative renal circulation. The various angiographic appearances following surgical treatment for renovascular hypertension were reported by EKELUND et al. (1978b) in 128 patients. Today, however, IVDSA has become the method of choice in evaluating these patients (HILLMAN 1983). ILLESCAS et al. (1987) reported on IVDSA in the evaluation of 28 patients following renal artery reconstruction. Satisfactory visualization of the renal artery was obtained in 26 cases and the clinical questions were adequately answered in these cases. If the diagnostic information from the intravenous study is insufficient, an intraarterial study can be added easily.

12.7 Radiologic Intervention in Renovascular Hypertension

12.7.1 Percutaneous Transluminal Renal Angioplasty

Whenever possible, the treatment of choice for renovascular hypertension should be correction of the renal artery stenosis. Surgical correction requires general anesthesia and many patients are poor risks because of severe atherosclerosis with renal insufficiency. For these reasons percutaneous transluminal renal angioplasty (PTRA) has attracted a great deal of attention in recent years. In 1978, GRÜNTZIG et al. successfully dilated a renal artery stenosis. Since then several reports describing the results of PTRA in large patient groups have been published (SCHWARTEN et al. 1980; SOS et al. 1983; LEVIN 1984; TEGTMEYER et al. 1984).

12.7.1.1 Technique

There have been continuous modifications of the technique and balloon catheters since Grüntzig's original description. PTRA is more complex than peripheral angioplasty and the procedure is far from harmless and should be performed only by experienced angiographers in collaboration with vascular surgeons.

The femoral approach can usually be used for dilatation of the renal artery and the axillary approach is only rarely needed. An abdominal aortography should always be obtained before the renal arteries are catheterized. The renal artery is entered with a diagnostic catheter of appropriate size which is carefully advanced across the stenosis. It is extremely important to keep the guidewire and catheter within the lumen when crossing the lesion. Larger diameter catheters usually select the vessels more easily but may be difficult to pass beyond the stenosis.

When the diagnostic catheter has crossed the lesion the catheter is exchanged for an appropriate di-

latation catheter. The three components of a successful dilatation in terms of balloon mechanics are the diameter of the balloon, the inflation pressure, and the time of inflation (SOS et al. 1986).

Several general principles have to be considered when choosing the balloon. The diameter is measured proximal and distal to the stenosis and the original size of the vessel is estimated in the area of the stenosis. The balloon chosen for angioplasty should be 1–2 mm greater in diameter than the diameter of the normal portion of the artery (SOS et al. 1986). Once a balloon of appropriate size has been selected, the pressure in the balloon becomes critical. In practice, normal renal arteries over 5 mm in diameter usually will not rupture if they are overdilated by 1–2 mm (TEGTMEYER and SOS 1986). This should be considered when choosing the length of the balloon. Two centimeter long balloons are usually employed for dilating renal lesions. Markers indicating the position of the balloon facilitate accurate placement. The balloon catheter is inflated with a mixture of contrast medium and saline, either with a pump or by hand. Inflation of the balloon should preferably be monitored with a pressure gauge. The larger the diameter of the balloon, the less pressure it takes to rupture it (ABELE 1980). Once the balloon has been properly positioned the pressure can be increased until the balloon expands completely. Between 4 and 10 atm are adequate to dilate most renal artery stenoses. The balloon should be inflated for 60 s (SOS et al. 1986) and then deflated slowly. Repeat dilatations should be kept to a minimum to avoid unnecessary trauma to the vessel and to prevent distal embolization. The pressures applied should not exceed 6 atm when polyethylene balloons larger than 6 mm in diameter are used (TEGTMEYER and SOS 1986).

In the case of very tight renal arterial stenoses, coaxial balloon catheter systems utilizing 8 or 9 French renal guiding catheters and 2 or 4.5 French coaxial balloon catheters can be used. The technique is more complex, but the advantage is that the fine coaxial catheter passes through a tight stenosis more readily than the femoral 7 French balloon catheter. It is also easy to maneuver this catheter out into the branches of the renal artery, especially over 0.014–0.018 in. steerable guidewires. In addition, the progress of the angioplasty can be monitored by injecting contrast medium either through the balloon catheter or through the larger guiding catheter. The disadvantages of the technique are (a) that the guiding catheter is stiff and may damage the aortic wall, and (b) balloon sizes above 4.2 mm are not available.

Coronary balloon catheters have been used with a coaxial system to dilate stenoses of branch arteries. Most recently, 3 and 4 French balloon catheters have become available that can be used for the same purpose.

Dilatation of osteal plaques by balloon catheters is difficult and often accompanied by complications. Vascular stents have been placed in the management of such osteal lesions. Both the Wall stent and the Palmaz stent have been successfully used for this purpose (Fig. 12.15).

Recently, percutaneous angioplasty has also been advocated as treatment for azotemia caused by renal artery stenosis (MARTIN et al. 1988). Salutary results have been noted in respect to the azotemia, although there is only rarely a concomitant response in blood pressure.

12.7.1.2 Results

In experienced hands renal angioplasty is a highly effective method of correcting renal artery lesions (Fig. 12.16). An initial technical success rate between 70% and 90% should be expected when dilating nonosteal arteriosclerotic and fibromuscular renal artery stenosis (COLAPINTO et al. 1982; MARTIN et al. 1986; TEGTMEYER and SOS 1986; KLINGE et al. 1989; TACK and SOS 1989; WILMS et al. 1989). A common denominator related to long-term success is the selection of a proper sized balloon with which the vessel is slightly overdilated. Follow-up studies have shown that this has reduced the incidence of recurrent stenoses in the renal artery, which are usually due to incomplete dilatation, atheroma formation around a residual stenosis, or vessel wall injury (SOS et al. 1986). Recurrent stenosis can be anticipated in 10%–15% of patients, the majority of whom will have at least 30% residual stenosis following dilatation (TEGTMEYER et al. 1984). Therefore, obtaining a good initial result is important. Recurrent stenoses will usually appear during the first year after PTRA and often respond well to repeat dilatation.

It has become clear that certain lesions are more amenable to PTRA than others. A good result can be anticipated in fibromuscular hyperplasia (TEGTMEYER et al. 1982). Short segmental atherosclerotic lesions also respond well to PTRA. Renal angioplasty is a clinically effective method of treating renovascular hypertension and good long-term results can be anticipated if the lesion is properly dilated. General anesthesia and major surgery are avoided and the morbidity is lower than from surgery.

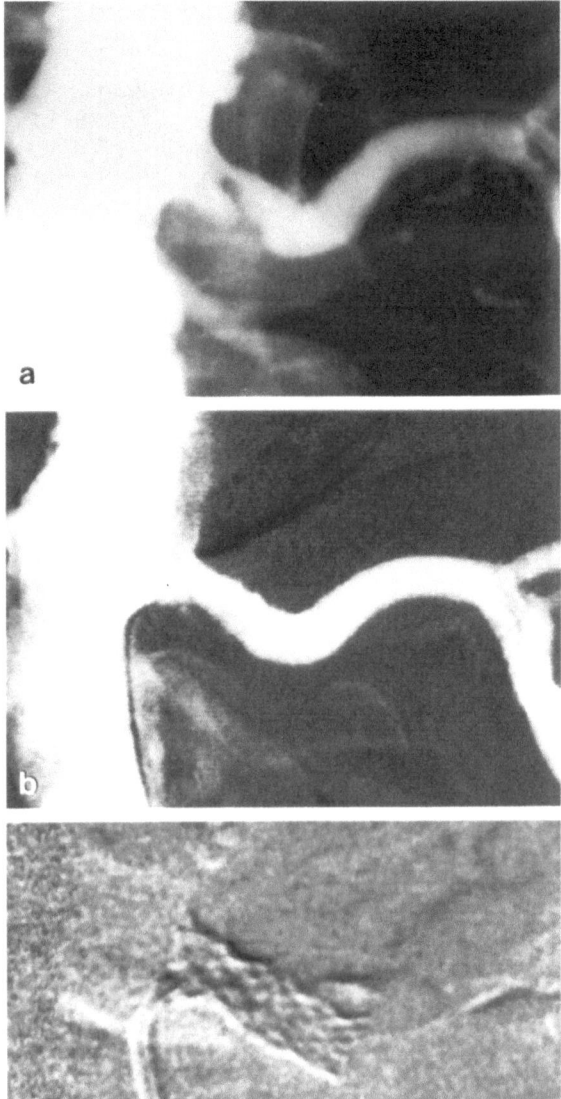

Fig. 12.15. a An aortogram shows an ulcerated artheroma in the proximal left renal artery producing a 90 percentile stenosis. **b** The lesion has been dilated and the Palmaz stent placed across the lesion. There is salutory response, the lumen is normalized. **c** A miss-registered DSA frame shows the stent in place. (Courtesy Dr. JULIO C. PALMAZ, San Antonio, TX)

12.7.1.3 Complications

Percutaneous transluminal renal angioplasty is not innocuous and the complication rate in renal arteries is over twice the rate in the iliofemoral arteries, being variously reported as between 6% and 15% (TEGTMEYER et al. 1984; GARDINER et al. 1986;

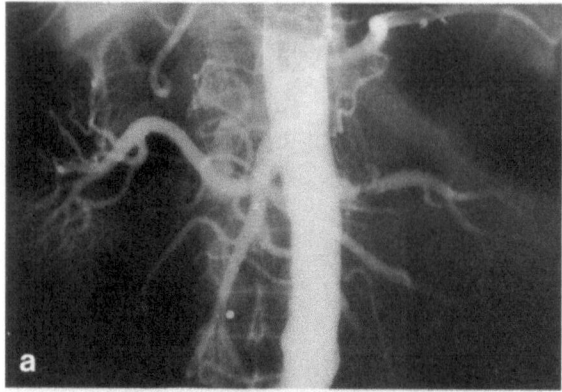
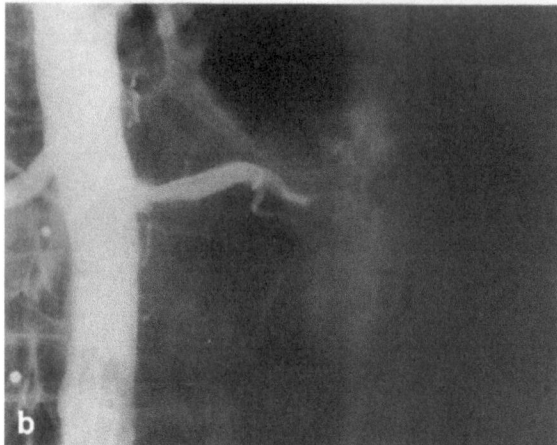
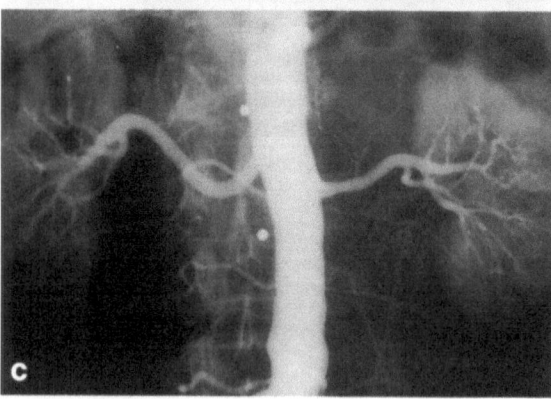

Fig. 12.16. a Abdominal aortogram showing atherosclerotic stenosis in the proximal part of the left renal artery (same patient as in Fig. 12.4). **b** Repeat aortogram immediately following PTRA. **c** Follow-up at 6 months reveals only mild residual stenosis. Patient normotensive

BERGQUIST et al. 1987; BILLSTRÖM et al. 1988). Minor complications are reversible while major complications are either irreversible or necessitate extended hospitalization or surgery. Major complications include perforation of the renal artery, intimal dissection with possible occlusion, and intramural hematoma. An atraumatic technique using soft flexible guidewires, properly sized catheters, and balloons should, in experienced hands, minimize the complication rate.

12.7.2 Transcatheter Embolization of Renovascular Malformations

There are instances of renal hypertension when percutaneous dilatation of a vessel may not be appropriate but when other types of radiologic interventional procedure may prove sufficient and advantageous relative to surgery. Transcatheter embolization may be an alternative treatment in patients with malignant hypertension and end-stage renal disease. This technique can also be used for the infarction of a renin hypersecreting renal segment distal to a branch stenosis, or for the occlusion of a renovascular malformation. These arteriovenous malformations may be of the capillary or cavernous type (EKELUND and GÖTHLIN 1975). Ischemia distal to the lesion is usually the cause of hypertension due to stimulation of the renin-angiotensin system.

Casting of the arteriovenous malformation with occlusive material such as surgical glue (avacryl, 6-cyanoacrylate) will eliminate the siphoning effect and normalize perfusion of distal and peripheral renal tissues. Total infarction of the compromised renal tissue is one other modality to break the renin-angiotensin cycle and attain normalization of blood pressure (SCHLOSSBERG et al. 1986; LANG 1982; LAMMERT et al. 1989).

References

Abele JE (1980) Balloon catheters and transluminal dilatation; technical considerations. AJR 135: 901–906

Allan TN, Davies ER (1970) Neurofibromatosis of the renal artery. Br J Radiol 43: 906–908

Andersson I (1976) Renal artery lesions after pyelolithotomy. A potential cause of renovascular hypertension. Acta Radiol [Diagn] (Stockh) 17: 685–695

Avasthi PS, Voyles WF, Greene ER (1984) Noninvasive diagnosis of renal artery stenosis by echo-Doppler velocimetry. Kidney Int 25: 824–829

Barth MO, Gagnadoux MF, Mareschal JL et al. (1989) Angioplasty of renal transplant artery stenosis in children. Pediatr Radiol 19: 383–387

Bech K, Hilden T (1975) The frequency of secondary hypertension. Acta Med Scand 197: 65–69

Bergquist D, Jonsson K, Weibull H (1987) Complication after percutaneous transluminal angioplasty of peripheral and renal arteries. Acta Radiol 28: 3–16

Billström Å, Ekelund L, Hietala S-O (1988) Complications of percutaneous transluminal renal angioplasty. J Interventional Radiol 3: 45–51

Blaufox MD, Freeman LM (1988) Renewed role of nuclear medicine in renovascular hypertension. Urol Radiol 10: 35–38

Blythe WB (1983) Captopril and renal autoregulation. N Engl J Med 308: 390–391

Boijsen E (1959) Angiographic studies of the anatomy of single and multiple renal arteries. Acta Radiol [Diagn] (Stockh) [Suppl] 183

Bookstein JJ (1966) Appraisal of arteriography in estimating the hemodynamic significance of renal artery stenosis. Invest Radiol 1: 281–294

Bookstein JJ, Abrams HL, Buenger RE et al. (1972a) Radiologic aspects of renovascular hypertension. 2. The role of urography in unilateral renovascular disease. JAMA 220: 1225–1230

Bookstein JJ, Abrams HL, Buenger RE et al. (1972b) Radiologic aspects of renovascular hypertension. 3. Appraisal of arteriography. JAMA 221: 368–374

Buonocore E, Meaney TF, Borkowski GP, Pavlicek W, Gallagher J (1981) Digital subtraction angiography of the abdominal aorta and renal arteries. Radiology 139: 281–286

Clayman AS, Bookstein JJ (1973) The role of renal arteriography in pediatric hypertension. Radiology 108: 107–110

Colapinto RF, Stronell RD, Harries-Jones EP et al. (1982) Percutaneous transluminal dilatation of the renal artery: follow-up studies on renovascular hypertension. AJR 139: 727–732

Cummings KB, Lecky JW, Kaufman JJ (1973) Renal artery aneurysms and hypertension. J Urol 109: 144–148

DeBakey ME, Lefrak EA, Garcia-Rinaldi R, Noon GP (1973) Aneurysm of the renal artery. Arch Surg 106: 438–443

Doyle TJ, McGregor WR, Fox PS, Maddison FE, Rodgers RE, Kauffman HM (1975) Homotransplant renal artery stenosis. Surgery 77: 53–60

Edsman G (1957) Angionephrography and suprarenal angiography. A roentgenologic study of the normal kidney. Expansive renal and suprarenal lesions and renal aneurysms. Acta Radiol [Diagn] (Stockh) [Suppl] 155: 104–116

Ekelund L, Göthlin J (1975) Renal hemangiomas. An analysis of 13 cases diagnosed by angiography. AJR 125: 788–794

Ekelund L, Lindholm T (1971) Arteriovenous fistulae following percutaneous renal biopsy. Acta Radiol [Diagn] (Stockh) 11: 38–48

Ekelund L, Lindholm T (1974) Angiography in collagenous disease of the kidney. Acta Radiol [Diagn] (Stockh) 15: 413–422

Ekelund L, Gerlock J Jr, Molin J, Smith C (1978a) Roentgenologic appearance of fibromuscular dysplasia. Acta Radiol [Diagn] (Stockh) 19: 433–446

Ekelund L, Gerlock J Jr, Goncharenko V, Foster J (1978b) Angiographic findings following surgical treatment for renovascular hypertension. Radiology 126: 345–349

Eskridge JM, Becker GJ, Rabe FE, Holden RW, Klatte EC (1983) Digital vascular imaging: practical aspects. Radiology 148: 703–705

Foster JH, Dean RH, Pinkerton JA, Rhamy RK (1973) Ten years' experience with the surgical management of renovascular hypertension. Ann Surg 177: 755–766

Gardiner JR GA, Meyerovitz MF, Stolles KR, Clouse ME, Harrington DP, Bettman MA (1986) Complications of transluminal angioplasty. Radiology 159: 201–208

Gardiner GA Jr, et al. (1988) Percutaneous transluminal angioplasty: delayed response in neurofibromatosis. Radiology 169: 79–87

Geyshes GG, Oei HY, Faber JAJ (1986) Prediction of blood pressure after dilatation of renal artery stenosis. Nephron 44 [Suppl 1]: 54–59

Grüntzig A, Vetter W, Meier B (1978) Treatment of renovascular hypertension within percutaneous transluminal dilatation of a renal artery stenosis. Lancet I: 801–802

Hillman B (1983) Imaging and hypertension. W. B. Saunders, Philadelphia

Horne ML, Conklin VM, Keenan RE, Varady PD, DiNardo J (1979) Angiotensin II profiling with saralasin: summary of Eaton collaborative study. Kidney Int 15: S-115–S-122

Hunt JC, Strong CG (1983) Renovascular hypertension. Mechanisms, natural history and treatment. Am J Cardiol 32: 562–574

Hunt JC, Harrison EG, Kincaid OW, Bernatz PE, Davis GD (1962) Idiopathic fibrous and fibromuscular stenosis of renal arteries associated with hypertension. Proc Mayo Clin 37: 181–216

Illescas FF, Sussman SK, McCann RL, Dunnick NR (1987) Digital intravenous subtraction angiography in the evaluation of reconstructed renal arteries. Cardiovasc Intervent Radiol 10: 205–209

Kaufman JJ (1979) Renovascular hypertension: the UCLA experience. J Urol 112: 139–144

Klinge J, Hali W, Puijlaert C et al. (1989) Percutaneous transluminal renal angioplasty: initial and long-term results. Radiology 171: 501–509

Kohler TR, Zierler RE, Martin RL, et al. (1986) Noninvasive diagnosis of renal artery stenosis by ultrasonic duplex scanning. J Vasc Surg 4: 450–456

Lacombe M (1975) Arterial stenosis complicating renal allotransplantation in man. A study of 38 cases. Ann Surg 181: 283–288

Lacombe M (1980) Les sténoses artérielles des reins transplantés. Acta Chir Belg 1: 1–8

Lammert GK, Merine D, White RJ et al. (1989) Embolotherapy of a high flow false aneurysm by using an occlusive balloon, thrombin, steel coils and the detachable balloon. AJR 152: 382–385

Lang EK (1982) Transcatheter Embolization Success depends on material Urol. Times 10 (2): 41

Lang EK (1975) Arteriography in the assessment of renal trauma. The impact of arteriographic diagnosis on preservation of renal function and parenchyma. J Trauma 15: 553–566

Levin DC (1984) Percutaneous transluminal angioplasty of the renal arteries. JAMA 251: 759–763

Marks LS, Maxwell MH (1975) Renal vein renin. Value and limitations in the prediction of operative results. Urol Clin North Am 2: 311–325

Martin LG, Casarella WJ, Alspaugh JP, Chuang VP (1986) Renal artery angioplasty: increased technical success and decreased complications in the second 100 patients. Radiology 159: 631–634

Martin LG, Casarella WJ, Gaylord GM (1988) Azotemia caused by renal artery stenosis: treatment by percutaneous angioplasty. AJR 150: 839–845

Maxwell MH, Gonick HC, Wiita R, Kaufman JJ (1964) Use of the rapid sequence intravenous pyelogram in the diagnosis of renovascular hypertension. N Engl J Med 270: 213–220

Morris PJ, Yadav RVS, Kincaid-Smith P et al. (1971) Renal artery stenosis in renal transplantation. Med J Aust 1: 1255–1257

Muller FB, Sealey JE, Case DB et al. (1986) The captopril test for identifying renovascular disease in hypertensive patients. Am J Med 80: 633–644

Munda R, Alexander JW, Miller S, First MR, Fidler JP (1977) Renal allograft artery stenosis. Am J Surg 134: 400–403

O'Connell TX, Mowbray JF (1973) Arterial intimal thickening produced by alloantibody and xenoantibody. Transplantation 15: 262–263

Orzel JA, Coldwell DM, Eskridge JM (1988) Superselective embolization for renal hemorrhage with a new co-axial catheter and steerable guide wire. Cardiovasc Intervent Radiol 11: 343-346

Ricotta JJ, Schaff HV, Williams GM, Rolley RT, Whelton PK, Harrington DM (1978) Renal artery stenosis following transplantation. Etiology, diagnosis and prevention. Surgery 84: 595-602

Robins JM, Bookstein JJ (1972) Regressing aneurysms in periarteritis nodosa. Radiology 104: 39-42

Rose GA (1957) The natural history of polyarteritis. Br Med J II: 1148-1152

Schlossberg P, Rosen RJ, Roven SJ (1986) Transcatheter embolisation of small vessel renal vascular malformations. J Intern Radiol 1: 25-27

Schwarten DE, Heun HY, Klatte EC, Grim CE, Weinberger HH (1980) Clinical experience with percutaneous transluminal angioplasty (PTA) of stenotic renal arteries. Radiology 135: 601-604

Sfakianakis G, Kyriakides G, Jaffe D et al. (1985) Single visit captopril renography for the diagnosis of curable renovascular hypertension. J Nucl Med 26: 133

Simon N, Franklin S, Bleifer K, Maxwell M (1972) Clinical characteristics of renovascular hypertension. JAMA 220: 1209-1218

Smith RB, Cosimi AB, Lordon R, Thompson AL, Ehrlich RM (1976) Diagnosis and management of arterial stenosis causing hypertension after successful renal transplantation. J Urol 115: 639-642

Sonda LP III, Konnak JW, Diokno AC (1982) Clinical aspects of non-vascular renal causes of hypertension. Urol Radiol 3: 257-260

Sos TA, Pickering TG, Sniderman K et al. (1983) Percutaneous transluminal renal angioplasty in renovascular hypertension due to atheroma or fibromuscular dysplasia. N Engl J Med 309: 274-279

Sos TA, Saddekini S, Pickering TG, Laragh JH (1986) Technical aspects of percutaneous transluminal angioplasty in renovascular disease. Nephron 4 [Suppl 1]: 45-50

Stanley P, Gyepes MT, Olson DL, Gates FG (1978) Renovascular hypertension in children and adolescents. Radiology 129: 123-131

Tack C, Sos TA (1989) Radiologic diagnosis of renal vascular hypertension and percutaneous transluminal angioplasty. Semin Nucl Med 19: 89-98

Talner LB, Stone RA, Coel MN, Levy SB, Emarine CW (1978) Furosemide-augmented intravenous urography: results in essential hypertension. AJR 130: 257-260

Tegtmeyer CJ, Sos TA (1986) Techniques of renal angioplasty. Radiology 161: 577-586

Tegtmeyer CJ, Elson J, Glass TA, Ayers CR, Chevalier RL, Wellons HA, Studdard WE (1982) Percutaneous transluminal angioplasty: the treatment of choice for renovascular hypertension due to fibromuscular dysplasia. Radiology 143: 631-637

Tegtmeyer CJ, Kellman CD, Ayes C (1984) Percutaneous transluminal angioplasty of the renal artery. Results and long term follow up. Radiology 153: 77-84

Tham G, Ekelund L, Herrlin K, Lindstedt E, Olin T, Bergentz SE (1983) Renal artery aneurysms. Natural history and prognosis. Ann Surg 197: 348-352

Thornbury JR, Stanley JC, Fryback DG (1982) Hypertensive urogram: a nondiscriminatory test for renovascular hypertension. AJR 138: 43-49

Tilford DL, Kelsch RC (1973) Renal artery stenosis in childhood neurofibromatosis. Am J Dis Child 126: 665-668

Tucker RM, Labarthe DR (1977) Frequency of surgical treatment for hypertension in adults at the Mayo Clinic from 1973 through 1975. Mayo Clin Proc 52: 549-555

Wilms GE, Baert AL, Staessen JA, Amery AK (1986) Renal artery stenosis: evaluation with intravenous digital subtraction angiography. Radiology 160: 713-715

Wilms GE, Baert AL, Amery AK et al. (1989) Short-term morphologic results of percutaneous transluminal renal angioplasty as determined by angiography. Radiology 170: 1019-1026

Wolf GL (1973) Rationale and use of vasodilated excretory urography in screening for renovascular hypertension. AJR 119: 692-700

13 Radiology of the Transplant Kidney

Sven Dorph, Jan Kofod Larsen, Thorkild Mygind, and Henrik S. Thomsen

CONTENTS

13.1 Introduction 311
13.1.1 Nephrologic Complications 312
13.1.2 Urologic Complications 312
13.1.3 Imaging of the Renal Allograft 313
13.2 Radionuclide Imaging 313
13.2.1 Monitoring 313
13.2.1.1 Radionuclear Angiography (Bolus Transit) .. 314
13.2.1.2 Renography 315
13.2.2 Complications 317
13.2.2.1 Vascular Occlusion 317
13.2.2.2 Arterial Stenosis 318
13.2.2.3 Hyperacute Rejection 318
13.2.2.4 Acute Tubular Necrosis 318
13.2.2.5 Acute Cyclosporine Nephrotoxicity 318
13.2.2.6 Acute Rejection 319
13.2.2.7 Infarcts 319
13.2.2.8 Chronic Diseases 319
13.2.2.9 Miscellaneous (Renal) 319
13.2.2.10 Urinary Leakage 320
13.2.2.11 Obstruction 320
13.3 Ultrasonography 320
13.3.1 Technique 320
13.3.2 Ultrasound Monitoring 320
13.3.2.1 Normal Appearance 320
13.3.2.2 Graft Size 321
13.3.2.3 Intrarenal Parenchymal Structures 321
13.3.2.4 Urologic Complications 322
13.3.3 Doppler Investigation 323
13.4 Conventional Radiography 324
13.4.1 Contrast Media in Kidney Transplantation .. 324
13.4.2 Intravenous Urography 324
13.4.3 Direct Pyelography 325
13.4.4 Cystography 326
13.4.5 Angiography 326
13.5 Computed Tomography 326
13.5.1 Technique 326
13.5.2 Imaging 327
13.6 Magnetic Resonance Imaging 328
13.6.1 Normal Renal Allografts 328
13.6.2 Graft Parenchymal Disease 328
13.6.3 Urologic Disease 329
13.7 Interventional Radiology 329
13.7.1 Urinary Leakage 329
13.7.2 Perirenal Fluid Collection 330
13.7.3 Ureteral Obstruction 330
13.7.4 Arterial Stenosis 333
13.7.5 Miscellaneous Complications 334
References 335

13.1 Introduction

Imaging of the transplanted kidney poses a number of specific problems and challenges for the radiologist. The graft is threatened by two major groups of complications, nephrologic and urologic. Any of these complications may cause graft dysfunction due to ischemia, rejection, drug toxicity, infection, leakage, fluid collection, or obstruction. Since two or more complications may be simultaneously at work, the clinical picture is often ambiguous.

Nuclear medical imaging, ultrasound, intravenous urography, cystography, direct pyelography, angiography, and computed tomography are all well-established imaging techniques in kidney transplant recipients, while digital subtraction angiography and magnetic resonance imaging are relatively new techniques with evolving roles in the diagnostic armamentarium for posttransplant dysfunction. Interventional procedures using imaging techniques have proven to be particularly useful in the management of a number of urologic posttransplant complications. It is the purpose of the present chapter to assess the impact of imaging on renal transplantation and to describe the role and significance of the many imaging modalities and interventional procedures in the diagnosis and management of posttransplant complications.

The use of renal allograft transplantation in the treatment of chronic renal failure is now well established and widespread. Since the early 1980s the number of renal transplants in the United States has increased from about 5000 to 7500 per year (Hanto and Simmons 1987). In Scandinavia the transplantation activity has generally been relatively high, but in recent years it has been somewhat restricted by insufficient donor kidney supply.

Sven Dorph, M.D. PhD., Associate Professor and Chairman, Department of Radiology; Jan Kofod Larsen M.D.; Thorkild Mygind, M.D., PhD., Professor of Diagnostic Radiology; Henrik S. Thomsen, M.D., PhD.; Department of Nuclear Medicine, Herlev Hospital, University of Copenhagen, Herlev Ringvej 75, 2730 Herlev, Denmark

Improvements in organ matching, surgical technique, and immunosuppressive medication have led to a steady increase in graft survival, which is currently reported to be about 90% at 1 year with live-related donors and 80% using cadaveric kidneys. The single most important factor contributing to the recent improvement in allograft survival has been the introduction of cyclosporine, which has reduced the number and severity of rejection episodes and the need for other immunosuppressive treatment (Canadian Multicenter Transplant Study Group 1983; European Multicenter Study Group 1983). Cyclosporine nephrotoxicity, on the other hand, has been added to the long list of posttransplant complications, many of which require early recognition and handling.

13.1.1 Nephrologic Complications

Nephrologic complications include rejection, acute tubular necrosis (ATN), and immunosuppressive therapy toxicity.

Episodes of rejection occur in about 50% of cadaveric allografts, mainly within the first 3 months after operation, and represent the chief cause of failing allograft function. Rejection can be divided into hyperacute, accelerated acute, early cell mediated, chronic, and acute/chronic (BECKER and KUTCHER 1978).

Hyperacute and accelerated acute rejection are humorally mediated and often give rise to alarming symptoms either at the time of surgery (edema, hemorrhage) or immediately thereafter. Kidney rupture may occur. There is rarely the time or need for elaborate diagnostic procedures. In the other forms of rejection the symptoms accompanying the reduction in renal function are generally uncharacteristic and similar regardless of whether the incidence occurs early or late after surgery.

Acute tubular necrosis may occur as a result of the ischemic damage to the kidney graft during the total transplantation procedure. It is therefore obvious that ATN occurs primarily in cadaveric allografts. Approximately 30%–50% of cadaveric grafts do not show immediate function due to ischemic damage. Most of these grafts will begin functioning in 1 or 2 weeks (KIRCHNER and ROSENTHALL 1982).

Cyclosporine, which is now almost universally used as an effective immunosuppressive agent, has nephrotoxic effects which may add to the frequency of delayed onset of function and dysfunction at later stages (DIEPERINK et al. 1986).

13.1.2 Urologic Complications

Urologic complications include extravasation, perirenal fluid collections, obstruction, and vascular complications. The overall incidence has been reported to be up to 20%, but in most centers it is now 10% or less (BENNETT et al. 1986). It is paramount that these conditions be diagnosed promptly and differentiated from other forms of failing graft function. Delay in treatment of urologic complications may result in graft loss and has been associated with high mortality (MUNDY et al. 1981).

Urinary leakage usually occurs during the first 4 weeks after surgery, most commonly at the ureterneocystostomy (BECKER and KUTCHER 1980; HUNTER et al. 1983; KUMAR et al. 1984) (Fig. 13.25). Leaks more proximal in the ureter may occur due to local ischemia (Fig. 13.26). The urine collection is usually extraperitoneal. The chief symptom is decreased urinary output, usually accompanied by obstruction. In the absence of treatment the mortality is high (GOLDSTEIN et al. 1981; MUNDY et al. 1981; LIEBERMAN et al. 1982; BENNETT et al. 1986).

Perirenal fluid collections include hematomas, urinomas, lymphoceles, and abscesses. Small asymptomatic hematomas are often demonstrated by ultrasonography in the early postoperative period (Fig. 13.13). Larger hematomas, which may be due to graft rupture or injury to larger vessels of the graft, will cause a palpable mass, fever, and obstruction.

Urinomas are the result of urinary leakage, which may no longer be ongoing at the time of diagnosis. Not every small urinoma detected needs treatment.

Abscesses may also present with fever and septicemia in the early or later postoperative period. They may be derived from urinomas or hematomas.

Lymphocele is the most common significant posttransplant fluid collection (2%–20%) (BECKER and KUTCHER 1980; LERUT et al. 1980; ZAONTZ and FIRLIT 1988) (Fig. 13.27). It is usually a late complication, often appearing after one or several episodes of graft rejection (ZINKE et al. 1975; BECKER and KUTCHER 1980). Its pathogenesis is not clear. Lymph accumulation due to intraoperative division of lymphatics and lymph leakage from the graft surface have been proposed. Another possible cause is rejection, which decreases lymph absorption by compression due to edema or increases lymph production due to venous compression (MEYERS et al. 1977; BENNETT et al. 1986). Lymphoceles often present with decreasing kidney function associated with compression symptoms such as swelling over the graft and leg edema. Obstruction may result (BROCKIS et al. 1978) (Fig. 13.27).

Ureteral obstruction may result from compression by fluid collections (Fig. 13.27), ureteral stones or clots, and stricture. Stricture formation is the most common (Figs. 13.28–13.30). The principal site is the ureterovesical junction (UVJ), although midureteric and ureteropelvic junction (UPJ) obstruction also occur. The technique of ureteroneocystostomy is the most common cause, but local inflammation due to rejection with resulting fibrosis, and ischemia caused by stripping of the vascular supply to the ureter during harvesting of the donor kidney may also result in stricture formation (GLANZ et al. 1983). Ureteral kinking and torsion occur very rarely (PALESTRANT and DEWOLF 1982).

Vascular complications: Stenosis of the graft artery causing hypertension or graft failure is reported in 1%–25% of cases (Figs. 13.19, 13.31); an overall estimate may be about 8% (DIAMOND et al. 1979; SNIDERMAN et al. 1980a, b; GROSSMAN et al. 1982; ZAJKO et al. 1982; LAASONEN et al. 1985; THOMSEN et al. 1985; CLEMENTS et al. 1987; GEDROYC et al. 1987; STANLEY et al. 1987; TAYLOR et al. 1987). Intrinsic vascular obstruction is usually surgical or arteriosclerotic in origin. Rare cases of pseudoaneurysm have been described. Areas of narrowing of the renal artery or its branches distal to the anastomosis can be seen associated with rejection and are caused by intramural proliferation.

Arterial stenosis should be suspected when a transplanted patient develops severe hypertension with or without impairment of renal function. An audible bruit may be demonstrable over the graft (LEE et al. 1978). Renin analyses are generally less reliable indicators of significant stenosis in graft kidneys than in native kidneys (SNIDERMAN et al. 1980a, b; LAASONEN et al. 1985; CLEMENTS et al. 1987). However, when severe stenosis is accompanied by a decrease in kidney function and/or arterial hypertension, attempts to relieve the stenosis should be considered, since progression usually occurs and may lead to total occlusion. The obstruction is usually seen within the 1st year following surgery and rarely after the 3rd year.

Renal vein occlusion is a rare finding, which can be caused by thrombosis or more commonly by external compression of the vein by a fluid collection (HANTO and SIMMONS 1987). Clinically, it presents as a nephrotic syndrome.

13.1.3 Imaging of the Renal Allograft

The long list of potential early posttransplant complications necessitates very careful postoperative monitoring based on the patient's clinical condition and kidney function (serum creatinine). However, the clinical presentation of increasing serum creatinine, fever, and kidney tenderness can cross over from one causative factor to another, and two or more complications can be simultaneously at work.

Imaging procedures are extremely useful to identify the potential cause of renal failure. Nuclear medical studies and ultrasonography represent the standard imaging procedures used for the routine monitoring of the graft, but conventional radiography, computed tomography (CT), and magnetic resonance imaging (MRI) can be useful to clarify specific problems. Furthermore it is possible to handle many urologic complications by interventional procedures using imaging techniques.

13.2 Radionuclide Imaging

The most frequent and important complications of renal transplantation – ATN, acute rejection, and cyclosporine nephropathy – are diffuse processes. Their functional and perfusional consequences are usually more prominent than their structural effects. For this reason radionuclide studies, being able to quantify perfusion and function, have assumed a dominant role in control of renal transplants. None of the radionuclide agents are specific enough to demonstrate a particular cause of renal impairment with certainty. Serial quantitative studies are needed in order to document improvement or deterioration in perfusion and/or function (Fig. 13.1). Radionuclide investigations have the advantage of being noninvasive and can be repeated frequently; this is important in a situation where the clinical condition may change rapidly.

13.2.1 Monitoring

At some transplantation centers the monitoring is limited to the periods during which biochemical parameters are few (SALVATIERRA et al. 1974; HALASZ et al. 1987). At other centers radionuclide examinations are performed routinely three times a week until discharge and thereafter only when clinical problems arise (THOMSEN et al. 1988). The most commonly used examinations are radionuclear angiography, which is a perfusion study, and renography, which is essentially a functional study. Deterioration in perfusion/function as judged from the radionuclide examinations may precede biochemical manifestations by 24–48 h (ROSENTHALL et al.

Acute rejection

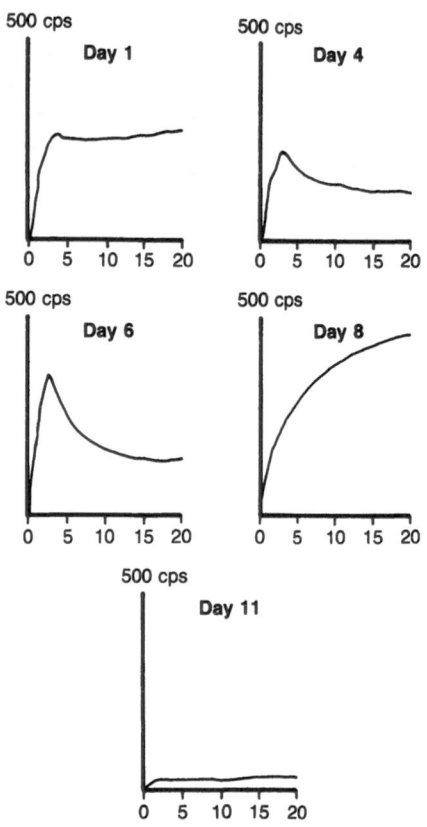

Fig. 13.1. Sequential renograms from a patient suffering irreversible acute rejection despite increased steroid treatment from day 8. For grading see Fig. 13.7. At the first three examinations the graft had a flow peak on the first passage curve, whereas at the two last no flow peak was present (Fig. 13.2)

1974). A single isolated radionuclide study is of little value except in the presence of specific conditions such as vascular thrombosis and urinary leakage. What is important is change in uptake/perfusion from one study to another (CLORIUS et al. 1979; KIM et al. 1986; THOMSEN et al. 1988).

13.2.1.1 Radionuclear Angiography (Bolus Transit)

Radionuclear angiography gives a histogram of count rates over the graft (first passage curve) which depends on the vascular transit of the radiotracer and the total vascular volume within the kidney. It can, in principle, be performed with any ^{99m}Tc- or ^{123}I-labeled radiopharmaceutical. Since the renal handling of ^{99m}Tc-mercaptoacetyltriglycine (MAG3), ^{99m}Tc-diethylenetriamine pentaacetic acid (DTPA), ^{123}I-hippuran, and ^{123}I-iothalamate influen-

ces the downslope of the first passage curve, these pharmaceuticals may be less useful in poorly or nonfunctioning kidneys (THOMSEN et al. 1987a). For simple routine investigations ^{99m}Tc-pertechnetate is preferable due to its low price, high vascular transit, and low kidney radiation.

The gamma camera is positioned over the kidney in the iliac fossa. The lower abdominal aorta and the external iliac artery should be in the field of view. The antecubical vein chosen for injection of the bolus should be as large as possible. When the bolus reaches the lower abdominal aorta seen on the persistence scope of the gamma camera, storage of 0.5-s frames for 60 s is started. Two regions of interest are chosen, one being the graft without underlying major vessels, the other the iliac artery (Fig. 13.2a). The iliac histogram is used to establish that a proper bolus has been given; $T^1/_2$ of the downslope should be less than 10 s.

Renal blood flow can be assessed both qualitatively and quantitatively by angioscintigraphy if a good bolus injection has been given. By visual inspection of the "normalized" first passage curve it can be determined whether the graft has a well-defined flow peak (= normal perfusion) (Fig. 13.2b), a poorly defined flow peak (= reduced perfusion), or no flow peak (= severely reduced perfusion) (Fig. 13.2c). This estimation is often sufficient for clinical purposes (THOMSEN and MUNCK 1987; THOMSEN et al. 1988; THOMSEN and NIELSEN 1988). Several methods of quantifying perfusion have been proposed over the years (DUBOVSKY and RUSSELL 1988). From normalized first passage curves a perfusion index (Fig. 13.3) (HILSON et al. 1978) can be calculated. Determination of $T^1/_2$ of the downslope of the graft curve (Fig. 13.4) has also been proposed (PRESTON and LUKE 1979; JACKSON et al. 1986). With both methods, however, there is overlap between normal grafts and those with complications causing reduced perfusion. In addition the individual mean vascular (arteriovenous) transit time of renal transplants varies too widely to be of practical value (SCHMIDLIN et al. 1986). BAILLET et al. (1986) evaluated several perfusion indices and found that all of the indices studied could discriminate between normal perfusion and impaired perfusion caused by rejection but that only one approach (WASHIDA et al. 1982) could differentiate between acute rejection and ATN. However, renal arterial stenosis may lead to a false diagnosis of acute rejection owing to its effect on renal washout and consequently on any of the indices (NIELSEN et al. 1987). Cyclosporine, with its vasoconstrictive effect (DIEPERINK et al. 1986), has introduced another hemodynamic factor which

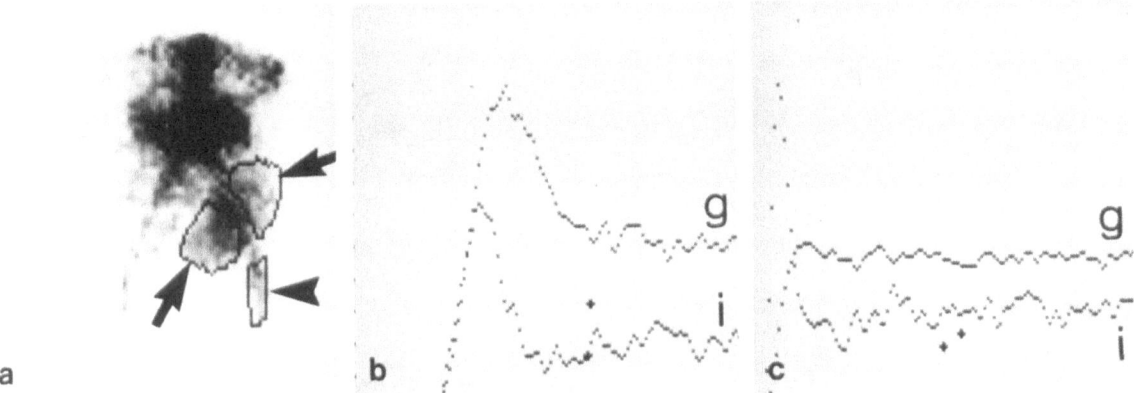

Fig. 13.2. a Image with regions of interest over the graft without the underlying iliac artery and over the iliac artery. **b** Histogram showing a well-defined flow peak on both the graft *(g)* and the iliac artery *(i)*. **c** Histogram from the graft *(g)* region of interest without a flow peak despite a well-defined flow peak on the iliac histogram *(i)*

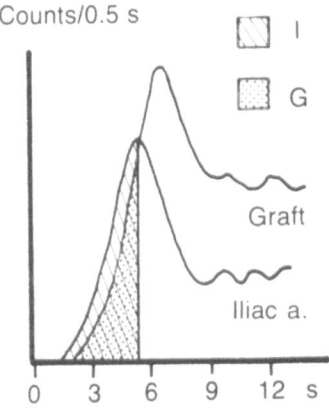

Fig. 13.3. Hilson's perfusion index (area under arterial curve to peak/area under renal curve). (HILSON et al. 1978)

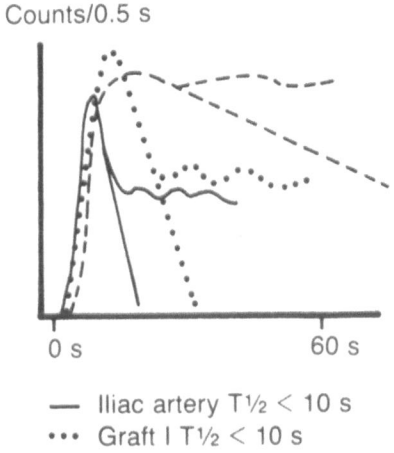

— Iliac artery T½ < 10 s
••• Graft I T½ < 10 s
--- Graft II T½ > 30 s

Fig. 13.4. $T^{1}/_{2}$ of the downslope. A bolus with an artery $T^{1}/_{2}$ lasting longer than 10 s should not be accepted. A graft $T^{1}/_{2}$ lasting longer than 28 s indicates abnormal perfusion (= rejection). (PRESTON and LUKE 1979; JACKSON et al. 1986)

may influence the interpretation of perfusion indices.

13.2.1.2 Renography

Most authors prefer gamma camera renography, which can be performed with ^{131}I-hippuran, ^{123}I-hippuran ^{99m}Tc-MAG3, or ^{99m}Tc-DTPA. Probe renography with ^{131}I-hippuran is a cheap but insufficient alternative. ^{99m}Tc-DTPA is mainly filtered by the glomeruli, whereas renal clearance of the other three radiopharmaceuticals occurs predominantly by tubular extraction. The physical properties of ^{131}I-hippuran are inferior to those of the other three radiopharmaceuticals, but it is cheap and easily available and the image contrast is suitable. Both ^{123}I-hippuran and ^{99m}Tc-MAG3 have the same favorable biologic properties as ^{131}I-hippuran and give excellent scans, but ^{123}I-hippuran is expensive and not readily available; experience with the newly introduced ^{99m}Tc-MAG3 (Fig. 13.5) is promising (TAYLOR et al. 1987 a, b; BUBECK et al. 1988). However, its use will be limited by the difficulties of performing two ^{99m}Tc studies in a row, especially in poorly or nonfunctioning grafts. The chosen radiopharmaceutical is injected intravenously and sequential frames for 20 or 30 min are stored in the computer. For background subtraction a symmetrical region of interest in the contralateral side of the pelvis is used.

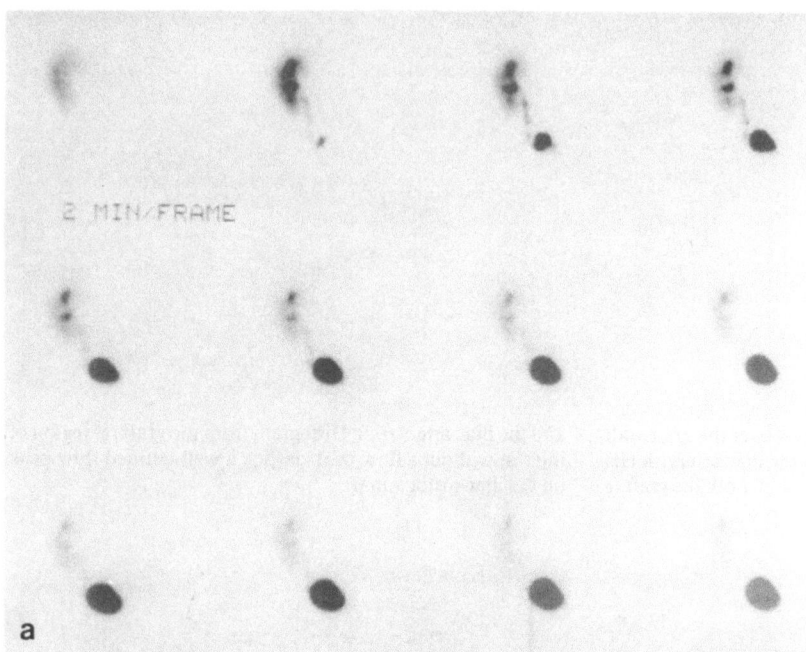

Fig. 13.5 a, b. ⁹⁹ᵐTc-MAG3 image
of **a** a normal and **b** a non-functioning graft 2 min/frame. (Courtesy of
Andrew Taylor, Jr., M. D., Atlanta,
GA)

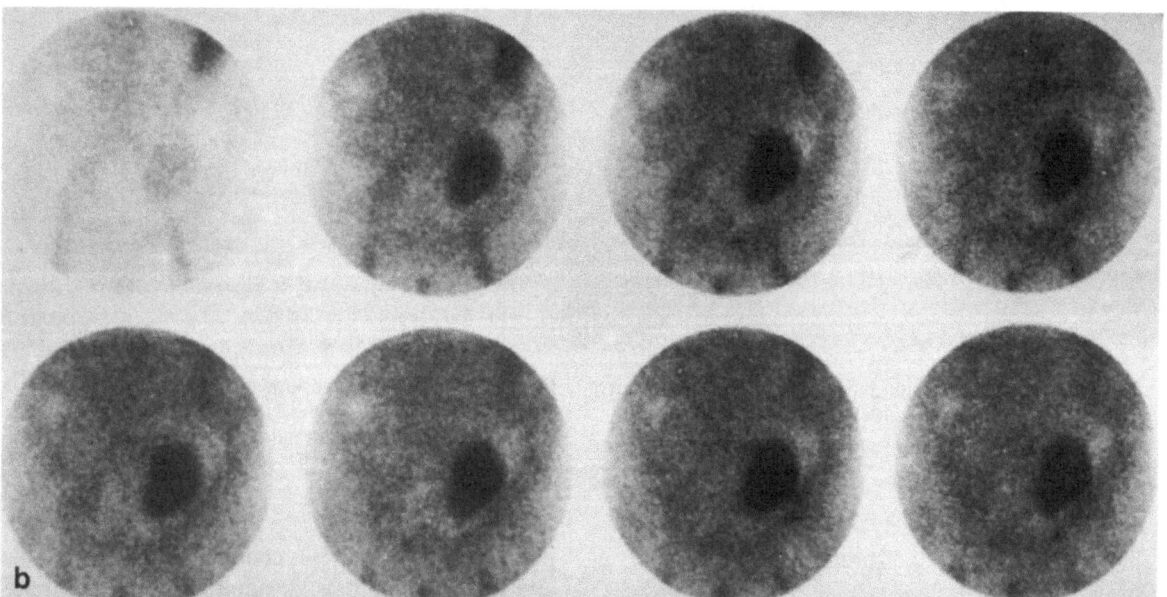

On scintigraphic images a normal graft has a
rapid uptake and the radiopharmaceutical is demonstrable in the bladder within the first 5 min.
After 20 min most of the activity is in the bladder
(Fig. 13.6). In cyclosporine nephrotoxicity, acute rejection, and ATN the scintigram will show decreased uptake in the graft, prolonged accumulation, and delayed appearance in the bladder
(Fig. 13.6). When ¹³¹I-hippuran is used, an ominous
sign is activity remaining from a study performed
24–48 h previously (Thomsen et al. 1985).

The method of evaluating the graft renogram is
adapted from that used for "normal" kidneys. Many
different parameters of the renogram have been
quantified with varying success. They include: time
to peak of the renogram, half-time of the elimination
phase, blood clearance curve, ratio of bladder/kid-
ney curve height, bladder appearance time, kidney
to background ratio, and bladder to kidney ratio
(Staab et al. 1969; Weiss et al. 1972; Moore and
Hayes 1974; Dubovsky et al. 1975). Thomsen et al.
(1985) have proposed a simple grading system

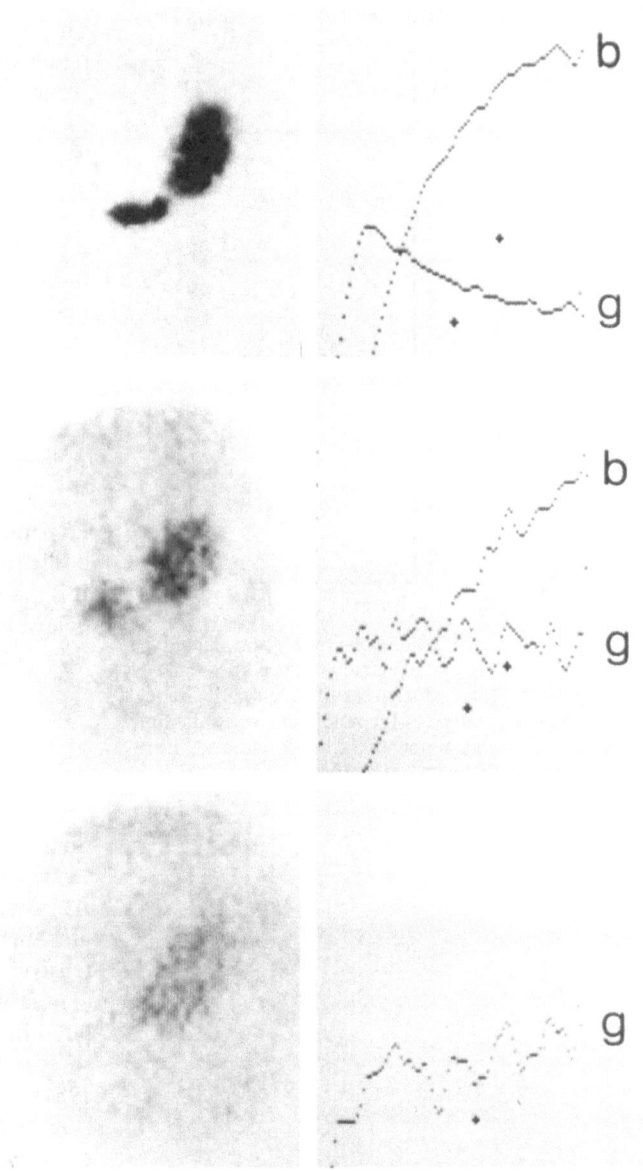

Fig. 13.6. ^{131}I-Hippuran scintigram and renogram from *(top)* a well-functioning graft, *(middle)* an adequately functioning graft, and *(bottom)* a poorly functioning graft. *g*, graft curve; *b*, bladder curve

(Fig. 13.7) for quantifying graft function from renograms. It seems to be sensitive enough to detect complications and is easy to communicate to the clinicians.

13.2.2 Complications

Immediately after transplantation (within 36 h) a study of the vascular supply to the graft should be performed; excellent perfusion is nearly always found and if it is not, a vascular complication must be present. Based on the knowledge of good perfusion immediately after operation the monitoring can

start. By performing serial radionuclide studies in the early postoperative phase and by interpreting them in relation to time and clinical circumstances, an acceptable level of diagnostic accuracy can be obtained.

13.2.2.1 Vascular Occlusion

In the early postoperative phase the angioscintigraphic diagnosis of vascular occlusion is very reliable (Fig. 13.8). Later (after months or years) the well-vascularized fibrotic tissue around the graft renders the diagnosis difficult.

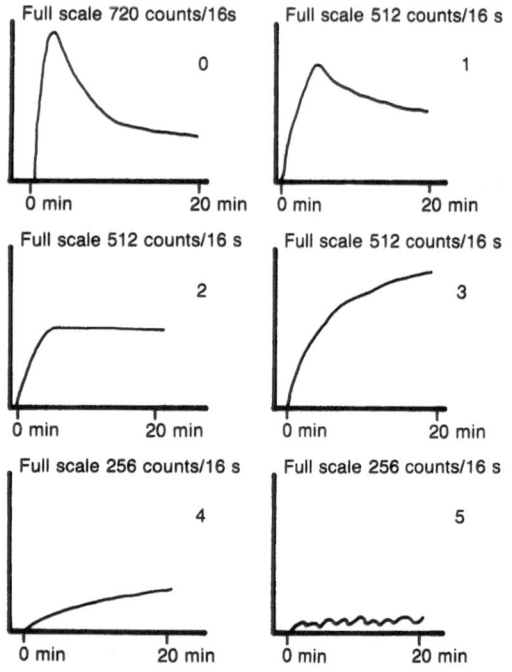

Fig. 13.7. ^{131}I-Hippuran renograms from transplanted patients graded according to the function of the graft: Grade 0 is from a graft with normal glomerular filtration rate. Grades 1 through 4 show the pattern of the renograms when the function decreases. The flat renogram, grade 5, indicates nearly abolished function. (THOMSEN et al. 1985)

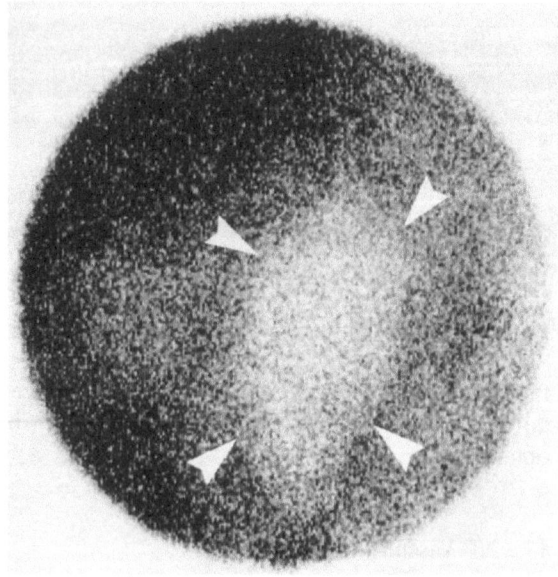

Fig. 13.8. Intravenous angiography with ^{99m}Tc-pertechnetate, performed with a mobile gamma camera and showing a photon-deficient region at the site of the graft *(arrowheads).* Such a finding indicates vascular occlusion and excision of the graft should be performed; radiologic confirmation by angiography is unnecessary

13.2.2.2 Arterial Stenosis

The effect of arterial stenosis on the renogram depends on its severity. Typically slow uptake and excretion are demonstrated. On the perfusion study there tends to be slow flow into the kidney; once activity reaches the kidney, good vascularization is generally demonstrated, but minor infarcts may be found on the scintigram. Scintigraphy before and immediately after angiotensin converting enzyme inhibition, which seems promising in native kidneys, may also be helpful in transplanted patients (DUBOVSKY et al. 1987) by distinguishing between functional and nonfunctional stenosis.

13.2.2.3 Hyperacute Rejection

Hyperacute rejection is caused by preformed antibodies leading to fulminant thrombosis of the vein. It is mainly a peroperative diagnosis. In the event of delayed reaction the radionuclide examination may show a photon-deficient area (Fig. 13.8).

13.2.2.4 Acute Tubular Necrosis

The ischemic demage leading to ATN is present in many cadaveric kidneys (KIRCHNER and ROSENTHALL 1982) and mainly resolves without therapy. Application of radiographic contrast media immediately before explantation (SZPIRT et al. 1984), hypotensive episodes during the initial reperfusion (THOMSEN et al. 1987b), and cyclosporine administered in high doses (CHOW et al. 1986) increase the severity of ATN. Good perfusion (SHANAHAN et al. 1981) and an increasing uptake curve (grade 3–4) (Fig. 13.7) unchanged at the first postoperative examinations indicate ATN.

13.2.2.5 Acute Cyclosporine Nephrotoxicity

Cyclosporine has a constrictive effect on the efferent arteriole (DIEPERINK et al. 1986) which may lead to secondary tubular dysfunction. Nephrotoxic levels of cyclosporine, which vary between individuals and decrease with age (LARSEN et al. 1988), result in decreased radionuclide perfusion and uptake. If severely ischemic grafts (e.g., kidneys obtained from non-beating-heart donors) are used, high dose cyclosporine may result in nonfunctioning grafts and a fall in radionuclide perfusion and uptake 48–96 h posttransplantation, followed by stabilization at a low level (THOMSEN and MUNCK 1987; THOMSEN et al. 1987c). This can be avoided by reducing the dose of cyclosporine and postponing its administration for a couple of days (THOMSEN et al. 1988).

13.2.2.6 Acute Rejection

Usually acute rejection first occurs from late in the first postoperative week, allowing two baseline examinations to be performed. If the renogram is studied in conjunction with a radionuclide angiogram it may help to distinguish ATN from acute rejection since classical ATN has good hippuran uptake but no elimination, a good circulation, and a good blood pool image. Acute rejection may have a similar hippuran appearance but reduced perfusion and a patchy blood pool image. A worsening of the perfusion and uptake from one radionuclide study to another performed with intervals up to 3 days indicates a rejection episode. A severe decrease in renal uptake (e.g., full grade or more) (Fig. 13.7) combined with a loss of peak on the graft histogram (Fig. 13.1) is a very strong indicator of rejection (THOMSEN et al. 1988). Similar changes found immediately after transplantation are likely to be due to synergistic potentiation between ischemia and cyclosporine nephrotoxicity, or superimposition of cyclosporine nephrotoxicity on the recovering ischemic kidney. If the decrease in renographic function is less than a full grade and the peak also disappears, the likelihood of acute rejection is high, but it is not certain to occur. In such cases a graft biopsy should be obtained and/or a repeat radionuclide examination should be performed within 24 h to demonstrate further deterioration. After antirejection therapy with steroids and/or murine monoclonal antibody to the surface antigen of human T lymphocytes (OKT3), its effect can be followed by the radionuclide examinations. A repeat study should always be performed following antirejection therapy – and during therapy when there is inadequate response to treatment

Over the years several radiopharmaceuticals have been proposed for the specific diagnosis of acute rejection. Three agents which have been studied in some detail are ^{125}I-fibrinogen (SALAMAN 1972; GEORGE et al. 1976), ^{99m}Tc-sulfur colloid (FRICK et al. 1976; GEORGE et al. 1976; PETERDY et al. 1981), and ^{67}Ga-citrate (GEORGE et al. 1976; FAWWAZ and JOHNSON 1979); none of these have gained wide acceptance due to a high rate of false-positives. Labeling of platelets, lymphocytes, and leukocytes has also been tested for the same purpose (FRICK et al.

1979; CHANDLER et al. 1983; MARTIN-COMIN 1986), but in each case there is again a high frequency of false-positives. All the above methods will give false-negative results when rejection is accompanied by severely impaired blood flow. Hope has now turned to labeled monoclonal antibodies as future specific indicators of acute rejection.

13.2.2.7 Infarcts

Ligation of a pole artery is the most frequent cause of graft infarct, but the latter may also be seen in arterial stenosis. At radionuclide angiography a small photon-deficient area will be found. Better visualization of the infarct can be obtained with ^{99m}Tc-dimercaptosuccinic acid scintigraphy. This is, however, not suitable for serial scanning due to the high radiation dose to the graft.

13.2.2.8 Chronic Diseases

Chronic cyclosporine nephrotoxicity, transplant disease, de novo kidney disease, and chronic rejection are all slow processes which can only be distinguished by a graft biopsy. In all four diseases, radionuclide studies performed at intervals of 1 or 2 months will show a gradual deterioration of perfusion/uptake, and there will also be shrinkage of the kidney on scintigrams.

13.2.2.9 Miscellaneous (Renal)

There is seldom time for radionuclide diagnosis of graft rupture and bleeding. In cases of arteriovenous fistula, rapid perfusion and a localized area with increased isotope activity are found. If the recipient's own kidney function is just above the limit for dialysis and the graft function is poor, the split function may be determined by ^{99m}Tc-DMSA scintigraphy (Fig. 13.9).

$$G = \frac{\sqrt{A_G \times P_G}}{\sqrt{A_G \times P_G} + \sqrt{A_{OK} \times P_{OK}}}$$

Fig. 13.9. Formula for determination of divided kidney function between own kidney *(OK)* and graft *(G)* according to the geometric mean method (HARTLING et al. 1987). A_G, anterior view, graft; P_G, posterior view, graft; A_{OK}, anterior view, own kidneys; P_{OK}, posterior view, own kidneys. The fractional function of own kidneys is: $OK = 1 - G$

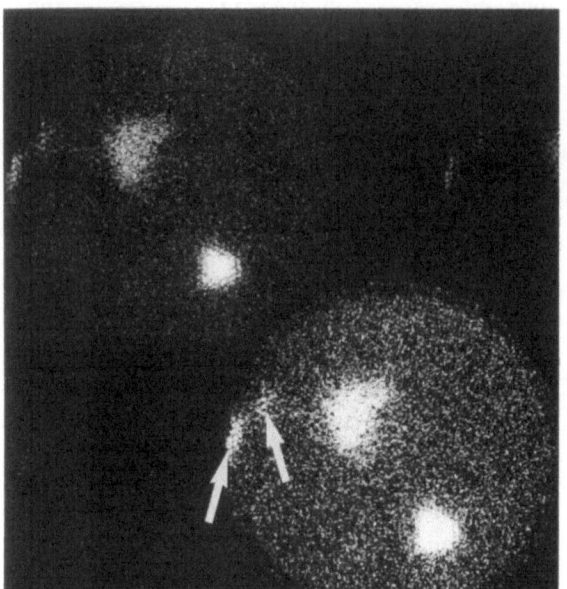

Fig. 13.10. ^{131}I-Hippuran image showing urinary leakage *(arrows)*. Such a finding requires radiologic and/or surgical intervention

13.2.2.10 Urinary Leakage

Scintigraphy is a sensitive method of diagnosing urinary leakage by demonstrating abnormal isotope accumulation outside the urinary tract (Fig. 13.10) (SPIGOS et al. 1977; DeLANGE et al. 1982). This should be followed by radiographic demonstration of its location and severity.

13.2.2.11 Obstruction

Ureteral obstruction causes a rising renogram and sometimes a prominent pelvis on the images, but in the early phase no change in perfusion. A prominent pelvis does not in itself indicate obstruction, but the appearance of a pelvis previously unseen is strongly suggestive of obstruction. In this setting it should be remembered that a poorly functioning graft may be unable to dilate the pelvic cavity even if there is severe obstruction (KIRCHNER and ROSENTHALL 1982). Radionuclide examinations are of no help in distinguishing the various causes of obstruction.

13.3 Ultrasonography

Ultrasonography (US) as an imaging modality has the advantages of being harmless, noninvasive, fast, and cheap. The renal transplant is especially well suited for US investigation due to its position in the pelvis just under the abdominal wall. Today US is used routinely in most centers for postoperative follow-up. It is useful in the management of perirenal collections and hydronephrosis and for the monitoring of graft size, relative echogenicity of intrarenal structures, and intrarenal vascular resistance.

13.3.1 Technique

Two basically different ultrasound investigations are used, a gray-scale B-scan and a Doppler investigation. The common US equipment yields what is termed a gray-scale B-scan picture, which is a representation of the acoustic properties in a section of the patient. The picture is obtained by emitting a very short pulse in a certain direction and recording the echoes, moving the direction a little, and repeating the process. Several hundred pulses make up an image.

In Doppler US, a sound wave with a well-defined frequency is emitted, and any deviation from this frequency is monitored in the received signal. Such deviations are recorded if the ultrasound is reflected from a moving object, and depend on the speed of the object and the angle between the ultrasound beam and the track of the moving object. The Doppler may be either continuous wave or pulsed. In the latter case, the Doppler pulse may be "gated" to include only a small part of the picture, e.g., a well-defined vascular structure. The result is presented as a time-velocity graph.

Recent technical developments have made it possible to combine these techniques into one picture. The direction and velocity are presented on the screen in colors - so-called color Doppler US.

The modern US apparatus includes powerful microprocessors which are able to calculate areas and circumferences on the B-scan picture and to perform calculations on the Doppler. Future developments will probably enable us to make comprehensive statistical analyses of the single elements in the picture - so-called tissue characteristics.

13.3.2 Ultrasound Monitoring

13.3.2.1 Normal Appearance

The US appearance of the renal transplant is essentially the same as that of native kidneys except that a better resolution is obtained due to the superficial position of the kidney (Fig. 13.11).

The US investigation of the renal transplant should be carried out in a standardized manner, and the following noted: graft size, cortical thickness, intrarenal parenchymal structures, and the presence of perirenal fluid collections and hydronephrosis. The first scan should be performed within a few days after surgery to establish a baseline against which later scans can be compared.

13.3.2.2 Graft Size

The size of the transplant should be evaluated by comparison with the early baseline scan. The volume of the graft normally increases moderately during the first 6–9 months after surgery and then slowly decreases (ABSY et al. 1987; LACHANCE et al. 1988). The volume of the graft may be calculated by the formula:

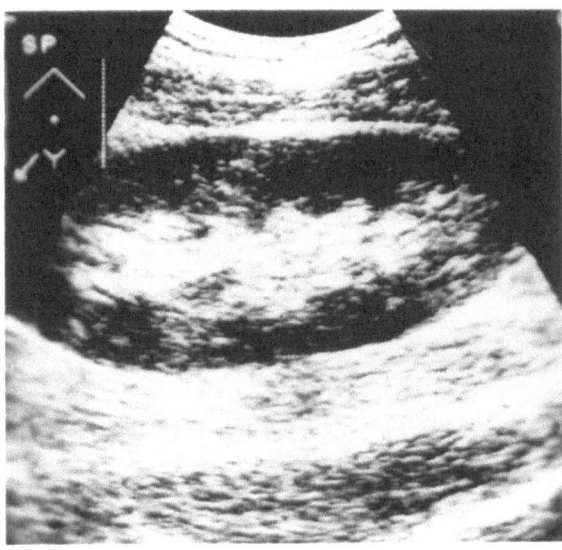

Fig. 13.11. Ultrasound scan of a normal kidney graft

$$L\,(\text{length}) \times H\,(\text{height}) \times W\,(\text{width}) \times 0.523$$

where 0.523 is $\pi/6$ (HRICAK and LIETO 1983).

Modern ultrasound scanners with calculating facilities compute the volume from the maximum length and the cross-section at the hilus level.

Rapid increase in size is associated with acute rejection and is ascribed to medullary and interstitial edema (HRICAK et al. 1979; FRICK et al. 1981; LINKOWSKI et al. 1987; COCHLIN et al. 1988). If the kidney is smaller than expected, this may be the result of chronic disease (HRICAK et al. 1979) or graft arterial stenosis (HRICAK et al. 1981).

13.3.2.3 Intrarenal Parenchymal Structures

During rejection episodes, changes in the intrarenal parenchymal structures may be seen (Fig. 13.12). Again, it is mandatory to compare these findings with the baseline scan.

The most common signs are: (a) increase in the corticomedullary relative echogenicity, (b) enlarged pyramids, and (c) decrease in sinus echoes (HRICAK et al. 1979, 1982; MAKLAD et al. 1979; FRICK et al. 1981; JAFRI et al. 1981; HECKEMANN et al. 1982; FRIED et al. 1983; SLOVIS et al. 1984; LINKOWSKI et al. 1987; COCHLIN et al. 1988). The enlargement of the pyramids is an absolute sign and is probably due to local edema. It may be combined with the cortical thickness to form the "medullary pyramid index" (MPI) (FRIED et al. 1983):

$$\text{MPI} = \frac{1/2\,(\text{pyramid length} \times \text{pyramid width})}{\text{cortical thickness}}$$

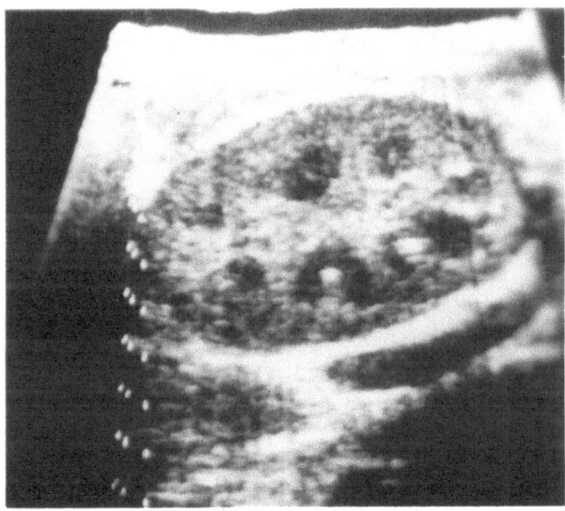

Fig. 13.12. Ultrasound scan of a graft undergoing acute rejection. There is increased relative corticomedullary echogenicity, prominent and enlarged pyramids, and a decrease in sinus echoes as compared with the normal graft (Fig. 13.11)

An increase in MPI is related to a decrease in graft function.

The decrease in sinus echoes occurs later than the other two common signs and is ascribed to degeneration of renal sinus fat to fibrous tissue. All these internal parenchymal parameters as signs of rejection have in common the drawback that while their specificity may be acceptable there are many false-negatives. Hence, we still need a noninvasive sensitive test for rejection. A possible future contribution from ultrasound may be tissue characterization.

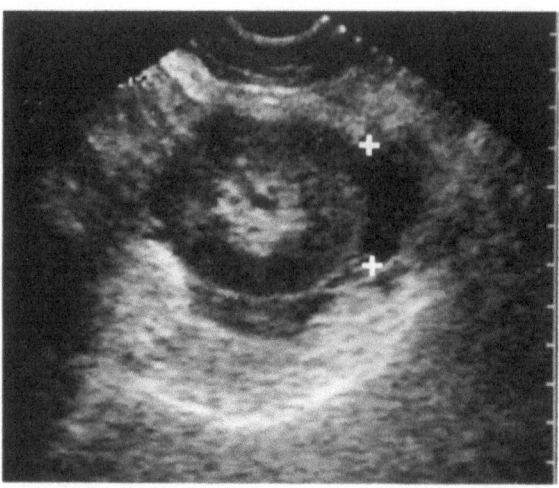

Fig. 13.13. Ultrasound scan of a fluid collection close to the graft surface containing some internal echoes. Puncture verified hematoma

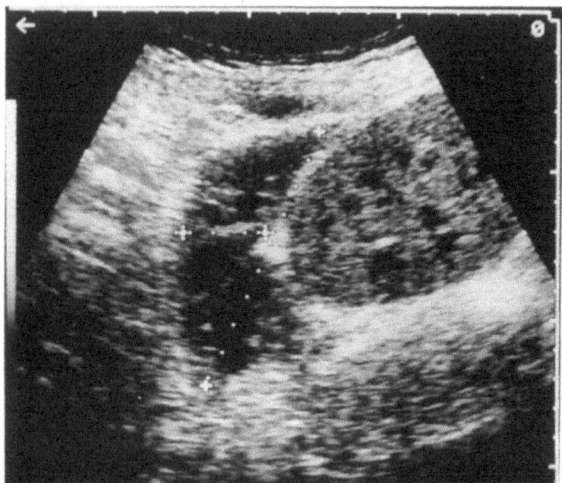

Fig. 13.14. Ultrasound scan of large collection at lower pole of graft with areas containing echoes. Lymphoceles with internal septa

In ATN the graft usually shows no sonographic abnormalities. Hence, it has been stated that a normal US examination in a nonfunctioning graft is highly suggestive of ATN (HRICAK et al. 1981; THOMSEN et al. 1985). However, overlap between sonographic features in ATN and acute rejection has been noted (JAFRI et al. 1981). Little is known about sonographic features in cyclosporine nephrotoxicity. One larger series indicates difficulty in differentiating this complication from acute rejection (LINKOWSKI et al. 1987).

In conclusion, US parenchymal changes are best demonstrated by repeated scanning. They may be of some help in differentiating the various causes of graft dysfunction, but should always be evaluated together with clinical, laboratory, and nuclear medical data.

13.3.2.4 Urologic Complications

While urinary leak is best demonstrated by scintigraphic or radiographic methods, ultrasound is extremely useful in both the diagnosis and the management of perirenal fluid collections and hydronephrosis.

Perirenal Fluid Collections. Normally, fluid collections will appear hypoechoic, except for hematomas, which may be more echogenic and thus evade detection (Fig. 13.13) (EICKS et al. 1978). Lymphoceles are usually larger than other collections and are often associated with compression or dislocation of adjacent structures. A lymphocele is frequently septated and often shows some internal echogenicity (Fig. 13.14) (COYNE et al. 1981; SILVER et al. 1981). Urinomas have no distinct appearance on US (NOVICK et al. 1981). Abscesses may be septated and show internal echogenicity (SILVER et al. 1981; STREEM and NOVICK 1983). Hematomas tend to be rather echogenic, but the ultrasonic appearance is variable (COYNE et al. 1981; SILVER et al. 1981). Thus, ultrasound is sensitive but not very specific in the diagnosis of perirenal fluid collections. When evaluated together with the clinical symptoms, differential diagnosis is sometimes possible. Often however, ultrasonically guided aspiration is performed for diagnostic and/or therapeutic purposes (SPIGOS and CAPEK 1975; BERNARDINO and BAUMGARTNER 1986; CASOLA and VAN SONNENBERG 1987).

Hydronephrosis. A dilated renal pelvis and calyces are readily demonstrated by US (KOEHLER et al. 1976; ROSENFIELD and TAYLOR 1976; COYNE et al. 1981), and in hydronephrosis these sonolucent structures will displace the central sinus echoes peripherally (Fig. 13.15). Due to the favorable position of the graft a dilated ureter can usually be traced to the point of obstruction (Fig. 13.15). As with native kidneys, the presence of dilatation does not necessarily indicate obstruction. Also significant obstruction can be present without dilatation. (BALCHUNAS et al. 1982; HUNTER et al. 1983; BENNETT et al. 1986). Since US examination is easy, rapid, and noninvasive, it is especially well suited for the follow-up of a suspected obstruction. Also ultrasound guidance is highly recommendable for any diagnostic or therapeutic intervention in hydronephrosis.

13.3.3 Doppler Investigation

The Doppler signal reflects the velocity of the blood flow, and the relative strength of the signal is dependent on the angle of the vessel with respect to the ultrasound beam. If the flow is perpendicular to the beam, a maximum Doppler signal is obtained. Due to the obvious difficulties in determining the direction of a small vessel, relative measures of velocity in the systolic and diastolic periods are used instead of absolute velocity values. Different mathematical approaches to achieve this end have been tried (TAYLOR and BURNS 1985), the simplest being the AB ratio, which is maximum frequency shift divided by minimum frequency shift in a cardiac cycle, bearing in mind that the measured frequency shift is directly proportional to the relative velocity. This method is very sensitive for precise measurement of the B value, which is often very low. A more sophisticated formula is the pulsatility index (PI), which is derived as $(A-B)/\text{mean}$, where mean is the mean frequency shift in one cardiac cycle (TAYLOR and BURNS 1985) (Fig. 13.16).

The PI may be derived from a hard copy of the time/velocity graph. However, modern instruments incorporate programs which greatly facilitate the calculation. A fully automatic PI calculation program has been implemented on one commercial Doppler apparatus (Quantascope). The kidney is essentially a vascular low resistance organ, resulting in a low PI (1.1–1.2) in grafts with a normal function. During rejection periods, the vascular resistance increases and the diastolic flow is diminished and

sometimes even reversed; hence PI is elevated during rejection periods (RIGSBY et al. 1987). At present, Doppler investigation alone cannot differentiate rejection from cyclosporine toxicity. At PI $\geqslant 1.5$, specificity is 90% and sensitivity approximately 75%. As would be expected, vascular obstruction produces a substantial increase in PI.

A vascular stenosis may be detected by a high velocity jet, followed by distal turbulence (TAYLOR et al. 1987). This is especially well demonstrated on the color Doppler where the jet (frequency shift $\geqslant 7.5$ kHz) is clearly seen, and the turbulence is depicted with color shifts. Apart from this, the color

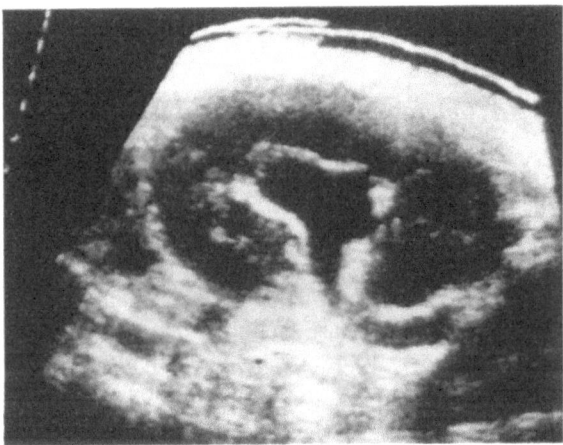

Fig. 13.15. Longitudinal scan of graft with hydronephrosis due to distal ureteral stricture. Dilated, sonolucent pelvicalyceal system with central sinus echoes displaced peripherally

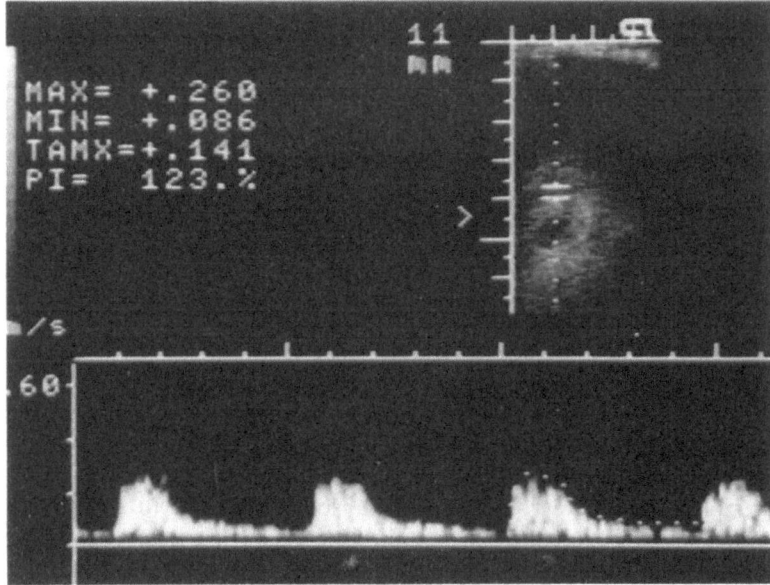

Fig. 13.16. Doppler investigation of a graft with calculation of pulsatility index. Index on the renal artery (PI = 1.23)

Doppler greatly facilitates the identification and clarifies the nature of vascular structures in the transplant, thus allowing a qualitative assessment of the overall vascularization of the transplant. Use of the color Doppler as a quantitative tool still remains to be demonstrated.

13.4 Conventional Radiography

A kidney graft located in the pelvis is less obscured by overlying bowel contents than kidneys in situ, but underlying bone and lack of fat capsule make the pelvic graft more difficult to see on plain films. Stones, arterial calcifications, and nephrocalcinosis can be readily seen. Air within the collecting system indicates emphysematous pyelonephritis.

13.4.1 Contrast Media in Kidney Transplantation

The early days of kidney transplantation overlapped the time when "high dose urography" gained worldwide acceptance as *the* method to visualize the kidney and collecting system in patients with severely impaired kidney function. Consequently ionic water-soluble contrast media in high doses were given to recently transplanted patients with no major hesitation. During the 1970s, however, it was recognized that contrast media could induce reversible or even permanent renal damage (DIAZ-BUXO et al. 1975; BYRD and SHERMAN 1979). A number of high risk groups were soon identified, among which patients with diabetes, dehydration, and nephropathy seem to be the most important (WEINRAUCH et al. 1977; VAN ZEE et al. 1978; EISENBERG et al. 1981).

Improvement in ultrasound technique, providing detailed visualization of the graft, and the development of nuclear medical methods to test the graft's vascular integrity and functional capacity have gradually reduced the need for graft urography and angiography. However, both methods are still occasionally indicated, and CT scanning has been added to the list of examinations that may involve the use of contrast media.

The problem of exposure of the kidney graft to contrast media, is therefore still of current interest. It may seem surprising that a final answer has not yet been obtained as to whether the graft is particularly susceptible to contrast media. However, many potential causes of graft failure may be at work, especially during the early phase after transplantation, and any possible extra strain on graft function from contrast media is therefore difficult to prove. Infor-

mation on this issue can only be compiled from the time when ionic contrast media were used, as summarized by THOMSEN et al. (1985).

In conclusion, ionic contrast media do not seem to be particularly harmful to the kidney graft. However, the transplanted patient has only one functioning kidney, which is threatened by a number of serious complications. Therefore, contrast media should be used only when the same information cannot be derived from noninvasive imaging. Use of more than 1 ml (300-400 mg I/ml)/kg body weight is not advisable.

While there is good clinical evidence that nonionic contrast media have fewer adverse generalized and cardiovascular effects compared with ionic media, the evidence for relative protection of kidney function by use of nonionic media is only indirect (DAWSON 1985).

We use nonionic media in patients with markedly reduced kidney function and in transplanted patients, mainly because such patients are generally fragile.

13.4.2 Intravenous Urography

Urography was the standard imaging procedure during the early days of transplantation. In many centers it was performed as soon as kidney function allowed it in order to detect early urologic complications such as urinary leak or obstruction (Fig. 13.27) and particularly to serve as a baseline study in case of later complications. This role has been taken over by ultrasound scanning, which is noninvasive, easy, fast, independent of kidney function, and can be repeated without risk. Urography can be a useful supplement in the event of equivocal ultrasound findings, especially when obstruction or urinary leak is suspected. It can be very precise in localizing these conditions.

Urography in transplanted patients differs from the usual urographic procedure in some respects. The anterior location of the graft gives a slightly greater magnification on supine films. Abdominal compression is not possible. Lack of fat capsule and underlying bone tend to obscure the outline of the graft. A liberal use of body section radiography throughout the examination and exposures in the early nephrographic phase can be of great help in overcoming some of these difficulties. We have used thin section hypocycloid radiography combined with subtraction to produce an excellent nephrogram (Fig. 13.17) (THOMSEN et al. 1984). This rather troublesome and time-consuming technique can be

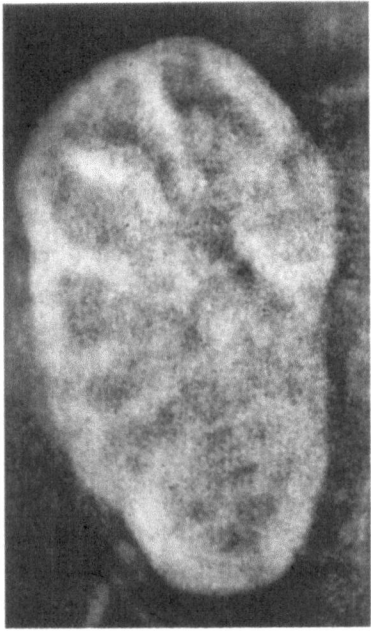

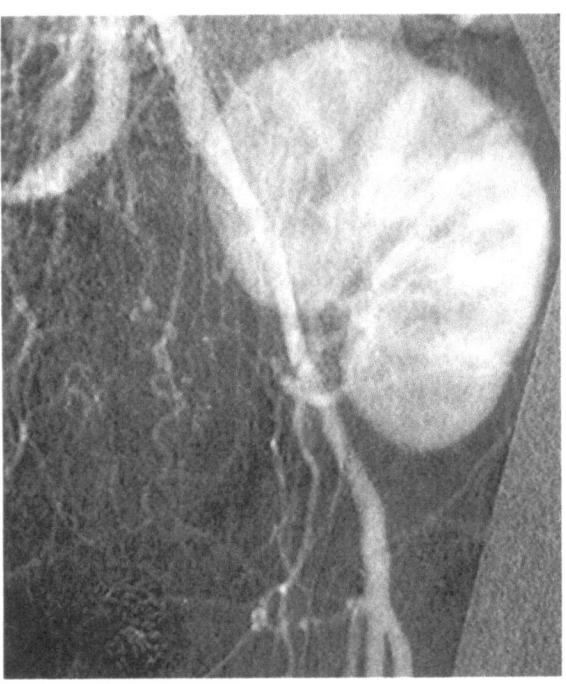

Fig. 13.17. Nephrographic phase of intravenous urography in normal graft. Hypocycloid, thin section radiography and subtraction. Exposure obtained 30 s after a rapid contrast bolus. Note the distinct demarcation between cortex and medulla

Fig. 13.18. Intravenous DSA in a normal graft. Arteriogram and nephrogram at the same time

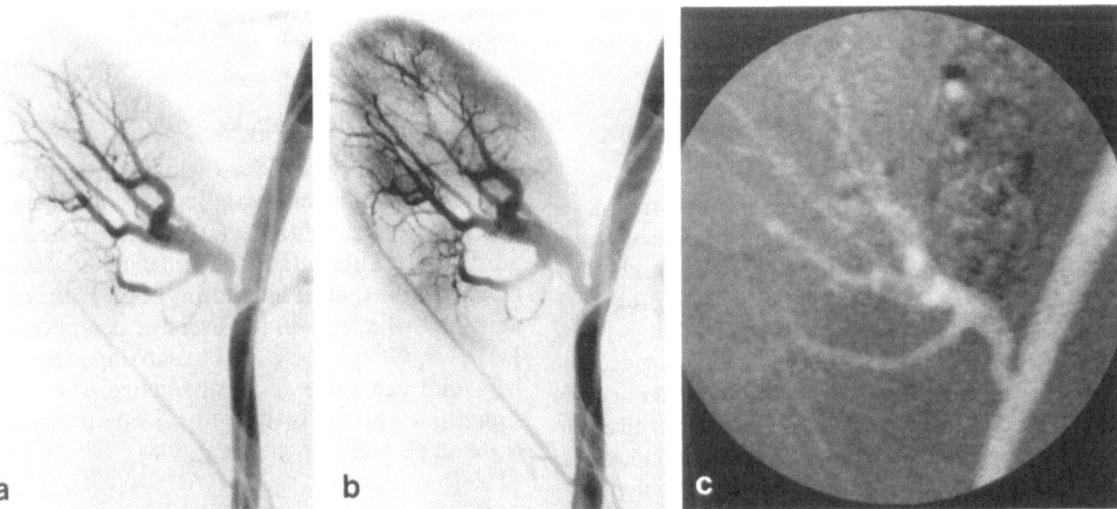

Fig. 13.19 a-c. Stenosis of renal artery at the end to side anastomosis with recipient external iliac artery. Pressure gradient across the stenosis, 100 mmHg. **a, b** Arterial DSA before and after percutaneous angioplasty. Gradient reduced to

5-10 mmHg. **c** Intravenous DSA 3 months later shows persistent result of angioplasty with no evidence of recurrent stenosis

excellently substituted by peripheral intravenous digital subtraction angiography (DSA) for the first exposures during urography. It can provide not only an excellent nephrogram but very often a diagnostic arteriogram (Figs. 13.18, 13.19 c).

13.4.3 Direct Pyelography

Since it is very often impossible to identify the orifice of a neoimplanted ureter by cystoscopy, direct pyelography is mainly performed via the antegrade

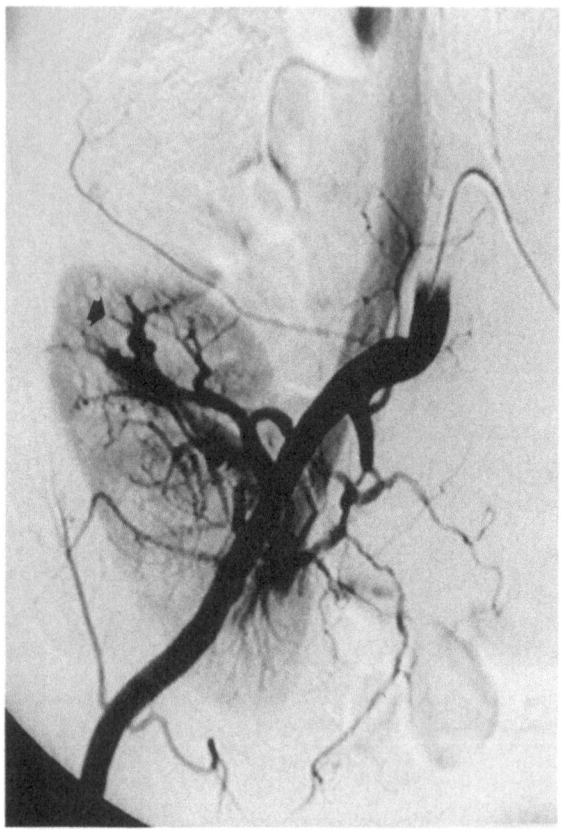

Fig. 13.20. Arterial DSA of kidney graft in patient who developed arterial hypertension and audible bruit over the graft after percutaneous graft biopsy. Arteriovenous fistula in upper pole *(arrow)* with simultaneous visualization of iliac and renal artery and vein

route (LIEBERMAN et al. 1981, 1982; HUNTER et al. 1983; CURRY et al. 1984; BENNETT et al. 1986). Antegrade needle puncture of the renal pelvis, preferably guided by ultrasound, is an easy and safe procedure in cases of obstruction with dilatation of the pelvicalyceal system (SCHMELLER et al. 1985), while technical difficulties may arise when no such dilatation is present. The puncture may be performed with a fine needle for purely diagnostic purposes and may also serve as a pathway for the placement of a nephrostomy catheter, a dilating balloon, or a stent (Figs. 13.26, 13.28–13.30).

13.4.4 Cystography

Cystography is a simple procedure to demonstrate urinary leakage involving the bladder wall. Oblique and postvoid films should be routinely used, since small leaks may otherwise pass undetected (HUNTER et al. 1983; STREEM and NOVICK 1983).

13.4.5 Angiography

In the early days of transplantation, angiography was used extensively to detect early vascular complications and especially to diagnose acute rejection and distinguish this entity from other causes of renal failure. Angiography for the last-mentioned purpose has been completely replaced by nuclear medical tests. Also in many cases the question of vascular patency can be answered without angiography, especially when nuclear medicine is combined with Doppler ultrasound (TAYLOR et al. 1987).

The major indication for angiography is now suspicion of renovascular hypertension. Arterial stenosis can be diagnosed by intravenous urography when supplied with digital subtraction in the early phase after contrast medium injection (Fig. 13.19 c). However, arterial injection is needed to demonstrate arterial detail when vascular reconstruction is considered. DSA is then a good choice, since the amount of contrast medium can be reduced (PICUS et al. 1985; ROEREN et al. 1986) (Fig. 13.19 a, b). Anteroposterior, oblique, or near lateral projections are usually required for the demonstration of the entire artery (STANLEY et al. 1987). Selective catheterization is usually unnecessary. Arteriovenous fistula, which is often a result of graft biopsy and may cause severe hypertension, is also readily diagnosed by DSA (Fig. 13.20).

13.5 Computed Tomography

Compared with the overwhelming literature on ultrasound in posttransplant patients, the literature on CT is limited. This reflects the generally accepted attitude that ultrasound is the imaging modality of choice for the routine monitoring of the kidney graft and the first choice in the event of complications. However, CT may be useful to solve specific problems and can serve as an alternative when ultrasound is equivocal or fails to provide a diagnosis (LOVE et al. 1979; NOVICK et al. 1981).

13.5.1 Technique

A complete examination of the lower abdomen and pelvis with 5 mm thin sections and 1 cm intervals after oral contrast is recommended. Rectal, vaginal, and/or bladder contrast may occasionally be helpful. Intravenous contrast may be used for specific indications such as urinary leak or renal infarcts, but should no longer be routinely employed in a category of patients whose main problem is failing kidney function (LETOURNEAU et al. 1987).

13.5.2 Imaging

The nonenhanced CT scan can readily demonstrate pelvic anatomy and the size and shape of the graft (Fig. 13.21). Parenchymal density values differing markedly from the usual 60-80 HU may indicate disease. An edematous graft undergoing acute rejection may appear normal but is typically low attenuating, while the density may be increased in some cases of chronic rejection (NOVICK et al. 1981; THOMSEN et al. 1985), occasionally due to parenchymal calcifications (LAMKI et al. 1981). Repeated CT scans through one selected level of the graft during the passage of intravenous contrast were introduced in the early 1980s in rather enthusiastic reports (sequential or dynamic CT scanning) (TREUGUT and MOLDE 1981; TREUGUT et al. 1983; FULD et al. 1984). This technique has been used to differentiate grafts undergoing rejection from normal grafts and grafts with ATN. The typical finding in acute rejection is poor or absent demarcation between cortex and medulla. This has also been observed during angiography and during the nephrographic phase of intravenous urography using thin section radiography and subtraction (THOMSEN et al. 1984). Using dynamic CT the contrast passage through the graft and the distribution between cortex and medulla related to time can be estimated in a more exact and convenient way by recording absolute attenuation values. However, the method has not gained widespread use for differential diagnosis of graft parenchymal disease, probably because it is time-consuming and requires intravenous contrast.

Nonenhanced CT is a reliable and specific method of diagnosing fresh hematoma or abscess containing air (STREEM and NOVICK 1983), while other fluid collections can be readily seen but not differentiated (KITTREDGE et al. 1978; STREEM and NOVICK 1983). Their identity must be established by uroradiologic techniques or aspiration (COYNE et al. 1981; HUNTER et al. 1983). CT is also sensitive in detecting air within or around the graft in cases of emphysematous pyelonephritis (BALSARA et al. 1985; POTTER et al. 1985).

A dilated renal pelvis and calyceal system is easily seen on CT, but, as with ultrasound, the functional significance may be difficult to evaluate. Also, it is important to be aware that significant obstruction can occasionally be missed by both methods (RASCOFF et al. 1983). Even though intravenous contrast medium injection should not be a routine procedure when scanning transplanted patients for urologic complications, it may be indicated, especially when renal infarction or extravasation due to ureteral leakage is suspected (Fig. 13.22).

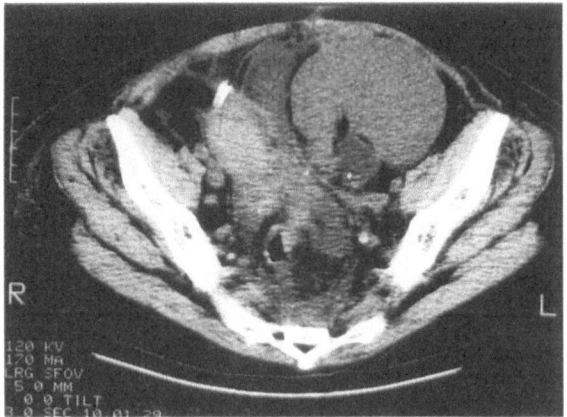

Fig. 13.21. CT scan (nonenhanced) of normal kidney graft

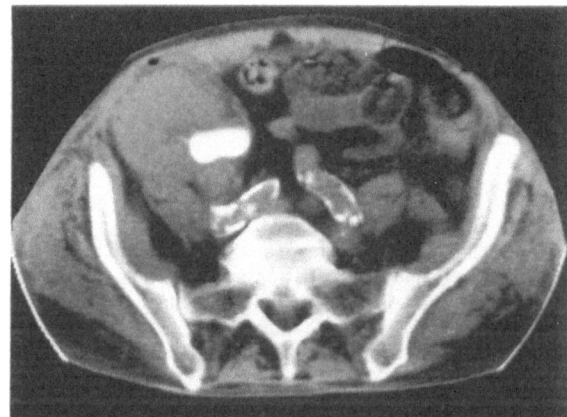

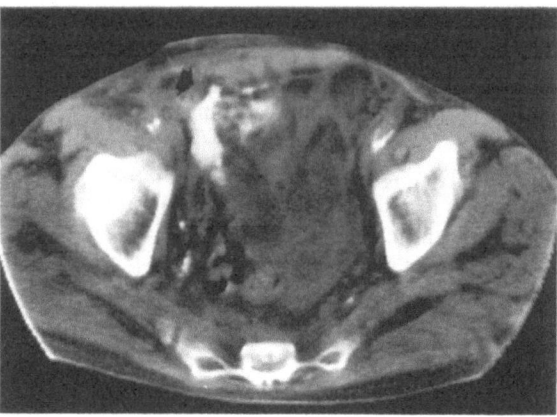

Fig. 13.22. *Above:* CT scan through graft 20 min after intravenous contrast. No sign of extravasation. *Below:* Leak into perivascular space *(arrow)* on scan 6 cm below

Computed tomography can be used in guiding needle passage for biopsy, fluid aspiration, or approach to the collecting system. However, ultrasound is preferred by most, since it is easier, quicker, and offers the advantage of continuous monitoring of the needle tip position.

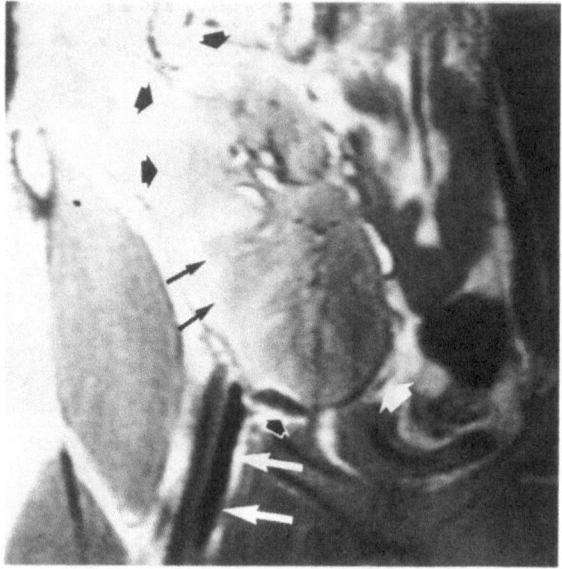

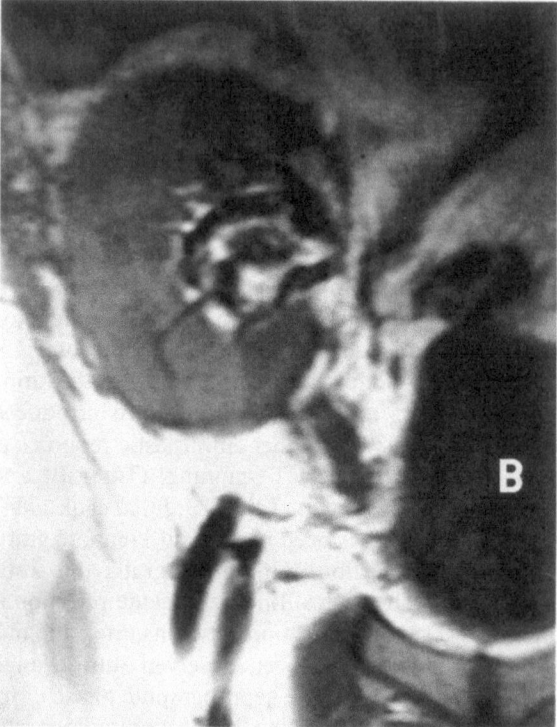

Fig. 13.23. MRI of normal renal transplant. Surface coil; spin-echo technique; TR 600 ms/TE 25 ms; field strength 1.5 T. This T1-weighted image demonstrates the allograft in the renal fossa *(arrowheads)*. The corticomedullary demarcation is well preserved *(arrows)*. A few intrarenal branch vessels can be identified in the upper pole. The femoral vessels can be seen *(white arrows)*. The kidney is not enlarged and there is no evidence of a pelvic fluid accumulation. There is no evidence of hydronephrosis. (Courtesy of Dr. HOWARD M. POLLACK)

Fig. 13.24. MRI of acute renal transplant rejection. Surface coil; spin-echo technique; TR 600 ms/TE 25 ms; field strength 1.5 T. A T1-weighted image using a receive-only surface coil demonstrates a loss of corticomedullary demarcation. The kidney is increased in transverse diameter subsequent to edema. Only the main renal vessels can be seen; the intrarenal branches are attenuated secondary to interstitial edema. *B*, urinary bladder. (Courtesy of Dr. HOWARD M. POLLACK)

13.6 Magnetic Resonance Imaging

Experience with magnetic resonance imaging (MRI) of renal allografts is still limited. Reports available indicate that MRI may be useful in the evaluation of both graft parenchymal disease and urologic complications (LUND et al. 1987).

13.6.1 Normal Renal Allografts

The morphologic features revealed by MRI in native kidneys are readily reproduced in kidney grafts (GEISINGER et al. 1984; BAUMGARTNER et al. 1986; HRICAK et al. 1986) (Fig. 13.23). The effect of respiration and bowel motion on image quality is insignificant and no respiratory gating is necessary. The relatively superficial location of the renal allografts allows the use of surface coils, which gives pictures with higher spatial resolution than those obtained with current body coils. The allograft surface is delineated by surrounding extraperitoneal fat and renal sinus fat is clearly seen. A characteristic feature of a normally functioning graft is the contrast between the high signal intensity of the cortex and the lower signal intensity of the medulla on T1-weighted images, reflecting differences in relaxation times (Fig. 13.23). On T2-weighted images such differentiation is not possible.

13.6.2 Graft Parenchymal Disease

In 1983 TODD et al. reported a correlation between T1 relaxation times and creatinine clearance in transplanted kidneys. In clinical reports on MRI of the failing graft the most consistent finding has been loss of corticomedullary contrast in the graft (Fig. 13.24). The largest case material has been reported by HRICAK et al. (1986) in a prospective study of 45 transplanted patients. Decreased or absent corticomedullary contrast, reflecting a prolonged relaxation time for cortex, was found in 27 out of 29 biopsy-proven cases of acute rejection, while nine normally functioning grafts all showed high corticomedullary contrast. Other, more inconsistent findings in acute rejection were globular shape, indistinct outline, and loss of renal sinus fat. Five patients with histologic and clinical findings compatible with cyclosporine nephrotoxicity all had normal morphology on MRI. Three out of four allografts with ATN showed normal morphology, while one was swollen and had obliterated corticomedullary contrast. Compared with quantitative scintigraphy and ultrasound the same group found MRI to be far more accurate in diagnosing rejection (HRICAK et al. 1987). Other reports show cases of obliterated corticomedullary contrast in ATN and in patients with cyclosporine nephrotoxicity (GEISINGER et al. 1984; BAUMGARTNER et al. 1986; LUND et al. 1987; STEINBERG et al. 1987; GOLDSMITH et al. 1988; WINSETT et al. 1988), and the overlap seems sufficient to indicate that corticomedullary contrast should not be depended upon to identify the nature of parenchymal graft failure (HALASZ 1986).

13.6.3 Urologic Disease

Caliectasis can be recognized as dilated collecting structures filled with urine in contrast to surrounding renal parenchyma and sinus fat, and even a dilated ureter may be seen to the level of the obstruction on coronal images. In some of these cases the cause of obstruction may be identified as an intraluminal filling defect (blood clot) or compression from a fluid collection.

Peritransplant fluid collections are demonstrated with high sensitivity (GEISINGER et al. 1984; HRICAK et al. 1986). Urinomas and lymphoceles typically show low signal intensity on T1-weighted images and intermediate or high signal intensity on T2-weighted images. Hematomas and perirenal abscesses, because of their higher signal intensity on T1-weighted images, may be differentiated from other fluid collections.

Multiplanar imaging may also be useful in the assessment of renal transplant vascular patency, and especially a renal vein thrombosis should be easy to recognize.

13.7 Interventional Radiology

Percutaneous radiologic technique has proven of value in a number of surgical complications in the kidney transplant recipient, either as definitive therapy or as a temporary measure to improve the patient's condition prior to surgical correction.

The most serious early complications after kidney transplantation other than rejection and wound infection include urine leakage, significant perirenal fluid collection with or without ureteral obstruction, and thrombotic vascular occlusion. Lymphoceles or ureteral strictures do not usually occur until several weeks after transplantation, and arterial stenosis is typically a much later complication. Any of these complications carry a risk of irreversible loss of graft function, and may become life threatening.

Vigilance towards such conditions is essential for early diagnosis and treatment, the more so since the symptoms and signs may simulate rejection, and since the intricate coincidence of surgical complications and rejection is a distinct possibility.

Surgical intervention on a renal transplant may be very difficult because of abundant fibrous tissue around the allograft, and is bound up with an added risk due to the immunosuppressed state of the patient. Usually both the physical and the psychological trauma to the patient are less with radiologic than with surgical intervention and some results of definitive percutaneous therapy are comparable or superior to those of surgery. In many cases, therefore, percutaneous radiologic interventions as described in the following are attractive therapeutic alternatives, and, whenever feasible, should be applied.

13.7.1 Urinary Leakage

A renal scintigram is probably the most sensitive diagnostic test for demonstrating urinary leakage. Intravenous urography may be useful, but a detailed definition of the lesion requires direct contrast radiography, cystography, or antegrade pyelography, depending on the site of the lesion (Fig. 13.25).

Earlier results of attempted primary surgical repair were poor until the procedure was combined with temporary surgical nephrostomy drainage, preferably in a two-stage intervention (GOLDSTEIN et al. 1981; STREEM et al. 1986). This observation led to the use of percutaneous nephrostomy in urinary graft leakage. Percutaneous drainage of the renal pelvis consistently reduces the leak and should at

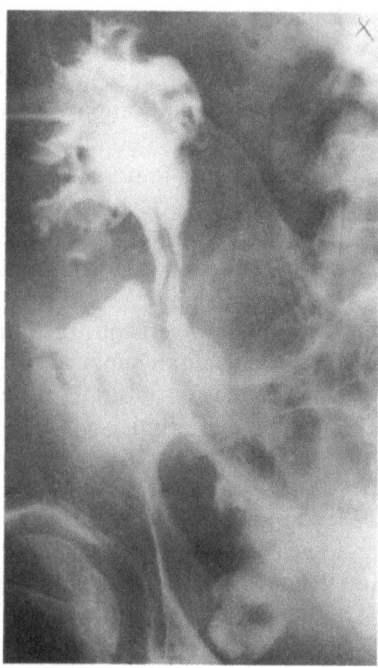

Fig. 13.25. Urine leak from ureterovesical junction, mid ureter, and upper calyces. Antegrade pyelogram by fine needle puncture

least be attempted as a preoperative measure (HUNTER et al. 1983; JAROWENKO et al. 1985). If at all possible the nephrostomy puncture should be completed with antegrade catheterization of the ureter, advancing a multiperforated catheter into the bladder for combined external/internal drainage (LANG 1981; LIEBERMAN et al. 1982; KUMAR et al. 1984; BENNETT et al. 1986; STREEM et al. 1986). This procedure, while maintaining the normal urinary pathway, eliminates the high fluid pressure in the ureter, and may, in many instances, lead to closure of the leak within 3–8 weeks, thus obviating the need for surgical intervention (Fig. 13.26).

13.7.2 Perirenal Fluid Collection

Larger collections in the early postoperative period may be the result of significant bleeding or urine leak. Ultrasonically guided aspiration will provide the differential diagnosis (BECKER and KUTCHER 1980; CURRY et al. 1984; KUMAR et al. 1984; JAROWENKO et al. 1985; BENNETT et al. 1986; LETOURNEAU et al. 1988; POLLAK et al. 1988) and may be the only therapy needed if the patient is stable and the urine output is unimpaired. If a urinoma is present, antegrade pyelography is important for finding out whether urine is still leaking, in which

case percutaneous ureteral stenting and/or pyelonephrostomy is indicated. Urinomas, hematomas, and abscesses can be drained by percutaneous catherization (LIEBERMAN et al. 1982; HUNTER et al. 1983; CURRY et al. 1984; LETOURNEAU et al. 1988), although it has been proposed that a urinoma need not be drained unless the urine is infected (STREEM et al. 1986) or the urinoma is symptomatic (POLLAK et al. 1988). Most perirenal fluid accumulations in the late postoperative phase are lymphoceles.

A lymphocele can be punctured and aspirated with ultrasound guidance for diagnostic and therapeutic purposes (BECKER and KUTCHER 1980; CURRY et al. 1984; KUMAR et al. 1984; GREENBERG et al. 1985; WHITE et al. 1985; BENNETT et al. 1986; LETOURNEAU et al. 1988) (Fig. 13.27), but tends to recur. In that case, repeated aspiration or long-term (1 to several weeks) percutaneous catheter drainage will usually be curative (WHITE et al. 1985; JENSEN et al. 1986; VAN SONNENBERG et al. 1986; COHAN et al. 1987). Sclerosing agents have been used in combination with drainage in some series (TERNEL et al. 1983; VAN SONNENBERG et al. 1986; COHAN et al. 1987), but they are not widely recommended. Some lymphoceles continue to recur, eventually requiring surgical intervention with marsupialization of the collection into the peritoneal cavity (BECKER and KUTCHER 1980; GREENBERG et al. 1985; VAN SONNENBERG et al. 1986; COHAN et al. 1987).

13.7.3 Ureteral Obstruction

Most obstructions are unequivocally identified with renal scintigraphy and ultrasonography in combination, although both examinations may sometimes be misleading (HUNTER et al. 1983; BENNETT et al. 1986) since the collecting system may be dilated without being obstructed and vice versa. Intravenous urography is of little use when renal function is impaired. Correct diagnosis of obstruction and determination of the level of obstruction are best achieved by direct puncture starting with a 22 gauge needle for antegrade pyelography (WHITAKER 1979; MITCHELL et al. 1981; GLANZ et al. 1983; LIST et al. 1983; BENNETT et al. 1986) (Figs. 13.28, 13.29). If there is doubt as to the significance of pelvicalyceal dilation, the antegrade approach can be combined with Whitaker testing for evaluating the need for decompression.

Following 1 or 2 days of percutaneous nephrostomy drainage, negotiating the stricture can be attempted (LIEBERMAN et al. 1982; BENNETT et al. 1986; STREEM et al. 1986) after passing a guidewire

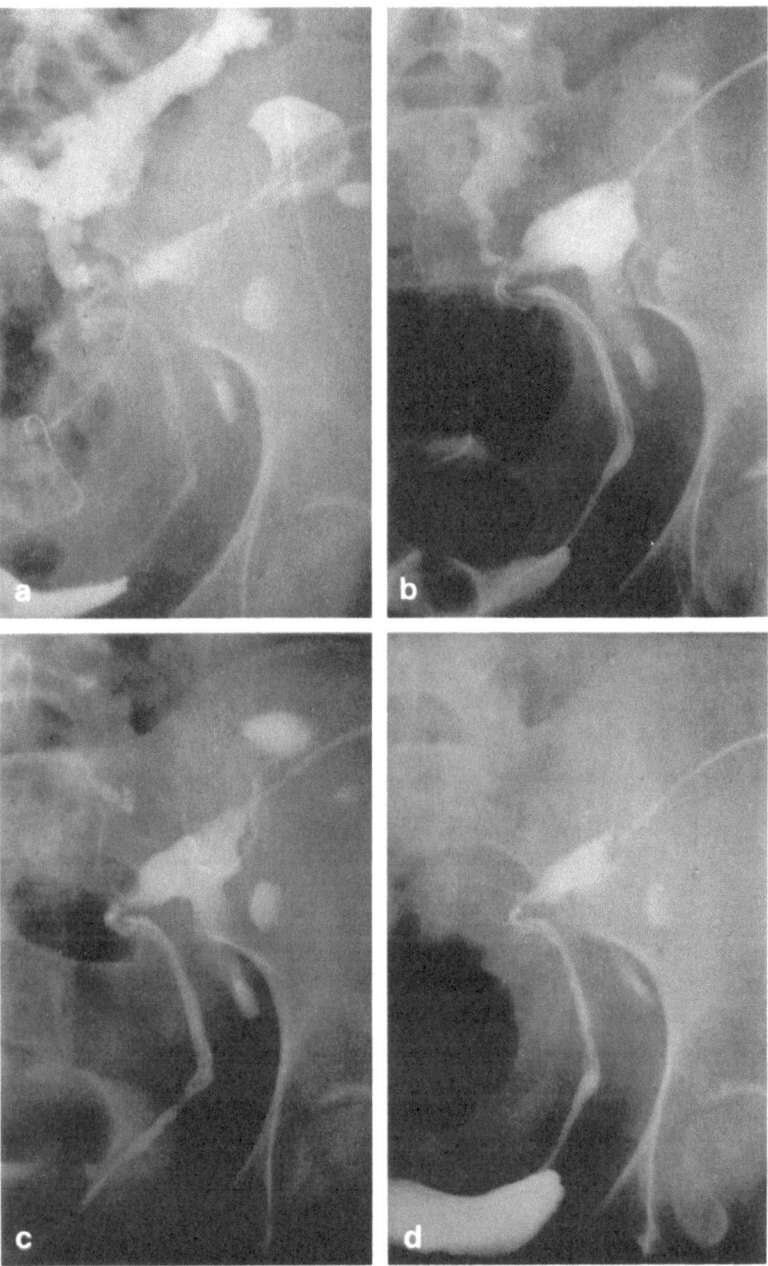

through the nephrostomy catheter to the bladder. When necessary, balloon dilatation in one or several stages has sufficed as definitive therapy to replace surgical correction in many cases (LIEBERMAN et al. 1982; GLANZ et al. 1983; LIST et al. 1983; STREEM et al. 1986) (Fig. 13.30). The procedure should be followed by introducing an internal/external ureteral stent to be left in place for 6–8 weeks (BENNETT et al. 1986). Alternatively, the ureter could be drained internally with a double pigtail endoprosthetic stent (GLANZ et al. 1983; BENNETT et al. 1986)

Fig. 13.26a–d. Urine leak from proximal ureter. Percutaneous nephrostomy with antegrade catheterization of upper ureter past the point of leakage. **a** At the time of diagnosis, 4 days after transplantation. **b** Six days later: regression of leakage. **c** After 2 weeks: furter improvement. **d** After 4 weeks: leak healed

(Figs. 13.28–13.30), in which case a nephrostomy catheter should be left in place for a couple of days until stent function is eventually ascertained by a secondary nephrostogram.

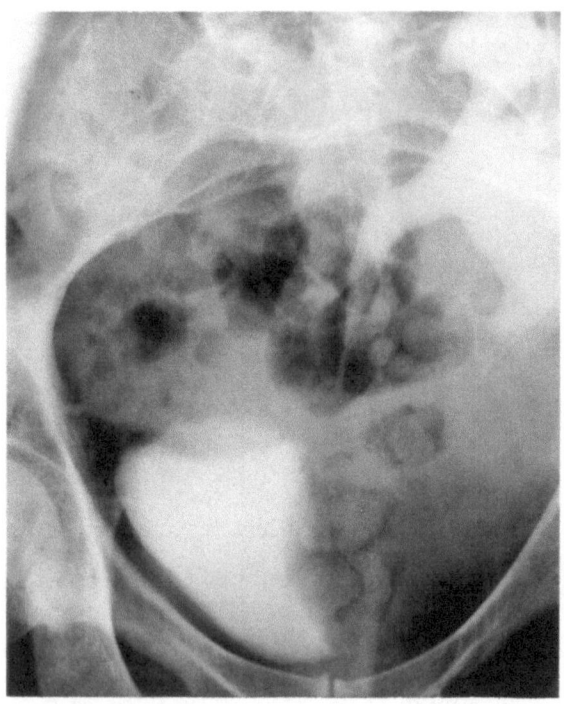

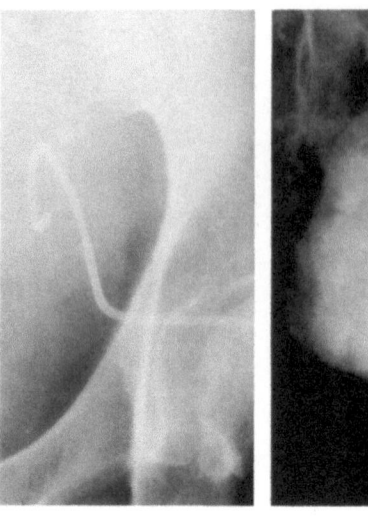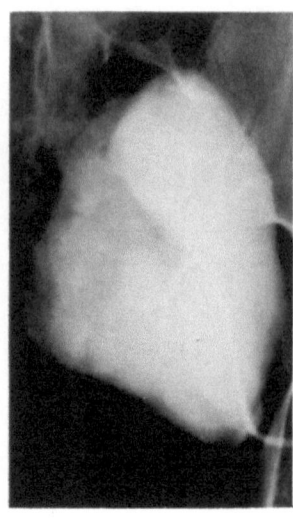

Fig. 13.27. Lymphocele compressing bladder and dislocating ureter with some obstruction. *Left:* intravenous urography. *Middle:* percutaneous catheter drainage. *Right:* direct visualization of lymphocele by contrast medium injection through drainage catheter

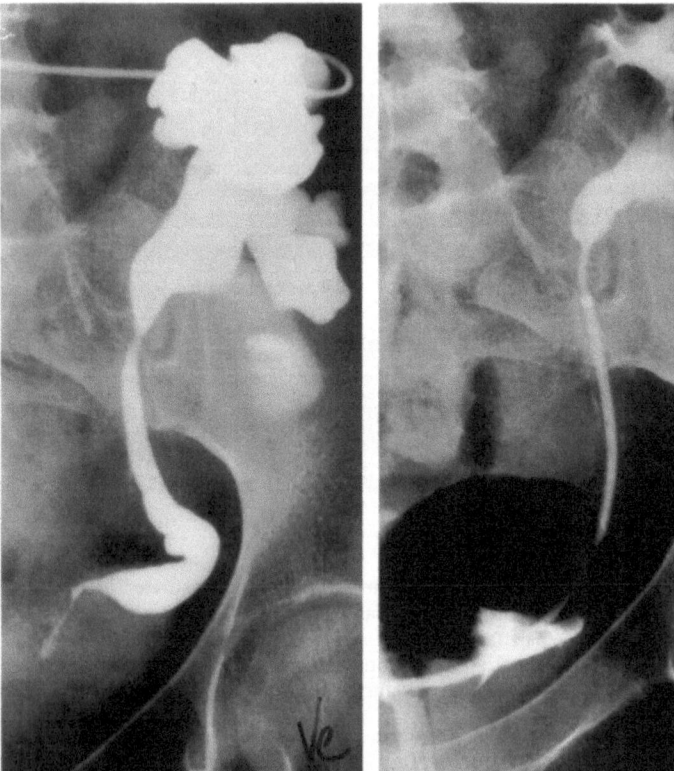

Fig. 13.28. Short distal ureteral stricture. *Left:* antegrade pyelogram. *Right:* double pigtail stent inserted

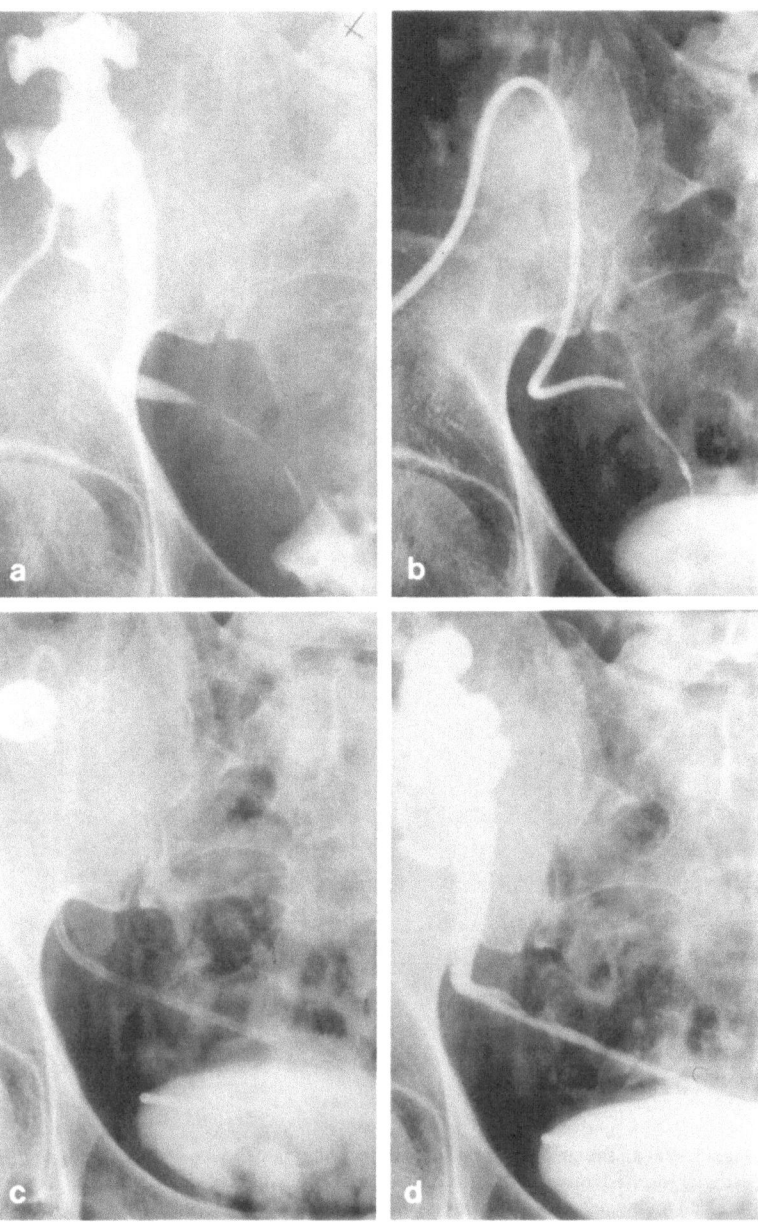

Fig. 13.29 a–d. Long distal ureteral stricture. **a** Antegrade pyelogram through nephrostomy catheter. **b** Catheter inserted for passing a guidewire to the bladder. **c** Double pigtail stent inserted. **d** Antegrade pyelogram shows function of the stent

13.7.4 Arterial Stenosis

Surgical correction of a renal arterial stenosis in a transplant patient with reanastomosis carries a relatively high risk of graft loss, although several series have shown acceptable results of vascular surgery. Since 1979 increasing evidence has favored the use of percutaneous transluminal angioplasty (PTA) as an alternative therapeutic approach comparing favorably with vascular surgery (DIAMOND et al. 1979; SNIDERMAN et al. 1980a; TEGTMEYER et al. 1981; GROSSMAN et al. 1982; RUSSELL 1982; ZAJKO et al. 1982; GERLOCH et al. 1983; LAASONEN et al. 1985; RAYNEAUD et al. 1986; CLEMENTS et al. 1987; GEDROYC et al. 1987) (Figs. 13.19, 13.31). In about 20% of patients the stenosed arterial segment proves inaccessible for selective catheterization and/or the insertion of a balloon catheter, because of either sharp angulation or small dimension of the artery.

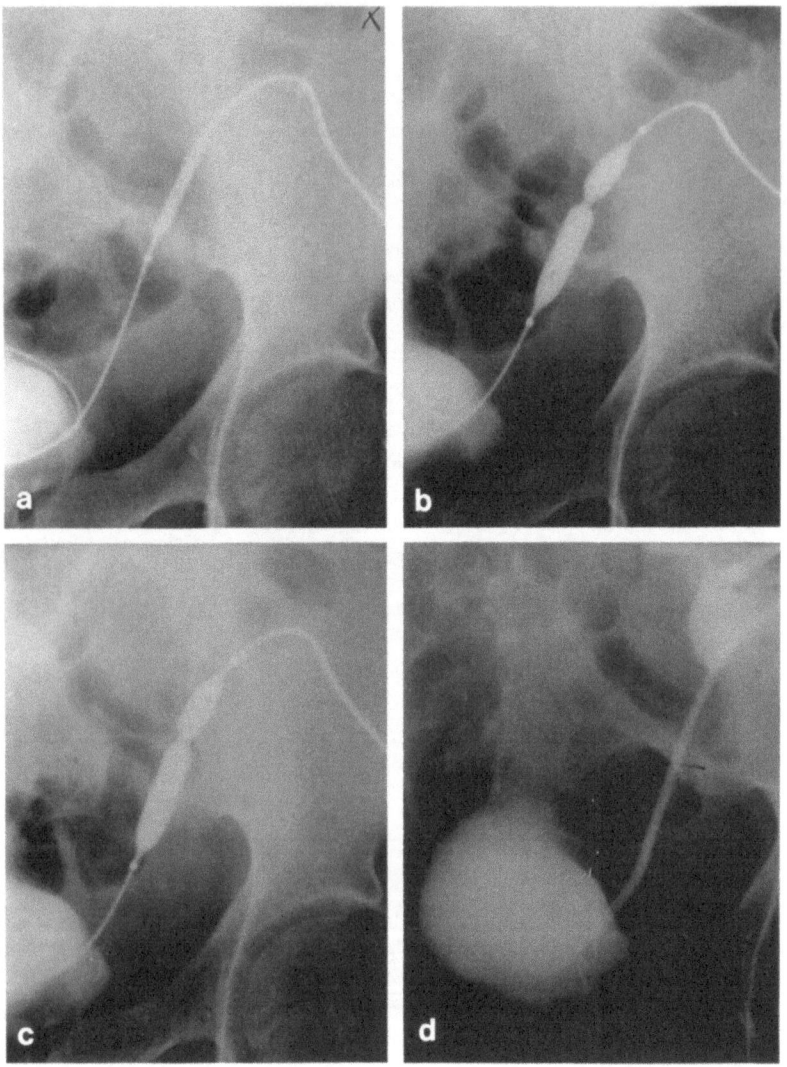

Fig. 13.30 a–d. Proximal ureteral stricture. **a** Dilating balloon catheter inserted through nephrostomy. **b, c** Dilating the stricture. **d** Double pigtail stent inserted temporarily

However, the rate of technically successful dilatation with clinical improvement ranges from 45% to 100% of attempted procedures in various reports, and very few complications have been encountered (SNIDERMAN et al. 1980a, b; MAJESKI and MUNDA 1981; MEDINA et al. 1981; GROSSMAN et al. 1982; CURRY et al. 1984). Recurrent stenosis is most frequently seen in the first 5 months following PTA (RAYNAUD et al. 1986). The recurrence rate in the largest recent study was 20%. However, most recurrent stenoses have been accessible for repeated PTA.

13.7.5 Miscellaneous Complications

Interventional radiologic procedures have been applied with success in other occasional complications of kidney transplantation, e.g.: selective arterial embolization in hematuria following graft biopsy (HO-ROWIZ et al. 1984), in renal allograft arteriovenous fistula (GEDROYC et al. 1987), and in renin-producing genuine kidneys in a transplant recipient (RUSSELL 1982); selective streptokinase infusion in acute transplant venous or arterial thrombosis (ZAJKO et al. 1982; ROBINSON et al. 1986); and percutaneous stone extraction from a renal transplant pelvis or ureter (FISHER et al. 1982; JAROWENKO et al. 1985; STREEM et al. 1986).

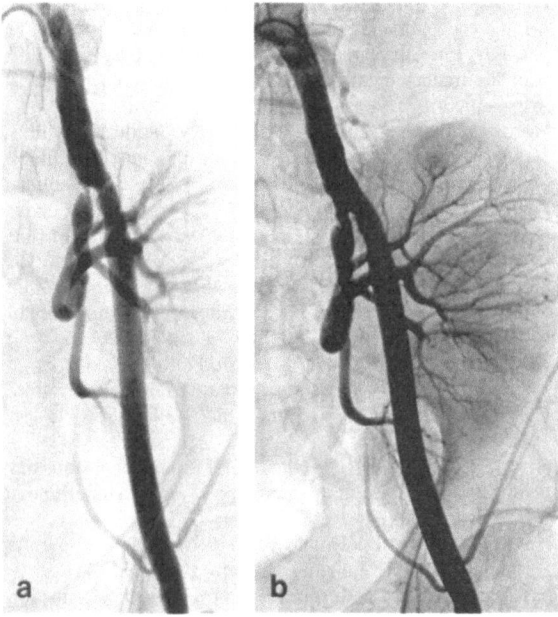

Fig. 13.31. a Marked stenosis of recipient internal iliac artery serving kidney transplant artery in a patient who developed severe hypertension 3 months after transplantation. **b** After successful PTA the artery has assumed normal diameter. Normal blood pressure resulted

References

Absy M, Metrewelli C, Matthews C, Al Khader A (1987) Changes in transplanted kidney volume measured by ultrasound. Br J Radiol 60: 525–529

Baillet G, Ballarin J, Urdaneta N et al. (1986) Evaluation of allograft perfusion by radionuclide first-pass study in renal failure following renal transplantation. Eur J Nucl Med 11: 463–469

Balchunas WR, Hill MC, Isikoff MB, Morillo G (1982) The clinical significance of dilatation of the collecting system in the transplanted kidney. J Clin Ultrasound 10: 221–225

Balsara VJ, Raval B, Maklad NF (1985) Emphysematous pyelonephritis in a renal transplant: sonographic and computed tomographic features. J Ultrasound Med 4: 97–99

Baumgartner BR, Nelson RC, Ball TI, Wyly JB, Bourke E, Delaney V, Bernardino ME (1986) MR imaging of renal transplants. AJR 147: 949–953

Becker JA, Kutcher R (1978) The renal transplant: rejection and acute tubular necrosis. Semin Roentgenol 13: 352–362

Becker JA, Kutcher R (1980) Renal transplantation. In: Elkin M (ed) Radiology of the urinary system. Little, Brown and Co, Boston

Bennett LN, Voegeli DR, Crummy AB, McDermott JC, Jensen SR, Sollinger HW (1986) Urologic complications following renal transplation. Radiology 160: 531–536

Bernardino ME, Baumgartner BR (1986) Abscess drainage in the genitourinary tract. Radiol Clin North Am 24: 539–549

Brockis JG, Hulbert JC, Patel AS et al. (1978) The diagnosis and treatment of lymphoceles associated with renal transplantation: a report of 6 cases and a review of the literature. Br J Urol 50: 307–312

Bubeck B, Brandau W, Steinbäcker M, Reinbold F, Dreikorn K, Eisenhut M, Georgi P (1988) Technetium-99m labeled renal function and imaging agents: II. Clinical evaluation of ^{99m}Tc MAG$_3$ (^{99m}Tc mercaptoacetglycylglycylglycine). Nucl Med Biol 15: 109–118

Byrd L, Sherman RL (1979) Radiocontrast-induced acute renal failure: a clinical and pathophysiologic review. Medicine 58: 270–279

Canadian Multicenter Transplant Study Group (1983) A randomized clinical trial of cyclosporine in cadaveric renal transplantation. N Engl J Med 399: 809–815

Casola G, van Sonnenberg E (1987) Sonographic guidance for percutaneous drainage of abscesses and fluid collections. Clin Diagn Ultrasound 21: 151–172

Chandler ST, Buckels J, Hawker RJ, Smith N, Barnes AD, McCollum CN (1983) Indium-labeled platelet uptake in rejecting renal transplants. Surg Gynecol Obstet 157: 242–246

Chow SS, Thorner P, Baumal R, Wilson DR (1986) Cyclosporin and experimental renal ischemic injury. Transplantation 41: 147–151

Clements R, Evans C, Salaman JR (1987) Percutaneous transluminal angioplasty of renal transplant artery stenosis. Clin Radiol 38: 235–237

Clorius JH, Dreikorn K, Zelt J et al. (1979) Renal graft evaluation with pertechnetate and I-131 hippuran. A comparative clinical study. J Nucl Med 20: 1029–1037

Cochlin DLL, Wake A, Salaman JR, Griffin JA (1988) Ultrasound changes in the transplant kidney. Clin Radiol 39: 373–376

Cohan RH, Saeed M, Sussman SK, Perlmutt LM, Schwab SJ, Bowie JD, Dunnick NR (1987) Percutaneous drainage of pelvic lymphatic fluid collections in the renal transplant patient. Invest Radiol 22: 864–867

Coyne SC, Walsh JW, Tisuado J et al. (1981) Surgically correctable renal transplant complications: an integrated clinical and radiologic approach. AJR 136: 1113–1119

Curry NS, Cochran, Barbaric ZL et al. (1984) Interventional radiologic procedures in the renal transplant. Radiology 152: 647–653

Dawson P (1985) Contrast agent nephrotoxicity. An appraisal. Br J Radiol 58: 121–124

DeLange EE, Pauwels EKJ, Lobatto S, Tjon Pian Gi-van Loon CE, Van Hoof JP (1982) Scintigraphic detection of urinary leakage after kidney transplantation. Eur J Nucl Med 7: 55–57

Diamond NG, Casarella WJ, Hardy MA, Appel GB (1979) Dilatation of critical transplant renal artery stenosis by percutaneous transluminal angioplasty. AJR 133: 1167–1169

Diaz-Buxo JA, Wagner RD, Hattery RR, Palumbo PJ (1975) Acute renal failure after excretory urography in diabetic patients. Ann Intern Med 83: 155–158

Dieperink H, Leyssac PP, Starklint H, Kemp E (1986) The nephrotoxicity of cyclosporin A. A lithium clearance and micropuncture study. Eur J Clin Invest 16: 69–77

Dubovsky EV, Russell CD (1988) Radionuclide evaluation of renal transplants. Semin Nucl Med 18: 181–188

Dubovsky EV, Logic JR, Diethelm AG, Balch CM, Tauxe WN (1975) Comprehensive evaluation of renal function in the transplanted kidney. J Nucl Med 16: 1115–1120

Dubovsky EV, Curtis JJ, Luke RG et al. (1987) Captopril as a predictor of curable hypertension in renal transplant recipients. Contrib Nephrol 56: 117–123

Eicks JD, Silver TM, Bree RL (1978) Gray scale features of hematomas. An ultrasonic spectrum. AJR 131: 977

Eisenberg RL, Bank WO, Hedgcock MW (1981) Renal failure after major angiography. AJR 136: 859–861

European Multicenter Study Group (1983) Cyclosporine in cadaveric renal transplantation: one year follow-up of a multicenter trial. Lancet II: 986–989

Fawwaz RA, Johnson PM (1979) Localization of gallium-67 in the normally functioning allografted kidney: concise communication. J Nucl Med 20: 207–209

Fisher MF, Haga JR, Persky L, Eckel RE, LiPuma J (1982) Renal stone extraction through a percutaneous nephrostomy in a renal transplant patient. Radiology 144: 95–96

Frick MP, Loken MK, Goldberg ME, Simmons RL (1976) Use of ^{99m}Tc-sulfur colloid in evaluation of renal transplant complications. J Nucl Med 17: 181–183

Frick MP, Henke CE, Forstrom LA, Simmons RA, McCullough J, Loken MK (1979) Use of ^{111}In-labeled leukocytes in evaluation of renal transplant rejection. A preliminary report. Clin Nucl Med 4: 24–25

Frick MP, Feinberg SB, Sibley R, Idstrom ME (1981) Ultrasound in acute renal transplant rejection. Radiology 138: 657–660

Fried AM, Woodring JH, Loh FK, Lucas BA, Kryscio RJ (1983) The medullary pyramid index: an objective assessment of prominence in renal transplant rejection. Radiology 149: 787–791

Fuld IL, Matalon TA, Vogelzang RL, Neiman HL, Kowal LE, Hitchins WW, Soper W (1984) Dynamic CT in the evaluation of physiologic status of renal transplants. AJR 142: 1157–1160

Gedroyc WMW, Reidy JF, Saxton HM (1987) Arteriography of renal transplantation. Clin Radiol 38: 239–243

Geisinger MA, Risius B, Jordan ML, Zelch MG, Novick AC, George CR (1984) Magnetic resonance imaging of renal transplants. AJR 143: 1229–1234

George EA, Cood JE, Newton WT, Haibach H, Donati RM (1976) Comparative evaluation of renal transplant rejection with radioiodinated fibrinogen ^{99m}Tc-sulfur colloid, and ^{67}Ga-citrate. J Nucl Med 17: 175–180

Gerloch AJ Jr, MacDonell RC Jr, Smith CW et al. (1983) Renal transplant arterial stenosis: percutaneous transluminal angioplasty. AJR 140: 325–331

Glanz S, Gordon DH, Butt K, Rubin B, Hong J, Sclafani SJA (1983) Percutaneous transrenal balloon dilatation of the ureter. Radiology 149: 101–104

Goldsmith MS, Tanasescu DE, Waxman AD, Crues JV (1988) Comparison of magnetic resonance imaging and radionuclide imaging in the evaluation of renal transplant failure. Clin Nucl Med 13: 250–257

Goldstein I, Cho SI, Olsson CA (1981) Nephrostomy drainage for renal transplant complications. J Urol 126: 159–163

Greenberg BM, Perloff LJ, Grossman RA, Naji A, Barker CF (1985) Treatment of lymphocele in renal allograft recipients. Arch Surg 120: 501–504

Grossman RA, Dafoe DC, Shoenfeld RB et al. (1982) Percutaneous transluminal angioplasty treatment of renal transplant artery stenosis. Transplantation 34: 339–343

Halasz NA (1986) Differential diagnosis of renal transplant rejection: Is MR imaging the answer? AJR 147: 954–955

Halasz NA, Gamboa EA, Ward DM, Steiner RW, Bronsther OL (1987) Kidney transplantation in the cyclosporine era. Arch Surg 122: 1001–1004

Hanto DW, Simmons RL (1987) Renal transplantation: clinical considerations. Radiol Clin North Am 25: 239–247

Hartling OL, Narving J, Munk O (1987) Scintigraphy of kidneys located at different dephts: the geometric mean method for determination of differential renal function. Case report. Clin Nucl Med 12: 956–957

Heckemann R, Rehwald U, Jakubowski HD, Donhuijsen K (1982) Sonographic criteria for renal allograft rejection. Urol Radiol 4: 15–18

Hilson AJW, Maisey MN, Brown CB, Ogg CS, Bewich MS (1978) Dynamic renal transplant imaging with Tc-99m DTPA (Sn) supplemented by a transplant perfusion index in the management of renal transplants. J Nucl Med 19: 994–1000

Horowiz MD, Russell E, Abitbol C, Kyriakides G, Miller J (1984) Massive hematuria following percutaneous biopsy of renal allograft: selective control by selective embolization. Arch Surg 119: 1430–1433

Hricak H, Lieto R (1983) Sonographic determination of renal volume. Radiology 148: 311–312

Hricak H, Toledo-Pereyra LH, Eyler WR, Madrazo BL, Zammit M (1979) The role of ultrasound in the diagnosis of kidney allograft rejection. Radiology 132: 667–672

Hricak H, Cruz C, Eyler W, Madrozo B, Romanski R, Sandler M (1981) Acute post-transplantation renal failure: differential diagnosis by ultrasound. Radiology 139: 441–449

Hricak H, Romanski RN, Eyler W (1982) The renal sinus during allograft rejection: sonographic and histopathologic findings. Radiology 142: 693–699

Hricak H, Terrier F, Demas BE (1986) Renal allografts: evaluation by MR imaging. Radiology 159: 435–441

Hricak H, Terrier F, Marotti M et al. (1987) Posttransplant renal rejection: comparison of quantitative scintigraphy, US and MR imaging. Radiology 162: 685–688

Hunter DW, Castaneda-Zuniga WR, Coleman CC, Herrera M, Amplatz K (1983) Percutaneous technique in the management of urological complications in renal transplant patients. Radiology 148: 407–412

Jackson SA, Ehrlich L, Martin RH (1986) The renal washout parameter as an indicator of transplant rejection. Eur J Nucl Med 12: 86–90

Jafri SZH, Kaude JV, Wright PG (1981) Ultrasound findings in renal transplant rejection. Acta Radiol 22: 245–253

Jarowenko MV, Flechner SM, Sandler CM, Van Buren CT, Kahan BD (1985) Salvage of difficult transplant complications by percutaneous techniques. J Urol 133: 840–843

Jensen SR, Voegeli DR, McDermott JC, Crummy AB (1986) Percutaneous management of lymphatic fluid collections. Cardiovasc Intervent Radiol 9: 202–204

Kim EE, Pjura G, Lowry P, Verani R, Sandler C, Flechner S, Kahan B (1986) Cyclosporin-A nephrotoxicity and acute cellular rejection in renal transplant recipients: correlation between radionuclide and histologic findings. Radiology 159: 443–446

Kirchner PT, Rosenthall L (1982) Renal transplant evaluation. Semin Nucl Med 12: 370–378

Kittredge RD, Brensilver J, Pierce JC (1978). Computed tomography in renal transplant problems. Radiology 127: 165–169

Koehler PR, Kanemoto HH, Maxwell JG (1976) Ultrasonic "B" scanning in the diagnosis of complications in renal transplant patients. Radiology 119: 661–664

Kumar R, Wilson DD, Santa-Cruz FR (1984) Postoperative urological complications of renal transplantation. Radiographics 4: 531–547

Laasonen L, Edgren J, Forslund T, Eklund B (1985) Renal transplant artery stenosis and percutaneous transluminal angioplasty. Acta Radiol 26: 609–613

Lachance SL, Adamson D, Barry JM (1988) Ultrasonically determined kidney transplant hypertrophy. Urology 139: 497–498

Lamki N, Raval B, Carey LS (1981) CT appearance of long-term renal transplant rejection. CT 5: 340–342

Lang EK (1981) Diagnosis and management of ureteral fistulas by percutaneous nephrostomy and antegrade stent catheter. Radiology 138: 311-317

Larsen S, Brun C, Dunn S, Løkkegaard H, Thomsen HS (1988) Early arteriolopathy following "high-dose" cyclosporine in kidney transplantation. APMIS [Suppl] 4: 75-82

Lee HM, Madge GE, Mendez-Picon G, Chatterjee SN (1978) Surgical complications in renal transplant recipients. Surg Clin North Am 58: 285-304

Lerut T, Lerut J, Broos P, Gruwez, Michielsen P (1980) Lymphatic complications in renal transplantation. Eur Urol 6: 83-89

Letourneau JG, Day DL, Feinberg SB (1987) Ultrasound and computed tomographic evaluation of renal transplantation. Radiol Clin North Am 25: 267-279

Letourneau JG, Day DL, Ascher NL, Castaneda-Zungia WR (1988) Imaging of renal transplants. AJR 150: 833-838

Lieberman RP, Crummy AB, Glass NR, Belzer FO (1981) Fine needle antegrade pyelography in the renal transplant. J Urol 126: 155-158

Lieberman RP, Glass NR, Crummy AB, Sollinger HW, Belzer FO (1982) Nonoperative percutaneous management of urinary fistulas and strictures in renal transplantation. Surg Gynecol Obstet 155: 667-672

Lieberman SF, Keller SF, Barry JM, Rösch J (1982) Percutaneous antegrade transluminal ureteroplasty for renal allograft ureteral stenosis. J Urol 128: 122-124

Linkowski GD, Warvariv V, Filly RA, Vincenti F (1987) Sonography in the diagnosis of acute renal allograft rejection and cyclosporine nephrotoxicity. AJR 148: 291-295

List AR, Blohmè I, Brynger H, Nilson AE (1983) Balloon dilatation for ureteral strictures in graft kidneys; a viable alternative to further surgery. Transplantation 33: 105

Love L, Revnes CJ, Churchill P, Moncada R (1979) Third generation CT-scanning in renal disease. Radiol Clin North Am 1: 77-90

Lund G, Letourneau JG, Day DL, Crass JR (1987) MRI in organ transplantation. Radiol Clin North Am 25: 281-288

Majeski JA, Munda R (1981) Hazard of percutaneous transluminal dilatation in renal arterial stenosis. Arch Surg 116: 1225-1226

Maklad NF, Wright CH, Rosenthal S (1979) Gray scale ultrasonic appearances of renal transplant rejection. Radiology 131: 711-717

Martin-Comin J (1986) Kidney graft rejection studies with labeled platelets and lymphocytes. Nucl Med Biol 13: 173-181

Medina M, Butt KMH, Gordon DH, Thanawala S, Solomon N (1981) A complication of percutaneous transluminal angioplasty in the transplanted kidney. Urol Radiol 3: 59-61

Meyers AM, Levine E, Myburgh JA, Goudie E (1977) Diagnosis and management of lymphoceles after renal transplantation. Urology 10: 497-502

Mitchell A, Fellows GJ, Wright FW, Morris PJ (1981) Hydronephrosis in a transplanted kidney; the use of pressure flow studies to exclude ureteric obstruction. Transplantation 32: 152-153

Moore TC, Hayes M (1974) Combined use of ^{131}I hippurate blood clearance and bladder/kidney ratio data in the early detection, classification, and management of accelerated rejection of human renal transplants. Surgery 76: 587-600

Mundy AR, Podesta ML, Bewick M, Rudge CJ, Ellis FG (1981) The urological complications of 1000 renal transplants. Br J Urol 53: 397-402

Nielsen SL, Hvid-Jacobsen K, Thomsen HS, Munck O (1987) Renal washout and vascular resistances. Eur J Nucl Med 12: 629-630

Novick AC, Irish C, Steinmüller D, Buonocoze E, Chen C (1981) The role of computerized tomography in renal transplant patients. J Urol 125: 15-18

Palestrant AM, DeWolf WC (1982) The pseudostricture of transplant ureteral torsion. Radiology 145: 49-50

Peterdy AE, Sutherland JB, Jeffery J, Benediktsson H, Greenberg ID (1981) Renal transplant uptake of technetium-99m sulfur colloid in various time periods after transplantation. Canad Assoc Radiol 32: 144-148

Picus D, Neeley JP, McClennan BL, Weyman PJ, Heiken JP (1985) Intraarterial digital subtraction angiography of renal transplants. AJR 145: 93-96

Pollak R, Veremis SA, Maddux MS, Mozes MF (1988) The natural history and the therapy for perirenal fluid collections following renal transplantation. J Urol 140: 716-720

Potter JL, Sullivan BM, Fluornoy JG, Guza C (1985) Emphysema in the renal allograft. Radiology 155: 51-52

Preston DF, Luke RG (1979) Radionuclide evaluation of renal transplants. J Nucl Med 20: 1095-1097

Rascoff JH, Golden RA, Spinowitz BS, Charyton C (1983) Nondilated obstructive nephropathy. Arch Intern Med 143: 696-698

Raynaud A, Bedrossian J, Remy P, Brisset J-M, Angel C-Y, Gaux J-C (1986) Percutaneous transluminal angioplasty of renal transplant arterial stenoses. AJR 146: 853-857

Rigsby CM, Burns PN, Weltin GG, Chen B, Bia M, Taylor KJ (1987) Doppler signal quantitation in renal allografts: comparison in normal and rejecting transplants, with pathologic correlation. Radiology 162: 39-42

Robinson JM, Cockrell CH, Tisnado J, Beachley MC, Posner MP, Tracy TF (1986) Selective low-dose streptokinase infusion in the treatment of acute transplant renal vein thrombosis. Cardiovasc Intervent Radiol 9: 86-89

Roeren T, Hauenstein K, Dinkel E, Kirste G (1986) Intraarterial digital subtraction angiography of renal transplants. Urol Radiol 8: 77-80

Rosenfield AT, Taylor KJW (1976) Obstructive uropathy in the transplanted kidney: evaluation by grey scale sonography. J Urol 116: 101-102

Rosenthall L, Mangel R, Lisbona R, Lacourciere Y (1974) Diagnostic applications of radiopertechnetate and radiohippurate imaging in post-renal transplant complications. Radiology 111: 347-358

Russell RD (1982) Embolization and angioplasty to relieve malignant hypertension and azotemia in a renal transplant patient. Cardiovasc Intervent Radiol 5: 307-311

Salaman JR (1972) A technique for detecting rejection episodes in human transplant recipients using radioactive fibrinogen. Br J Surg 59: 138-142

Salvatierra O Jr, Powell MR, Price DC, Kountz SL, Belzer FO (1974) The advantages of ^{131}I-orthoiodohippurate scintiphotography in the management of patients after renal transplantation. Ann Surg 180: 336-342

Schmeller NT, Schüller J, Hofsletter A, Land W (1985) Fine needle antegrade pyelography of transplanted kidneys. Urol Radiol 7: 19-22

Schmidlin P, Clorius JH, Lubosch E-M, Siems H, Boehm M, Dreikorn K (1986) Renal perfusion and mean vascular transit time. Eur J Nucl Med 11: 69-72

Shanahan WSM, Klingensmith WC III, Weil R III (1981) ^{99m}Tc-DTPA renal studies for acute tubular necrosis: specificity of dissociation between perfusion and clearance. AJR 136: 249-256

Silver TM, Campbell D, Jeffrey DW, Lorber MI, Surace P, Turcotte J (1981) Peritransplant fluid collections. Radiology 138: 145-151

Slovis TL, Babcok DS, Hricak H et al. (1984) Renal transplant rejection: sonographic evaluation in children. Radiology 153: 659-665

Sniderman KW, Sos TA, Sprayregen S et al. (1980a) Percutaneous transluminal angioplasty in renal transplant arterial stenosis for relief of hypertension. Radiology 135: 23-26

Sniderman KW, Sprayregen S, Sos TA et al. (1980b) Percutaneous transluminal dilatation in renal transplant arterial stenosis. Transplantation 30: 440-444

Spigos D, Capek V (1975) Ultrasonically guided percutaneous aspiration of lymphoceles following renal transplantation: a diagnostic and therapeutic method. J Clin Ultrasound 4: 45-46

Spigos DG, Tan W, Pavel DG, Mozes M, Jonasson O, Capek V (1977) Diagnosis of urine extravasation after renal transplantation. AJR 129: 409-413

Staab EV, Kelly WD, Loken MK (1969) Prognostic value of radioisotope renograms in kidney transplantation. J Nucl Med 10: 133-135

Stanley P, Maleksadeh M, Diament M (1987) Posttransplant renal artery stenosis: angiographic study in 32 children. AJR 148: 487-490

Steinberg HV, Nelson RC, Murphy FB et al. (1987) Renal allograft rejection: evaluation by Doppler US and MR imaging. Radiology 162: 337-342

Streem BH, Novick AC (1983) Pelvic imaging techniques in renal transplantation. Urol Clin North Am 10: 301-313

Streem SB, Novick AC, Steinmuller DR, Musselman PW (1986) Percutaneous techniques for the management of urological renal transplant complications. J Urol 135: 456-459

Szpirt W, Ekelund B, Ryder L (1984) Effect of exposure of donor kidney to X-ray contrast media on graft function and survival. Poster, The 9th International Congress of Nephrology, Los Angeles

Taylor KJ, Burns PN (1985) Duplex Doppler scanning in the pelvis and abdomen. Ultrasound Med Biol 11: 643-658

Taylor A Jr, Eshima D, Alazraki N (1987a) ^{99m}Tc-MAG$_3$, a new renal imaging agent: preliminary results in patients. Eur J Nucl Med 12: 510-514

Taylor A Jr, Eshima D, Christian PE, Milton W (1987b) Evaluation of Tc-99m mercaptoacetyltriglycine in patients with impaired renal function. Radiology 162: 365-370

Taylor KJW, Morse SS, Rigsby CM, Bia M, Sciff M (1987) Vascular complications in renal allografts: detection with duplex Doppler US. Radiology 162: 31-38

Tegtmeyer CJ, Teates CD, Crigler N, Gandee RW, Ayers CR, Stoddard M, Wellons HA Jr (1981) Percutaneous transluminal angioplasty in patients with renal artery stenosis. Radiology 140: 323-330

Ternel JL, Escobar EM, Quereda C, Mayayo T, Ortuno J (1983) A simple and safe method for management of lymphocele after renal transplantation. J Urol 130: 1058-1059

Thomsen HS, Munck O (1987) Use of ^{99}Tc^m radionuclides to show nephrotoxicity of cyclosporin A in transplanted kidneys. Acta Radiol 28: 59-61

Thomsen HS, Nielsen SL (1988) Triple therapy and initial graft perfusion. Dan Med Bull 35: 393-395

Thomsen HS, Dorph S, Mygind T (1984) Subtraction nephrotomography during urography of transplanted kidneys. Acta Radiol 25: 495-500

Thomsen HS, Dorph S, Mygind T, Holm HH, Munck O, Damgaard-Pedersen K (1985) The transplanted kidney. Di-

agnostic and interventional radiology. Acta Radiol 26: 353-367

Thomsen HS, Hvid-Jacobsen K, Nielsen SL (1987a) Alternating use of ^{123}I and ^{131}I hippuran for routine postoperative monitoring of transplanted kidneys is impracticable. Acta Radiol 28: 365-367

Thomsen HS, Løkkegaard H, Munck O (1987b) Influence of normal central venous pressure on onset of function in renal allografts. Scand J Urol Nephrol 21: 143-145

Thomsen HS, Nielsen SL, Larsen S, Løkkegaard H (1987c) Renography and biopsy-verified acute rejection in renal allotransplanted patients receiving cyclosporin A. Eur J Nucl Med 12: 473-476

Thomsen HS, Løkkegaard H, Nielsen SL, Larsen S (1988) Postoperative radionuclide monitoring of renal allografts on triple therapy. Dan Med Bull 35: 395-397

Todd LE, Perez JL, Elizondo G, Hazlewood CF (1983) In vivo T1 relaxation times in transplanted kidneys of human subjects. Physiol Chem Phys Med NMR 15: 27-29

Treugut H, Molde A (1981) Funktionskontrolle des Nierentransplantats durch Sequenz-CT. Fortschr Röntgenstr 135: 133-142

Treugut H, Nyman U, Hildell J, Husberg B (1983) Control of renal transplant function by diagnostic imaging. In: Heuck FHW, Donner MW (eds) Radiology today. Springer, New York Berlin Heidelberg, p 67

Van Sonnenberg E, Wittich GR, Casola G, Wing VW, Halasz NA, Lee AS, Winthers C (1986) Lymphoceles: imaging characteristics and percutaneous management: Radiology 161: 593-596

Van Zee B, Hoy W, Talley TE, Jaenike JR (1978) Renal injury associated with i.v. pyelography in nondiabetic and diabetic patients. Ann Intern Med 89: 51-54

Washida H, Tsugaya H, Fushimi N, Watanabe H, Tanaka F (1982) Evaluation of intensity of first perfusion of renoscintigram using ^{99m}Tc DTPA in practical urology. In: Raynaud C (ed) Proceedings of the IIIrd World congress of nuclear medicine and biology. Pergamon, Paris, pp 1556-1559

Weinrauch LA, Healy RW, Leland OS et al. (1977) Coronary angiography and acute renal failure in diabetic azotemic nephropathy. Ann Intern Med 86: 56-59

Weiss ER, Bladh WH, Krishnamurthy GT, Winston MA (1972) The diagnosis of renal transplant rejection in association with acute tubular necrosis using the scintillation camera. J Urol 107: 917-921

Whitaker RH (1979) An evaluation of 170 diagnostic pressure flow studies of the upper urinary tract. J Urol 121: 602-604

White M, Mueller PR, Ferrucci JT et al. (1985) Percutaneous drainage of postoperative abdominal and pelvic lymphoceles. AJR 145: 1065-1069

Winsett MZ, Amparo EG, Fawcett HD, Kumar R, Johnsen RF Jr, Bedi DG, Winsett OE (1988) Renal transplant dysfunction. MR evaluation. AJR 150: 319-323

Zajko AB, McLean GK, Grossman RA, Barker CF, Freiman DB, Ring EJ, Alavi A (1982) Percutaneous transluminal angioplasty and fibrinolytic therapy for renal allograft arterial stenosis and thrombosis. Transplantation 33: 447-449

Zaontz MR, Firlit CF (1988) Pelvic lymphocele after pediatric renal transplantation: a successful technique for prevention. J Urol 139: 557-559

Zinke H, Woods JE, Aguilo JJ, Leary IJ, DeWeerd JH, Frohnert PP, Hattery RR (1975) Experience with lymphoceles after renal transplantation. Surgery 77: 444-450

14 Ultrasound Diagnosis of Neonatal Conditions of the Genitourinary Tract

JANE CLAYTON and WILLIAM WELLS

CONTENTS

14.1   Introduction 339
14.2   Normal Kidney 339
14.3   Renal Agenesis 340
14.4   Obstructive Conditions 340
14.4.1 Multicystic Dysplastic Kidney 340
14.4.2 Ureteropelvic Junction Obstruction 341
14.4.3 Ureterovesical Junction Obstruction 342
14.4.4 Duplication Upper Pole Moiety
        with Ectopic Ureterocele 343
14.4.5 Posterior Urethral Valves 344
14.5   Infantile Polycystic Kidney Diseases 345
14.6   Urinary Tract Infection 346
14.7   Renal Calculi with Furosemide Therapy 347
14.8   Conclusion 347
        References 348

14.1 Introduction

Ultrasound evaluation of suspected neonatal genitourinary abnormalities is readily accomplished. The newer real-time high resolution (transducer frequencies of 5, 7.5, and 10 MHz) scanners have made the examination rapid, requiring no sedation, and portable to examine newborns in the nursery. Ultrasound is the procedure of first choice for identification of neonatal genitourinary conditions.

In the neonate an intravenous pyelogram is difficult to use for evaluation of the urinary tract because the neonatal kidney has a limited ability to filter and concentrate intravenous contrast (HALLER and COHEN 1987). The outer cortical nephrons are immature and the glomerular filtration rate is reduced (SHERMAN et al. 1988). Renal vascular resistance is increased, and total renal blood flow is decreased with preferential flow to the juxtamedullary areas (GONZALES 1985). Ultrasound examination requires no contrast. However, it does not evaluate renal function. Renal scintigraphy with technetium 99m-

JANE CLAYTON, M.D., Assistant Professor; WILLIAM WELLS, M.D., Assistant Professor; Department of Radiology, LSU Medical Center, 1542 Tulane Avenue, New Orleans, LA 70112, USA

DTPA is suggested for information about function (HAYDEN and SWISCHUK 1987).

The following examples of renal abnormalities seen in neonates demonstrate their ultrasound appearance, and comments are supplied regarding embryologic origin and clinical presentation. The majority of examinations in our ultrasound laboratory are performed for urinary tract infection and abdominal masses.

14.2 Normal Kidney

The normal kidney (Fig. 14.1) in the term infant is 4–5 cm long. The premature infant may have kidneys 3 cm or less in length (SHERMAN et al. 1988). Neonatal kidneys are different in appearance from adult kidneys. The renal cortex is more echogenic, the medullary pyramids are more prominent, and the central renal sinus echoes are less dense. The neonatal kidney assumes a more adult appearance by 6 months of age (HAN and BABCOCK 1985).

The increased echogenicity of the cortex, equal to the echogenicity of liver, is caused by glomeruli occupying a greater volume of renal cortex during the first few months of life, a glomerular tuft with a greater cellular component, and loops of Henle in the renal cortex. The glomeruli occupy 18% of renal cortical volume as compared with 8.6% in the adult kidney. The epithelial cells are prominent in the glomerular tuft. Twenty percent of the loops of Henle are in the renal cortex (HRICAK et al. 1983).

The medullary pyramids occupy a larger volume of the corticomedullary volume than later in life. Dilute fluid is present in the collecting tubules. This may account for their prominence. The distinction of the medulla may be a relative impression because of the increased echogenicity of the cortex (HRICAK et al. 1983).

The decreased density of the central sinus echoes is because of lack of fat in the newborn renal sinus. It gradually increases in echogenicity with age (HAN and BABCOCK 1985).

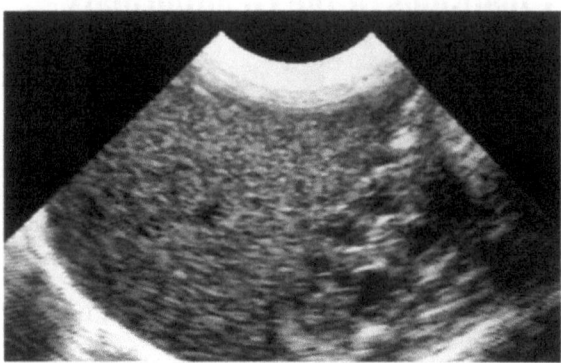

Fig. 14.1. Normal neonatal kidney. Note the cortical echogenicity equal to liver echogenicity, the prominent medullary pyramids, and the decreased amount of central sinus fat

Embryologically, development of the normal kidney begins at the end of the 5th week, when the ureteric bud originates from the mesonephric duct. The ureteric bud joins the nephrogenic blastema in the 6th week, and the definitive kidney begins to form. The kidneys ascend during the 6th and 7th weeks (GRAY and SKANDALAKIS 1972). The ureteric bud induces formation of nephrons as it branches. The first three to five branches form the renal pelvis. The next generations of branches form the calyces and papillae, and the next branches form the collecting tubules. Nephron induction continues until 32–36 weeks (POTTER and CRAIG 1975).

14.3 Renal Agenesis

Renal agenesis is the absence of formation of either one or both kidneys. The ureteric bud fails to make contact with the nephrogenic blastema (GRAY and SKANDALAKIS 1972).

Bilateral renal agenesis is a lethal anomaly with an incidence of 0.3/1000 births. It is transmitted in a polygenic pattern with a recurrence rate of 2%–5%. Infants with bilateral renal agenesis also have pulmonary hypoplasia, typical facies, and aberrant hand and foot positioning, the Potter syndrome. Ultrasound diagnosis is made by failing to see renal tissue, and the absence of a bladder. The adrenal glands adopt an oval disk shape because they have not been compressed by adjacent renal tissue. This appearance may simulate a kidney. The ultrasound examiner must be careful to identify a renal capsule and renal pelvis (ROMERO et al. 1985).

Unilateral renal agenesis is more common on the left. It is associated with genital anomalies such as agenesis of the fallopian tube, more often in the female. It is usually an incidental finding if the remaining kidney is normal (GRAY and SKANDALAKIS 1972).

14.4 Obstructive Conditions

Hydronephrosis in the neonate is usually detected as an abdominal mass. The most common abdominal mass is a hydronephrotic kidney. Causes include ureteropelvic junction obstruction (22%), posterior urethral valves (18%), ectopic ureterocele (14%), prune-belly syndrome (12%), and ureterovesical junction obstruction (8%) (KIRKS et al. 1985). Multicystic dysplastic kidney is the second most common neonatal abdominal mass, and is thought to result from early in utero obstruction.

14.4.1 Multicystic Dysplastic Kidney

A multicystic dysplastic kidney (Fig. 14.2) results from pelvic or ureteral atresia usually before 8–10 weeks of life. Complete obstruction or atresia of the ureteric bud causes impaired ureteral development, and resultant decreased division of collecting tubules and inhibition of induction and maturation of nephrons (KLEINER et al. 1986). Multicystic dysplastic kidney is associated with contralateral renal anomalies in 20%–45% of cases. If generalized multicystic dysplastic kidney disease is bilateral, it is a lethal abnormalitiy (Fig. 14.3).

Pathologically, the collecting tubules and nephrons are abnormal in form, and fewer in number. The diameter of the collecting tubules is increased, and the end of the tubules are cystic, with kidney size determined by the size of the cysts (POTTER and CRAIG 1975). The renal parenchyma is replaced by cysts of varying sizes, intervening stroma with scattered fetal tubules encircled by layers of fibromuscular tissue. Islets of cartilage are often present. The ureter distal to the area of atresia is small but patent (VINOCUR et al. 1988).

The ultrasound examination shows multiple cysts varying in size and shape with the largest located in the periphery of the kidney. The cysts do not communicate, and no renal parenchyma surrounds the cysts. Areas of increased echogenicity corresponding to tiny cysts are located eccentrically, scattered between the cysts (SANDERS and HARTMAN 1984). A hydronephrotic variant of multicystic dysplastic kidney will have moderate to severe corticomedullary dysplasia, but will have residual renal tissue (VINO-

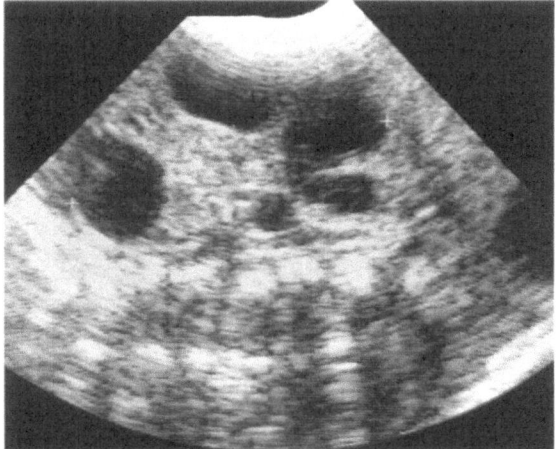

Fig. 14.2. Unilateral multicystic dysplastic kidney. Sagittal view

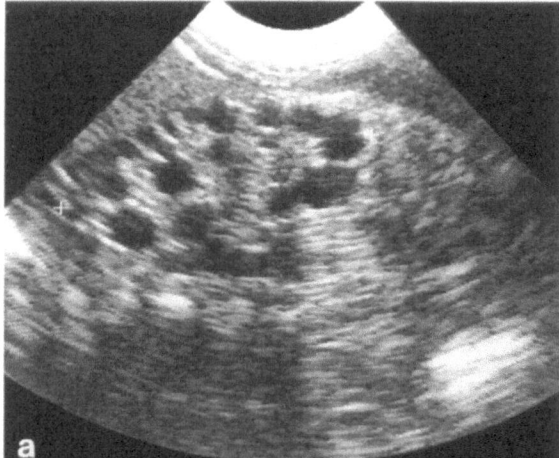

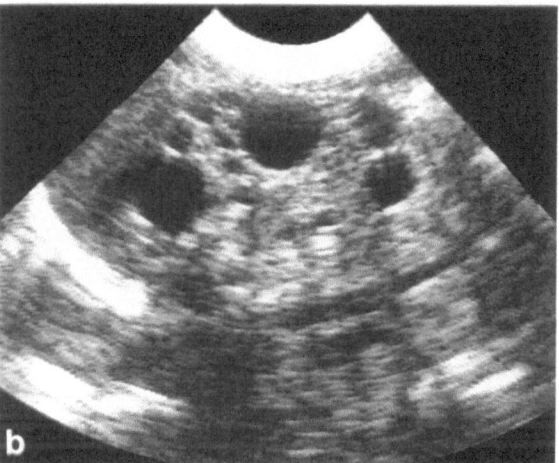

Fig. 14.3 a, b. Bilateral multicystic dysplastic kidneys. The anomaly was lethal. **a** Sagittal right. **b** Sagittal left

VUR et al. 1988). Small peripheral cysts may bud from a large central cyst (HAYDEN et al. 1986b).

Mistakes in diagnosis may occur with a medially located cyst mimicking a dilated ureter, megaureter, large central solitary cysts mimicking a dilated renal pelvis, prominent gallbladder adjacent to a hydronephrotic renal pelvis, and connections between the cysts (SANDERS and HARTMAN 1984). If questions about the diagnosis of multicystic dysplastic kidney occur, a technetium 99m-DTPA renal scan will show a nonfunctioning kidney. Cyst puncture and opacification will show noncommunicating cysts in multicystic dysplastic kidney.

14.4.2 Ureteropelvic Junction Obstruction

Ureteropelvic junction obstruction (Fig. 14.4) is the most common cause of neonatal hydronephrosis. It is bilateral in approximately one-third of cases (LEBOWITZ and TEELE 1983). The cause of the obstruction at the junction of the ureter and the renal pelvis may be either muscular hypertrophy, a partial or complete membrane, or an actual atresia (POTTER and CRAIG 1975).

Sonography shows hydronephrosis with a disproportionately dilated renal pelvis. Renal parenchyma surrounds the dilated calyces. The calyces and renal pelvis communicate. The calyceal cystic spaces are of uniform size. No dilated ureter can be seen to leave the renal pelvis. Mild ureteropelvic junction obstruction may be more difficult to diagnose ultrasonographically because it may be mistaken for transient dilatation of the upper tracts. Approximately one-third of cases of neonatal hydrone-

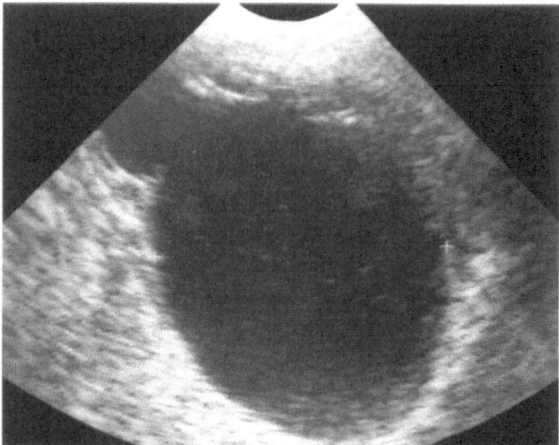

Fig. 14.4. Ureteropelvic junction obstruction. The renal pelvis is the most dilated portion of the intrarenal collecting system. Sagittal view

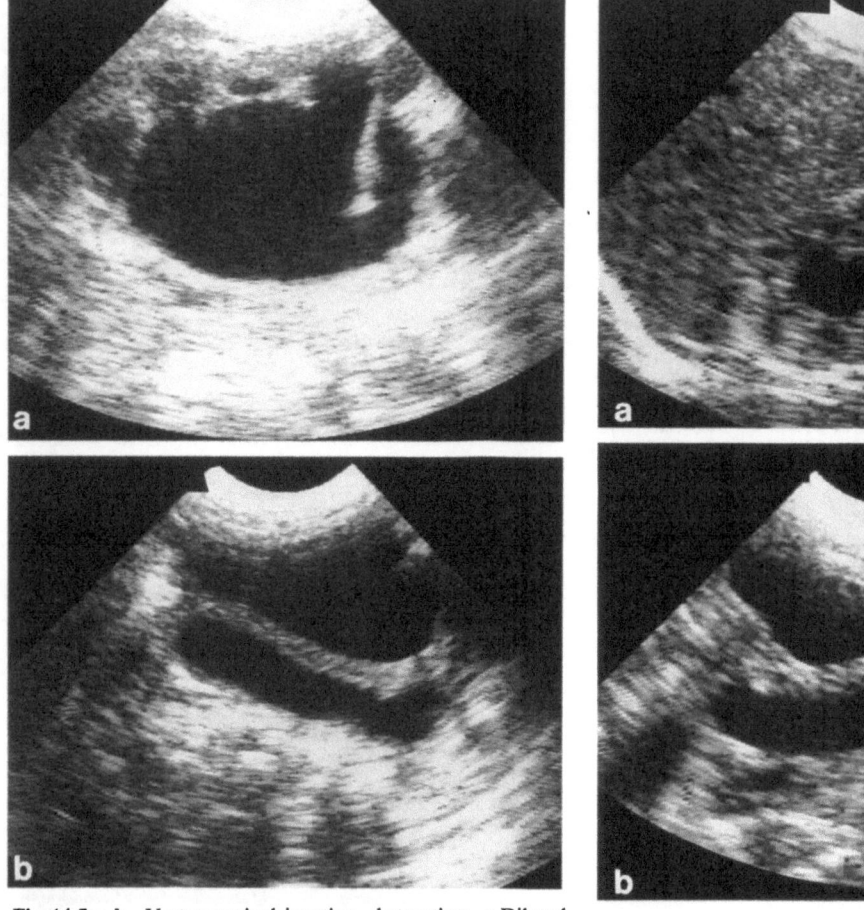

Fig. 14.5 a, b. Ureterovesical junction obstruction. **a** Dilated intrarenal collecting system, renal pelvis, and proximal ureter, sagittal view. **b** Dilated distal ureter, sagittal view

phrosis may be caused by an immature ureteropelvic junction. Increasing urinary output after birth results in dilatation of the upper tracts if the ureteropelvic junction has not fully matured. The renal blood flow increases to 18 times the in utero flow as renal resistance to arterial blood flow decreases in the first 2–3 weeks of life. The glomerular filtration rate increases by two to three times. Serial observations of a mildly dilated renal collecting system are suggested before surgery (HOMSY et al. 1986). A technetium 99m-DTPA scan will aid in the differentiation between ureteropelvic junction obstruction and multicystic dysplastic kidney (GIBBONS 1985).

14.4.3 Ureterovesical Junction Obstruction

Ureterovesical junction obstruction (Fig. 14.5) is caused by local muscular hypertrophy, or a dysplastic poorly innervated segment of ureter just before it

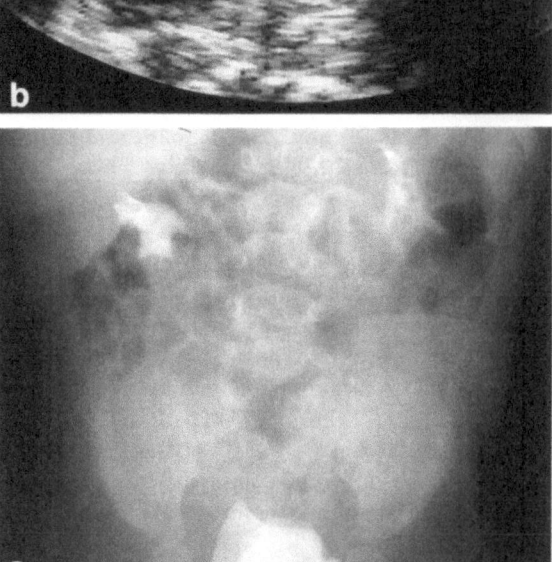

Fig. 14.6 a–c. Duplication anomaly of upper pole with ectopic ureterocele distally. **a** Sagittal view of right kidney showing dilated upper pole calyces. **b** Sagittal view of dilated distal right ureter. The ureterocele is outlined by cursors. **c** Intravenous pyelogram showing "drooping lily" sign of obstructed upper pole duplication

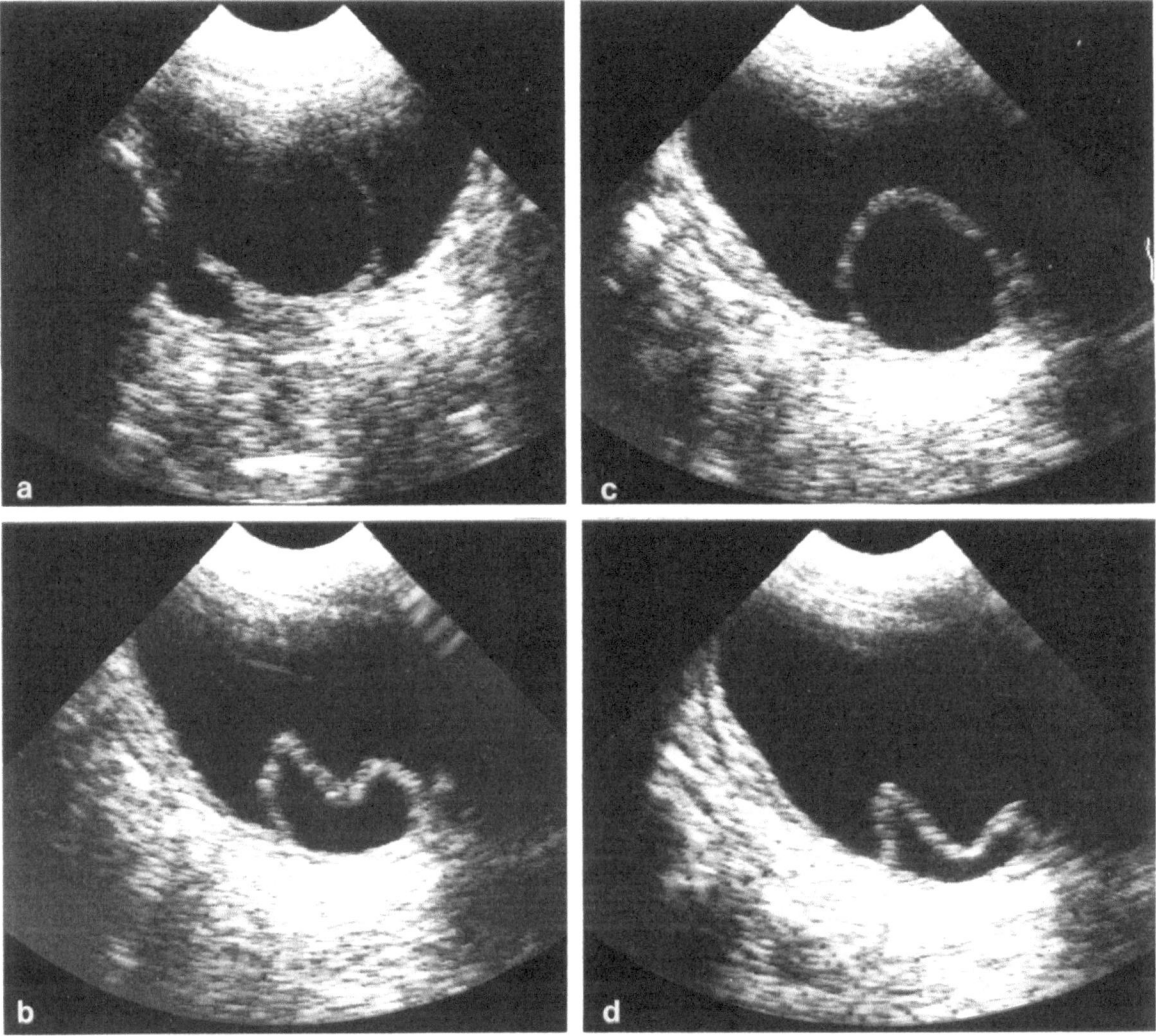

Fig. 14.7 a–d. A ureterocele may change in appearance during real-time observation. These images were obtained during 1 min

enters the bladder (HALLER and COHEN 1987). It is usually partial and can occur either unilaterally or bilaterally. As the ureters ascend from the bladder, they become more dilated, with the renal pelvis the area of maximum enlargement (POTTER and CRAIG 1975).

The ultrasound examination shows dilated calyces, renal pelvis, and ureter. The ureter can be followed to the ureterovesical junction with careful scanning. The ureter may be rather tortuous.

14.4.4 Duplication Upper Pole Moiety with Ectopic Ureterocele (Fig. 14.6)

Duplication anomalies arise when two metanephric ureteric buds develop, either by splitting at the tip of the ureteric bud or by growth of an accessory bud. The extent of the duplication depends on when the initial separation occurred. The degree of divergence of the ureteric buds before they reach the metanephric blastema determines the extent of renal duplication. Complete ureteral duplication tends to allow vesicoureteral reflux. The ureter from the lower pole enters the bladder above the one from the upper pole, and has a short intramural segment which allows reflux (GRAY and SKANDALAKIS 1972).

If the second ureteric bud arises at a more cranial point from the mesonephric duct, the orifice will be in an ectopic location. When the ureteral orifice is in the urethra, the bladder neck, or the trigone, part of

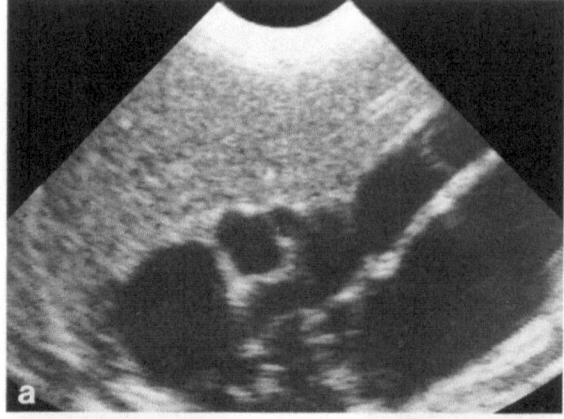

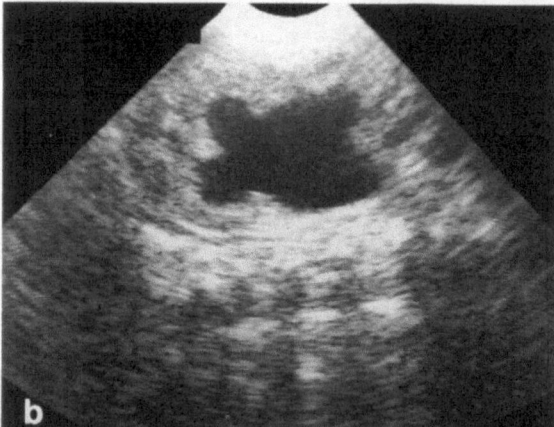

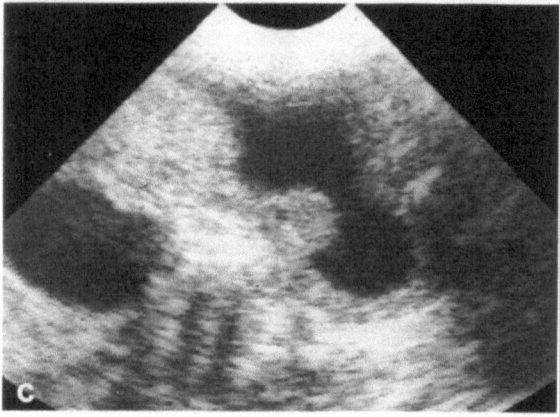

Fig. 14.8 a–c. Posterior urethral valves. **a** Sagittal view of massively dilated upper tract on right. **b** Sagittal view of moderately dilated upper tract on left. **c** Sagittal view of thick-walled bladder and dilated posterior urethra

The upper pole duplication with an ectopic ureterocele usually manifests in a urinary tract infection in the first few months of life (CALDAMONE 1985).

Sonographically, the collecting system in the upper pole of the kidney is dilated, and the draining duplicated ureter is also dilated and may be tortuous. The central sinus echoes in the lower pole are evident, with no dilatation seen. When the ureter is followed to the bladder, the ectopic ureterocele may be seen protruding into the bladder. It is a rounded thin-walled urine-filled structure at the base of the bladder. During real-time scanning, the ureterocele will change appearance depending upon the degree of distention with urine (Fig. 14.7).

14.4.5 Posterior Urethral Valves

Posterior urethral valves (Fig. 14.8) result when a membrane is formed by anterior fusion of two abnormal folds descending from the sides of the verumontanum in male children (CREMIN 1986). Embryologically the wolffian duct orifices migrate posterolaterally as the urorectal septum divides the cloaca into bladder and rectum. When division is complete, the wolffian duct orifices lie posteriorly in the urethra at the verumontanum as ejaculatory ducts. According to Young's classification, in type 1 urethral valves the wolffian ducts are located too far anteriorly, with mucosal folds extending anteroinferiorly from the verumontanum, often fusing anteriorly at the lower level. Type 1 is the most common form of posterior urethral valves. Type 2 is rare, and has mucosal folds extending anterosuperiorly from the verumontanum. Type 3 is the result of faulty perforation of the urogenital membrane with disk-like membranes located below the verumontanum and unrelated to it (MACPHERSON et al. 1986).

The posterior urethral valves obstruct the flow of urine. Consequently the detrusor muscles of the bladder become hypertrophied; the bladder walls thicken and have trabeculations, sacculations, and diverticula formation. The urethra proximal to the valves dilates. Hydroureteronephrosis results from either vesicoureteral reflux or from vesicoureteral obstruction caused by detrusor hypertrophy. Urinoma, urine ascites, and urothorax are further consequences. If the obstruction occurs early, cystic dysplastic changes may be seen in the kidneys (MACPHERSON et al. 1986).

Clinically neonates have signs and symptoms related to obstruction. Bilateral renal masses may be palpated on examination. The abdomen may be distended from urine ascites.

the distal ureter lies under the bladder mucosa (NUSSBAUM et al. 1987). A ureterocele may result if the distal ureteral orifice is obstructed. The distal ureter is closed during the 6th embryonic week, and the membrane resorbs by the 8th week. With partial resorption the distal ureter may balloon into the bladder, resulting in a ureterocele.

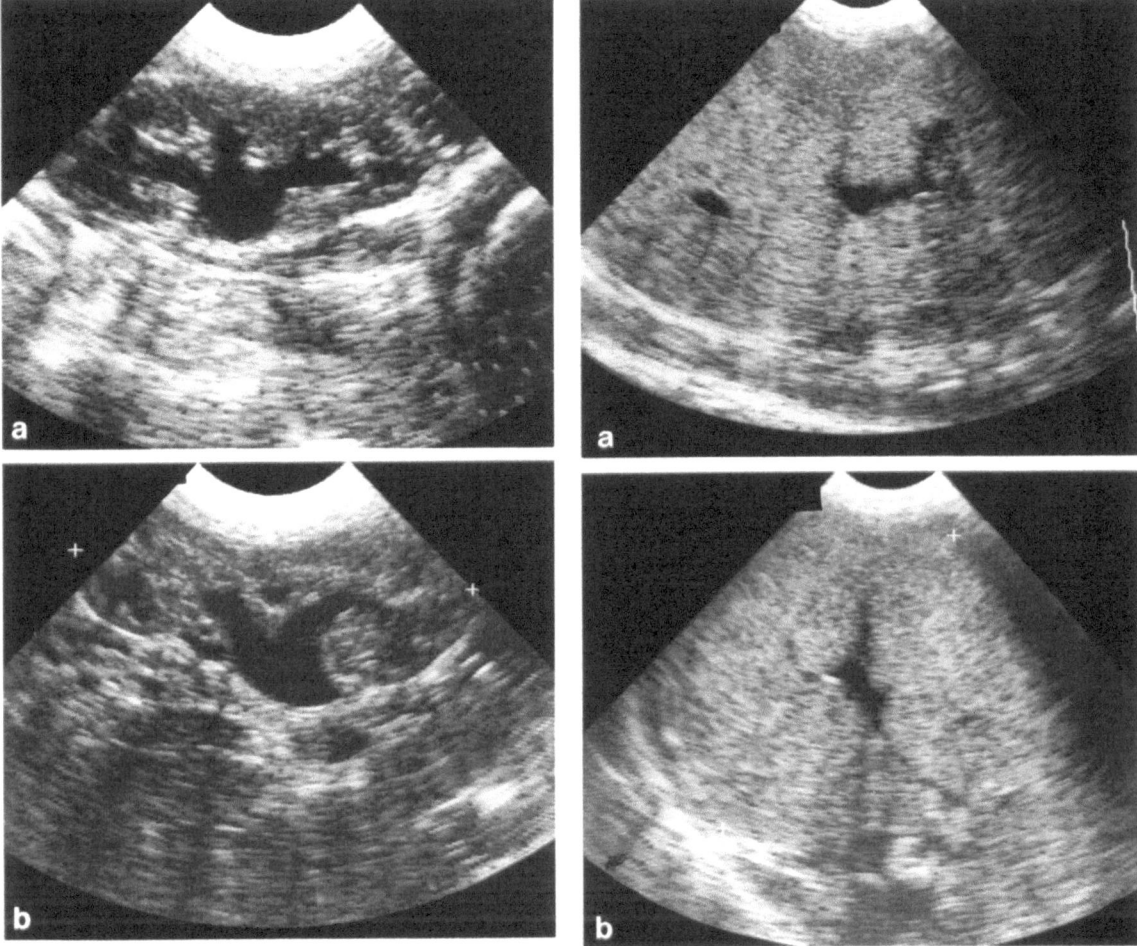

Fig. 14.9 a, b. Prune-belly syndrome. The upper tracts are dilated bilaterally. **a** Sagittal right. **b** Sagittal left

Fig. 14.10 a, b. Infantile polycystic kidney disease. Note the massively enlarged kidney with very echogenic parenchyma. **a** Sagittal right. **b** Transverse right

Ultrasound examination shows a massively dilated bladder with a thickened trabeculated wall. A dilated bladder is also associated with bladder neck obstruction caused by ectopic ureterocele, prune-belly syndrome, neurogenic bladder, and urethral stricture (CREMIN 1986). With urethral valves, the posterior urethra is dilated. Bilateral hydroureteronephrosis is present, and the ureters can be tortuous. Both urinomas and urine ascites can be imaged with ultrasound. Three types of urinoma can be found: subcapsular, localized perirenal, and diffuse perirenal (MACPHERSON et al. 1986).

Prune-belly syndrome (Fig. 14.9) can have a similar appearance ultrasonographically. Hydronephrosis, dilated tortuous ureters, and a distended bladder are seen. However, to distinguish prune-belly syndrome from posterior urethral valves on a clinical basis, partial or complete absence of abdominal wall musculature is demonstrated.

14.5 Infantile Polycystic Kidney Disease

The kidneys of infantile polycystic kidney disease (Fig. 14.10) or Potter I kidneys are bilaterally enlarged and symmetrically involved. Pathologically, the collecting tubules in the kidneys are diffusely enlarged. The cortex of these kidneys has greatly enlarged terminal branches of collecting tubules with normal nephrons interspersed. The medulla has variable sized collecting tubules with sacculations and diverticula (POTTER and CRAIG 1975). The inheritance of the disorder is autosomal recessive, with an incidence of 2/100,000 births (ROMERO et al. 1984). The embryologic insult has not been found. Infantile polycystic kidney disease also is associated with varying degrees of periportal fibrosis in the liver.

The disease is suspected in a neonate with bilateral flank masses, abdominal distention, and progressive renal failure. Infantile polycystic kidney disease has been divided into four groups by BLYTH and OCKENDEN:

1. Perinatal: more than 90% renal tubule involvement; little periportal hepatic fibrosis; rapid neonatal death from renal failure
2. Neonatal: kidneys are smaller with 60% renal involvement; mild hepatic fibrosis and death within 1 year
3. Infantile: 20% renal involvement; presentation at 3–6 months; moderate hepatic fibrosis with hepatosplenomegaly; progression to chronic renal failure and portal hypertension
4. Juvenile: less renal involvement than in the infantile form; manifestation at 6 months to 1 year; hepatic fibrosis and portal hypertension (ROMERO et al. 1984; BOAL and TEELE 1980).

Sonographically, the kidneys are bilaterally enlarged and have echogenic parenchyma, thought to be from the myriad of interfaces with the dilated collecting tubules. The reniform shape of the kidneys is maintained. The calyces are poorly defined, and the renal margins are not well delineated from surrounding tissues, especially liver (BOAL and TEELE 1980).

14.6 Urinary Tract Infection

Urinary tract infection is the most common urinary tract disease in children and is the most common reason for the imaging evaluation of the urinary tract in children. Bacterial infection of the urinary tract frequently causes a systemic illness in neonates. Bacteremia occurs in 30%–40% and life-threatening sepsis and meningitis can result. In the 1-month-old to 2-year-old sepsis and severe illness are less common, although urinary tract infection continues to cause systemic illness (STY et al. 1987).

An ultrasound examination has become the accepted test of first choice for evaluation of a child with a urinary tract infection (STY et al. 1987; KANGARLOO et al. 1985; HAYDEN et al. 1986a; JEQUIER et al. 1985; LEONIDAS et al. 1985). An ultrasound examination defines the anatomy of the kidneys and bladder without ionizing radiation, sedation, or limitation of detail because of glomerular function. The major area poorly imaged by ultrasound is vesicoureteral reflux. The current approach is to perform an ultrasound examination at the time of initial diagnosis of a urinary tract infection. If the ultrasound scan is normal, a voiding cystourethrogram is done in approximately 6 weeks to evaluate the child for

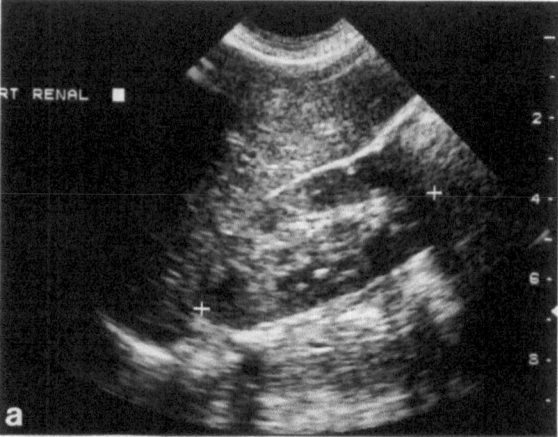
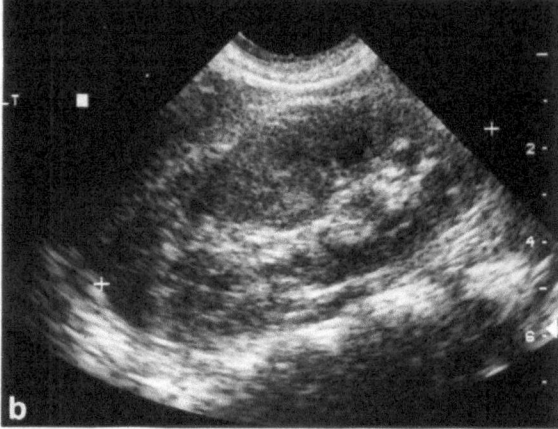

Fig. 14.11 a, b. Left acute pyelonephritis, normal right kidney. The left kidney is much larger than the right. **a** Sagittal right, 6.7 cm long. **b** Sagittal left, 9.2 cm long

reflux. If the ultrasound examination shows an anatomic abnormality, e.g., ureteropelvic junction obstruction, appropriate therapy is undertaken at the time of diagnosis.

Changes associated with urinary tract infection that are seen on an ultrasound examination include: enlargement of a kidney with pyelonephritis (Fig. 14.11), decrease in parenchymal echogenicity, increased renal sound transmission, mild dilatation of the renal pelvis, loss of delineation of the boundary between the cortex and medulla, mass associated with focal pyelonephritis, debris in the collecting system, and bladder wall thickening (STY et al. 1987; DINKEL et al. 1986).

In infants who have a history of therapy with broad spectrum antibiotics or have vascular catheters, *Candida* can infect the urinary tract. The baby has anuria or a flank mass or oliguria or hypertension. An ultrasound examination shows pyonephrosis with dilated calyces and debris in the collecting system (Fig. 14.12), parenchymal lesions, and

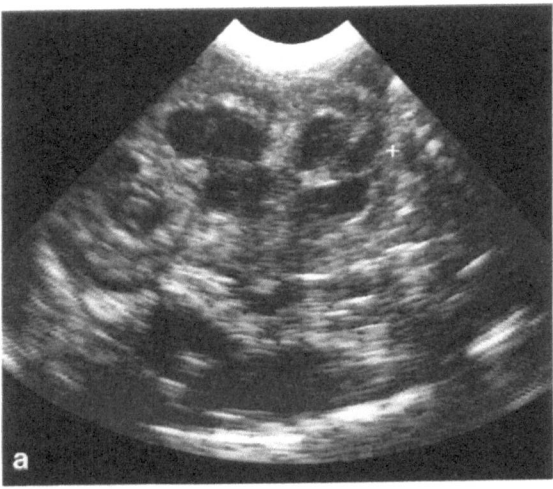

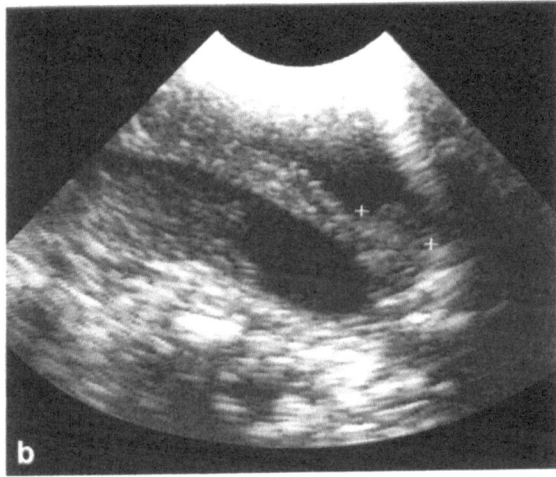

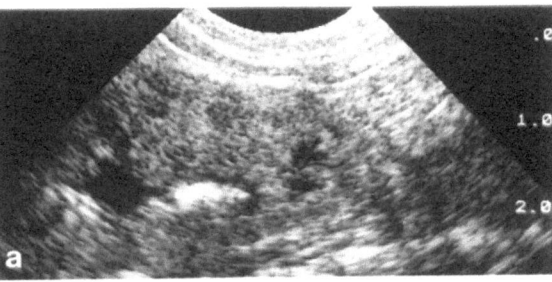

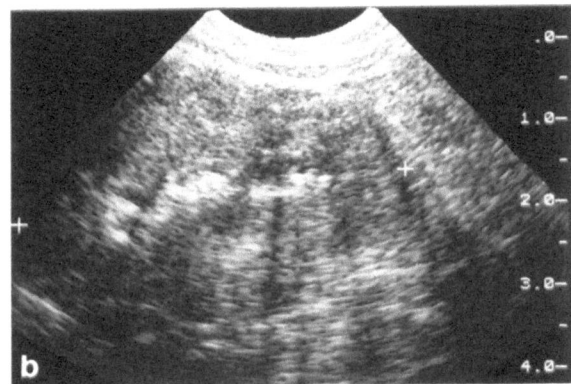

Fig. 14.13 a, b. Renal calculi after furosemide therapy. Note brightly echogenic stones centrally in both kidneys. **a** Sagittal right. **b** Sagittal left

◁

Fig. 14.12 a, b. Yeast infection of obstructed right collecting system. **a** Sagittal right kidney showing debris in dilated calyces. **b** Sagittal right distal ureter with debris in ureter and edematous ureteral orifice between the cursors

fungal bezoars in the collecting system (KINTANAR et al. 1986; COHEN et al. 1986).

14.7 Renal Calculi with Furosemide Therapy

Infants receiving chronic furosemide therapy tend to develop renal calculi (Fig. 14.13). The furosemide may be adminstered for chronic lung disease associated with complication of pulmonary hypertension, for congestive heart failure, for hypertension, or for neonatal asphyxia. It is administered daily for 3–6 weeks before the calcifications develop. Urinary calcium excretion is increased by furosemide's action in the medullary loop of Henle. It decreases calcium and sodium reabsorption in this segment with a resultant 10- to 20-fold increase in calcium excretion (MYRACLE et al. 1986; PEARSE et al. 1984).

The renal calculi may be demonstrated on ultrasound examination. They are rounded echogenic foci greater than 3 mm in diameter located in either the papillary area or the renal collecting system. The collecting system may have gravity-dependent echogenic debris.

14.8 Conclusion

Ultrasound evaluation of the neonatal genitourinary tract is rapid and requires no sedation and no ionizing radiation. It delineates the anatomy of the kidney and bladder and defines anatomic abnormalities. Because ultrasound examination has these characteristics, it is recommended as the first imaging procedure to be performed in an infant with a suspected genitourinary abnormality. The findings seen on an ultrasound scan can be used to direct further evaluation.

References

Alon U, Pery M, Davidai G, Berant M (1986) Ultrasonography in the radiologic evaluation of children with urinary tract infection. Pediatrics 78: 58–64

Amundson GM, Trevenen CL, Mueller DL, Rubin SZ, Wesenberg RL (1987) Neuroblastoma: a specific sonographic tissue pattern. AJR 148: 943–945

Avni EF, Brion LE (1983) Ultrasound of the neonatal urinary tract. Urol Radiol 5: 177–183

Boal DK, Teele RL (1980) Sonography of infantile polycystic kidney disease. AJR 135: 575–580

Bove KE, McAdams AJ (1976) The nephroblastomatosis complex and its relationship to Wilms' tumor: a clinicopathologic treatise. Perspect Pediatr Pathol 3: 185–222

Brenbridge AN, Chevalier RL, Kaiser DL (1986) Increased renal cortical echogenicity in pediatric renal disease: histopathologic correlations. J Clin Ultrasound 14: 595–600

Brown T, Mandell J, Lebowitz RL (1987) Neonatal hydronephrosis in the era of sonography. AJR 148: 959–963

Caldamone AA (1985) Duplication anomalies of the upper tract in infants and children. Urol Clin North Am 12: 75–91

Cohen HL, Haller JO, Schechter S, Slovis T, Merola R, Eaton DH (1986) Renal candidiasis of the infant: ultrasound evaluation. Urol Radiol 8: 17–21

Cremin BJ (1986) A review of the ultrasonic appearances of posterior urethral valve and ureteroceles. Pediatr Radiol 16: 357–364

Cremin BJ, Aaronson IA (1983) Ultrasonic diagnosis of posterior urethral valve in neonates. Br J Radiol 56: 435–438

Davidson AJ (1985) Radiology of the kidney. W. B. Saunders, Philadelphia, pp 71–74

Davies CH, Stringer DA, Whyte H, Daneman A, Mancer K (1986) Congenital hepatic fibrosis with saccular dilatation of intrahepatic bile ducts and infantile polycystic kidneys. Pediatr Radiol 16: 302–305

Diament MJ, Takasugi J, Kangarloo H (1984) Hydronephrosis in childhood – reliability of ultrasound screening. Pediatr Radiol 14: 31–36

Diard F, LeDosseur P, Cadier L, Calabet A, Bondonny JM (1984) Multicystic dysplasia in the upper component of the complete duplex kidney. Pediatr Radiol 14: 310–313

Dinkel E, Orth S, Dittrich M, Schulte-Wisserman H (1986) Renal sonography in the differentiation of upper from lower urinary tract infection. AJR 146: 775–780

Fenelon MJ, Alton DJ (1981) Prolapsing ectopic ureteroceles in boys. Radiology 140: 373–376

Fong KW, Rahmani MR, Rose TH, Skidmore MB, Connor TP (1986) Fetal renal cystic disease: sonographic-pathologic correlation. AJR 146: 767–773

Franken EA, Yiu-Chiu V, Smith WL, Chiu LC (1982) Nephroblastomatosis: clinicopathologic significance and imaging characteristics. AJR 138: 950–952

Gibbons MD (1985) Postnatal management of UPJ obstruction detected antenatally. Dialogues in Pediatric Urology 8: 2–8

Gonzales ET (1985) Urologic considerations in the newborn. Urol Clin North Am 12: 43–51

Goodman JD, Norton KI, Carr L, Yeh HC (1986) Crossed fused renal ectopia: sonographic diagnosis. Urol Radiol 8: 13–16

Gray SW, Skandalakis JE (1972) Embryology for surgeons. W. B. Saunders, Philadelphia, pp 443–552

Haller JO, Cohen HL (1987) Pediatric urosonography: an update. Urol Radiol 9: 99–109

Han BK, Babcock DS (1985) Sonographic measurements and appearance of normal kidneys in children. AJR 145: 611–616

Hayden CK, Swischuk LE (1987) Pediatric ultrasonography. Williams and Wilkins, Baltimore, pp 263–345

Hayden CK, Santa-Cruz FR, Amparo EG, Brouhard B, Swischuk LE, Ahrendt DK (1984) Ultrasonographic evaluation of the renal parenchyma in infancy and childhood. Radiology 152: 413–417

Hayden CK, Swischuk LE, Fawcett HD, Rytting JE, McCord G (1986 a) Urinary tract infections in childhood: a current imaging approach. Radiographics 6: 1023–1038

Hayden CK, Swischuk LE, Smith TH, Armstrong EA (1986 b) Renal cystic disease in childhood. Radiographics 6: 97–116

Homsy YL, Williot P, Danais S (1986) Transitional neonatal hydronephrosis: fact or fantasy? J Urol 136: 339–341

Hricak H, Slovis TI, Callen CW, Callen PW, Romanski RN (1983) Neonatal kidneys: sonographic anatomic correlation. Radiology 147: 699–702

Jequier S, Forbes PA, Nogrady MB (1985) The value of ultrasonography as a screening procedure in a first-documented urinary tract infection in children. J Ultrasound Med 4: 393–400

Kangarloo H, Gold RH, Fine RN, Diament MJ, Boechat MI (1985) Urinary tract infection in infants and children evaluated by ultrasound. Radiology 154: 367–373

Kenney PJ, Spirt BA, Leeson MD (1984) Genitourinary anomalies: radiologic-anatomic correlations. Radiographics 4: 233–260

Kintanar C, Cramer BC, Reid WD, Andrews WL (1986) Neonatal renal candidiasis: sonographic diagnosis. AJR 147: 801–805

Kirks DR, Rosenberg ER, Johnson DG, King LR (1985) Integrated imaging of neonatal renal masses. Pediatr Radiol 15: 147–156

Kirpekar M, Abiri MM, Hilfer C, Enerson R (1986) Ultrasound in the diagnosis of systemic candidiasis (renal and cranial) in very low birth weight premature infants. Pediatr Radiol 16: 17–20

Kleiner B, Filly RA, Mack L, Callen PW (1986) Multicystic dysplastic kidney: observations of contralateral disease in the fetal population. Radiology 161: 27–29

Lebowitz RL, Teele RL (1983) Fetal and neonatal hydronephrosis. Urol Radiol 5: 185–188

Leonidas JC, McCauley RGK, Klauber GC, Fretzayas AM (1985) Sonography as a substitute for excretory urography in children with urinary tract infection. AJR 144: 815–819

Macpherson RI, Gordon L, Bradford BF (1984) Neonatal urinomas: imaging considerations. Pediatr Radiol 14: 396–399

Macpherson RI, Leithiser RE, Gordon L, Turner WR (1986) Posterior urethral valves: an update and review. Radiographics 6: 753–791

Mason WG (1984) Urinary tract infections in children: renal ultrasound evaluation. Radiology 153: 109–111

Melson GL, Shackelford GD, Cole BR (1985) The spectrum of sonographic findings in infantile polycystic kidney disease with urographic and clinical implications. J Clin Ultrasound 13: 113–119

Myracle MR, McGahan JP, Goetzman BW, Adelman RD (1986) Ultrasound diagnosis of renal calcification in infants on chronic furosemide therapy. J Clin Ultrasound 14: 281–287

Nussbaum AR, Dorst JP, Jeffs RD, Gearhart JP, Sanders RC (1986) Ectopic ureter and ureterocele: their varied sonographic manifestations. Radiology 159: 227–235

Nussbaum AR, Hartman DS, Whitley N, McCauley RGK, Sanders RC (1987) Multicystic dysplasia and crossed renal ectopia. AJR 149: 407-410

Pearse DM, Kaude JV, Williams JL, Bush D, Wright PG (1984) Sonographic diagnosis of furosemide-induced nephrocalcinosis in newborn infants. Journal of Ultrasound in Medicine 3: 553-556

Pedicelli G, Jequier S, Bowen AD, Boisvert J (1986) Multicystic dysplastic kidneys: spontaneous regression demonstrated with US. Radiology 160: 23-26

Potter EL, Craig JM (1975) Pathology of the fetus and infant, 3rd edn. Year Book Medical Publishers, Chicago, pp 434-475

Romero R, Cullen M, Jeanty P, Grannum P, Reece EA, Venus I, Hobbins JC (1984) The diagnosis of congenital renal anomalies with ultrasound II. Infantile polycystic kidney disease. Am J Obstet Gynecol 150: 259-262

Romero R, Cullen M, Grannum P, Jeanty P, Reece EA, Venus I, Hobbins JC (1985) Antenatal diagnosis of renal anomalies with ultrasound III. Bilateral renal agenesis. Am J Obstet Gynecol 151: 38-43

Rosenbaum DM, Korngold E, Teele RL (1984) Sonographic assessment of renal length in normal children. AJR 142: 467-469

Sanders RC, Hartman DS (1984) The sonographic distinction between neonatal multicystic kidney and hydronephrosis. Radiology 151: 621-625

Sanders RC, Nussbaum AR, Solez K (1988) Renal dysplasia: sonographic findings. Radiology 167: 623-626

Schneider K, Jablonski C, Wiessner M, Kohn M, Fendel H (1984) Screening for vesicoureteral reflux in children using real-time sonography. Pediatr Radiol 14: 400-403

Sherman NH, Boyle GK, Rosenberg HK (1988) Sonography in the neonate. Ultrasound Q 6: 91-149

Stuck KJ, Koff SA, Silver TM (1982) Ultrasonic features of multicystic dysplastic kidney: expanded diagnostic criteria. Radiology 143: 217-221

Sty JR, Wells RG, Starshak RJ, Schroeder BA (1987) Imaging in acute renal infection in children. AJR 148: 471-477

Vinocur L, Slovis TL, Perlmutter AD, Watts FB, Chang CH (1988) Followup studies of multicystic dysplastic kidneys. Radiology 167: 311-315

Wernecke K, Heckemann R, Bachman H, Peters PE (1985) Sonography of infantile polycystic kidney disease. Urol Radiol 7: 138-145

Subject Index

abdominal musculature, loss, prune-belly syndrome 66, 168
- calculus disease 177, 179
abdominal plain film
- adrenal diseases 2
- brucellosis 127
- calcifications, renal cyst 233, 235
- carcinoma, renal pelvis 266
- congenital renal solitary cyst 44
- echinococcosis 125
- horseshoe kidney 53
- medullary sponge kidney, calcifications 51
- nephrolithiasis 177, 179
- papillary necrosis, calcifications 140
- pheochromocytoma 2
- radiolucent (cystine) renal stones 163
- renal sarcoma 253
- tuberculosis, renal 117
abdominal trauma, renal injury 190, 209
abscess
- actinomycosis 125
- adrenal 15
- amebiasis 129
- candidiasis 126, 127
- coccidioidomycosis 130
- cryptococcosis 129
- drainage, CT-, ultrasound control 133
- infrarenal
- - AIDS, CT 97
- - clinical background, radiology 131-133
- kidney transplantation 312, 322
- psoas, tuberculosis, CT 120
- renal
- - pararenal, perinephritic 131-136
- - predisposing factors 131
- - pyramids 41
- - subcapsular gas bubbles, CT 200
- - tuberculosis 118
- - xanthomatous pyelonephritis 121, 123
ACTH producing tumor, Cushing's syndrome 19
actinomicosis, renal 128, 129
acute
- chronic
- - glomerulonephritis, diagnosis, clinical picture 76, 77
- - interstitial nephritis, clinical picture, pathology, radiology 85, 87

- ureteral obstruction, pathophysiology 151, 152
Addison's syndrome
- adrenal insufficiency, CT 16, 17
- amyloidosis 17
- autoimmune adrenalitis 17
- hemochromatosis 17
- hemorrhage 17
- histoplasmosis 17
- inflammation 15
- lymphoma 17
- metastases 17
- necrosis 17
- tuberculosis 15
- Waterhouse-Friedrichsen syndrome 16, 17
adenoma
- adrenal 2, 3, 5, 7, 9, 10, 17-22, 27
- - biopsy, CT-guided 4, 5
- - calcifications .2, 7, 9, 16, 18, 20, 22
- - hormonal characterization 5
- - hyperfunctioning, MRI 3
- biopsy, CT guided 4
- cortical, Conn's syndrome, CT 18
- - dynamic CT 2
- Cushing, imaging characteristics 11
- nonfunctioning, CT 8
- renal 217, 218
- - carcinoma 277
- sebaceum, angiomyolipoma 219
adrenal hormones
- excess secretion, differential diagnosis 17-27
adrenalitis, autoimmune, Addison's disease, CT 16, 17
adrenals
- adenoma, bilateral, dynamic CT 4
- - biopsy, CT-guided 4, 5
- - cortical, Conn's syndrome, CT 18
- - Cushing, imaging characteristics 11, 19-21
- - dynamic CT 2
- - hormonal characterization 5
- - nonfunctioning CT 8
- adrenalitis, autoimmune, Addison's disease, CT 7, 16
- AIDS, Kaposi sarcoma, necrosis 9, 16
- arteriography 5, 25
- atrophy 15

- bleeding, differential diagnosis 14, 15
- calcifications, pseudocysts 8, 9
- - teratoma 12
- - tuberculosis, CT 16
- - Wolman disease (familial xanthomatosis) 17
- carcinoma, MRI 3
- Conn's syndrome, plain film, urography 2
- cysts, classification 7
- - diagnostic imaging 8, 9
- function, history 1
- hamartoma, renal angiomyolipoma 219
- hemangioma, CT 12, 14
- hyperfunction 17-27
- imaging characteristics, differential diagnosis 11
- inflammatory diseases, diagnostic imaging 15, 16
- insufficiency, Addison's disease, Waterhouse-Friedrichsen syndrome 17
- Kaposi sarcoma infiltration 9
- lipoma, dynamic CT 2
- lymphoma, CT 9, 10, 12
- medulla, ^{131}I-MIBG imaging 4
- metastases, dynamic CT 2, 9, 10
- myelolipoma, diagnostic imaging 2, 10, 11, 12
- necrosis, etiology 7, 16
- neuroblastoma, diagnostic imaging 10, 11
- normal
- - anatomy, topography 1-3, 6
- - arteriography 5
- - CT, mean attenuation value 2, 6
- - MRI 3
- - ultrasound 3, 6
- pheochromocytoma, imaging 2, 10, 11, 22-25
- teratoma, CT 11, 13
- tuberculosis, insufficiency, CT 16, 17
- vein thrombosis 16
- venography, complications, necrosis, thrombosis 7, 16
adrenogenital syndrome
- congenital adrenal hyperplasia, feminization, masculinization 21
- ultrasound 21
agenesis, adrenal 7

AIDS
- adrenal 15-17
- Kaposi sarcoma, adrenals 9
- nephropathy 94-97
aldosterone/cortisol ratio, Conn's syndrome 19
aldosteronoma
- adrenocortical radionuclide scanning 3, 18
- Conn's syndrome 2, 17-19
- dynamic CT 2, 18
- imaging characteristics 11
- selective venous blood sampling 5, 18, 19
allergy
- acute tubular necrosis 85
- anaphylactoid purpura, Henoch-Schönlein syndrome 80
amebiasis, renal 129
amyloidosis
- adrenal insufficiency 7, 17
- see Addison's syndrome
- renal carcinoma 276
analgetic abuse, clinical background, pathology, radiology 88, 89
anatomy
- adrenals, normal 1-3, 6
- renal 72, 73
- - arteries 299
aneurysms
- angiomyolipoma 221
- circle of Willis 48
- mycotic, renal 141
- pseudoaneurysm, renal artery, stab wound 204
- renal artery 64, 65
- - angiography 299, 300, 301
- - rupture, hematoma 78
angiography
- abscess, intrarenal, perinephric, pararenal 133, 134
- acute bacterial nephritis 108
- adrenal 5, 25
- aneurysm, mycotic, renal 141, 142
- angiomyolipoma 222
- arteriovenous fistulas, congenital 65
- autosomal dominant polycystic kidney disease (Swiss cheese appearance) 49, 239
- carcinoma, renal pelvis 267
- chronic pyelonephritis 115
- crossed ectopic kidney 57
- digital subtraction
- - normal renal 75
- - renovascular hypertension, sensitivity, specifity 298, 305
- echinococcosis 126
- kidney graft, arteriovenous fistula 326
- malacoplakia 128
- medullary cystic renal disease 52
- multilocular cystic nephroma 46, 47
- obstructive uropathy 162, 163
- pyelonephritis, xanthomatosis 123
- radiation nephritis 94

- radionuclear, kidney transplantation 313, 314, 318
- renal
- - artery
- - - before and after angioplasty 325
- - - hypertension 298, 299
- - - intimal flap 203
- - - pseudoaneurysm 204
- - - stenosis
- - - - hypertension 83
- - - - iliac artery anastomosis 325
- - carcinoma 276, 277, 286-288
- - chronic glomerulonephritis 77
- - hypoplasia 36
- - infected cysts 232
- - metastases 258
- - microaneurysms 71, 78
- - oncocytoma 217
- - parenchymal diseases 71, 75
- - perfusion differences, cortex, medulla 73
- - sarcoma 253, 255
- - sclerosis, cortical 83
- - transplantation 304
- - trauma 203
- selective, renal abscess 132, 133
- tuberculosis, renal 119
angiomyolipoma
- coexistent, renal trauma 202
- renal 218-222
angioplasty
- control, Doppler ultrasonography 305
- renal artery, technique, results, complications 306-308, 325
angiotensin - renin mechanism
- hypertension, arteriovenous fistula 65
- - Ask-Upmark kidney 52
- - breaking, embolization 308
- - renovascular 295
- renal
- - infarct 308
- - trauma 200
- renovascular hypertension 295
anomalies see developmental anomalies
aortic coarctation, hypertension 303, 304
- renal
- - arteriography, technique 299
- - artery
- - - fibromuscular hyperplasia 301
- - - stenosis, atherosclerotic, angioplasty
- - - - before and after 308
- - - - stent in place 307
arteriovenous fistulae
- congenital 65
- kidney graft 326
- within renal carcinoma 275
- renal, embolization 308
- renovascular hypertension 299
aspergillosis, renal 130

atherosclerosis, renovascular hypertension 300, 307, 308
atrophy, renal 15
autosomal
- dominant polycystic disease
- - renal
- - - association with hepatic, pancreatic cysts 228, 238
- - - etiology, diagnosis 237
- - - high density cysts 240
- - - rupture into the perinephric space 240
- recessive polycystic disease
- - increased hepatic echogenicity 241
- - renal
- - - characterization 241
- - - classification 228
- - - contrast medium retention in tubules 241
- - - CT 241
- - - histopathology 241
- - - neonatal form 241
- - - radionuclide findings 241
- - - urogram 241
- - - in utero diagnosis 241

Beckwith-Wiedemann syndrome
- adrenal carcinoma 21
- renal cystic disease 228
biopsy
- CT-guided
- - adrenals 4, 5, 7, 16, 17, 27
- - infrarenal abscess 97
- renal
- - graft, arteriovenosis fistula 326
- - Henoch-Schönlein syndrome 80
- - Wegener's granulomatosis 81
bladder
- carcinoma, ilial loop urinary diversion 167
- malacoplakia 128
- pressure, renal pressure, step-off pressure, mild, severe obstruction 169
blastomycosis
- adrenal 15
- renal 130
bleeding
- adrenal
- - calcification 14, 16
- - differential diagnosis 14-17
- splenic artery, CT 193
- traumatic, renal arteries, radionuclide imaging 205
bone, metabolic diseases, Fanconi's syndrome 91
Bourneville's disease
- angiomyolipoma 219, 248
- renal
- - cyst, tuberous sclerosis 246
- - cystic disease 228
Bright's disease, clinical background, pathology, radiology 76, 77
brucellosis, renal 127

Burkitt's lymphoma, differential diagnosis 265

Calcifications
- adrenals 2, 8, 9, 11, 14–17, 21, 26
- - Addison's disease 16
- - bleeding 14
- - carcinoma 21
- - computed tomography 2
- - differential diagnosis 16, 17
- - ganglioneuroma 16
- see calculus disease
- - hemangioma 16
- - histoplasmosis 16
- - inflammatory disease 15, 16
- - metastases 9
- - myelolipoma 11, 16
- - neuroblastoma 10, 26, 28
- - pheochromocytoma 16
- - tuberculosis, CT 16
- - Wolman disease (familial xanthomatosis) 17
- angiomyolipoma 219
- brucellosis 127
- carcinoma renal pelvis 266, 270, 271
- coccidioidomycosis 130
- Fanconi's syndrome 92
- hemorrhagic renal cyst 233
- horseshoe kidney 54
- medullary sponge kidney 51
- multilocular cystic nephroma 46, 47, 222
- nephrocalcinosis 246
- papillary necrosis 140
- polycystic renal disease 46
- pseudocysts 8, 9
- renal
- - carcinoma 279, 281
- - cystic disease 235
- - necrosis, bilateral, cortical 83
- - pelvis 265–270
- - sarcoma 253
- - teratoma 11, 13, 16
- - tuberculosis, renal 116, 117
- - Wolman disease (familial xanthomatosis) 17
calcitriol deficiency, renal osteodystrophy, manifestations 84
calculus disease
- lithotripsy, extracorporal 180, 181, 182
- see nephrolithiasis
- renal, neonates, ultrasound 347
- stone
- - fragmentation, problems 181
- - removal
- - - percutaneous 184, 185
- - - transurethral ureteroscopy 180
- - type, CT density range 179
- transurethral ureteroscopy 182–184
- ureter
- - extracorporal lithotripsy, technique, applications 180, 181
- - "Steinstrasse", ureteroscopy 181
- - ultrasonic lithotrypsy 183

- ureteroscopy, stone fragmentation, extraction 182, 183
candidiasis, renal 126, 127
Captopril
- angiotensin converting enzyme inhibitor 296
- interstitial nephritis 85
- renography, hypertension 297
Carcinoids, ^{131}I-MIBG storage 4
carcinoma
- adrenal 5, 21–22
- - arteriography 5
- - Beckwith-Wiedemann syndrome 21
- - calcifications 16, 21
- - Conn's syndrome 18
- - CT 21
- - Cushing's syndrome 21
- - imaging characteristics 3, 11
- - magnetic resonance imaging 10, 22
- - ultrasound 21, 22
- bladder, ilial loop urinary diversion 167
- colon, ureteral obstruction, CT 162
- hyperaldosteronism 21
- renal
- - cells
- - - CT 57
- - - oncocytoma, coexisting 215
- - - renal trauma 202
- - cystic disease, differential diagnosis 233
- - sarcomatoid 252
- - schistosomiasis 121
- ureteropelvic junction 268
Caroli's disease
- medullary sponge kidney 50, 51
- renal cystic disease 228, 241
cavography, malacoplakia, renal vein thrombosis 128
cephalosporins, acute interstitial nephritis 85
cerebral vascular system, berry aneurysms 48
cerebrohepatorenal syndrome, Zellweger, renal cystic disease 228
chest, scan, metastases, renal carcinoma 285
childhood
- adrenals
- - bacterial infections, necrosis 16
- - normal, anatomy, topography 6
- Ask-Upmark kidney 52, 53
- autosomal recessive polycystic kidney disease 46, 47
- chronic granulomatosis disease 131
- congenital
- - hydronephrosis 66
- - megaureter 168
- echinococcosis 125
- ectopic ureter 168
- Fanconis' syndrome 91
- fetal lobation, renal, CT 58
- Henoch-Schönlein syndrome 80

- hypertension, neurofibromatosis 304
- infantile polycystic kidney disease 345, 346
- intussusception, Henoch-Schönlein purpurea 80
- juxtaglomerular cell tumor (reninoma) 218
- malacoplakia 127, 128
- prune belly syndrome 168
- reflux nephropathy 104
- Riley-Newhouse syndrome 48
- ultrasound, abdominal pathology 2, 3
- ureteropelvic junction obstruction 167
- urinary
- - infection 104
- - obstruction 156
- Wilm's tumor, differential diagnosis, ultrasound 3
cholesteatoma, renal 142
chyloma, renal, traumatic 199
circulatory disturbances, adrenal 17
classification
- adrenal diseases 7
- autosomal
- - dominant polycystic kidney disease 228
- - recessive polycystic kidney disease 46
- cystic disease, kidney 227, 228
- hydronephrosis, congenital 66
- inflammatory renal disease 104
- lupus erythematosus 78
- multicystic dysplastic kidney 43
- renal
- - anomalies 34
- - carcinoma 277
- - injuries 189
- - traumatic tears, renal parenchyma 194, 195
- tubulointerstitial renal diseases 84
clinical results
- extracorporal lithotrypsy 182
- renal
- - angioplasty 307
- - trauma 210
coccidioidomycosis, renal 130
complications
- acute glomerulonephritis 76, 77
- adrenal venography 5
- AIDS 95
- biopsy, fine needle aspiration 6
- cyst puncture 231, 232
- extracorporal lithotripsy 182, 183
- Henoch-Schönlein syndrome 80
- horseshoe kidney 53
- iatrogenic, adrenal venography, necrosis 16
- kidney transplantation 311, 312, 322, 334
- malacoplakia 128
- nephrosclerosis 83
- obstructive uropathy 151

complications
- pulmonary embolism, renal vein thrombosis 80
- radiation nephritis 93, 94
- renal
- - angioplasty 307, 308
- - arteriography 300
- - artery microaneurysms, rupture, hematoma 78
- - carcinoma 278
- schistosomiasis 121
- transurethral ureteroscopy 184
Conn's syndrome
- adenoma 18, 19
- carcinoma 18
- diagnosis 2, 17–19
- hyperplasia 18, 19
contrast
- enhancement
- - adrenal, CT 8, 10
- - renal, CT, injuries 198, 200, 202
- medium
- - excretion, unilateral absence, renal trauma 191
- - extravasation, renal contusion, dynamic CT 191, 194, 196, 197, 202
- - heterotopic liver excretion, ureteral obstruction 155
- - kidney transplantation 324
- - to-and-fro motion, duplex kidneys, ureters 39
cortisol
- aldosterone/cortisol ratio, Conn's syndrome 19
- determination, venous blood sampling 5
crush injuries, acute tubular necrosis 85
cryptococcosis
- adrenal 15
- renal 129, 130
CT
- abscess
- - adrenal 15
- - infrarenal, AIDS 97
- - intra-, pararenal, perinephric 133, 134, 136
- actinomycosis, retroperitoneal 129
- acute glomerulonephritis, complications 76, 77
- adenoma 2, 7, 9, 17–21
- - biopsy 4
- - Conn's syndrome, hyperaldosteronism 18
- - cortical, Cushing's disease 20
- adrenal, normal 1, 2, 6
- adrenalitis, autoimmune, Addison's disease 16
- adrenogenital syndrome 21
- AIDS, retroperitoneal lymphoma 96
- angiography
- - renal 74
- - traumatic renal hematoma, urinoma 198
- angiomyolipoma 218, 220
- autosomal

- - dominant renal polycystic disease 239, 240
- - recessive renal polycystic disease 241
- bilateral acute pyelonephritis, striated nephrogram 107
- bleeding, adrenals 15
- calcifications, renal cysts 236, 237
- calculus disease, renal, ureteral 178
- candidiasis 126, 127
- carcinoma
- - adrenal 11, 21, 22
- - renal 280–285
- - - pelvis 269, 270
- Conn's syndrome 18, 19, 21
- control, abscess drainage 133, 134
- Cushing's syndrome 11, 19–21
- cysts
- - adrenal 2, 8, 9, 11
- - renal 230, 232, 235
- density range, various stone types 179
- differential enhancement pattern, renal cortex, medulla 192, 280
- duodenal rupture, perinephric abscess 135
- duplex kidney 38
- see dynamic CT
- echinococcosis 126, 228
- ectopic fused kidneys 56
- fetal renal lobation, dysmorphisms 58
- follow up, perirenal hematoma, healing 196
- free air, intraperitoneal, trauma 192
- guided
- - biopsy
- - - adrenals 4, 5, 7, 16
- - - inflammatory cystic disease 233
- - - infrarenal abscess 97
- - - renal transplant 327
- - - renal cyst puncture, double contrast 233, 237
- hemangioma 12, 14
- hematoma
- - after lithotripsy 183
- - renal trauma 192, 197, 199
- hemorrhagic renal cyst 234
- horseshoe kidney 55
- hydronephrosis, ureter compression 157, 162
- hyperplasia 20
- inflammatory renal cyst, attenuation coefficients 232
- intracalyceal, intraparenchymal air 111
- kidneys
- - calculus disease 178
- - ectopic fused 56
- - malrotation 63, 64
- - perfusion differences, cortex, medulla 73, 75
- lipoma, adrenal 2
- malacoplakia, renal vein thrombosis 128

- malignant lymphoma 263, 264
- mean attenuation value 2
- medullary sponge kidney 246
- mesoblastic nephroma 223
- metastases, adrenals 2, 9, 11
- multilocular cystic nephroma 222
- myelolipoma 2, 11, 12
- nephrosclerosis, complications 83
- neuroblastoma 10, 11, 26, 27
- nodularity, adrenals 20
- normal
- - kidney graft 327
- - renal parenchyma, density 280
- oncocytoma 216, 217
- parenchymal kidney diseases 71, 74, 75, 76, 79, 80, 81, 82, 83, 87, 90, 96, 97
- pheochromocytoma 2, 10, 11, 22–25
- polycystic
- - dysplastic kidney 243
- - renal disease 45, 234
- - - criteria 235
- post enhancement, renal trauma 193, 199
- pyelonephritis
- - acute 107, 109
- - chronic 114
- - emphysematosis 110, 111
- - xanthomatosis 123, 124, 125
- pyonephrosis 137, 139
- renal
- - agenesis 35
- - cell carcinoma 57, 276, 280–285
- - cyst, criteria 230
- - haemorrhage, polyarthritis nodosa 78
- - insufficiency 77
- - metastases 259, 260
- - necrosis, cortical 83
- - pelvis fracture 194
- - polycystic disease 234
- - sarcoma 254–256
- - stones, radiolucent (cystine) 163
- - transplantion 326, 327
- - trauma
- - - associated injuries 191
- - - categorization 191, 194, 210
- - - contusion 189, 194
- - - thrombosis 200, 201
- - reninoma 218
- - residual stone fragments after lithotripsy 183
- - retroperitoneal hemorrhage, non-Hodgkin's lymphoma 91
- - scleroderma 82
- - technique 2, 191, 280, 326
- - teratoma 13
- - thrombosis, renal vein, traumatic 200
- - traumatic
- - - chyloma, attenuation coefficient 199
- - - renal infarct 200
- - tuberculosis
- - - adrenal 16

- - renal 118, 120
- ureteral
- - compression, renal atrophy 157
- - obstruction, colon carcinoma 162
- - urinoma, perinephric 161
- Wegener's granulomatosis 81
Cushing's adenoma, imaging characteristics 11
Cushing's syndrome
- ACH producing tumor 19
- adrenal carcinoma 21
cyclosporine
- immunosuppressive therapy, kidney transplantation 312
- nephrotoxicity 312, 313, 318
cystic disease
- chronic interstitial nephritis 87
- echinococcosis 125, 126
- infantile, renal 345, 346
- megacystic interstitial nephritis, malacoplakia 127, 128
- multilocular nephroma 46, 47
- renal
- - acquired 241, 242
- - angiography 52
- - autosomal
- - - dominant 238
- - - recessive 241
- - hydronephrosis, differential diagnosis 168
- - medullary 242, 243
- - multicystic dysplasia 43
cystography
- pyelotubular backflow 156
- urinary leakage 326
cystoscopy, brucellosis 127
cysts
- adrenal
- - calcifications 8, 16
- - diagnostic imaging 8, 9, 11, 16
- - lymphangioma, CT 14
- - tumor classification 7
- angiomyolipoma 219
- calcifications, multilocular cystic nephroma 47
- congenital renal solitary cyst 44
- differential diagnosis, solid tumor, CT 280
- double contrast study 231
- glomerulocystic disease 228
- guided puncture, inflammatory disease 233
- hemorrhagic
- - etiology, pathology 234
- - ultrasound criteria 234, 235
- hepatic, pancreatic 48
- infected, abscesses, renal, differential diagnosis 143
- inflammatory
- - guided puncture 233
- - LDH content 233
- lump kidney 54
- medullary cystic kidney disease 50, 51
- multicystic dysplastic kidney 43-45

- multilocular 237
- - cystic nephroma 45, 46, 47
- neoplastic cysts, differential diagnosis 233
- parapelvic
- - aspiration 242, 246
- - interventional radiology management 246
- - puncture, ultrasound guided 341
- pyelitis cystica 138
- renal
- - classification 227
- - CT diagnosis 281
- - cystic disease 227-250
- - puncture, double contrast 230, 231, 237
- - sinus 242, 245
- - - classification 227, 228
- - tuberous sclerosis (Bourneville's disease) 246
cytology, fine needle aspiration, sensitivity 6
cytomegaly virus
- acute interstitial nephritis 85
- adrenal, diagnosis, CT 7

Deceleration trauma, renal injury 204
definition
- corticomedullary junction, MRI 208
- hepatorenal syndrome 94
- hypertension 295
- multiloculated renal cyst 228
- radionuclide renogram 164
developmental anomalies
- adrenal agenesis, hypoplasia, heterotopia 7
- adrenogenital syndrome 21
- congenital mesoblastic nephroma 276
- extrarenal 64-66
- hamartoma 50, 52, 223, 248, 281
- lymphangiatresia, parapelvic 242
- medullary sponge kidney 246
- obstructive uropathy 341-345
- pelvioinfundibular atresia 242
- renal
- - abortive (blind ending) calyx 40
- - adult polycystic disease 48, 49
- - agenesis 34, 35, 40, 340
- - Ash-Upmark kidney 52, 53
- - autosomal recessive polycystic disease 46, 47
- - bifid, trifid pelvis 38
- - calyceal anomalies 40-42
- - classication 34
- - clear cell sarcoma 52
- - column of Bertin 58, 59
- - congenital mesoblastic nephroma 223
- - crossed ectopy 54-58
- - disk kidney 55
- - dromedary hump 58
- - duplex kidney, hydronephrosis 37-39
- - ectopic fused kidneys 56

- - ectopy 54, 55, 56, 60, 64, 340
- - extrarenal pelvis 40
- - fetal lobation, dysmorphism 58, 59
- - hamartoma 50, 52, 223, 248
- - horseshoe kidney 53, 54
- - hydronephrosis 37, 39, 66
- - hydronephrosis, multicystic dysplastic kidney 43
- - hypoplasia 36
- - infantile polycystic disease 46, 47
- - leiomyomatous hamartoma 50, 52
- - lump kidney 54
- - malrotation 37, 53, 54, 60, 62-64
- - medullary
- - - cystic kidney disease 50, 51
- - - sponge kidney 50
- - megacalyces 41, 42
- - mesoplastic nephroma 50, 52
- - multicystic dysplastic kidney 43-- 45
- - neonates 345, 346
- - nephroptosis 60-62
- - pelvic infundibular diverticulum 40, 41
- - polycystic
- - - dysplastic segmental malformations 243
- - - kidney disease 39, 227-250
- - - pseudotumors, classification, differential diagnosis 38, 58
- - - Riley-Newhouse syndrome 48
- - - supernumerary kidneys 37
- - - thoracic kidney 61, 62
- renovascular, embolization 308
- ureteral, obstructed megaureter 153
- ureteropelvic junction obstruction 153, 158
dexamethason suppression test, adrenocortical scintigraphy, specifity 3
diabetes mellitus
- acute bacterial nephritis 108
- emphysematous pyelonephritis 109
- papillary necrosis, renal 141
- pyelitis, interstitial nephritis 86
diagnosis
- adrenal insufficiency 17
- aldosteronoma (Conn's syndrome) 2, 17-19
- Cushing's syndrome 20, 21
- early
- - failing renal graft function 312
- - obstructive uropathy 151, 153
- echinococcosis 125
- false-positive, hydronephrosis 161
- hypertension, renovascular 296
- mistakes, obstructive uropathies 341
- multilocular cysts 237
- neonatal conditions, ultrasound 339-349
- nephrocalcinosis 246
- papillary necrosis 88
- polyarthritis nodosa 77
- poorly functionating renal graft 313-318
- renal trauma 190

diagnosis
- shattered kidney 197, 199
- tuberculosis renal 116
- tubulointerstitial renal diseases 84,
  85
- ureteral obstruction 330
diagnostic imaging
- carcinoma, renal pelvis 266
- malignant lymphoma 263
- renal
- - metastases 258
- - sarcoma 253
differential diagnosis
- acute tubular necrosis 73
- adenoma, malignancy, nephrogram 8
- adrenal
- - hormones, excess secretion 17–27
- - lesions, imaging characteristics 11
- appendicitis, perinephric abscess,
  cholecystitis 134
- bleeding, adrenals 14, 15
- brucellosis 127
- Burkitt's lymphoma 265
- calcifications 8, 9, 11, 16, 17
- - cyst, tumor 235, 236
- carcinoma, renal pelvis 266
- cystic, neoplastic disease 233, 280
- failing renal graft function 312
- fluid collection, perirenal 330
- focal pyelonephritis, traumatic infarct 200
- hematoma, urinoma, ultrasound
  206, 207
- hydronephrosis 160
- - renal cysts 168
- hydroureter 158
- hypertension, renovascular 297
- legionnaires' disease 80
- malacoplakia 128
- neuroblastoma, ultrasound 3
- perinephric abscess, appendicitis,
  cholecystitis 134
- polycystic dysplastic kidney 342
- pyelonephritis, emphysematous,
  CT 111
- renal
- - abscess, cysts 132, 133
- - calyces, anomalies 41
- - cell carcinoma 222
- - cysts, inflammatory, hemorrhagic
  233
- - parenchymal diseases 71, 72
- - pseudotumors, scintigraphy 58, 59
- - transplant rejection 73
- - traumatic infarct 200
- - tumors, benign, malignant 215
- traumatic renal infarct 200
- tuberculosis, renal 120
- tubulointerstitial renal diseases 84
- unilateral large, unilateral small kidneys 72
- ureteral reflux 158
- ureteropelvic junction obstruction
  342
- Wilms' tumor 3, 222, 223

DiGeorge syndrome, renal cystic disease 228
dioctophyma renale, parasitic infection
  131
diuretic renogram
- evaluation 164, 297
- false-positive, hydronephrosis 165
Doppler ultrasonography
- control of angioplasty 305
- renal
- - carcinoma 285
- - cyst 229, 231
- - graft, pulsatility index 323
- - trauma 207
- - renovascular hypertension 297
Down syndrome (trisomy 21), renal cystic disease 228
drug abuse, intravenous, parenchymal
  lesions of kidney 71, 94
drugs
- associated with interstitial nephritis
  85, 88
- cytotoxic, uric acid nephropathy 92
duodenum
- hematoma, renal trauma 191
- injury, renal trauma 202
- rupture, perinephric abscess,
  emphysema 135
dynamic CT
- aldosteronoma 2
- benign renal cyst 231, 232, 237
- bilateral adenomas 4
- lack of enhancement, renal trauma
  201
- pancreas, body fracture 196
- postenhancement-, intrarenal abscess 132
- renal
- - artery
- - - avulsion 202
- - - intimal flaps 201
- - - thrombus 201
- - carcinoma 280, 282
- - -, staging 280, 282
- - contusion 195, 196, 197, 202
- - hematoma, subcapsular 203, 204
- - trauma 192–197
- - - parenchymal tears 202
- - - tissue viability 192
- - tumor thrombus, renal vein, vena
  cava 285
- traumatic renal infarct 200
- stileto renal injury 196

Echinococcus
- pseudocysts 8
- renal 125, 126, 228
Ehlers-Danlos syndrome
- medullary sponge kidney 50, 51
- renal cystic disease 228
embolism
- pulmonary, renal vein thrombosis 80
- septic 141, 142
embolization
- adrenals, malignancies 5

- renal
- - artery 303
- - carcinoma 291
- - trauma 205
- - renovascular malformations 308
embolus, pulmonary, renal carcinoma
  278
embryology
- crossed ectopy, renal 56
- genitourinary tract 339, 340
- kidney 339, 340
- metanephric blastoma, fusion, horseshoe kidney 53
- nephrogenesis 228
- renal
- - carcinoma 276
- - development 33
- ureter 340
epididymis, blastomycosis 130
erythromycin, interstitial nephritis 85
etiology
- adrenal diseases 7
- crossed ectopy, renal 56
- Page kidney 304
- renovascular hypertension 295
- - renal transplantation 304, 305
experimental work, ureteral obstruction 152
extracorporal lithotripsy
- advantages, disadvantages 182
- long term studies 182
- technique, applications 180, 181

Fanconi's syndrome, clinical background, radiology 91, 92
fistulas
- actinomycosis 125
- aortocaval, renal trauma 202
- arteriovenous
- - congenital 65
- - embolization 308
- - kidney graft 326
- - renal
- - - carcinoma 275
- - - injury 202, 205
- - renovascular hypertension 299
- jejunal-calyceal, urogram 209
- renal-duodenal, xanthomatous
  pyelonephritis 124
fluid collections, percutaneous drainage 173
follow up examinations, renal trauma 210
fracture
- renal
- - parenchyma, scintigram 206
- - pelvis, CT 194, 196
fungus infections
- actinomycosis 128
- aspergillosis 130
- brucellosis 127
- candidiasis 126
- coccidioidomycosis 130
- cryptococcosis 129
- mycotic aneurysms, renal 141, 142
- yeast infection, neonates 347

Ganglioneuroma
- adrenal medulla
- - calcifications 16
- - CT 7, 12, 13, 16
genitourinary tract conditions, neonates, ultrasound diagnosis 339-349
Gerota's fascia
- resection, radical nephrectomy 278
- thickening
- - malignant lymphoma 265
- - renal carcinoma, CT 281
Gianturco coil, renal interlobar artery, occlusion 205
glomerular
- filtration
- - decrease, urinary obstruction 151, 154
- - rate, neonates 339
- nephritis, focal atrophic 52
gold, interstitial nephritis 85
Goldenhar's syndrome, renal cystic disease 228
Goodpasture's syndrome, clinical background, pathology, radiology 79, 80
graft, renal
- dysfunction, rejection 311, 312
- implantation, radiology 311-338
- parenchymal disease 328, 329

Hajdu-Cheney syndrome, renal cystic disease 228
hamartoma, renal 50, 52, 223, 248, 281
hematoma
- adrenal
- - calcifications 16
- - CT 2, 7, 12, 14
- dissecting splenorenal ligament, CT 193
- duodenum, liver, spleen, renal trauma 191
- intra-, peri-, pararenal, location, size, CT 199
- kidney transplantation 312, 322
- perirenal, follow up CT 196
- renal
- - Page kidney 304
- - subcapsular, CT 281, 304
- - trauma 192, 197, 199
- - urinoma, coexisting 197
- small, renal trauma, MRI 207
hemochromatosis, adrenal insufficiency 17
hemodialysis, long-term, renal carcinoma 275
hemorrhage
- angiomyolipoma 229, 281
- bladder, scrotum, Henoch-Schönlein purpura 80
- see bleeding
- cystic disease
- - LDH content 235
- - puncture, aspiration 234, 235
- intracerebral, juvenile polycystic kidney disease 49

- perirenal space, CT, lupus erythematosus 79
- pseudocysts 8
- pulmonary, Goodpasture syndrome 79
- renal
- - artery microaneurysms, rupture 78
- - polyarthritis nodosa, CT 78
- retroperitoneal, CT, non-Hodgkin's lymphoma 91
hemosiderosis, Goodpasture's syndrome 79
Henoch-Schönlein syndrome, clinical background, pathology, radiology 80
hepatorenal syndrome, definition, clinical picture, radiography 94
hereditary renal diseases, principal causes 84
heterotopia, adrenal, localizations 7
Hippel-Lindau's disease
- pheochromocytoma 246
- renal
- - adenoma 217
- - carcinoma 275
- - cysts 228
histogram, renal transplant 315
histology
- autosomal recessive renal polycystic disease 241
- hemangiopericytoma 252
- liposarcoma 252
- oncocytoma 216
- pelvioinfundibular atresia 242
- renal
- - carcinoma 266
- - cyst 229
- - parenchyma 73
histoplasmosis
- adrenal
- - calcifications 16
- - insufficiency 15-17
- renal 130, 131
history
- adrenals, function 1
- surgical calculus therapy 179, 180
- tuberculosis 116
Hodgkin's disease
- adrenal lymphoma, CT 9
- pathology 261
horseshoe kidneys
- renal carcinoma 275
- Turner's syndrome 53
- ultrasound 54
hydatide disease, renal 125, 126
hydronephrosis
- chronic, pathophysiology 151
- crossed ectopic kidney 57
- differential diagnosis, renal cystic disease 168
- diuretic renogram 164
- - false-positive 165
- false-positive diagnosis 161
- giant, congenital ureteropelvic junction obstruction 158, 159

- horseshoe kidney 53, 54
- lump kidney 54
- multicystic dysplastic kidney 43, 228
- neonates 340, 341
- obstructing megaureter, reimplantation 169
- polycystic dysplastic kidney 242
- pyonephrosis 137
- tuberculosis 118, 119
- ultrasound 74, 178, 179, 340
- upper hole, duplex kidneys 37, 39
- ureteral
- - stone, ultrasound 178, 179
- - structure 322, 323
- urinary obstruction, CT 157
hydroureter, lower ureteral obstruction 158
hygroma, renal trauma 199
hyperaldosteronism
- adrenal carcinoma 21
- Conn's syndrome 2, 17-19
- reninoma 218
hyperfunction
- adrenal 17-21
- - medullary 22
hyperplasia
- adrenal 7, 18-22
- adrenocortical 19, 21
hypertension
- aortic coarctation 303, 304
- chronic glomerulonephritis 77
- congenital mesoblastic nephroma 223
- definition 295
- juxtaglomerular cell tumor (reninoma) 218
- malignant, transcatheter embolization 308
- pheochromocytoma 5
- renal
- - artery stenosis, arteriography 83
- - carcinoma 276
- - cyst 229
- - graft, arteriovenous fistula 326
- renin-, angiotensin production renal trauma 200
- renovascular
- - angiography, findings 298, 299, 300, 304
- - angioplasty 306
- - angiotensin-renin mechanism 295
- - diagnosis 296
- - digital subtraction angiography 298
- - Doppler ultrasonography 297, 298, 305
- - etiology, pathophysiology 295, 296, 304
- - nuclear medicine 297, 305
- - pheochromocytoma 296, 303
- - radiologic
- - - intervention 306-308
- - - screening methods 296-300
- - renal transplantation 304, 305
- - urography 296, 297

hypertension
- scleroderma 81
- stenosis, renal graft artery 304, 305, 313
- Takayasu's arteritis 303
- Wegener's granulomatosis 81
hypofunction, adrenal, see Addison's syndrome

[131]I-hippuran scan, renal, obstructive uropathy 76
^{131}I-MIBG, adrenergic tissue localizing agent 4
ileal loopogram, bladder carcinoma 167
imaging modalities
- adrenal 2-6
- carcinoma, renal pelvis 266
- kidney transplantation 313-320
- malignant lymphoma 263
- renal
- - AIDS patients 95
- - calculus disease 177, 178
- - carcinoma 279-292
- - medullary cystic disease 242
- - metastases 258
- - sarcoma 253
- - transplant 326
- - trauma 189
- - tumors
- - - benign, malignant 215
- - - small 218
- - value, limitations 74
- revascularization procedures 305, 306
immunautoradiography, Tamm-Horsfall protein, chronic bacterial pyelonephritis 111, 112
immune
- disorders
- - acute chronic interstitial nephritis 85, 87
- - tubulointerstitial nephropathy, causes 84
- - xanthomatous pyelonephritis 122
- suppression
- - aspergillosis-, coccidioidomycosis infection 130
- - - kidney transplantation 312
incidence
- Addison's disease 17
- adult polycystic kidney disease 48
- aldosteronoma 18
- autosomal recessive polycystic kidney disease 46
- bifid renal pelvis 39
- crossed renal ectopy 54
- duplex kidneys 37
- horseshoe kidney 53
- renal
- - agenesis 36, 340
- - cortical tumors 217
- - graft survival 312
- - sarcoma 251

- - transplantation, complications 312
- renovascular hypertension 295
- systemic lupus erythematosus 78
- tuberculosis, renal 116
incidentaloma, adrenal 7, 8
indications
- arteriography
- - adrenals 5
- - kidney transplantation 326
- CT, kidneys 74
- extracorporal lithotripsy 181
- radioisotope scanning 3, 4
- radionuclide
- - imaging, renal trauma 205
- - renography 163
- renal angiography 298, 299
- retrograde pyelography 74
- surgery
- - calculus disease 179
- - congenital hydronephrosis 66
- - renal trauma 189, 190, 210
- ultrasound, renal parenchyma, evaluation 178
- urography 178
infantile polycystic kidney disease, ultrasound diagnosis 345, 346
infarct
- adrenal 16
- renal
- - renin-angiotensin hypertension, embolization 308
- - traumatic 200
infectious disease
- tuberculosis, renal 85, 116-120
- urinary tract
- - neonates 339, 346
- - pregnancy 142
inflammation
- acute interstitial nephritis 85
- adrenal 15
- - calcification 15, 16
- necrotizing vasculitis 85
inflammatory diseases, renal
- clinical background, diagnosis, therapy 103-149
- cysts 232
injury, renal, see renal trauma
insufficiency, adrenal 16, 17
interferon, therapy, renal carcinoma 291

juvenile polycystic disease, renal 228

Kaposi sarcoma, adrenal involvement 9
Kaufman McKusick syndrome, renal cystic disease 228
kidneys
- abscess
- - clinical background, diagnosis, therapy 131-133
- - gas bubbles, subcapsular fluid collection 200
- actinomycosis 128, 129
- adult polycystic disease 48, 49

- agenesis 33, 34, 35, 340
- AIDS nephropathy 94-97
- amebiasis 129
- anatomy, histology 72, 73
- aneurysm, mycotic 141, 142
- Ask-Upmark 52, 53
- aspergillosis 130
- autonephrectomized, tuberculosis 117
- autosomal
- - dominant polycystic disease 238
- - recessive polycystic disease 46, 47, 241
- blastomycosis 130
- brucellosis 127
- calcified, nonfunctionating, tuberculosis 118, 119
- calculus disease, therapy 177-188
- calyx en face 41
- carcinoma
- - see renal carcinoma, tumors
- - schistostomiasis 121
- Caroli's disease 228, 241
- cerebrohepatorenal syndrome of Zellweger 228
- cholesteatoma 142
- coccidioidomycosis 130
- collagenous disease 302
- compensatory hypertrophy, renal agenesis 36
- contusion 194-197
- cortical
- - epithelial tumors 217
- - vascular anatomy 73
- cryptococcosis 129, 130
- cystic disease 227-250
- destruction, dioctophyma renale 131
- developmental anomalies 33-69, 339-349
- see developmental anomalies, nephritis, nephrotic syndrome, pyelonephritis, nephrolithiasis
- disk kidney, pyelogram 55
- displacement
- - abscess 134
- - fluid collections 190
- donor supply, transplantation 311
- drug abuse nephropathy 71, 94-97
- duplex 37-39
- dysplasia, hypoplasia 33, 34, 36, 228
- echinococcosis 125, 126, 228
- ectopy 54, 55, 56, 60
- embryology 339, 340
- fetal lobation 58
- fracture, scintigram 206
- fungal infections 95, 116, 130, 141, 142
- glomerular
- - diseases
- - - acute, chronic glomerulonephritis 72, 76, 77
- - - clinical picture 72, 76, 79, 81, 82
- - - Goodpasture's syndrome 72, 79
- - - Henoch-Schönlein syndrome 72, 80

- - - nephrosclerosis 82
- - - pathology 72, 76, 77, 78, 80, 81, 82
- - - polyarthritis nodosa 72, 76
- - - radiology 72, 76, 77, 79, 80, 82
- - - scleroderma 81, 82
- - - systemic lupus erythematosus 72, 78
- - - Wegener's granulomatosis 80, 81
- - filtration rate, neonates 339
- glomerulocystic disease 228
- graft, radiology 324-335
- granulomatosis disease 131
- hamartoma 50, 52, 223, 248
- Hippel-Lindau disease 217, 228
- histoplasmosis 130, 131
- horseshoe- 53, 54
- infantile polycystic disease 345, 346
- inflammatory
- - cystic disease 232
- - diseases 103-149
- - neovascularity CT 199
- lump kidney 54
- lymphatic drainage 277
- malrotation 37, 53, 54, 60, 62-64
- medullary
- - cystic disease 242, 243
- - necrosis 41
- - sponge, cystic kidney diseases 50, 51, 228, 246
- multicystic, dysplastic 43-45, 341
- multilocular cystic nephroma 45
- necrosis, acute tubular 85-87
- nephrectomy, congenital mesoplastic nephroma 52
- nephritis, acute, chronic interstitial, causes, drug induced 85, 87
- nephron, basic functional unit 72
- nephroptosis 60-62
- nephrosclerosis 82, 83
- non-Hodgkin's lymphoma, CT 10
- normal, neonates 339
- obstructive uropathy 151-175
- Page- 304
- pancreatitic involvement 136
- papillary necrosis
- - etiology, pathology, radiology 88, 138-141
- - tuberculosis 118
- parenchyma, traumatic tears, categorization 194, 195
- parenchymal diseases
- - AIDS, drug abuse nephropathy 94-97
- - bilateral cortical necrosis 83, 84
- - tubulo-interstitial diseases 84-94
- polycystic
- - disease 39, 227-250
- - - acquired 241
- - displastic 242
- pseudotumors, classification, differential diagnosis 58
- pyelonephritis, interstitial nephritis 85

- renal cortex, blood supply 73
- renin hypersecreting segment, embolization 308
- rupture, graft rejection 312
- scans
- - reflux nephropathy 52
- - tuberculosis 116
- schistosomiasis 120, 121
- shattered, trauma 199
- stab wound, angiography, pseudoaneurysm 204
- stileto injury, dynamic CT 196
- supernumerary
- - ectopic ureteroceles 37
- - fused 56
- thoracic 61, 62
- tomography, polycystic renal disease 45
- transplant
- - candida abscess 127
- - coccidioidomycosis 130
- - function, renogram 318
- - malacoplakia 128
- - rejection 85, 311, 312, 318, 319, 328
- transplantation
- - angiography 313, 314, 318
- - complications 311, 312, 317, 322
- - fluid collection, ultrasound 322
- - graft rejection 311, 312, 318, 319
- - hypertension, imaging 304, 305
- - immunosuppressive therapy 312
- - radiology 311-338
- - radionuclide imaging 313, 314
- - rejection, pathogenesis 312
- - renographic control 315, 316
- - trauma, see renal trauma
- - tuberculosis 85, 116-120
- - tubular necrosis, graft rejection 312, 318
- - tubulointerstitial diseases
- - acute
- - - chronic interstitial nephritis 85, 87
- - - tubular necrosis
- - AIDS nephropathy 94
- - drug abuse nephropathy 94
- - Fanconi's syndrome 91
- - hepatorenal syndrome 94
- - leukemia, lymphoma 90
- - multiple myeloma 90
- - papillary necrosis 88
- - radiation nephritis 93
- - sickle cell hemoglobinopathies 89
- - uric acid nephropathy 92
- - tumors, see tumors
- - Wegener's granulomatosis 80, 81
- - xanthomatous pyelonephritis 121-125

Lead poisoning, chronic, tubulointerstitial nephritis 93
legionnaires' disease
- acute interstitial nephritis 85
- differential diagnosis 80

lesions
- adrenal 27
- - with hyperfunction 17-21
- - with hypofunction 17
- causing renovascular hypertension 299
- renal
- - drug abuse 71
- - parenchymal, lupus erythematodes 71, 78
leukoplakia, renal 142
lipoma, adrenal, CT 2, 11
liposarcoma
- adrenal, retroperitoneal 11
- tumor classification 7
lithotripsy
- extracorporal
- - advantages, disadvantages 182
- - long term results 182
- - techniques, applications 180, 181
- - ureteroscopy, transurethral 180, 182, 183
lithotriptor, shock wave devices 181
liver
- cerebrohepatorenal syndrome of Zellweger 228
- cysts 48
- hematoma, renal trauma 191
- hepatic fibrosis, portal hypertension, Riley-Newhouse syndrome 48
- hepatopathy, Stauffer's syndrome, renal carcinoma 276, 278
- hepatorenal syndrome 94
- heterotopic excretion, contrast material 155
- increased sonographic echogenicity, renal polycystic disease 241
- injury, renal trauma 202, 209
- metastases, MRI 3, 285, 289
- periportal fibrosis, juvenil polycystic disease 228
lupus erythematosus
- interstitial nephritis 85
- parenchymal lesions of kidneys 71, 78
lymphangiatresia, parapelvic 242
lymphangioma, adrenal 11, 12
lymphangiomatosis, angiomyolipoma 219
lymphocele, kidney transplantation 312, 322, 332
lymphoma
- adrenal, dynamic CT 7, 9, 10, 12
- AIDS, CT 96
- perirenal, CT 264
- renal, malignant 261-265
- ureteral compression
- - nephrostomy tube placement 170
- - renal atrophy 157

Magnetic resonance imaging
- abscess, renal, peri-, pararenal 133, 134
- acute pyelonephritis 107

magnetic resonance imaging
- adrenals 1-3, 5-7, 9-12, 14, 17, 18, 20-22, 24-27
- - adenoma 3, 5, 7, 10, 18, 20, 21, 27
- - carcinoma 3, 10, 22
- - Conn's syndrome 18
- - ganglioneuroma 13
- - metastases 3, 10
- - myelolipoma 10, 11, 12
- - neuroblastoma 10, 11, 26
- - normal 1, 3
- - pheochromocytoma 3, 10, 24
- - tuberculosis 15, 16
- autosomal dominant polycystic kidney disease 49, 50, 240
- calculus disease, renal, ureteral 179
- corticomedullary junction, definition 208
- Cushing's syndrome 20
- giant hydronephrosis 166
- kidneys
- - corticomedullary definition 73
- - hemorrhagic cyst 235
- - hyperplasia 20
- - parenchymal diseases 71, 75, 77, 78, 79, 80, 87, 89, 91, 96, 97
- liver metastases 3
- malacoplakia, renal vein thrombosis 128
- medullary fibroma 224
- nephrosclerosis, complications 83
- oncocytoma 216
- pheochromocytoma 3, 10, 24
- polycystic disease, renal 208
- pyelonephritis, xanthomatous 125
- pyonephrosis 137, 139
- renal
- - artery microaneurysms, rupture, hematoma 78
- - carcinoma 288-291
- - cysts 233, 235, 238
- - graft function 321
- - sarcoma 256, 257
- - transplant
- - - acute rejection 328
- - - normal 328
- - trauma 207
- - vein thrombosis 284
- - urinary obstruction 166
- venous anatomy 289
- Wegener's granulomatosis 81
malakoplakia, renal 127, 128
malformations
- adrenal agenesis, hypoplasia, ectopia 7
- adrenogenital syndrome 21
- see developmental anomalies
- medullary sponge kidney 246
- renal hamartoma 50, 52, 223, 248
- renovascular, embolization 308
Malta fever, brucellosis 127
medullary
- fibroma, diagnosis therapy 223, 224
- sponge kidney, associated malformations 246

megaureter
- lower ureteral obstruction 158
- obstructing, reimplantation, Whitaker test 169
mesonephric (Wolffian) duct, renal development 33
metabolic toxins, tubulointerstitial renal diseases 84
metanephric blastoma
- fusion: horseshoe kidney 53
- lump kidney 54
metaplasia, renal 142
metastases
- adrenals 2, 3, 7, 9, 10, 17, 27, 285
- biopsy, CT-guided 5, 6
- calcifications 9
- dynamic CT, non-contrast enhanced scans 2, 8, 9, 10
- ^{131}I-MIBG imaging 4
- liver, MRI 3
- lymph notes, renal hilus, CT 281, 283
- renal 251, 252, 256-261
- - adenoma, cut-off point 218
- - carcinoma, diagnosis, therapy 291
- - cortical, diameter 275, 277, 278, 285
- teratoma, testicular 11
methyldopa, interstitial nephritis 85
Michaelis-Gutmann body, malacoplakia 127
microaneurysms, renal artery, polyarthritis nodosa 71
microcystic disease, renal, classification 227
Miranda syndrome, renal cystic disease 228
mortality
- abscess, perirenal 134
- kidney transplantation 312
MR spectroscopy
- adrenal adenomas 3
- renal parenchymal diseases 76
multilocular
- cystic nephroma, diagnosis, therapy 222, 223
- renal cysts
- - classification 227
- - etiology, diagnosis 237
multiple endocrine neoplasia syndrome (MEN), adrenal 22
mycobacteriosis, adrenal 15
myelolipoma
- adrenal 2, 10, 11, 16
- - calcifications 11, 16
- classification, diagnostic imaging 2, 7, 10, 11, 12
myeloma, multiple, tubulointerstitial nephritis 90

Necrosis
- acute tubular, clinical background, pathology, radiology 85-87
- adrenal 16
- renal papillary 138-141

neonates
- adrenal bleedings, CT 14
- autosomal recessive polycystic kidney disease 46, 47, 241
- candidiasis 126, 127
- fetal renal hamartoma 223
- genitourinary tract diseases, ultrasound 339-349
- kidney, normal 339, 340
- mesoplastic nephroma 50, 52, 223
- obstructive uropathy 340-345
- posterior urethral valves 344
- pyelonephritis 346
- renal blood flow 339
- ultrasound
- - abdominal pathology 2, 3
- - adrenals 6, 15
- Wolman disease (familial xanthomatosis) 17
- yeast infection 347
nephrectomy
- Ash-Upmark kidney 53
- congenital mesoplastic nephroma 52
- radical, renal carcinoma 278
nephritis
- abacterial 111
- acute, chronic
- - glomerulonephritis 76, 77
- - interstitial 85, 87
- bacterial 103, 107, 108
- hereditary 84
- interstitial, malacoplakia 127, 128
- lupus erythematosus 78
- papillary necrosis 88, 138-141
- polyarthritis nodosa 76
- radiation induced 93, 94
nephrocalcinosis, diagnosis 246
nephrogenic cord, renal development 33
nephrogram
- absent, renal trauma 194
- acute
- - pyelonephritis 106, 107
- - ureteral obstruction 153
- adenoma, malignancy, differential diagnosis 8
- angiomyolipoma 221
- disruption, renal laceration 190, 191
- horseshoe kidney 53
- nephrosclerosis 82
- normal, corticomedullary differentiation 154
- patchy, spotty, renal trauma 290, 294
- renal
- - graft 325
- - necrosis, bilateral, cortical 83
- urinary obstruction 154
nephrolithiasis
- see calculus disease
- Franconi's syndrome 92
- pregnancy, nephrostomy 143
- radiolucent (cystine) stones, plain film, CT 163
- Tamm-Horsfall protein 111
- therapy 177-188

- xanthomatous pyelonephritis 122, 124
nephroma
- congenital mesoblastic (fetal renal hamartoma) 50, 52, 223, 276
- mulilocular cystic, CT 45, 46, 222
nephron
- damage, acute ureteral obstruction 151, 152
- destruction, tubuculosis 116
nephronia, focal, lobar 103, 108
nephrosclerosis, clinical background, pathology, radiology 82
nephrostomy
- catheter placement, technique 170, 171
- nephrolithiasis, pregnancy 142, 143
- ureteral urine leak 331
nephrotic syndrome
- drug abuse 95
- lupus erythematosus 78
- vena cava infiltration, renal carcinoma 278
nephrotomography
- abscess, intrarenal 131, 132
- acute ureteral obstruction 154
- angiomyolipoma 220
- chronic urinary tract obstruction 157
- echinococcosis 125
- malacoplakia 128
- polycystic renal disease 45, 229
- renal
- - necrosis, cortical 83
- - trauma 191
nephrotomy, candidiasis 127
nephrotoxicity, cyclosporine 312, 313, 318
nephrotoxins
- chronic interstitial nephritis 87
- heavy metal, Fanconi's syndrome 91
neuroblastoma
- adrenals
- - calcifications 16, 26, 28
- - diagnostic imaging 10, 11, 16, 25–27
- differential diagnosis, ultrasound 3
- imaging characteristics 11
- ^{131}I-MIBG imaging 4
neurocutaneous syndrome, adrenal medullary hyperfunction 22
neurofibromatosis, renal artery stenosis, hypertension 303, 304
newborn, renal sinus, lack of fat 339
nodularity
- adrenal 20, 54
- renal, malignant lymphoma 262
- Wegener's granulomatosis 81
non-Hodgkin lymphoma
- adrenals, CT 9, 10
- renal
- - infiltration 90
- - CT 263, 264
Noonan's syndrome, renal cystic disease 228
nuclear medical examinations

- abscess, renal 132
- autosomal
- - dominant renal polycystic disease 240
- - recessive renal polycystic disease 241
- gadolinium - DTPA, tumor thrombus 289
- kidney
- - multicystic dysplastic 342
- - transplantation 313, 314
- nephrosclerosis 82
- parenchymal kidney diseases 71, 75
- see radioisotope scanning, scintigraphy
- renal trauma 205
- renovascular hypertension 297, 304, 305
- septic emboli 141, 142
- urinary obstruction 163-166, 342

Obstructive uropathy
- AIDS 95
- antegrade pyelography, pressure-flow study (Whiteaker test) 167-169
- computed tomography 161, 162
- fluid collections, percutaneous drainage 173
- hereditary 84
- ^{131}I-hippuran scan, renogram 76
- magnetic resonance imaging 166
- neonates 340-345
- nephrostomy placement, percutaneous 171
- pathophysiology 151-153
- percutaneous nephrostomy tube placement 170, 171
- pressure flow studies (Whiteaker test) 168, 169
- pyelogram antegrade, retrograde 159, 167
- radionuclide renography 163-166
- retrograde ureter stenting 169, 172, 173
- sonography 159-161, 340, 345
- step-off pressure, mild, severe obstruction 169
- ureteral stenting, percutaneous 172, 173
- urography 153-159
osteomalacia, Franconi's syndrome 91

Page kidney, etiology 304
Palmaz stent, renal artery, angioplasty 307
pancreas
- body fracture, dynamic CT 196
- injury, renal trauma 202, 209
- pancreatitis
- - pararenal abscess, CT 135, 136
- - renal involvement 136
- polycystic disease 48, 228
papillary necrosis
- etiology, pathology, radiology 88, 138-141

- tuberculosis 118
paraganglioma, ^{131}I-MIBG imaging 4
pararenal space, abscess drainage, daughter abscess 135, 137
parasites
- amebiasis 129
- dioctophyma renale 131
- echinococcosis 125, 126, 228
- histoplasmosis 130, 131
- schistosomiasis 120, 121
Patau's syndrome (trisomy 13-15), renal cystic disease 228
pathogenesis, renal transplant rejection 312
pathology
- acute, chronic glomerulonephritis 72, 76, 77
- adrenals, classification of diseases 7
- analgetic abuse 89
- cholesteatoma 142
- Goodpasture's syndrome 80
- hemorrhagic cysts 234
- Henoch-Schönlein syndrome 80
- interstitial nephritis 86
- malignant lymphoma 261
- multicystic dysplastic kidney 340
- nephrosclerosis 82
- oncocytoma 216
- papillary necrosis 139
- polyarteritis nodosa 72, 77
- pyelonephritis, necrotizing 109
- renal
- - adenoma 218
- - carcinoma 276, 277
- - metastases 256, 257
- - necrosis, bilateral, cortical 83
- - parenchymal diseases, categories 72
- - pelvis carcinoma 265, 266
- - sarcoma 251, 252
- - schistosomiasis 121
- - scleroderma 81, 82
- - xanthomatous pyelonephritis 121
pathophysiology
- obstructive uropathy 151-153
- renovascular hypertension 295
pelviolithotomy, calculus disease 180
penicillins, interstitial nephritis 85
percutaneous
- nephrostomy tube placement, indications, technique 170, 171
- stone removal, indications, technique 184, 185
- ureteral stenting, indications, technique 169, 172, 173
pheochromocytoma
- abdominal plain film 1, 2, 22-25
- adrenal/extraadrenal 2, 5, 10, 16, 22-25
- arteriography 5
- CT 10, 11, 22-25
- von Hippel-Lindau disease 246
- hypertension, renovascular 296, 303
- hypertensive crises, induction by forceful injection 5

pheochromocytoma
- ^{131}I-MIBG imaging 4
- magnetic resonance imaging 3
- nephrogram 8
- percutaneous biopsy, fatal hypertensive crisis 6
- renovascular hypertension 296, 303
- selective venous blood sampling 5
phlebography, see venography
physiology, ureteral peristalsis 152
pituitary
- adenoma 19
- - venous sampling 20
plain film
- abdominal
- - arterial hypertension 2
- - brucellosis 127
- - calcifications, renal cyst 233, 235
- - calculus disease 177, 179
- - Conn's syndrome 2
- - cystic nephroma 222
- - echinococcosis 125
- - horseshoe kidney 53
- - indications 1
- - medullary sponge kidney 51
- - papillary necrosis, calcifications 140
- - pheochromocytoma 2
- - radiolucent (cystine) renal stones 163
- - - pelvis carcinoma 266
- - - sarcoma 253
- - - solitary cyst, congenital 44
- - - tuberculosis 117
pneumography, retroperitoneal 1
polyarteritis nodosa
- microaneurysms, renal artery 71
- Page kidney 304
- pathology 72, 77
- radiology 72, 77, 78
polycystic disease
- angiomyolipoma 219
- see cystic disease
- multilocular cystic nephroma 222, 223
- pancreas 48, 228
- renal
- - cell carcinoma 219
- - classification 227
- - diagnosis, treatment 227-258
- - dialysis, carcinoma 275
- - dysplasia 228
- - pelvioinfundibular atresia 242
- - trauma 202
Potter syndrome, ultrasound diagnosis 340
pregnancy
- nephrolithiasis, nephrostomy 143
- urinary tract infection 105, 142
pressure flow studies
- step-off pressure, mild, severe obstruction 169
- Whiteaker test, urinary obstruction 167-169
prognosis

- lupus erythematosus 78, 79
- renal
- - carcinoma 277
- - pelvis carcinoma 266
- - traumatic renal hematoma, urinoma, CT 198
pronephros, renal development 33
prostate, blastomycosis 130
prune belly syndrome, ureteral obstruction 66, 168, 345
pseudocysts
- hemorrhagic, parasitic 8
- malignant lymphoma 264, 265
- perinephric 229
pseudohepatorenal syndrome, definition, causes 94
pseudotumors
- chronic pyelonephritis, pyelogram 112
- definition, dynamic CT 13
- duplex kidney, duplex ureters 38
- renal, classification 58
pulmonary embolus, renal carcinoma 278
pyelitis cystica, radiography 138
pyelogram
- antegrade
- - bladder carcinoma, ileal loop urinary diversion 167
- - giant hydronephrosis 159
- - neoimplantation of ureter 325
- - pressure flow study (Whitaker test), urinary obstruction 167-169
- - pyonephrosis 137, 138
- - ureteral stricture 332, 333
- - urinary leakage 330
- neonates 339
- retrograde
- - atretic ureter 45
- - candidiasis 126, 127
- - crossed fused ectopia 55
- - disk kidney 55
- - ectopic kidney 61
- - polycystic disease 48
- - pyelonephritis
- - - acuta 105, 106
- - - chronica, follow up 115
- - - xanthomatous 122, 123
- - renal
- - - parenchymal diseases 71, 74
- - - pelvis carcinoma 266, 267
- - - trauma 206
- - tuberculosis 119
- - ureteric obstruction, pyonephrosis 139
- - urinary tract obstruction 159
pyelonephritis
- actinomycosis 128
- acute
- - bacterial, focal, interstitial 104-108
- - chronic 136-138
- - interstitial nephritis 85
- - severe 107-109
- atrophic 104, 107, 109, 111, 116
- chronic 111-115

- - Tamm-Horsfall protein 111, 112
- cryptococcosis 129
- emphysematous 109-111
- neonates, ultrasound diagnosis 346
- xantogranulomatous 121-125
pyonephrosis
- acute, chronic 136, 137
- obstructive uropathy 151

radiation
- exposure, adrenal scintigraphy 4
- nephritis, clinical background, radiology 93, 94
radioisotope scanning
- adrenal 1, 3-5, 17-21, 24-26
- - adenoma 3, 4, 17-21
- - aldosteronoma (Conn's syndrome) 3, 18, 19
- - Cushing's syndrome 4
- - indications 3, 4
- - metastases, pheochromocytoma 4, 24, 25
- - neuroblastoma 4, 26
- - paraganglioma 4
- - pheochromocytoma 4, 24
- renal
- - autosomal
- - - dominant polycystic disease 240
- - - recessive polycystic disease 241
- - gallium, indium, abscess 132
- - hippuran renogram, nephrosclerosis 82
- - transplantation 305
- see scintigraphy
radiology
- abscess, intrarenal, perinephritic, pararenal 131-133, 134, 135
- actinomycosis 128, 129
- acute, chronic
- - glomerulonephritis 72, 76, 77
- - interstitial nephritis 86, 87
- algorism, renal trauma assessment 209, 210
- analgetic abuse 89
- aspergillosis 130
- brucellosis 127
- calculus
- - disease 177, 178
- - localization, lithotripsy 181
- candidiasis 126, 127
- cholesteatoma 142
- echinococcosis 125, 126
- Goodpasture's syndrome 80
- Henoch-Schönlein syndrome 80
- hypertension, renovascular 296
- - interventions 306-308
- nephrosclerosis 82
- malacoplakia 128
- parapelvic cysts 246
- polyarthritis nodosa 72, 77, 78
- pyelitis cystica 138
- pyelonephritis
- - chronic 112
- - emphysematous 110
- renal

- - carcinoma 279-292
- - cystic disease, categorization 227, 229
- - necrosis, bilateral, cortical 83, 84
- - transplantation 311-338
- - trauma 203, 205, 206
- schistosomiasis 121
- scleroderma 82
- tuberculosis, renal 117-120
- Wegener's granulomatosis 81
- xanthomatous pyelonephritis 122-125
radionuclide
- imaging
- - kidney transplantation 313, 314
- - see nuclear medical examinations, radioisotope scanning, scintigraphy
- - renal trauma 205
- renography
- - curves, obstructed, nonobstructed 164, 165
- - false-positive, hydronephrosis 165
- - renovascular hypertension 297
- - urinary
- - - leakage 320
- - - obstruction 163-166
radiopharmaceuticals, renography 315
Raynaud's phenomenon, scleroderma 81, 82
v. Recklinghausen's disease, renal artery stenosis, hypertension 303, 304
reflux nephropathy, clinical background, pathology, radiology 104, 111-115
rejection, renal graft 311, 312, 318, 319, 321, 328
renal
- abscess, gas bubbles, subcapsular fluid collection, CT 200
- agenesis
- - ultrasound 340
- - urogram, CT 33, 34
- angioplasty, renovascular hypertension 306, 307, 308
- artery
- - aneurysms 64, 65, 299, 300, 301
- - atherosclerosis 299, 300
- - avulsion, CT 202
- - collateral circulation 299
- - Doppler sonography, graft, pulsatility index 323
- - DSA before and after angioplasty 325
- - embolization 303
- - fibromuscular hyperplasia, "string of beads" 300, 301
- - microaneurysms, polyarteritis nodosa 71
- - perforation, angioplasty 308
- - stenosis
- - - angioplasty 306
- - - - stent in place 307
- - - hemodynamic aspects 299
- - - hypertension, angiography 83

- - - iliac artery anastomosis 325
- - - renal transplantation 304, 305, 313
- - - renogram 318
- - - renovascular hypertension 296, 297, 298, 304, 305
- - - thrombosis, traumatic, CT 201, 305
- - - traumatic severance 201
- atrophy, obstructive, ureter compression, CT 157
- blood flow
- - neonates 339
- - transplant, evaluation 314
- calculi
- - extracorporal lithotripsy 180
- - neonates, forosimide therapy 347
- carcinoma
- - angiography 276, 277, 286-288
- - arteriovenous fistulae 275
- - CT 57, 276, 280-285
- - cystic, CT 281
- - etiology 275
- - excessive gonadotropin production 276
- - magnetic resonance imaging 284, 288-291
- - metastases 275, 277, 278, 281, 283, 285
- - pathology 276, 277
- - prognosis 277
- - radical nephrectomy 278
- - radiologic imaging 279
- - Stauffer's syndrome 276
- - symptoms 275, 276
- - therapy 291
- - ultrasound 285, 286
- - urography 279, 280
- - venacavography 288, 289
- - vena cava infiltration 278
- - venography, vein thrombosis 284, 288
- cyst
- - associated with other diseases 228
- - classification 227
- - glomerulocystic disease 228
- - von Hippel-Lindau disease 228, 246
- - inflammatory, infected 232
- - microcystic disease 228
- - microdissection studies 227
- - perinephric pseudocyst 229
- - pyelogenic cyst 228
- - syndromes 228
- developmental anomalies
- - diagnosis, clinical features 33-69
- - hereditary diseases 84
- dysplasia, multicystic disease 228
- edema
- - acute ureteral obstruction 151
- - chronic pyelonephritis 111
- endocrine deficiencies, manifestations 84
- failure
- - acute tubular necrosis 85, 318

- - medullary cystic disease 50
- - obstructive uropathy 151
- - peritoneal dialysis, cystic mass 231
- - radiation nephritis 93
- - renal
- - - allograft transplantation 311
- - - cystic disease, carcinoma 275
- - scleroderma 81
- function
- - divided, determination, formula 329
- - irreversible loss, chronic urinary tract obstruction 157
- - neonates, ^{99m}Te-DTPA-scintigraphy 339
- - radionuclide renography, evaluation 163
- - recovery, after urinal obstruction 151
- graft, rejection 311, 312, 318, 319
- infarction, renin-angiotensin hypertonus, embolization 308, 319
- insufficiency
- - chronic glomerulonephritis 77
- - tuberculosis 117
- - uric acid nephropathy 92
- metastases, pathology, clinical findings, diagnosis 256-261
- necrosis, bilateral, cortical 83, 85
- osteodystrophy, tubulointerstitial disorder 84
- parenchyma, sonographic evaluation 178
- parenchymal
- - damage, ureteral obstruction, major factors 152
- - diseases
- - - differential diagnosis 71, 72
- - - see kidneys, glomerular, parenchymal diseases
- pelvis
- - carcinoma 265-270, 276
- - fracture, CT 194
- - needle puncture 326
- - pressure, elevated, extravasation of opacified urine 155, 156
- - uroepital striations 155
- - vascular impressions 65
- plasma flow rate, renal injury 205
- sarcoma, pathology, clinical findings, diagnosis 251-256
- segment, renin hypersecreting, embolization 308
- sinuses
- - newborn 339
- - peripheral fat sign 245
- transit time, urinary obstruction 164
- transplant, rejection 85, 311, 312, 318, 319, 328
- trauma
- - angiography 203
- - associated intraabdominal injury 190, 202, 209
- - autotransplantation of fragments into the pelvis 199

renal
- trauma
- - blood clot, temporary seal of tear, CT 196, 197
- - blunt, excretory urography 190
- - chyloma 199
- - collecting system violation 195
- - contrast medium
- - - excretion
- - - - diminished 190
- - - - unilateral absent 191
- - - extravasation 191, 196
- - contusion 189, 194
- - CT
- - - accuracy of diagnosis 209
- - - categorization of injury 191, 194
- - - dynamic, tissue viability 192
- - - patchy, spotty nephrogram 190, 194
- - - pelvis fracture 194
- - - post enhancement 193-200
- - deceleration injury 204
- - diagnosis, urography, accuracy 190
- - Doppler sonography 207
- - embolization 205
- - fistulae, arteriovenous, aortocaval 202, 205
- - free air, intraperitoneal, CT 192
- - gunshot wounds 190
- - hematoma 191, 197, 199
- - hygroma 199
- - infarct 200
- - laceration, corticomedullary 189, 192
- - liver, pancreas, spleen, associated injuries 202, 209
- - magnetic resonance imaging 207
- - management concepts 189
- - myoglobinuria 202
- - nephrogram
- - - absent 194
- - - patchy, spotty 190, 194
- - opacified urine extravasation 191, 196
- - parenchymal tears, categorization 195
- - pedicle injuries 189
- - pelvis fracture, CT 194
- - penetrating 189, 190
- - polycystic disease 202
- - radiologic examinations, sequence 210
- - radionuclide imaging 205
- - renal
- - - artery
- - - - avulsion 201
- - - - severance 201
- - - cell carcinoma, coexistent 202
- - - plasma flow rate 205
- - retrograde pyelography 206
- - severance of main renal artery 201
- - shattered kidney 199
- - surgery, indications 189, 190, 210
- - thrombosis, renal arteries, veins, CT 200, 201

- - ultrasound 206
- - urinoma 193, 197
- - - hematoma, drainage, CT 198
- - vascular injuries 201, 202
- vein
- - occlusion, kidney transplantation 313
- - renin sampling 298
- - retrograde filling, disruption of arterial flow 201
- - thrombosis, traumatic 200, 201
renin-angiotensin axis
- hypertension
- - arteriovenous fistula 65
- - Ash-Upmark kidney 52
- - breaking, embolization 308
- - renovascular 295
- renal
- - infarct 308
- - trauma 200
renin hypersecretion, renal segment, embolization 308
reninoma, hypertension, hyperaldosteronism 218
renogram
- Hilson's perfusion index, renal graft 315
- ^{131}I-Hippuran, renal graft function 318
- radionuclide, urinary obstruction 163-166
- rejection, kidney transplant 314
- renal
- - transplantation 304, 305
- - trauma, reduced perforation 206
- [99m]Tc, normal, non functionating renal graft 316
renovascular hypertension, pathophysiology, diagnosis, therapy 295-310
Riley-Newhouse syndrome, juvenile polycystic kidney disease 48
Robson, staging renal carcinoma 277

Salt loosing nephropathy, diagnosis, treatment 228
sarcoma, clear cell sarcoma, renal 52
scars
- chronic, atrophic pyelonephritis 111, 113, 115
- tuberculosis, renal 116
schistosomiasis
- egyptian mummies 120
- renal involvement 121
schwannoma, renal 252
scintigraphy
- aneurysms, mycotic 141, 142
- differential diagnosis, renal pseudotumors 58
- Franconi's syndrome 91
- Gadolinium-DTPA, tumor thrombus 289
- Gallium scan, non Hodgkin's lymphoma 91
- kidney, fracture 206

- see radioisotope scanning, nuclear medical examinations
- renal
- - ^{131}I-hippuran scan
- - - obstructive uropathy 76
- - - renal graft dysfunction 317
- - renovascular hypertension 297
- - transplantation 304, 305
- septic emboli 141
- ^{99m}Tc-DTPA-
- - multicystic dysplastic kidney, differential diagnosis 341, 342
- - renal function, neonates 339
- [99m]Tc glucoheptonate, acute pyelonephritis 107, 109, 111
- urinary leakage 329
scleroderma, clinical background, pathology, radiology 81, 82
sepsis
- bacterial, childhood, adrenal necrosis 16
- congenital hydronephrosis 66
- obstructive uropathy 151
shock, acute tubular necrosis 85
sickle cell heminoglobinopathies, renal lesions 89
Sipple's syndrome, multiple endocrine neoplasia (MEN II) 22
sonography
- Doppler
- - renal
- - - cyst 229
- - - trauma 207
- see ultrasound
specimen
- horseshoe kidney 53
- kidney, microradiograph 73
- multicystic dysplastic kidney 44
SPECT, resolution, small lesions 3
spectroscopy, adrenal 3
spleen
- hematoma, injury, renal trauma 191, 202, 209
- laceration, CT 193
splenic artery, bleeding, CT 193
splenomegaly, Riley-Newhouse syndrome 48
staging, Robson, TNM systems 277
Stauffer's syndrome, renal carcinoma 276
sulfonamides, interstitial nephritis 85
surgery
- calculus disease, therapy 179, 180
- congenital mesoplastic nephroma 52
- indications
- - congenital hydronephrosis 66
- - renal trauma 189, 190, 210
- kidney transplantation 311, 312
- multilocular cystic nephroma 223
- oncocytoma, nephrectomy 215
- renal
- - adenoma 218
- - carcinoma 278
- - graft excision, vascular occlusion 318

- - trauma, intraoperative urogram
  191
- revascularization procedures 305
- vena cava resection, renal carcinoma
  278
survival times, renal carcinoma 277
synonyma
- acute bacterial nephritis 103
- focal lobar nephronia 103
- multicystic dysplastic kidney 43
- multilocular cystic nephroma 45
- reflux nephropathy 104, 111
syphylis, adrenal 15
systemic lupus erythematosus (SLE)
- interstitial nephritis 85
- parenchymal lesions, kidneys 71, 78

Takayasu's arteritis, hypertension 303
technique
- CT 2, 191, 326
- extracorporal lithotripsy 180, 181
- percutaneous
- - nephrostomy catheter placement
  170, 171
- - stone removal 184
- - transluminal renal angioplasty
  306, 307
- - ureteral stenting 172, 173
- renography 315
- sonography 3, 339
- transurethral ureteroscopy 183, 184
- ultrasonography, renal transplant
  320
teratoma
- adrenal
- - calcification 11, 16
- - CT 11, 13, 16
therapy
- amebiasis 129
- blastomycosis 130
- brucellosis 127
- calculus disease
- - history 179, 180
- - kidney, ureter 177–188
- candidiasis 126
- conservative, renal trauma 189
- furosemide, renal calculi 347
- immunosuppressive, kidney transplantation 312
- pyelonephritis
- - chronic 112
- - emphysematous 110
- renal
- - adenoma 218
- - carcinoma 291
- - trauma, concepts 189
- schistosomiasis 121
- tuberculosis, renal 116
thrombosis
- adrenal
- - veins 16
- - venography 5
- inferior vena cava, CT 285
- renal
- - artery 305

- - - renal veins, trauma 200, 201,
  202
- - vein
- - - Goodpasture's syndrome 80
- - - malacoplakia 128
- - - venography, MRI 284
- - tumor
- - - gadolinium - DTPA scan 289
- - - ultrasound 285
- - - vena cava, renal vein 277
TNM system, renal carcinoma 277
tomography
- abscess, intrarenal 131, 132
- acute pyelonephritis 108
- angiomyolipoma 220
- kidneys 1
- - cortical necrosis 83
- - polycystic disease 45
- - trauma 191
topography, adrenals, normal 1–3, 6
toxoplasmosis, adrenal 15
transfusion, accidents, acute tubular necrosis 85
transplant
- rejection, interstitial nephritis 85
- renal
- - candida abscess 127
- - coccidioidomycosis 130
- - malacoplakia 128
- - radiology 311–338
transplantation, renal
- angiography 313, 314, 318
- hypertension 304, 305, 313
- radionuclide imaging 313, 314
- renogram 314, 316, 318
trauma
- acute interstitial nephritis 85, 86
- hepatorenal syndrome 94
- Page kidney 304
- renal, see renal trauma
traumatic infarct, renal, CT 200
trisomy 13–15
- Patau's syndrome, renal cystic disease 228
trisomy 16–18
- horseshoe kidney 53
- renal cystic disease 228
tuberculosis
- Addison's disease 15
- adrenalitis
- - adrenal insufficiency 7, 15, 16, 17
- - calcifications 16
- renal 85, 116–120
tuberous sclerosis
- oncocytoma coexisting 215
- renal cyst (Bourneville's disease)
  246
tuberous sclerosis
- syndrome, angiomyolipoma 218,
  219
tubular reabsorption, decrease, urinary
  obstruction 151, 154
tubulointerstitial diseases
- manifestations 84
- principal causes 84

tumors
- ACTH producing, Cushing's syndrome 19
- adrenal
- - carcinoma, Beckmann-Wiede-
  mann syndrome 18, 21
- - classification 7
- - neuroblastoma 25, 26
- - pheochromocytoma 22–25
- associated, renal cystic disease 246
- benign
- - angiomyolipoma 218–222, 281
- - congenital mesoplastic nephroma
  50, 52, 223
- - fetal renal hamartoma 223
- - hamartoma 50, 52, 223, 248, 281
- - juxtaglomerular cell tumor 218
- - medullary fibroma 223, 224
- - multilocular cystic nephroma 45,
  46, 222, 223
- - myelolipoma 10
- - oncocytoma 215–217
- - renal adenoma 217, 218
- - renal medullary interstitial cell
  tumor 223, 224
- - reninoma 218
- hormonal characterization, venous
  blood sampling 5
- malignant
- - adrenergic, ^{131}J-MIBG imaging 4,
  5
- - angiosarcoma 252
- - Burkitt's lymphoma 265
- - carcinoma, schistosomiasis 121
- - clear cell sarcoma, renal 52
- - embolization 5
- - fibrosarcoma 251
- - fibrous histiocytoma 256, 257
- - hemangiopericytoma 252
- - leiomyosarcoma 252
- - liposarcoma
- - - adrenal, retroperitoneal 7, 11
- - - renal 251, 252
- - lymphoma 261–265
- - metastases 256–261
- - osteogenic sarcoma 251
- - pheochromocytoma 2, 4, 22–25
- - renal
- - - cell carcinoma 57, 215, 217,
  219, 222
- - - metastases 258–261
- - - pelvis carcinoma 265–270
- - - reticulum cell sarcoma 261
- - - rhabdomyosarcoma 252
- - - sarcoma, sarcomatoid carcinoma
  251–256
- - - urothelial, urography 267
- - Wilms' tumor
- - - in adults 252, 256
- - - ultrasound
- nephroma
- - - congenital mesoblastic 50,
  52
- - multilocular cystic 45, 46
- paraganglioma 4

tumors
- polycystic disease, differential diagnosis 233
- pseudotumors, definition 13
- renal
- - angiography 75
- - lymphoma, AIDS, CT 90, 96
- - multiple myeloma 90
- - pseudotumors, differential diagnosis, scintigraphy 58, 59
- - staging, TNM system, Robson 277
- - tubulointerstitial, classification 84
- sarcoma, retroperitoneal, radiation nephritis 94
- thrombosis, vena cava 277, 278
- Tru-Cut biopsy 6
Turner's syndrome
- horseshoe kidney 53
- renal cystic disease 228

ultrasound
- abdominal pathology 2, 3
- abscess, intra-, pararenal, perinephric 133, 134, 136
- acute, chronic glomerulonephritis 76, 77
- adrenal 15, 18, 20–22, 24, 26
- - abscess 15
- - adenoma 3, 7, 18, 20, 22
- - aldosteronoma (Conn's syndrome) 18
- - bleeding 14, 15
- - carcinoma 21, 22
- - children, neonates 6
- - Cushing's syndrome 20
- - cysts 9, 11, 14
- - ganglioneuroblastoma 26
- - hyperplasia 20
- - metastases 10, 11
- - myelolipoma 11, 12
- - neuroblastoma 10, 11, 26
- - normal 1, 3, 9
- - pheochromocytoma 22, 24
- adrenogenital syndrome, bilateral adrenal hyperplasia 21
- angiomyolipoma 220
- autosomal
- - dominant polycystic kidney disease 49, 239
- - recessive
- - - renal polycystic disease 241
- - - polycystic kidney disease 47, 241
- benign renal cyst 230
- calculus
- - disease, renal 178
- - localization, lithotriptor 181
- candidiasis 126, 127
- carcinoma, renal pelvis 267, 268
- control, abscess drainage 133, 134
- criteria, cystic disease 234, 235
- diabetic pyelitis, interstitial nephritis 86
- Doppler sonogram
- - control of angioplasty 305
- - renal

- - - carcinoma 285
- - - graft, pulsatility index 323
- - renovascular hypertension 297
- - traumatic flap, thrombus 207
- echinococcosis 126
- ectopic kidney 61
- horseshoe kidney 54
- hydronephrosis 74, 159, 160, 340
- - occult 83
- - tuberculosis 118, 120
- - ureteral stone 178, 179
- infantile polycystic kidney disease 345, 346
- kidneys
- - AIDS 95
- - cortical necrosis 83
- - corticomedullary definition 73
- - cysts 229
- - malignant lymphoma 263
- - metastases 258, 259
- - nephrosclerosis 83
- - parenchymal diseases 71
- - sarcoma 253, 254, 255
- - scleroderma 82
- lithotripsy 183
- malacoplakia, renal vein thrombosis 128
- medullary sponge kidney 246
- mesoblastic nephroma 223
- multicystic dysplastic kidney, hydronephrotic form 44, 45
- multilocular cystic nephroma 45, 222
- neonates
- - genitourinary tract diseases 339–349
- - normal kidney 340
- - obstructive uropathy 340–345
- nephrocalcinosis 246
- oncocytoma 216
- polycystic
- - dysplastic kidney 242
- - renal disease 45, 46
- posterior urethral values 344
- prune belly syndrome 345
- pyelonephritis
- - acute 104, 105, 106
- - chronic 113
- - emphysematous 110, 111
- - xanthomatous 123
- pyonephrotic syndrome, tuberculous 120
- renal
- - agenesis 340
- - calcus localization, lithotriptor 181
- - carcinoma 285, 286
- - cyst 229
- - - inflammatory infected 232
- - transplant
- - - acute rejection 321
- - - fluid collection 322
- - - hydronephrosis 322, 323
- - - lymphocele 322
- - - normal 320, 321, 326
- - - trauma 206, 207

- - yeast infection 347
- reninoma 218
- "ring sign", congenital mesoblastic nephroma 52
- septum of Bertin 59
- supernumerary fused kidneys 56
- technique 3, 339
- tuberculosis, renal 118, 120
- ureter dilatation, obstruction pyonephrosis 138
- ureterocele 342, 343
- urinary obstruction 159–161
- in utero, postnatal, multicystic dysplastic kidney 44
uremia, chronic ureteral obstruction 152
ureter
- acute ureteral obstruction, pathophysiology 151, 152
- atresia
- - retrograde pyelogram 45
- - ultrasound 340
- atretic, multicystic dysplastic kidney 43
- blockage, dioctophyma renale 131
- calculi, spontaneous passage during urography 155
- calculus disease
- - sonography 178
- - therapy 177–188
- compression
- - lymphoma, percutaneous nephrostomy tube placement 170
- - stenting 169, 172, 173
- duplex, Weigert Mayer rule 37
- ectopic ureterocele 342
- embryology 340
- neoimplanted, pyelogram 325
- neoplasma, chronic obstruction, angiography 163
- obstructing megaureter, reimplantation, Whitaker test 169
- obstruction
- - kidney transplantation 312, 313, 330, 332
- - pyonephrosis 138, 139
- percutaneous ureteral stenting 172, 173
- peristalsis
- - acute urinary obstruction 153
- - normal physiology 152
- "Steinstrasse", retrograde ureteroscopy 181
- stenosis, schistosomiasis 121
- stent
- - after calculus extraction 205
- - stone localization 178
- stone
- - hydronephrosis, sonography 178, 179
- - obstruction, hydronephrosis 160
- - ultrasonic lithotripsy 183
- - ureteroscopic removal 180
- - urography 154, 178
- stricture, hydronephrosis 322, 323

- tuberculosis 116, 118, 119
- ureteral reflux, differential diagnosis 158
- ureteric bud, metanephric blastoma, renal development 33
- ureterocele, ectopic 37
- vesicoureteral reflux 66
ureterocele, extopic, ultrasound 342
ureterocystostomy, urine leak, kidney transplantation 312, 330
ureteroileal anastomosis, antegrade pyelogram 167
ureteroneocystostomy, cystography, pyelotubar backflow 156
ureteropelvic junction
- avulsion, opacified urine extravasation 191
- carcinoma 268
- obstruction, ultrasound 341
- stenosis, tuberculous 118
- stricture, congenital 66
ureteroscopy
- transurethral, stone
- - removal 180, 181, 182
- - - advantages, disadvantages 184
ureterovesical junction
- obstruction, kidney transplantation 313
- obstructive uropathy 151
- urine leak, pyelogram 330
urethra, posterior valves, ultrasound 344
uric acid nephropathy, clinical background, pathology, radiology 92, 93
urinary obstruction, see obstructive uropathy
urinoma
- calyceal fornix rupture 151, 156
- extent, contrast injection into drainage catheter 198
- kidney transplantation 312, 331
- perinephric 229
- renal trauma 193, 197
urography
- abortive (blind-ending) calyx 40
- abscess
- - intrarenal 131, 132
- - perinephritic, emphysema, air delineation, Gerota's fascia 135
- actinomycosis 129
- adrenals, morphology 1, 2
- angiomyolipoma 220, 221
- autosomal
- - dominant polycystic kidney disease 48, 238
- - recessive polycystic kidney disease 47, 241
- bifid renal pelvis 41
- calculus disease, renal, filling defects 117, 179

- calyceal diverticulum 41, 42
- candidiasis 126, 127
- carcinoma, renal pelvis 266, 267
- congenital
- - mesoblastic nephroma 223
- - renal solitary cyst 44
- crossed ectopic kidney 57
- cysts, renal sinuses, peripheral fat sign 245
- duplex kidneys, ureters 38
- echinococcosis 125
- extrarenal pelvis 40
- high dose, kidney transplantation 324
- horseshoe kidney 53, 54
- hydronephrosis, ureteral stone 178
- hypertension, renovascular 296, 297
- indications 178
- intraoperative, renal trauma 191
- jejunal-calyceal fistula 209
- leukemia 90
- malrotation, kidneys 63
- medullary cystic, sponge kidney diseases 50, 51
- megacalyces, congenital 42
- multilocular cystic nephroma 45, 46, 47
- nephroscrosis, complications 83
- nephroptosis 60
- normal renal graft 325
- obstructive uropathy 153-159
- oncocytoma 216
- papillary necrosis, tuberculous 118
- parenchymal diseases, kidneys 71
- pyelitis cystica 139
- pyelotubular backflow 156
- pyonephrosis
- - acute, chronic 136, 137
- - tuberculous 117
- renal
- - agenesis 35
- - carcinoma 279, 280
- - cyst 229, 230
- - hypoplasia 36
- - sarcoma 253, 254, 256, 258
- - trauma, accuracy 190
- rupture of calyceal fornices 156
- supernumerary kidney 37
- ureter stone 178
urosepsis
- congenital hydronephrosis 66
- urinary obstruction 151

V. cava
- inferior, tumor thrombus 277, 285, 290
- infiltration, renal carcinoma 278
vascular
- disorders, tubulointerstitial nephropathy, causes 84

- injuries, renal trauma 201, 202
- tumors, angiomyolipoma 218-222
vasculitis
- renal, necrotizing 85
- Wegner's granulomatosis 80
vasospasms, renal necrosis, bilateral, cortical 83
venography
- adrenals
- - complications 5, 16
- - Cushing's syndrome 20
- - pheochromocytoma 5
- - risk 5, 16
- renal
- - carcinoma, vein thrombosis 284, 288
- - chronic pyelonephritis 115
- - epinephrine, acute pyelonephritis 107
- - parenchymal diseases 75
venous sampling
- adrenal 5, 18, 20, 21
- - ACTH producing tumor 5
- - adrenogenital syndrome 21
- - aldosteronoma 5
- - Cushing's syndrome 5, 20
- - medullary hyperplasia 5
- - pheochromocytoma 5, 24, 25
- - pituitary adenoma 5
- - renal, renin values 298
- technique 17
virus infection, children, sepsis, adrenal necrosis 16

Waldenström's macroglobulinemia, chronic interstitial nephritis 87
Waterhouse-Friedrichsen syndrome, adrenal cortex destruction 16, 17
Wegener's granulomatosis, clinical picture, radiology 80, 81
Wilms' tumor
- in adults 252, 256
- cystic 228
- differential diagnosis 3, 222, 223
- microscopic foci, multilocular cystic nephroma 46
Wolman's disease, adrenal, calcification 17

xanthomatosis
- familial (Wolman disease) 7, 17
- xanthogranulomatous pyelonephritis 121-125

yeast infection, renal, neonates 347

Zellweger syndrome, renal cystic disease 228
Zuckerkandl, organ 22

List of Contributors

LAWRENCE R. BIGONGIARI, M.D.
Clinical Professor
Department of Radiology
St. Francis Regional Medical Center
University of Kansas
929 North St. Francis
Wichita, KS 67214, USA

JANE CLAYTON, M.D.
Assistant Professor
Department of Radiology
LSU Medical Center
1542 Tulane Avenue
New Orleans, LA 70112, USA

LUDOVICO DALLA-PALMA, M.D.
Professor and Chairman
Istituto di Radiologia dell' Università
Ospedale di Cattinara
Strada di Fiume
34149 Trieste, Italy

SVEN DORPH, M.D., PhD.
Associate Professor and Chairman
Department of Radiology
Herlev Hospital
University of Copenhagen
Herlev Ringvej 75
2730 Herlev, Denmark

LEIF EKELUND, M.D., PhD.
Professor and Chairman
Department of Diagnostic Radiology
University Hospital
90185 Umeå, Sweden

RICHARD M. FRIEDENBERG, M.D.
Professor and Chairman
Department of Radiological Sciences
University of California
Irvine Medical Center
101 City Drive
Orange, CA 92668, USA

STANFORD M. GOLDMAN, M.D.
Professor of Radiology and Urology
Johns Hopkins School of Medicine
Radiologist-in-Chief
Department of Radiology
Francis Scott Key Medical Center
4940 Eastern Avenue
Baltimore, MD 21224, USA

ROLF W. GÜNTHER, M.D.
Professor and Chairman
Department of Diagnostic Radiology
Medical School, RWTH Aachen
University of Technology
Pauwelsstraße 30
W-5100 Aachen FRG

SVEN-OLA HIETALA, M.D., PhD.
Associate Professor of Diagnostic Radiology
Department of Diagnostic Radiology
University Hospital
90185 Umeå, Sweden

ERICH K. LANG, M.D.
Professor and Chairman
Department of Radiology
School of Medicine in New Orleans
Louisiana State University
Medical Center
1542 Tulane Avenue
New Orleans, LA 70112-2822, USA

JAN KOFOD LARSEN, M.D.
Department of Nuclear Medicine
Herlev Hospital
University of Copenhagen
Herlev Ringvej 75
2730 Herlev, Denmark

ANDREW J. LEROY, M.D.
Associate Professor of Diagnostic Radiology
Mayo Medical School and Consultant in
Diagnostic Radiology, MAYO Clinic
200 1st Street, SW
Rochester, MN 55905, USA

W. Scott McDougal, M.D.
Professor and Chairman
Department of Urology
Vanderbilt University School of Medicine
Nashville, TN 37232-2730, USA

Christoph Müller-Leisse, M.D.
Department of Diagnostic Radiology
Medical School, RWTH Aachen
University of Technology
Pauwelsstraße 30
W-5100 Aachen, FRG

Thorkild Mygind, M.D., PhD.
Professor of Diagnostic Radiology
Department of Nuclear Medicine
Herlev Hospital
University of Copenhagen
Herlev Ringvej 75
2730 Herlev, Denmark

Jeffrey H. Newhouse, M.D.
Professor of Radiology
Columbia Presbyterian Medical Center
177 Ft. Washington Avenue
New York, NY 10032, USA

Nicholas Papanicolaou, M.D.
Associate Professor of Radiology
Harvard Medical School
Rockville, MD 20850, USA

Richard Pfister, M.D.
Professor of Radiology
University Medical Center
University of South Alabama
2451 Fillingim Street
Mobile, AL 36617, USA

Roberto Pozzi-Mucelli, M.D.
Assistant Professor
Istituto di Radiologia dell' Università
Ospedale di Cattinara
Strada di Fiume
34149 Trieste, Italy

Henrik S. Thomsen, M.D., PhD.
Department of Nuclear Medicine
Herlev Hospital
University of Copenhagen
Herlev Ringvej 75
2730 Herlev, Denmark

Felix Wang, M.D.
Assistant Clinical Professor
Department of Radiological Sciences
University of California
Irvine Medical Center
101 City Drive
Orange, CA 92668, USA

William Wells, M.D.
Assistant Professor
Department of Radiology
LSU Medical Center
1542 Tulane Avenue
New Orleans, LA 70112, USA

Alan C. Winfield, M.D.
Professor of Radiology
Department of Radiology and
Radiological Sciences
Vanderbilt University School of Medicine
Nashville, TN 37232-2730, USA

Hilary Zarnow, M.D. MS (Renal Pathology)
Clinical Associate Professor of Radiology
Department of Radiology
St. Francis Regional Medical Center
University of Kansas
929 North St. Francis
Wichita, KS 67214, USA

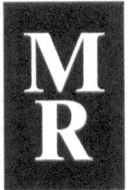

Medical Radiology

Diagnostic Imaging and Radiation Oncology

Series Editors:
L. W. Brady, M. W. Donner, H.-P. Heilmann, F. Heuck

This series recognizes the demand for an international state-of-the-art account of the developments reflecting the progress in the radiological sciences. Each volume conveys an overall picture of a topical theme so that it can be used as a reference work without taking recourse to other volumes.

The contents of the volumes concentrate on new and accepted developments in a manner appropriate for review by physicians engaged in the practice of radiology.

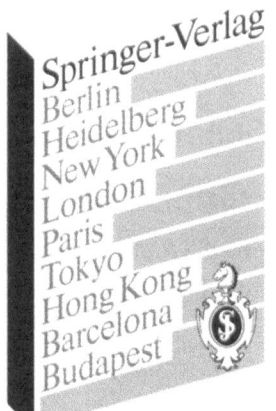

Springer-Verlag
Berlin
Heidelberg
New York
London
Paris
Tokyo
Hong Kong
Barcelona
Budapest

C. W. Scarantino (Ed.)

Lung Cancer
Diagnostic Procedures and Therapeutic Management with Special Reference to Radiotherapy

1985. XI, 173 pp. 42 figs. Hardcover.
ISBN 3-540-13176-0

H. R. Withers, University of California, Los Angeles, CA; L. J. Peters, University of Texas, Houston, TX (Eds.)

Innovations in Radiation Oncology

1987. XVII, 329 pp. 111 figs. Hardcover.
ISBN 3-540-17818-X

G. E. Laramore, University of Washington, Seattle, WA (Ed.)

Radiation Therapy of Head and Neck Cancer

1989. XII, 237 pp. 123 figs. Hardcover.
ISBN 3-540-19360-X

J. H. Anderson, The Johns Hopkins University, Baltimore, MD (Ed.)

Innovations in Diagnostic Radiology

1989. XIII, 213 pp. 144 figs. some in color.
Hardcover. ISBN 3-540-19093-7

R. R. Dobelbower Jr., Toledo, OH (Ed.)

Gastrointestinal Cancer
Radiation Therapy

1990. XV, 301 pp. 76 figs. 90 tabs. Hardcover.
ISBN 3-540-50505-9

E. Scherer, C. Streffer, University of Essen; K.-R. Trott, London (Eds.)

Radiation Exposure and Occupational Risks

1990. XI, 150 pp. 32 figs. 55 tabs. Hardcover.
ISBN 3-540-51174-1

S. E. Order, The Johns Hopkins University, Baltimore, MD; S. S. Donaldson, Stanford University, Stanford, CA

Radiation Therapy of Benign Diseases
A Clinical Guide

1990. VIII, 214 pp. 103 tabs. Hardcover.
ISBN 3-540-50901-1

R. Sauer, University of Erlangen-Nürnberg, Erlangen (Ed.)

Interventional Radiation Therapy Techniques – Brachytherapy

1991. XII, 388 pp. 193 figs. 162 tabs. Hardcover.
ISBN 3-540-52465-7

E. Scherer, C. Streffer, University of Essen; K.-R. Trott, Medical College of London (Eds.)

Radiopathology of Organs and Tissues

1991. X, 496 pp. 156 figs. 56 tabs.
Hardcover. ISBN 3-540-19094-5

M. Rotmann, C. J. Rosenthal, State University of New York, NY (Eds.)

Concomitant Continuous Infusion Chemotherapy and Radiation

1991. XIV, 304 pp. 42 figs.
Hardcover. ISBN 3-540-52545-9